# Human Communication Disorders
## An Introduction

Edited by

### George H. Shames
University of Pittsburgh

and

### Elisabeth H. Wiig
Professor Emeritus, Boston University

MERRILL PUBLISHING COMPANY

A Bell & Howell Information Company

Columbus Toronto London Melbourne

Cover Art: Gerald Richards, Southeast School, Columbus, Ohio

Published by Merrill Publishing Company
A Bell & Howell Information Company
Columbus, Ohio 43216

This book was set in Korinna.

Administrative Editor: Ann Castel
Production Coordinator: Linda Bayma
Art Coordinator: Raydelle Clement
Cover Designer: Russ Maselli
Photo Editors: Gail Meese and Terry L. Tietz

Photo Credits: All photos copyrighted by individuals or companies listed. Cleveland Speech and Hearing Center, pp. 35, 447, and 451. Caren Strock, pp. 48 and 60. Photos not credited within the text were supplied by the authors.

Library of Congress Catalog Card Number: 89-62570
International Standard Book Number: 0-675-20995-1
Printed in the United States of America
1  2  3  4  5  6  7  8  9—93  92  91  90

# PREFACE

$T$he purpose of the third edition of *Human Communication Disorders: An Introduction*, like the prior editions, is to lead you gradually into the world of the person who has problems communicating with other people. As guides for this journey, leading authorities in the fields of speech and hearing science, speech-language pathology, and audiology have contributed chapters that focus on individual facets of this multidimensional topic. While each author presents his or her own perspective, the perspectives of others are incorporated throughout. In this way, we have tried to blend the parts into a cohesive picture of a complex profession. A common thread is our interest in *serving people* with communication problems. This book is for the beginner, for whom it may well be the first venture into a rewarding career as a speech-language pathologist, audiologist, special educator, or classroom teacher. We hope the textbook will also help readers become informed citizens, whatever their profession.

The text is divided into five major parts. Part One, *Introduction*, develops a view of the profession—its history, philosophy, and ethics. Part Two, *Bases of Human Communication*, provides basic information that underlies our understanding of communication problems, and how they are studied and managed. Theoretical and scientific principles that help us understand human communication problems are reviewed. Separate chapters describe the communication process and what language is, and the physical aspects of the act of speaking.

The first chapter in Part Three, *Differences and Disorders of Language*, considers the types of language differences encountered in our society, and how these differences can contribute to special types of communication problems. The next chapters turn to developmental language disorders in preschool and school-age children and adolescents. For each age level, the authors discuss basic characteristics and types, theories of causation, and approaches to language assessment and language therapy.

Part Four, *Disorders of Articulation, Voice, and Fluency*, considers each of the major categories of disorders of speech. Each chapter places the disorder in perspective, discusses basic theories of causation, introduces identifying characteristics, and presents special procedures for evaluation and treatment.

Part Five, *Disorders of Special Populations*, focuses on children and adults that have certain unique, physical characteristics that are associated with or contribute to communication disorders. This section, like those preceding, focuses on the events that can facilitate your task of helping persons with communication handicaps. You are introduced to the philosophies of the clinician and how they mesh with the problems of the client.

Each chapter opens with a list of common myths, followed immediately by the corresponding realities of the situations. Each chapter in Parts Three through Five presents a concrete, real-life case history to help you better understand some of the human, social, and emotional aspects of the problems. To augment your understanding, marginal notes are featured in each chapter. For easy reference and review, a glossary at the end of the book defines key items, which are boldfaced in the text. Additionally, each chapter provides study questions for your review. Because people's speech and language problems cannot be easily categorized into chapters in a book, we have also included numerous cross-references from chapter to chapter.

Human communication and its disorders are part of the overall human condition. Each of us exists as a uniquely synthesized unit. We express ourselves to one another, not as a mouth or a tongue or an ear, but as an individual, thoughtful, caring person. The momentary focus on separate aspects of human communication in separate chapters reflects our own attempts to analyze a complex process to try to understand it. But when we communicate, the body and mind respond together as a unit; it is this synthesis that we are concerned with in this text.

The production of a third edition of a text requires constructive feedback from professionals who have used the prior editions in their teaching. We were fortunate to receive valuable suggestions from both survey respondents and reviewers among our colleagues.

The reviewers receive our gratitude for their in-depth evaluations of the second edition, constructive suggestions for editing and updating chapters, and final reviews for revised chapters. The reviews greatly influenced the process of revising individual chapters and integrating the final product. The reviewers were Rhoda Agin, California State University, Haywood; John Bernthal, University of Nebraska—Lincoln; Gordon Blood, Pennsylvania State University; Richard C. Folsom, University of Washington; Beth Hardaway, University of South Alabama; Nancy Helm-Estabrooks, Boston VA Medical Center; Raymond H. Hull, University of Northern Colorado; Roger N. Kasten, Wichita State University; Michael J. Morman, Auburn University; Wayne Secord, Ohio State University; Harry N. Seymour, University of Massachusetts at Amherst; Eugene Sheeley, University of Alabama; and Kim A. Wilcox, The University of Kansas at Lawrence.

The chapter authors deserve special commendations for their continued commitment to this text. Special thanks go to Fred Martin, who joined the list of authors by contributing the chapter on audiology. We also express our appreciation to Marilyn Condon, who joined the authors and contributors by preparing the teacher's manual and the computerized test bank.

Other people, in other roles, also deserve our expressions of appreciation: Vicki Smith, for the hours she spent on the word processor to assist one of the editors in developing the glossary, and Janet McCarthy, for organizing the list of references at the end of the book.

Last, but not least, the editors express mutual gratitude for the continued support and collaboration in carrying out the editorial responsibilities.

# CONTENTS

# PART THREE   DIFFERENCES AND DISORDERS OF LANGUAGE

# PART FOUR   DISORDERS OF ARTICULATION, VOICE, AND FLUENCY

# PART FIVE   DISORDERS OF SPECIAL POPULATIONS

*When we are children we learn to understand the nature of the world we live in and to accept love and caring from those who are around us.*

*When we are adults we learn to share those understandings and to care for those who are in need.*

*The mission of this book is to promote a special kind of understanding and caring for those children and adults and their families who live with communication problems.*

*It is to the achievement of this mission that the editors humbly dedicate this book.*

# PART ONE

# Introduction

# The Professions of Speech-Language Pathology and Audiology

## JACK MATTHEWS

### MYTHS AND REALITIES

- *Myth:* To become a professional helping children with communication disorders requires a certificate as a classroom teacher.
- *Reality:* Some take the route from classroom teaching to speech-language pathology, but many begin their masters' programs in speech-language pathology with a liberal arts/science undergraduate degree.
- *Myth:* An undergraduate degree in speech-language pathology qualifies you to work with children with communication disorders.
- *Reality:* The individual who is awarded a certificate of clinical competence must hold a master's degree or equivalent, with major emphasis in speech-language pathology, audiology, or speech-language and hearing science.

■ *Myth:* Like physical therapists and occupational therapists, speech-language pathologists and audiologists work on a prescription basis under the supervision of a physician.

■ *Reality:* Speech-language pathologists and audiologists cooperate as members of a total rehabilitation team; however, in the area of communication disorders, they operate as professionals rather than as workers carrying out a prescription from someone who is not trained in the area of communication disorders.

■ *Myth:* A master's degree in speech-language pathology limits you mostly to work with children in a school situation.

■ *Reality:* Training programs approved by the American Speech-Language Association prepare you to work with children and adults, in schools, hospitals, rehab centers, or private practice offices.

■ *Myth:* The field of communication disorders offers little opportunity for individuals interested in research.

■ *Reality:* Although the majority of speech-language pathologists work as clinicians, there are opportunities to pursue a career as a researcher in speech-language pathology and audiology.

■ *Myth:* The number of communicatively handicapped is small compared to those with other handicaps.

■ *Reality:* There are millions of communicatively handicapped people who seek help in schools, hospitals, rehabilitation centers, clinics, and offices of speech-language pathologists and audiologists in private practice throughout the country.

■ *Myth:* Unlike doctors or lawyers, speech-language pathologists and audiologists do not go into private practice.

■ *Reality:* Approximately 15% of speech-language pathologists and audiologists are in private practice.

■ *Myth:* The yellow pages are an adequate source of professionals competent to provide service to those with communication disorders.

■ *Reality:* American Speech-Language Association certification is the most reliable way for the general public, as well as for other professionals, to identify a professional who has been adequately trained as a speech-language pathologist or audiologist.

HOW many of these myths have you accepted in the past? You may be surprised to learn that many intelligent and caring people share one or more of these myths. We hope this book will give the reader a realistic perspective, one not based on myth.

This book is about people—people with communication disorders, the people speech-language pathologists and audiologists try to help. The problems these people face have various origins. Some stem from physical causes, such as cleft palate, brain damage, hearing loss. Some have roots in the childhood environment—a lack of language stimulation, for example. Many stem from the way people feel about themselves. Some may result from an unmeasurable combination of these factors. Regardless of the cause or causes of the problem, speech-language pathologists and audiologists try to help the *whole person* who is experiencing a communication difficulty. In some instances, the problem is "cured." In other cases, no cure is found but the person is helped to compensate and to reach maximum communicative potential.

As you become better acquainted with the work of speech-language pathologists and audiologists, you will find that they are caring people. But in addition to caring, they must know a good deal about people, how they communicate, and what breakdowns can occur in their communication. You will soon become acutely aware that becoming a professional involves much more than learning about communication disorders and how to alleviate them. In fact, sometimes we cannot restore certain lost or impaired functions. Instead we modify and train residual or retained abilities. You will see that speech-language pathologists and audiologists often work with other professionals in education, medicine, social work, psychology, rehabilitation, and dentistry to provide the necessary help for the person who has a communication disorder.

To begin, let us look at some people whose lives were changed by speech-language pathologists. The stories of Annabelle, Roger, and Jerry are dramatic and are intended to capture your attention and to suggest the great challenges and rewards of working in the field of speech-language pathology and audiology. Of course, few speech-language pathologists and audiologists are able to fill their practice entirely with the kinds of dramatic challenges presented by Annabelle, Roger, and Jerry. Much time is spent helping people with less dramatic but nevertheless important problems— children born with cleft palate who retain nasal voice quality following surgery; adults who must learn to speak following surgical removal of a portion of their vocal mechanism; children and adults who must learn to read lips and to use hearing aids; and the millions of communicatively handicapped people who seek help in schools, hospitals, rehabilitation centers, clinics, and offices of speech-language pathologists and audiologists in private practice throughout the country.

Let me start by telling you about Annabelle. Until she was about 5, she lived almost like a caged animal. The adults in her world hid her from society because she was illegitimate. Her grandparents, with whom she and her mother lived, believed that the family's "disgrace" would be concealed by keeping Annabelle out of sight. The little room she grew up in was more a closet than a child's nursery. She saw no sunshine. She had no friends. She was fed much like an animal. When the juvenile court authorities found her (early 1940s), Annabelle was malnourished, was not able to walk, and had no language or speech, even though she was almost 5 years old. In many ways she was more a little beast than a little girl. Because Annabelle's mother was thought to be mentally retarded and because Annabelle could not talk, some juvenile court workers assumed that Annabelle, too, was retarded and should be placed in the state institution, which in those days was known as the State School for the Feebleminded.

Annabelle was taken to Children's Hospital in Columbus, Ohio. While she was there, she was seen by a speech-language pathologist. Several graduate students played with her. They bounced and tossed a ball to each other, and, as they played with it, kept saying, "ball, ball, ball." After a few minutes of patient stimulation of this kind, Annabelle responded to the ball by uttering the sounds "ba-ba," as she, too, tossed the ball.

Annabelle smiled broadly when a wristwatch was held to her ear. She could hear. It was clear she could see the ball and other people and objects in her environment. While she was in Children's Hospital, physicians, psychologists, speech-language pathologists, and audiologists carried out a series of diagnostic examinations. They concluded that Annabelle had the necessary "equipment" to speak. What she needed was appropriate stimulation and training, in addition to general health care.

Because I subsequently married one of the graduate students who helped in Annabelle's training, I had the opportunity to watch her develop. To me it was almost a miracle to observe Annabelle as she grew from a near animal into a youngster who showed promise of leading a normal life. Annabelle has not proved to be a genius. She has not won a Nobel Prize. But she did grow into a healthy, attractive child and was adopted by a warm, loving family. She completed high school and entered nursing school. Annabelle did not spend the rest of her life in a state institution. She was given a chance to develop her potential. Both Annabelle and our society have profited from the efforts of a team of professionals, which included several knowledgeable and concerned speech-language pathologists. If you become a speech-language pathologist or audiologist, you will spend most of your time helping people with less dramatic problems than Annabelle's. Nonetheless, it can be rewarding to watch the smile of accomplishment on the face of a child who at long last is able to produce a speech sound you have taught her to make.

Next I want to describe Roger, a young man for whom speaking was unpleasant. When he spoke, he had severe blocks and many repetitions. People called him a stutterer. He finished college and, without a personal interview, was somehow hired as a teacher in a remote rural school. During the first few minutes of his first day of teaching, he avoided talking by writing the names of texts, assignments, and everything else on the blackboard.

Shortly after class began, the superintendent came into the classroom by the rear door. Roger immediately fled through the front door. A number of hours later, he was found near death from carbon monoxide poisoning. He had started the motor of his car and closed the garage doors. Fortunately, Roger was revived. He was encouraged to seek professional help for his speech problem at a clinic affiliated with a large university and was given an opportunity to talk through his problem with a speech-language pathologist. He learned some techniques for handling it and was helped to change his attitude toward his speech and himself. While he was doing all of this, Roger decided to enter graduate school to learn more about the nature of stuttering, communication disorders, and psychology. At the same time, he continued working on his own speech in the speech clinic. In a few years he completed his doctorate. His speech improved, and today he is successfully engaged in the profession of his choice. Speech-language pathology gave Roger an opportunity to develop many fine capabilities that he had never used—instead of becoming nothing more than a suicide statistic. Society is richer today because Roger was given a chance to develop his potential. Speech-language pathology played an important role in Roger's development, a role that involved much more than simply correcting a stutter.

Finally, let's look at Jerry, another example of the kind of person speech-language pathologists and audiologists try to help. He came to the clinic where I was working to get some vocational guidance. He told me he wanted to study sheet metal work. Everything he communicated to me was written on a slip of paper. The few times he tried to speak, he was difficult to understand. The tests Jerry took indicated that he had little aptitude for sheet metal work. I told him the test results, and he was upset. I finally succeeded in getting him to tell me his story. Jerry's speech had been a problem for as long as he was able to remember. He had managed to finish high school and begin college. Shortly after entering college, however, he dropped out and decided to get a job that would not require him to speak. He naively thought that, as a sheet metal worker, he would not have to talk to people. He thought he would be able to take an order for a furnace, deliver it, and install it. He hoped he might be able to do all of this without having to speak at all.

As Jerry returned for subsequent visits to the clinic, we helped him realize that sheet metal workers, like most people, have to communicate. With the aid of the clinic audiologist, we discovered that he had a hearing loss that contributed to his speech problem. He began a program in our clinic that helped him manage his hearing problem and also helped him speak more intelligibly. While we could not cure his hearing loss, Jerry was able to profit from the use of a hearing aid. As his speech began to improve, Jerry revealed many things about his earlier life and about some of his real ambitions. He told me that he had spent many rewarding hours coaching youth groups. That was what he really enjoyed doing best. As his speech continued to improve, we encouraged him to return to college, where he majored in physical education. Shortly before I saw Jerry for the last time, he had received a letter from the superintendent of a nearby school offering him a teaching and coaching job.

The three people I have just described were not geniuses; none of them made the cover of *Time* magazine. But Annabelle was saved from a useless existence as an inmate of an institution and instead became a successful nurse. Roger eventually earned a Ph.D. and has made an outstanding contribution to his profession. Jerry did not become the number one athletic coach in the United States, but he did not become a failure in work he was not suited for. Instead, he became a happy and useful teacher and greatly admired athletic coach. These three people have one thing in common— each was helped to develop unrealized potential that had been blocked because of communication problems.

These examples are obviously dramatic, and all have happy endings. Of course, not all of the people speech-language pathologists and audiologists work with have such dramatic appeal and provide us with such happy endings. I can assure you, however, having been in this field for almost 50 years, that the kinds of experiences I just reported do take place in the practice of speech-language pathologists and audiologists. Anyone who begins a career in this field can expect to experience similar satisfaction.

## HOW MANY PEOPLE HAVE COMMUNICATION DISORDERS?

The information we have about the exact number of people with communication disorders is not as accurate as I would like. While there have been many studies to determine the number of people with communication disorders, reliable figures are hard to come by. One problem is comparing a study done by one investigator with that by another. Not all studies employ exactly the same definition of *communication disorder.* Another problem is sampling. One report may be based on a population that is different from the population that another researcher studies. There are so many variables to consider that the best we can do is to make some estimates about the incidence and prevalence of communication disorders.

One of the early large-scale efforts to determine the prevalence of communication disorders was the 1950 White House Conference (ASHA Committee, 1952). The committee that studied the problem at the time estimated that 5% of the population between ages 5 and 21 had defective speech. Let me present a brief quotation from the White House Conference report.

Incidence *refers to the number of new cases of a condition identified within a group over a specific period of time;* prevalence, *to the total number of cases existing at a particular place or time.*

> It is to be stressed that the figures are presented as the lowest defensible estimate; they would be regarded as serious underestimates in certain respects by some authorities. They leave out of account an estimated additional 5% or 2,000,000 children who have minor speech and voice defects, unimportant for the most practical purposes but serious in their

effects on personal and social adjustment in some cases, and obviously significant for children destined for fields of work, such as teaching, requiring good speech. (p. 129)

This report concentrated on children, but not all individuals with communication disorders are between ages 5 and 21. In fact, some communication disorders are found more frequently in an older population. Robert Milisen, in *Handbook of Speech Pathology and Audiology* (1971, pp. 621–622), summarized the studies of the incidence and prevalence of communication disorders. Later in this book, the authors writing about various types of communication disorders will provide more specific information about the incidence and prevalence of particular communication disorders. For the time being, it is safe for us to say that communication disorders affect millions of people of all ages.

## SCOPE OF THIS BOOK

This book is only an introduction and therefore cannot include everything that is known about communication disorders. Although we deal with a variety of communication disorders, we concentrate on the oral-verbal part of communication. Other books and other professions may give greater emphasis to communication disorders related to reading, writing, spelling, and so on. In this chapter, we will focus on the professions of speech-language pathology and audiology, which specialize in the oral-verbal aspects of communication.

Throughout this book you will find discussions of many elements of disordered oral-verbal communication. Some specialists will tell you about children and adults who have difficulty producing certain sounds, that is, with articulation. In many instances, it's hard to understand what a person is saying. Sometimes you can understand what is being said, but the "defective" sound production is so noticeable that you concentrate on the unfamiliar sounds. In so doing, you can miss much of what the person is trying to say. Other specialists will describe speakers whose voices are not appropriate for their age and sex or who are not pleasant to listen to. You will learn about cases in which the problem is neither voice nor sound production, but the fluency with which the speech is produced. You will learn that in some instances the disorder of communication is related to how a speaker feels about the way he talks. You will learn about children who do not talk, or who at age 8 sound like a child of 3. We will discuss communication disorders associated with special problems such as hearing impairment, brain damage, cleft palate, and mental retardation. You will learn about communication problems in which sound production, voice, and fluency are not involved, but where the individual has trouble associating the appropriate word or sound with the object or the concept he wishes to talk about.

In addition to learning about problems, you will read about the processes used to help. You will learn about the diagnostic procedures speech-language pathologists and audiologists carry out, and how the information obtained by other professional workers can help you understand the nature and causes of the communication disorder. You will learn about remedial procedures employed directly by speech-language pathologists and audiologists and those carried out by parents, teachers, and a variety of others who are in contact with the person with a communication disorder. You will learn that, in some instances, it is possible to restore a lost or impaired function, as in the case of plastic surgery for a child with a cleft palate; in other cases, the most that can be done is to modify a residual function, as might be true with someone who has paralysis following a stroke. In still other cases, we prescribe adaptive equipment, such as a hearing aid, to help perform the function of a damaged or even missing body part.

You will also learn where speech-language pathologists and audiologists are employed and the variety of jobs—clinical service, research, teaching, administration, etc.—they perform. You will discover the kind of people who have been attracted to the profession and their satisfaction with their choice of profession. You will learn about the requirements to prepare yourself for a career in this field and the code of ethics members of the profession are expected to follow. You will have a chance to look ahead to what the profession is likely to be in the years ahead and to decide whether this is a profession you may wish to enter.

## OTHER PROFESSIONS CONCERNED WITH COMMUNICATION DISORDERS

It is important to realize that there are many professions that are concerned with certain communication disorders. Over 30 years ago, Dorothea McCarthy (1954) noted that increasingly large numbers of individuals with normal intelligence and intact senses have difficulty in acquiring facility in the various essential forms of communication.

> This phenomenon has in turn given rise to the several professions concerned with remediation, such as speech therapists and remedial reading teachers who together with clinical psychologists and psychiatrists are concerned with alleviating the various language disorders. . . . Whether a child is referred to a speech therapist, to a psychologist, or to a remedial reading teacher is largely a matter of timing. It is a question of when a particular symptom becomes intolerable to someone in the environment and what facilities are available in the community. (p. 514)

If McCarthy were writing today, she might add several additional specialists who are concerned with communication disorders: pediatricians, otolaryngologists, audiologists, neurologists, classroom teachers, and specialists in learning disabilities. Albert Murphy in the first edition of this book developed Figure 1.1 to show the variety of professions related to human communication disorders.

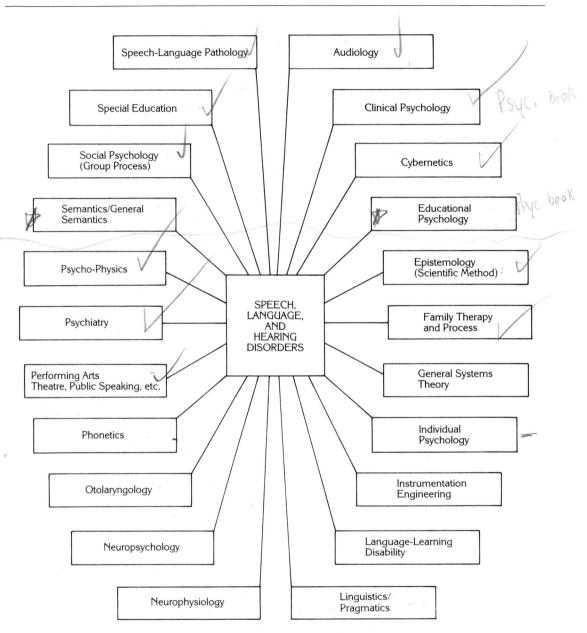

**Figure 1.1**  Professions related to human communications disorders

In a text directed to otolaryngologists and pediatricians, Matthews (1982) points out that the variety of specialists concerned with communication disorders can be a source of confusion to parents.

It can be confusing to the parents of a 3-year-old child who is not speaking to receive different and often conflicting opinions concerning the etiology of delayed language. The otolaryngologist may stress the role of hearing loss. The psychologist may attribute the problem to mental retardation. The psychiatrist may give major importance to emotional problems in the home. Other specialists may blame an environment lacking adequate language stimulation or confusion growing out of a bilingual background. The presence of one of these factors does not rule out the possible influences that may be exerted by the others. The incidence of hearing loss is, indeed, higher in the mentally retarded than in the nonretarded population (Birch & Matthews, 1951), and hearing loss can result in frustration and emotional problems. A physical disability can result in parents overly protecting a child so the child finds little need to learn to talk. The task of differential diagnosis in the child with a language disorder is difficult and goes beyond the scope of training of most pediatricians and otolaryngologists, even though the contributions of these physicians are important in the diagnosis and treatment of the disorders. (pp. 1484–1485)

In both diagnosing and treating a communication disorder, it is often desirable to involve specialists from speech-language pathology, audiology, special education, psychology, social work, neurology, psychiatry, pediatrics, otolaryngology, and other medical and dental specialties. But of all these professions, only speech-language pathology and audiology has communication disorders as its central concern. For this reason, we will begin our text on communication disorders with a discussion of the profession of speech-language pathology.

## WHAT DO SPECIALISTS IN COMMUNICATION DISORDERS CALL THEMSELVES?

In this book, we use the term *speech-language pathologist* as the title for specialists who diagnose and treat individuals with communication disorders. In a 1980 survey (Taylor, 1980), there were 19 professional titles applied by state departments of education to the speech-language pathologist working in the school setting. These titles included speech and language clinician, speech correctionist, communication disorders specialist, speech and hearing therapist, speech clinician, teacher of speech handicapped, and speech therapist. Some state departments of education do not use any of the 19 professional titles for the *specialists* in communication disorders, but instead designate the *specialty area* by employing one of 14 different terms, including speech correction, speech pathology, speech disorders, speech and hearing therapy, and speech and language pathology. To work as a speech-language pathologist in a school system, you must have a certificate issued by the state department of education. Speech-language pathologists in job settings outside the school system are expected to hold a certificate of clinical competence issued by the American Speech-Language-Hearing Association (see Appendix A). This certificate attests to the fact that certain prescribed education and training has been completed.

Although specialists in communication disorders use the term *speech-language pathologist* as the title for those who diagnose and treat individuals with communication disorders, the general public is much more likely to use the term *speech therapist*. Aronson (1987) has expressed concern that "65% of the general public know us as *speech therapists* but only 5% know us as *speech-language pathologists*." In this book we use the term *speech-language pathologist* to designate professionals who diagnose and treat individuals with communication disorders.

In contrast, *audiologists* are concerned with identification, measurement, and study of hearing and hearing impairments. The audiologist is usually the professional who prescribes the hearing aid, if necessary. Because hearing problems are often related to communication disorders, audiologists and speech-language pathologists work together to determine both the sources of a problem and a coordinated program of rehabilitation.

## WHERE DO SPEECH-LANGUAGE PATHOLOGISTS AND AUDIOLOGISTS WORK?

The profession of speech-language pathology is made up only in part of specialists who work in school systems. Many speech-language pathologists and audiologists work in hospitals, rehabilitation centers, university speech clinics, and community speech and hearing centers. In April 1969 Florida became the first state to issue a license to practice speech-language pathology. The license provides a legal right to practice your profession within the guidelines of the governmental unit that issues the license.

An estimated 50% of the working speech-language pathologists in the United States are members of the American Speech-Language-Hearing Association (ASHA). Cynthia Shewan (1988) examined several employment characteristics of the membership of the American Speech-Language-Hearing Association. Almost 75% of the members worked full-time, approximately 17% were employed part-time, and about 1% were unemployed and seeking employment. Fifty-five percent worked in educational facilities, 19% were in nonresidential health care facilities, and 6% were in residential health facilities. Fourteen percent of ASHA members were self-employed; 53% were employed by federal, state or local governments (including school districts); 13% were employed by a private for-profit company; and 20% by public or private nonprofit organizations. Fifty-five percent were in educational facilities —preschool, primary, secondary, and postsecondary settings. In the past 5 years, there has been a large increase in the number of speech-language pathologists/audiologists employed by private for-profit companies. More and more opportunities are becoming available in management because services are being provided to those with communication disorders in these firms.

Shewan (1987) compared the primary work setting of ASHA members who graduated between 1945 and 1949 and between 1980 and 1984. About 16% of the 1945–1949 graduates were employed in schools. Nearly 50% of the 1980–1984 graduates had their primary employment in schools. The college/university employment setting for 1945–1949 graduates was 57% and dropped to about 5% for 1980–1984 graduates. The figures for the category of hospital/government agency rose from 9% for 1945–1949 graduates to nearly 32% of the 1980–1984 group. The private practice setting doubled from 4.5% for the 1945–1949 graduates to 9.4% for the 1980–1984 group.

*[handwritten margin notes: More in public schools / college/univ ↓ / hospital/gov't ↑ / private practice ↑ x2]*

Kellum, Wylde, Dickerson, and Ulrich (1987) compared the primary employment setting of ASHA members and ASHA legislative councilors (elected representatives who constitute the government of the organization). Their findings are based on the September 1987 demographic profile of ASHA. About 45% of ASHA members worked in the school setting, 21% in clinics, 15% in hospitals, 10% in private practice, and 8% in college/university settings. Forty percent of the legislative councilors, as compared to 8% of the general ASHA members, worked in college/university settings. For the councilors, only 14% as opposed to 45% of the general ASHA members worked in schools.

Although the majority of speech-language pathologists and audiologists work as clinicians in schools, hospitals, and rehabilitation centers, about 10% are working as private practitioners who serve their clients in much the same way as doctors or lawyers who are in private practice. Still others are employed by a clinical facility, but also devote some time to private practice.

## WHAT ARE THE MAJOR WORK ACTIVITIES OF SPEECH-LANGUAGE PATHOLOGISTS AND AUDIOLOGISTS?

Shewan (1987) analyzed the primary professional activities of a group of ASHA members who graduated in the 1980s. Almost 86% reported that they were providing clinical services; 5% devoted most of their time to supervision, 2% to administration, and 1% to research. In contrast 48% of the graduates from the 1940s reported that they spent most of their time teaching in colleges/universities, 27% in providing clinical services, 16% in administration, and 2% in research. About 2% of both the 1940s and 1980s graduates work in special education teaching handicapped children in classroom settings. Speech-language pathologists and audiologists work in a variety of job settings and engage in a wide variety of work activities.

Public Law 99–457, which President Reagan signed into law on October 8, 1986, provides new opportunities for speech-language pathologists and audiologists to develop and implement programs and services for infants, toddlers, and children from birth through age 5. It is anticipated that by the 1990–1991 school year, all children ages 3 to 5 with communication disorders will be provided the services of qualified speech-language pathologists and audiologists.

## ESTABLISHING THE COMPETENCE OF SPEECH-LANGUAGE PATHOLOGISTS AND AUDIOLOGISTS

Approximately 50% of the specialists working in the field of communication disorders are members of ASHA. This association has over 50,000 members and maintains a national headquarters in Rockville, Maryland. ASHA sets standards for colleges and universities that train speech-language pathologists and audiologists as well as for facilities that provide services for people with communication disorders. ASHA issues a certificate of clinical competence (CCC) for individuals who have successfully completed a program of graduate study in speech-language pathology or speech-language and hearing science, have passed a national written examination, and have completed a year of full-time clinical experience under the supervision of someone holding a certificate of clinical competence. An equivalent certificate is available for audiologists. Although most holders of the certificate of clinical competence are members of ASHA, membership in the association is not required for certification. The certificate is not a membership card, but instead is proof of having completed both the graduate academic and the clinical experience to demonstrate competence in performing professional duties. The requirements for the ASHA certificates of clinical competence are often higher than those of the states that issue a license for speech-language pathologists or audiologists. ASHA certification has become the best way for members of the general public as well as for other professional workers to identify a professional who has been adequately trained as a speech-language pathologist, an audiologist, or both.

If you plan a career as a speech-language pathologist or an audiologist, you should be aware of the requirements for the certificates of competence issued by the American Speech-Language-Hearing Association. These requirements are revised periodically. The April 1985 revision is presented in Appendix A. Future revisions may be obtained by writing to the ASHA headquarters.

By writing to ASHA, you can also obtain a list of colleges and universities that offer accredited master's degree programs in speech-language pathology or audiology. The list includes programs that have applied for, but not yet received, accreditation. The most recent list includes more than 125 colleges and universities throughout the United States and Canada.

In addition to standards developed by the American Speech-Language-Hearing Association, most states have developed requirements to obtain a license to practice speech-language pathology and audiology. In most states, if you wish to work in a school system, you must obtain a certificate issued by the state department of education. Many state speech-language-hearing societies are working to upgrade state education department standards.

Public Law 99–457 will have the effect of upgrading state education and department certification standards for speech-language pathologists and audiologists. For employment in most settings other than school, ASHA certification and/or state license is required.

Taking a certain number of courses at "approved" training centers does not guarantee that you will be an effective professional, nor does the possession of a license to practice. The truly effective professional in the helping professions should have not only a certain level of information, knowledge, and skill, but also a desire to help others and an ability to relate to people seeking help.

As a further protection to the public, ASHA is encouraging the development of continuing education programs, which will help certified speech-language pathologists and audiologists to update their training continuously to keep up with new research findings and clinical procedures, not only in their own field but in other areas that relate directly to communication disorders. Examples would include special workshops, seminars, and conferences dealing with the use of computers by speech-language pathologists; procedures for evaluating the effectiveness of therapy programs; current status of legislation relating to requirements for providing special services to children, etc. Signer (1988) presented vignettes of four speech-language pathologists and audiologists who continued their learning and growing as they adjusted to challenges of their postgraduate careers. One has "found her 'niche' in computers." Another has "survived the hard times of taking over a private practice." Ten years ago few would have predicted that the lead book review in a 1987 issue of *Asha* (a monthly journal of the American Speech-Language-Hearing Association) would be of a book on the application of computers to speech-language services in the schools (Work, 1987). Nor would many have predicted that in 1988 almost an entire issue of *Asha* would be devoted to articles dealing with private practice (*ASHA,* 1988). This same issue of *Asha* also contains recommendations on competencies for speech-language pathologists providing augmentative communication services that employ technologies such as computers, telephones, speech synthesizers, speech recognition devices, etc. An increasing number of positions in private for-profit companies are becoming available in the supervision and management of providing services to those with communication disorders. These are concepts and procedures found in few training programs 5 years ago. As you begin your training, you should be prepared to continue to keep abreast of new developments in the field after you receive your certificate of clinical competence.

# AMERICAN SPEECH-LANGUAGE-HEARING ASSOCIATION

Because the American Speech-Language-Hearing Association is such an important part of the profession, you may be interested in looking back a few years to see how this organization came into being. In a sense this will give us a general picture of the history of speech-language pathology as a profession in the United States. A more detailed account of this history can be found in Elaine Paden's (1970) *A History of the American Speech and Hearing Association, 1925–1958.*

Of course, before ASHA was founded, there were people in the United States who were helping other people with hearing and communication disorders. Workers relied heavily on information available in writing that appeared in Germany, Austria, France, and England. Throughout Europe until World War II, most communication disorders were treated by members of the medical profession.

References to speech disorders go back to biblical times. Greek writers several centuries before the birth of Christ mentioned a variety of communication disorders. Perhaps the best known legend regarding speech disorders deals with a description of Demosthenes going down to the ocean and shouting over the waves as he attempted to talk with a mouth full of pebbles. Legend has it that this technique was recommended to cure his stuttering. Although our records of this story are not reliable, it has been suggested that the person who advised this treatment for Demosthenes was an actor named Satyrus.

Over the years, some people have made strong claims about their ability to cure communication disorders. These claims have not always proved to be true. Some of the worst offenders promised cures for stuttering, and founded schools for the cure of stuttering and stammering. They held out false hope to those with problems and on occasion extracted large sums of money from people who could ill afford their fees.

While all of this was going on, a number of concerned practitioners from a variety of fields were trying to apply the knowledge available in the field of communication disorders. These individuals by and large did not make wild claims for guaranteed cures. Their fees were reasonable—in fact, many of these professional workers were employed by universities and did not themselves receive fees for the services they rendered.

By the early 1900s, a number of ethical practitioners were actively engaged in the treatment of communication disorders. At that time there were no formal training programs in the United States for the individual who wished to concentrate in this field. Clinicians practicing in the United States in the early 1900s often went to Germany and Austria to learn from the workers there. It was not until well into the second decade of the 20th century that a number of Americans began to contribute to the literature in the field of communication disorders. Although Alexander Graham Bell is best known for his work in the development of the telephone, he must also be credited as one of the first people in the United States to write in the field of hearing and communication disorders. Among other early American writers in the field were Elmer Kenyon, Edward Scripture, Charles Blumel, and Knight Dunlap. Often these American writers repeated the theories that were prevalent in Europe. More often than not, their writing consisted of highly subjective reports and descriptions of observations of clients and treatment procedures.

Early in this century, American school systems began to employ specialists to work with children with communication disorders. Paden (1970) reports that, as early as 1910, the Chicago public schools employed 10 speech correction teachers. At that same time, the city of Detroit had two speech correctionists in the school system. Boston's schools began a program of speech correction in 1913, and New York and San Francisco had established programs by 1916. In the state of Wisconsin, eight cities had speech correction teachers in the public schools by 1916. This trend for school systems to establish programs of therapy for children with communication disorders developed to such an extent that in 1918 Dr. Walter B. Swift published a paper entitled "How to Begin Speech Correction in the Public Schools" (Paden, 1970).

By the early 1920s there was a considerable increase in the publication of scientifically based studies in the field of communication disorders. Along with this increase of scientific studies came the development of university courses concerned with the nature and treatment of communication disorders. Somewhere around 1915 the University of Wisconsin established what was probably the first speech clinic in any American university. The same university granted the first Ph.D. in the field of communication disorders to Sarah M. Stinchfield in 1921.

The University of Wisconsin was followed by other universities in establishing programs for training specialists in communication disorders. Included among these pioneer programs were Columbia University, the University of Pennsylvania, and the University of Iowa. There was continued development of university-level training programs dealing with communication disorders. This growth proved to be particularly strong throughout universities in the Midwest.

Although many clinicians working in the field of communication disorders came from university departments in the broad field of speech and communication, many of those contributing to the field of speech pathology in its early years in the United States were not academic teachers of speech but came from such fields as otolaryngology, psychology, neurology, and psychiatry. From the very beginning of speech-language pathology in the United States, the field has profited from the contributions of experts from a variety of disciplines.

During the first quarter of the 20th century, the National Association of Teachers of Speech (NATS) provided the opportunity for workers in the field of communication disorders to present papers and publish papers in the official journals of that association. By 1920 enough members of the National Association of Teachers of Speech were interested in communication disorders to form a small interest group. This group met with NATS to hold meetings concerned entirely with communication disorders. Of the 84 articles published from 1921 to 1923 in the *Quarterly Journal of Speech Education,* 10 dealt with speech correction and 7 were concerned with phonology and phonetics. During the 1920s, the *Quarterly Journal of Speech Education* showed a good deal of interest in the field of communication disorders. This can be seen in reviews of new books of concern to speech-language pathologists. It can also be seen by an examination of various reports of research in progress.

The increasing interest in the field of communication disorders grew to the point where, in 1925, a small group met in Iowa City and proposed the creation of an organization devoted entirely to the study and treatment of communication disorders. Credit for bringing this small group together is often given to Dean Carl E. Seashore of the University of Iowa Graduate School. By training, Seashore was a psychologist, and many of the early organizers of the group that eventually became ASHA came out of a strong background in psychology. December 29, 1925, is considered to be the date of the formal action that established an association devoted to the study of the field of communication disorders. Eleven individuals are mentioned in the official minutes of that first meeting. The group chose as a name the American Academy of Speech Correction and stated as its purpose "the promotion of scientific, organized work in the field of speech correction" (Paden, 1970). The membership of the new organization was limited to members of the National Association of Teachers of Speech who met certain requirements, which included working in the field of communication disorders, teaching others to become specialists in communication disorders, and conducting research dealing with the causes and treatment of communication disorders. In those early days, membership in the American Academy of Speech Correction required individuals to be involved not only in clinical activities but in teaching and research as well. For almost 25 years, the American Academy of Speech Correction continued to meet each year with the National Association of Teachers of Speech.

In 1935 the organization changed its name to American Speech Correction Association. It now had 87 members, who decided to begin a publication titled *Journal of Speech Disorders.* The first editor of the *Journal of Speech Disorders* was G. Oscar Russell, who served in this capacity for 7 years. Some indication of the rapid growth of the profession can be seen from the fact that within my own professional lifetime, the membership in the professional association devoted to communication disorders has grown from about 100 members to nearly 50,000. The increase in the number of association publications has increased in an equally dramatic fashion.

At the December 31, 1947, business meeting of the American Speech Correction Association held in Salt Lake City, a motion was passed to amend the constitution to change the name of the association to include reference to hearing rehabilitation. The new name became the American Speech and Hearing Association. This name continued until 1978, when the present name, American Speech-Language-Hearing Association, was adopted. This most recent name change recognized the large number of children and adults whose communication problem was in the area of language.

*1978*
*Amer Speech -*
*Lang-Hearing*
*Assoc.*

The inclusion of the term *hearing* in the name of the association recognized the rapid growth of interest in aural rehabilitation during World War II. Four retraining centers had been established during the war to serve the needs of military and navy personnel with hearing impairments. With the end of the war in 1945, the staff of the programs established for the hearing casualties of the war began applying their knowledge and skills to the needs of the civilian population. A new profession, audiology, began. Today the audiologist is one of several specialists serving the needs of those with communication disorders.

From the beginning, the members of the American Academy of Speech Correction had a deep commitment to a strong code of ethics. As early as 1926, one of the five qualifications for membership listed in the original constitution was

> Possession of a professional reputation untainted by a past record (or present record) of unethical practices such as latent commercialization of professional services or guaranteeing of "cures" for stated sums of money. (Paden, 1970)

As early as 1930, a section of the constitution was devoted to a statement of principles of ethics. Section III was devoted to a list of unethical practices. These unethical practices included

1. To guarantee to cure any disorder of speech
2. To offer in advance to refund any part of a person's tuition if his disorder of speech is not arrested
3. To make "rash promises" difficult of fulfillment to secure pupils or patients
4. To employ blatant or untruthful methods of self-advertising
5. To advertise to correct disorders of speech entirely by correspondence
6. To seek self-advancement by attacking the work of other members of the society in such a way as might injure their standing and reputation. Reproaches or criticisms should be sympathetically discussed with the member involved
7. For persons who do not hold a medical degree to attempt to deal exclusively with speech patients requiring medical treatment without the advice or the authority of a physician
8. To extend the time of treatment beyond the time when one should recognize his inability to effect further improvement
9. To charge exorbitant fees for treatment (Paden, 1970)

These same ethical concerns are incorporated in ASHA's present code of ethics (see Appendix B). Additional statements have been incorporated into the present-day code of ethics to provide further protection to the clients whom members of the profession serve. Upholding the code of ethics is one of the most valuable functions of ASHA. As Paden (1970) stated in concluding her chapter dealing with ethics in the history of the American Speech and Hearing Association,

> The stature which ASHA has held, however, is due in no small degree to its early and continued concerns for the high ethical principles which it has insisted be upheld in the relations to all members, to the public, and which has, in turn, brought substantial reward to the members themselves.

## YOU AND THE CODE OF ETHICS

As someone who is considering a career in speech-language pathology or audiology, you need to be aware of the ethical concerns leading to the formation of the professional society that eventually became the American Speech-Language-Hearing Association. You should also be aware of the ethical responsibilities you would be asked to assume as a practicing member of the profession today. For this reason, you should carefully read the most recent statement (1986) of the code of ethics of ASHA (Appendix B). The ASHA code of ethics includes the following six major principles, each of which involves certain ethical proscriptions or matters of professional propriety.

1. Individuals shall hold paramount the welfare of persons served professionally.
2. Individuals shall maintain high standards of professional competence.
3. Individuals' statements to persons served professionally and to the public shall provide accurate information about the nature and management of communicative disorders, and about the profession and services rendered by its practitioners.
4. Individuals shall maintain objectivity in all matters concerning the welfare of persons served professionally.
5. Individuals shall honor their responsibilities to the public, their profession, and their relationships with colleagues and members of allied professions.
6. Individuals shall uphold the dignity of the profession and freely accept the profession's self-imposed standards.

## Responsibility to Client

A code of ethics is more than a statement of "Thou shalt nots." The real basis of a code of ethics is giving highest priority to the welfare of the clients a profession is to serve. What is ethical or not ethical in one's behavior as a professional boils down to the kinds of choices one makes. The professional is confronted frequently with making choices that could be based on answers to three questions:

1. What is the appropriate decision as determined by the best interest of my client?
2. What is the best decision in terms of the organization I work for?
3. What is the best decision for me personally?

It is safe to say that any time a decision is made on the basis of "what is best for my organization" or "what is best for me personally" rather than *"what is best for my client,"* there is a real chance that the answer may be unethical. Speech-language pathologists and audiologists have an overriding responsibility for the welfare of people who have communication disorders. Part of the responsibility we believe speech-language pathologists should take is the responsibility to serve as advocates for the communicatively handicapped who are not receiving the services they should have and to which they are entitled under the law.

In trying to bring needed help to an individual with a communication disorder, you may occasionally encounter a situation where you seem to be in competition with a professional from another discipline who is also trying to help. This can lead to differences of opinion such as whether a child with a language problem should receive therapy from a speech-language pathologist, from a specialist in learning disabilities, or from a classroom teacher. There is no one right approach. In each instance you—as an ethical professional—will have to decide which type of service delivery will be best for the person with the communication disorder. Your decision cannot ethically be made on the basis of the status of your profession, income to the agency you work for, or your own financial or prestige enhancement.

There is also the possibility of a jurisdictional dispute between a speech-language pathologist and the physician who has the overall responsibility for the health of a child or adult who has a communication disorder. In this situation, the physician may become involved in decisions relating to speech-language therapy for which he has no training, or the speech-language pathologist may become involved in aspects of care that are clearly outside the realm of speech-language pathology. Again, ethics demand that decisions be made on the basis of what is best for the person with the communication problem.

Because it is difficult to completely separate and isolate a communication disorder from the health, educational, social, and psychological characteristics of the person with the disorder, speech-language pathologists and audiologists frequently work closely with teachers, physicians, dentists, psychologists, social workers, and other professionals equally committed to human service. Speech-language pathologists and audiologists are trained to work with representatives of many professions to be able to best treat the *person* with a problem rather than the communication disorder.

## Responsibility to Society

The profession also has a responsibility to society in general. As more and more questions are being raised about how our tax dollars are being spent, professionals will be subjected to public demands for accountability. We can point to Annabelle, Roger, and Jerry and say, "Look what speech-language pathology has accomplished by making it possible for these individuals to develop their potential." We can point to happier lives resulting from the correction of communication disorders. We can also show that the treatment of people with communication disorders results in economic benefits to the larger society, which in a real sense pays the cost of our treatment efforts. Spending a few hundred dollars for speech-language treatment for Annabelle helped her to develop into a normal, happy person who now earns a living and pays taxes. Without the help of speech-language pathology, Annabelle would have been supported in a state institution at taxpayers' expense for the rest of her life. We have ample evidence to show that, in the long run, our services contribute to the economic well-being of society by helping people with communication disorders become productive, tax-paying citizens. As more and more competition develops for the tax dollar that supports education and rehabilitation programs, our professions will have to inform the public that providing help for those with communication disorders not only enriches their individual lives, but also enriches the general society in economic and human terms.

Another part of our responsibility to society is to continuously evaluate our procedures. Do our treatment techniques accomplish their purposes? Is the system we use to deliver services the most effective? Does it reach the people who need our services? Is there a less costly way to provide the needed services? All of these questions will be raised by the general public as well as those responsible for allocating funds for education, health, and "the general welfare."

As we try to answer some of these questions of accountability, we may come to realize that certain of the traditional activities of speech-language pathologists and audiologists need to be modified or can be carried out more economically by other workers. This has already happened in some other professions. For example, prior to World War II, most shots were given by physicians. Now the majority of shots are administered by other members of the health professions who have had less training than physicians. X-ray technicians and a host of medical technicians carry out other procedures that once were handled exclusively by physicians. Today the cleaning of teeth is frequently done by dental hygienists rather than by graduate dentists.

Although the Legislative Council of ASHA approved guidelines for the employment and utilization of supportive personnel in 1969, the profession as a whole has not accepted this to the extent adopted by other providers of health care. The 1969 guidelines were revised by the Committee on Supportive Personnel, and the revision was approved by the Legislative Council in 1980. In December 1987 an addendum (ASHA, 1987) to these guidelines was proposed. The new guidelines in part are a response to growing concerns that we are not meeting our responsibilities to underserved populations: American Indians, the economically disadvantaged, people in remote/rural regions, linguistic minorities, the institutionalized, and people in developing regions. Part of our responsibility as professionals is to find the most effective ways of helping those with communication disorders, which could quite possibly involve using paraprofessionals—those with less training than that received by speech-language pathologists or audiologists.

You face the challenge of taking the information and skills presented in this book and evaluating their effectiveness in the settings in which you will be working. For this reason, we will not try to give you cookbook recipes for diagnosis and treatment, but instead will give you general principles. Where possible, we will explain the extent to which these principles are based on research findings or on clinical observations or impressions. As practicing speech-language pathologists and audiologists, we will try to tell you what we know, what we don't know, and how we have decided what we think we know. As the professional worker of tomorrow, you will be called upon to assume more responsibility and to be more directly accountable to the public than has been true for most of us in our careers. As a professional, you will need to know not only the procedures to follow in helping your students or clients, but also how to evaluate your own effectiveness and that of your profession as a whole. It is not enough to understand evaluation procedures; you must be honest and open to self-evaluation in the best interests of the individuals you are committed to help and of the society that pays for a large portion of that help.

## Prevention and Research

As we assume greater responsibility for accountability, we also have a responsibility to try to prevent communication disorders, which requires us to learn more about their causes. This knowledge will come from the research efforts of speech-language pathologists and of other professionals as well. In speech-language pathology research, we try to better understand normal communication to better understand disordered communication. In turn, our increasing knowledge of the disordered will contribute to our understanding of the normal.

Some research projects are carried out by speech-language pathologists and audiologists working in university and hospital laboratories, others in schools and clinics. As we seek better treatment procedures for individuals with communication disorders, we will try new approaches and compare them with the old in an effort to find the most effective therapies—effective both in terms of results and costs. A person about to embark on a career in speech-language pathology and audiology can look forward to stimulating work in research as well as clinical service.

For those with an interest in the teaching of a new generation of speech-language pathologists and audiologists, there will also be opportunities as college and university teachers and supervisors of clinic practice in the many training programs.

# A LOOK AT THE FUTURE OF
# SPEECH-LANGUAGE PATHOLOGY

It is difficult to predict how speech-language pathology and audiology in 5 years will differ from the profession as we know it today, but we can make a few educated guesses, based in part on some current federal legislation. One piece of legislation that has already affected speech-language pathology is Public Law 94–142, the Education for All Handicapped Children Act. In addition to providing more federal money to identify and treat children with communication disorders, this legislation requires that services to handicapped students be provided in "the least restrictive environment." This mandate is often referred to as "mainstreaming"; it means that, as much as possible, a child is not segregated from nonhandicapped peers but instead receives as much therapy and education as possible in the regular classroom. Many of the remedial procedures speech-language pathologists have historically carried out in special speech rooms are now carried out in the regular classroom—often by the classroom teacher with advice and consultation from the speech-language pathologist. To be effective in working in the classroom, the speech-language pathologist and audiologist will have to learn about classroom procedures, curriculum, how reading and spelling are taught, and so on. The speech-language pathologist and audiologist working in a school setting in the future will have to be able to work as part of a team concerned with more than the problem of a communication disorder. The speech-language pathologist and audiologist in tomorrow's schools will be more involved with the overall education of children with communication disorders.

Another effect of P.L. 94–142 was an increase in attention directed to identifying children with learning disabilities and designing programs of remediation for them. Speech-language pathologists and audiologists are particularly well qualified to work with those students whose primary learning disability is manifested by disorders of language acquisition, comprehension, and production. Speech-language pathologists and audiologists are being called upon to help assess children suspected of having learning disabilities to determine if there is a language disorder. Speech-language pathologists and audiologists on their own, and in cooperation with special educators, plan programs to assist children with language disorders and language-based learning disabilities (Gruenewald, 1980). Speech-language pathologists and audiologists in some instances carry out remedial procedures themselves. In other instances, they may design programs to be carried out by teachers or other specialists. Thus, speech-language pathologists and audiologists are providing consulting services as well as direct services to individuals. In keeping with the long-standing tradition of the profession as well as ASHA's code of ethics, any jurisdictional problems should again be resolved by making decisions that are in the best interest of the individual student. P.L. 94–142 requires that all placement and program decisions be made by a team comprised of at least the classroom and special teacher, the parents, an administrator, and all relevant specialists, which would include the speech-language pathologist. Thus, the school speech-language pathologist and audiologist of the future will need to be able to participate effectively both as a team member and as an expert in the field.

Another effect of P.L. 94–142 was the extension of services to previously unserved populations. The law mandated services to handicapped children between the ages of 3 and 21, which meant that more preschoolers are evaluated and, presumably, treated. Children with more severe handicaps, including the hearing impaired, the mentally retarded, and the physically handicapped, are moving into regular classrooms and regular schools—in some cases, from institutions. The public school speech-language pathologist and audiologist are likely to see students with a broader range of communication disorders than used to appear in that setting. It is also likely that audiologists will evaluate more children referred by the public schools.

Public Law 99–457 will provide new opportunities for speech-language pathologists and audiologists to develop and implement programs and services for infants and toddlers from birth to age 2. Increased financial support will be available for programs serving ages 3 through 5. States will be required to ensure the use of qualified personnel to provide special education and related services. We can anticipate that by school year 1990–1991, all children ages 3 to 5 with communication disorders will be receiving the services of qualified speech-language pathologists and audiologists.

Certain other shifts in emphasis are also likely. We will be called upon to serve more senior citizens as well as more preschoolers. We will be called upon to provide more services to the multiply and severely handicapped. Caseloads will probably shift from an emphasis on problems of articulation to language and learning disabilities. As speech-language and audiology services are integrated into students' total educational programs, we can expect to be more involved with team teaching and other cooperative activities with special education and classroom teachers. We can expect to see greater concern for providing services to populations now underserved: American Indians, the economically disadvantaged, linguistic minorities, etc.

It will become desirable for some speech-language pathologists and audiologists to supplement their ASHA membership with membership in other professional associations that have overlapping interests. Speech-language pathologists in public schools may become more active in the Council for Exceptional Children (CEC). Those who see many cleft palate patients will find value in affiliation with the American Cleft Palate Association (ACPA). The American Association for Mental Deficiency (AAMD) may be attractive to those working with retarded children and adults, The Association for the Severely Handicapped (TASH) to those working with the multiply handicapped.

Along with these developments, we can expect to see increasing opportunities for private practice. Donna R. Fox, president of the Academy of Private Practice, pointed out that "in the past 25 years, private practice has grown from a few isolated practitioners to thousands of practitioners in both full- and part-time practice" (1980, p. 383). She concluded a recent guest editorial in *Asha* with the following statement about the challenges and rewards of private practice.

> Clinicians in private practice understand the dilemma of serving two masters: the need to provide quality service at a reasonable price and the need to actively contribute to their profession through research and organizational affiliation. This dedication to serving both makes private practice an exciting and rewarding professional setting. (p. 384)

Fox's 1980 beliefs concerning the challenges and rewards of private practice are echoed by Feldman (1988), Dunn-Engel (1988), and Signer (1988).

With the growth of third-party payment for health services, we can expect to see an increase in the number of companies organized to provide speech-language pathology and audiology services in nursing homes, hospitals, and rehabilitation centers, as well as in the homes of patients. These companies are carrying out aggressive recruiting campaigns to attract personnel who can provide services for clients with communication disorders. Within these companies there will be opportunities for speech-language pathologists and audiologists to serve in a variety of supervisory and administrative roles.

## CONCLUSION

Speech-language pathology and audiology have been satisfying careers for many (Wisniewski & Shewan, 1987). Some of us have experienced satisfaction as clinicians, some as researchers, some as teachers and administrators. We have in our lifetime seen our professional association, ASHA, grow from fewer than 100 members to over 50,000. We have been able to observe the results of our efforts when people with communication disorders become happy and productive citizens. The future is equally bright for someone about to embark on a career in this field. We hope that the balance of this book will lead many of you to that rewarding career.

## SELECTED READINGS

Dunn-Engel, E. (1988). A quality-oriented solo private practice. *Asha, 30*(1) 33.

Matthews, J. (1964). Communicology and individual responsibility. *Asha, 6*(1).

Paden, E. P. (1970). *A history of the American Speech and Hearing Association, 1925–1958.* Washington, D.C.: American Speech and Hearing Association.

Perkins, W. H. (1978). *Human perspectives in speech and language disorders.* St. Louis: C. V. Mosby.

Shewan, C. M. (1987). ASHA members: You are a changin'! Part II. *Asha, 29*(11) 41.

Shewan, C. M. (1988). ASHA members at work. *Asha, 30*(1) 34.

Van Riper, C. (1979). *A career in speech pathology.* Englewood Cliffs, NJ: Prentice-Hall.

Wisniewski, A. T., & Shewan, C. M. (1987). There is joy in Mudville career satisfaction. *Asha, 29*(10) 30–31.

Work, R. S. (1987). Microcomputer applications for speech-language services in the schools. *Asha, 29*(11) 50.

# Bases of Human Communication

# CHAPTER TWO

# Development of Communication, Language, and Speech

## ROBERT E. OWENS, JR.

## MYTHS AND REALITIES

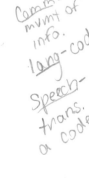

- *Myth:* The terms *communication, language,* and *speech* all mean the same thing.

- *Reality:* Communication is a process of moving information from the brain of one person to that of another. To be transmitted, the message must be coded in some form, called language, that both communication partners understand. Finally, this code is transmitted by some physical act, such as speech or writing. While all three terms—*communication, language,* and *speech*—are related, they describe different aspects of the process. In this chapter, we shall describe each term in detail and explore development in this area.

- *Myth:* Language develops prior to communication, which cannot occur without the use of language symbols.

- *Reality:* If we concentrate our study on only language and language rule acquisition, we miss the full context within which language develops. Language is a social tool used to accomplish our goals of influencing others, exchanging information, and the like. It is within this rich environment of communicative interaction that language first emerges. The newborn child and her caregiver act as communication partners almost from the moment of the child's birth. The caregiver treats the child as if she has something to communicate, and treats her behavior as if it is meaningful. The child gradually learns to communicate through gestures, and to attend to her caregiver to ensure that the caregiver is noticing. Through continued interactions, the child learns to request, point, give, and so on. Language symbols are then acquired to fulfill the uses of these gestures. Language is learned as a more effective manner of communicating.

- *Myth:* Children learn language through imitation.

- *Reality:* It is impossible to learn the rich, flexible, versatile language system of the average child or adult through imitation alone. In fact, most children cease imitating their caregivers shortly after age two. Rather, young children form their own language rules from the examples of language that they hear around them. These rules are then used by the child to construct novel sentences that he has neither heard nor said before.

- *Myth:* Children's language rule systems are versions of adult rule systems that are in error.

- *Reality:* Children's rule systems are valid within themselves. While adult rules do not permit "Mommy sock," this utterance is perfectly acceptable for a 2-year-old. Children devise their own rule systems based on the language that they hear. Since these children do not know the adult rules, their own rules could not possibly be errant versions of adult rules.

- *Myth:* Learning language consists of merely learning syntactic rules.

- *Reality:* When each of us attended elementary school, we learned about nouns, verbs, adjectives, and so on. We knew how to use these elements long before we learned the labels and the stated rules. This instruction left the impression with most of us that syntax, the aspect of language concerned with nouns, verbs, and the like, is all there is to language. Language is much more complex than just the word relationships specified in syntax. Language development involves acquisition of word meanings and categories, rules for the speech sound combinations used in transmission, and discourse skills for language use in conversation. Adult development continues to concentrate on semantics and pragmatics with increased vocabulary growth and versatility in use. Vocabulary growth and categorization continues throughout life. New words are added for specialized occupations, interests, and socialization. In addition, the adult becomes an even more adept user of language, able to adapt her language style to different social contexts and different communication goals.

*[handwritten margin note: Concerned w/ lang. use; communi- w/ th communication context]*

THERE are several persistent myths or misconceptions about the development of communication, language, and speech. In this chapter, we shall explore the nondisordered (normal) development of communication, language, and speech by middle-class children in the United States. I hope to provide the prospective speech-language pathologist with a model of development, and to dispel some of the persistent myths. As we discuss development of communication, language, and speech, the reader may encounter several ideas that challenge his or her notion of communication development. That is as it should be in a text. Further study will help to clarify questions raised. In the sections that follow, we shall explore the terms *communication, language,* and *speech,* and the development that occurs within each.

## COMMUNICATION

**Communication** is the process of exchanging information and ideas. An active process, it involves encoding, transmitting, and decoding the intended message. There are many means of communicating, and many different message systems. Therefore, the probability of message distortion is high, given the number of ways that a message can be formed and the connotations and perceptions of each participant. Each communication partner must be alert to the needs of the others, so that messages are conveyed effectively and intended meanings preserved.

Speech and language are only a portion of communication. Other aspects of communication may enhance or even eclipse the linguistic code. These aspects are **paralinguistic, nonlinguistic,** and **metalinguistic.** Paralinguistic mechanisms can change the form and meaning of a sentence by acting across individual sounds or words of a sentence. These mechanisms signal attitude or emotion, and include intonation, stress, rate of delivery, and pause or hesitation. Intonation patterns are changes in pitch, such as a rising pitch at the end of a sentence used to signal a question. Stress is employed for emphasis. At one point, as a child, each of us firmly asserted, "I *did* take a bath." Rate varies with the speaker's state of excitement, familiarity with the content, and perceived comprehension of the listener. Pauses may be used to emphasize a portion of the message or to replace it. Even young children recognize that a short maternal pause after a child's request usually signals a negative reply. Each of us has experienced the pause that followed, "Can Ray eat over tonight?"

Nonlinguistic cues include gestures, body posture, facial expression, eye contact, head and body movement, and physical distance or proxemics.

Each of these aspects of nonlinguistic behavior can influence communication. For example, gestures tend to enhance speech and language, and to set the rhythm for communication. Body posture and facial expression can convey the speaker's attitude toward a message, partner, or situation. The speaker who says, "Oh sure, I like that idea," but sits in a defensive, tight posture conveys a different attitude. Likewise, eye contact and physical distance can communicate the degree of involvement of two participants in the message or in the communicative interaction. A wink may convey more than a whole sentence.

Metalinguistic cues signal the status of communication based on our intuitions about the acceptability of utterances. In other words, metalinguistic skills enable us to talk about language, analyze it, think about it, separate it from its context, and judge it. Communication partners monitor both their own and their partner's communication. The focus is on what is transmitted, but also how this is accomplished.

# Development of Communication

Communication appears to be present at birth. The newborn and her mother begin communicating almost immediately. Within a few minutes of her birth, the child will move her body in synchrony with the human voice (Condon & Sanders, 1974). She will not move in synchrony to disconnected vowel sounds or to tapping. In addition, the newborn will search for the human voice and demonstrate pleasure or mild surprise when she finds the face that is the sound source. Both she and her mother will do almost anything to attend to the other's face and voice.

For us, the primary communication context of interest is the child-mother or child-caregiver pair. As caregivers respond to their infants' early reflexive behaviors, the infants learn to communicate their intentions. Gradually, through repeated interactions, the infants refine these communication skills. The process is not one-sided, nor is the child a passive participant (Bell, 1968; Moerk, 1972). Within the first few months of life, infants are able to discriminate contrasting phonemes, different intonational patterns, and speech from nonspeech (Eimas, 1974; Hirschman & Katkin, 1974; Kearsley, 1973; Moffitt, 1971; Turnure, 1971). Infants are also able to discriminate different voices and to demonstrate a preference for the human face and human speech sounds (Richards, 1974). In addition, the infant learns different gaze patterns used in communication (Bateson, 1979; Collis, 1977). The infant also learns the signal value of head movements. Both the face and head are important for early communication because these structures are relatively advanced in their maturation (Stern, 1977). These discrimination abilities and preferences provide the bases for early communication.

Caregivers respond to these infant behaviors and treat them as meaningful social communication. The degree of caregiver responsiveness appears to be positively correlated with later language abilities (Bell & Ainsworth, 1972). In addition, such responsiveness forges an attachment bond between mother and child that fosters communication (Ainsworth, Bell, & Slayton, 1974; Blehar, Lieberman, & Ainsworth, 1977). By 3 to 4 months, interactions based on eye gaze form early dialogues that evolve into conversational exchanges.

Infants receive highly selective language input within the routines of child-parent interactions (Bruner, 1975). Two routines, *joint action* and *joint references,* are particularly noteworthy. Within joint action routines, such as "peek-a-boo" and "this little piggy," children learn turn-taking skills. Mothers provide a consistent set of behaviors that enable their children to predict the outcome and later to anticipate. Children learn to signal their intention to play.

Caregivers systematically train children to differentiate between objects by joint reference, or the focusing of attention by both partners on objects. Once the referent has been established, mothers provide linguistic input relative to it. This process is important for early meaning development (Wells, 1974). Maternal speech is modified systematically so that it is comprehensible to the child (Mahoney, 1975; Snow, 1977a, 1977b).

For their part, children progress from reflexive, nonintentional communication to conventional, verbal intentions by the second year of life. There appear to be three developmental stages of early communication intentions (Bates, 1976). Initially, the child's behaviors are undifferentiated and his intentions unknown. Next, the child uses gestures and vocalization to express intent. This stage is significant because of the child's demonstrated intention to communicate specific information through his persistent use of gestures and vocalizations accompanied by eye contact (Scoville, 1983). Finally, words are used to convey intentions previously expressed in gestures (Dore, 1974; Owens, 1978). Language structure is acquired as a more efficient means of communicating these intentions.

Even at the single-word level, however, the child demonstrates considerable communication skill. For example, the child exhibits presupposition, or the assumption that her listener knows or does not know certain information that will affect her message. The preschooler learns to use emphasis and stress to improve her message quality. She also adjusts her manner of delivery for her prospective listener. Even 4-year-old children can modify their speech and language when conversing with much younger language-learning children. In general, preschool communication gives the impression of greater intimacy. Communication distance is much closer than that of adults. Even young school-age children do not exhibit the greater social space of adults.

It is in the school-age period that the child makes the greatest advances in the use of paralinguistic, nonlinguistic, and metalinguistic aspects of communication. The older child can use his communication skills to create a mood, role play, or express sarcasm. He learns to use timing or rate to heighten his delivery or to create curiosity. Gestures are used to enhance or

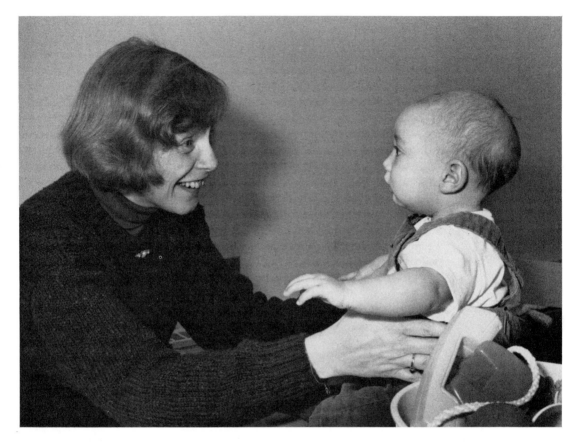

Parental expressiveness and attention enhance the development of communication in children.

to add emphasis to the message. He adjusts his message and its manner of delivery to his listener, and tries to predict the effects of his transmission.

Although metalinguistic abilities appear in the preschool years, full awareness does not occur until about age 7 or 8 (Saywitz & Cherry-Wilkinson, 1982). The preschool child tends to make judgments of utterance acceptability based on the content rather than on the grammatical structure. A 4-year-old might judge "Daddy painted a picture" as unacceptable because "Daddies don't paint pictures, pictures come from cameras." By kindergarten, the child is just beginning to separate what is said from how it is said, separate referents from words, and notice structure. The school-age child demonstrates an increasing ability to judge the grammatical acceptability of sentences, reflecting a growing knowledge of language structure. Metalinguistic abilities usually emerge after the child has mastered a linguistic form. For example, it is some time after the child both comprehends and produces passives that she can judge passive and active sentences as synonymous (Beilin & Spontak, 1969).

The preschool child attempts to repair her erroneous or misinterpreted utterances and adjusts her speech and language for her intended listener. She also corrects others and comments on the effectiveness of communication (Clark, 1978). By school age, she can use intonation to signal new words in the conversation; correct utterances inappropriate for the setting or specific listener; identify linguistic units, such as syllables and sentences; provide definitions; and construct humor (Clark, 1978). In addition, she is able to explain why a sentence is appropriate or impossible and how it should be interpreted.

Metalinguistic abilities depend on development of language. With increased skill, the child is freed from the immediate linguistic context to attend to how a message is communicated (Brown, 1978; Flavell, 1977; Flavell & Wellman, 1977). Saywitz and Cherry-Wilkinson (1982) found metalinguistic skill development to be related to cognitive development, reading ability, academic achievement, IQ, environmental stimulation, and play.

## Summary

The child communicates from the time of birth. Early communication does not depend on the use of language or speech. In fact, communication provides the vehicle within which initial language develops. As language skills improve, there is also a corresponding improvement in overall communication abilities.

## LANGUAGE

**Language** can be defined as a socially shared code or conventional system for representing concepts through the use of arbitrary symbols and rule-governed combinations of those symbols. English is a language, as is French or Farsi. Each has its own symbols and rules for symbol combination. Dialects are subcategories of these parent languages that use similar but not identical rules. Languages exist because language users have agreed on the symbols and the rules to be used. This agreement is demonstrated through language usage. Since users can agree to follow the rules of a language, they can also agree to change the rules. New words and rules can be added, while others fall into disuse. The conventional or socially shared code allows language users to exchange information. The code is a device that enables each to represent one thing with another. Each user encodes and decodes according to his concept of a given object, event, or relationship. Thus, coding is a factor of the speaker's and listener's shared meanings, the linguistic skills of each, and the context.

Individual symbols communicate little. Most of the information is contained in symbol combinations. For example, *chemist Tom a is* seems to be a meaningless jumble of words. By shifting a few words, we can create *Tom is a chemist* or *Is Tom a chemist?* Language is a "system of relationships" (Dever, 1978, p. 11), and it is the rules for these relationships that give language order and permit language to be used creatively. A finite set of symbols and a finite set of rules governing symbol use are used to create and interpret an infinite number of sentences. Language is not limited to the rules, however, but also includes the process of rule usage.

A language user's underlying knowledge about the system of rules is called **linguistic competence.** It consists of knowledge of the operating principles needed to be a language user. As you know, you do not always observe the linguistic rules. In fact, much of what you say is ungrammatical. Linguistic knowledge translated into your usage is called **linguistic performance.** It is from performance that linguists must deduce the language rules.

Even though much that is said is ungrammatical, native speakers have little difficulty decoding new or novel utterances. If a native speaker knows the words being used, she can apply the rules and understand any sentence encountered. In addition, comprehension is influenced by the intent of the speaker, and by the context (Bloom, 1974; Bransford & Johnson, 1972; Ingram, 1974b; Lakoff, 1972; Schank, 1972; Winograd, 1972). In summary, native speakers of a language do not learn all possible word combinations. Rather, they learn the linguistic rules that enable each language user to understand and to create an infinite variety of sentences.

## Components of Language

Language is a complex combination of several component rule systems. Bloom and Lahey (1978) have divided language into three major components; form, content, and use. *Form* includes **syntax, morphology,** and **phonology,** those components that connect sounds or symbols with meaning. *Content* encompasses meaning or **semantics,** and the *use* component includes **pragmatics.** These five components—syntax, morphology, phonology, semantics, and pragmatics—are the basic rule systems found in language.

The five components are distinct but interrelated. *Syntax* is a rule system governing the ordering of words in sentences. *Morphological rules* govern changes that modify meaning at the word level. For example, *dog* can be modified by the addition of *s* to form *dogs*. *Phonological rules* determine which sounds may appear together and where sounds may appear. For example, the plural *s* on *cats* sounds like an *s*, but that on *dogs* sounds like a *z*. Some sounds may not be placed together. There are, for example, no English words that begin with *dm*. These two sounds are not combined at the beginning of English words, but may appear in the middle, as in *madman. Semantic rules* govern meaning and the relationships between meaning units. They help language users to distinguish sense from nonsense. Finally, *pragmatics* is a set of rules for language use. These rules govern the manner of communication, how to enter and exit a conversation, adoption of roles, sequencing of sentences, and anticipation of listener needs, to name a few functions. All of these rule systems are used simultaneously in communication.

## Syntax

The rules of syntax govern the form or structure of a sentence. They specify word order; sentence organization; relationships between words, word classes or types; and other sentence constituents. Syntax specifies which word combinations are acceptable, or grammatical, and which are not. Word sequences follow definite word-order rules. In addition, syntax specifies which word classes may appear in noun and verb phrases, and the relationship of these two. Each sentence must contain a noun phrase and a verb phrase that include a noun and a verb, respectively. Therefore, a sentence must contain a noun and a verb. Within noun and verb phrases, certain word classes appear. For example, articles appear before nouns and adverbs modify verbs.

Knowledge of the language rules enables language users to understand and generate language. Thus, there is a link between language form and cognitive processing. **Psycholinguistic theory** attempts to explain this relationship. The leading proponent of the psycholinguistic view is Noam Chomsky. Chomsky described language from a psychological perspective. He concentrated on the linguistic process instead of the grammatical products. Although human languages differ, Chomsky claimed that they differ only superficially, and that underlying principles are universal.

According to Chomsky, there are two levels of linguistic processing, characterized by the use of **phrase structure rules** and **transformational rules.** *Phrase structure rules* delineate the basic relationships underlying sentence organization. Units within each sentence are organized hierarchically, which means that each, in turn, may be broken into its parts. In all languages, a sentence, containing at least a noun and a verb, is the basic unit. This basic relationship is written as follows:

$$S \rightarrow NP + VP$$

This formula is read as, "A sentence can be rewritten as a noun phrase and a verb phrase." A noun phrase contains a noun and associated words, such as articles and adjectives. Verb phrases consist of a verb, plus adverbs, prepositional phrases, and possibly a noun phrase (an object of the verb). Using these rules, a tree diagram can be constructed, such as the one in Figure 2.1. The variety of sentences that can be produced is limited only by

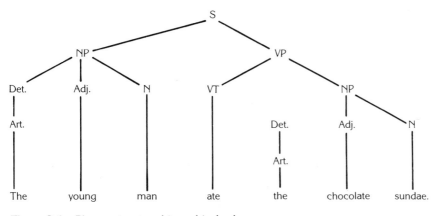

**Figure 2.1** Phrase structure hierarchical rules

the number or words available for each category. Unfortunately, phrase structure rules do not create language, and really concern only the relationship of concepts with one another.

Transformational rules rearrange the basic phrase structure units to create general sentence types, such as questions, negatives, passives, and more complex sentences. A transformational rule is a formula. For example, a rule for passive sentences might read:

$$NP_2 + be + V + ed + by + NP_1$$

This rule can be read as, "Noun phrase 2, followed by the verb *to be,* followed by the verb plus *-ed,* followed by *by,* followed by noun phrase 1." This rule is a transformation of the phrase structure $NP_1 + V + NP_2$. Applying the rule, the sentence *The dog chases the cat* becomes *The cat is chased by the dog.*

Each sentence has both a *deep structure* and a *surface structure* (Figure 2.2). The **deep structure** contains the basic meaning of the sentence. The actual sentence produced is called the **surface structure.** The relationship between the deep and surface structures is determined by the transformational rules. By changing, reordering, and modifying the deep structure elements, these transformational operations create the surface structure.

## Morphology

Morphology, considered by some linguists to be a subcategory of syntax, is concerned with the internal organization of words. Words consist of one or more smaller units called *morphemes.* The smallest unit of meaning, a **morpheme,** is indivisible without violating the meaning or producing mean-

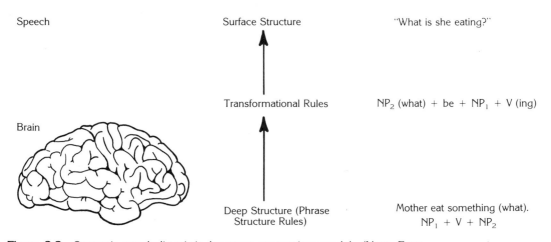

Speech                          Surface Structure                     "What is she eating?"

Brain                           Transformational Rules              $NP_2$ (what) + be + $NP_1$ + V (ing)

                                Deep Structure (Phrase                Mother eat something (what).
                                Structure Rules)                      $NP_1$ + V + $NP_2$

**Figure 2.2**  Syntactic psycholinguistic language-processing model. *(Note: From Language Development: An Introduction (2nd ed.) by R. E. Owens, Jr., 1988. Columbus, OH: Merrill. Copyright 1988 by Merrill Publishing Company. Reprinted by permission.)*

ingless units. Morphology enables the language user to modify word meanings and produce semantic distinctions, such as number (dog, dog*s*), verb tense (talk, talk*ed*), and possession (Mary, Mary*'s*); extend word meanings (*dis*interested, *un*interested); and derive word classes (quick, quick*ness*, quick*ly*).

There are two varieties of morphemes, *free* and *bound.* Free morphemes can be used independently. They form words or parts of words. Examples of free morphemes are *dog, big,* and *happy.* Bound morphemes are grammatical markers that cannot function independently and must be attached to free morphemes or to other bound morphemes. Examples include *'s, er, un-,* and *-ly* (meaning possession, more, negative, and manner, respectively). By combining the free and bound morphemes mentioned above, we can create *dog's, bigger,* and *unhappily.* Bound or grammatical morphemes are attached to words in the noun, verb, and adjective classes to accomplish changes in meaning.

## Phonology

Each language has specific speech sounds or *phonemes* and sound combinations that are characteristic of that language. **Phonemes,** the smallest meaningful units of speech sound, are combined in specific ways to form language units known as *words.* Phonological rules govern the distribution and sequencing of phonemes within a language. Distributional rules describe which sounds can be employed in various positions in words.

For example, in English, the /ŋ/, found in *ring,* may not appear at the beginning of a word. Likewise, the /h/ may not appear at the end. Sequencing rules determine which sounds may appear in combination. For example, the word *bring* is perfectly acceptable in English. *Bling* is not an English word, but would be acceptable. *Bning* could never be an acceptable English word. In addition, sequencing rules concern the sound modifications made when two phonemes appear next to each other. The distributional and sequencing rules may both apply. For example, the combination *nd* will not appear at the beginning of a word, but may appear elsewhere, as in *window.*

*[handwritten margin note: sequencing— in combo]*

## Semantics

Meaning is an arbitrary system for dividing reality into categories and units (Bolinger, 1975). These categories and units group similar objects, actions, and relationships, and distinguish dissimilar ones. Some units are mutually exclusive, such as *walk* and *ride.* A human being can't do both. Other units overlap somewhat, as do *walk, run,* and *jog. Semantics* is concerned with the relationship of language form to objects, events, and relationships, and with words and word combinations.

Words or symbols do not represent reality, but rather each language user's ideas or concepts of reality. A concept is related to a whole class of experiences rather than to any single one. It is the result of a cognitive categorization process. Each word meaning contains two portions drawn from the concept, the semantic features and selection restrictions (Katz, 1966). *Semantic features* characterize the word. For example, the semantic features of *bachelor* include "unwed" and "male." *Selection restrictions* are based on specific features and prohibit certain word combinations as meaningless. For example, *bachelor's wife* is meaningless; *unwed bachelor* is redundant. In addition to objective features, there is also a connotative meaning of subjective features or feelings. Throughout life, language users acquire new features, delete old features, and reorganize the remainder to sharpen word meanings.

The more features two words share, the more they are alike. Words with identical features are *synonyms.* Some examples of synonyms are *big* and *large,* and *little* and *small.* Words with opposite polarity of features, or opposite meanings, are *antonyms.* Examples include *long* and *short, happy* and *sad,* and *black* and *white.*

Words may have several meanings; therefore, users must rely on additional cues, such as selection restrictions, linguistic context, and nonlinguistic context (Brown, 1958; Olson, 1970). Sentences represent a meaning greater than the sum of the individual words because they include relationships between those words that go beyond the individual symbols used.

Early multiword utterances that appear around 18 months of age may represent semantic rather than syntactic relationships. Children's speech contains consistent relationships that are expressed by simple word-order rules such as "agent precedes action," rather than through abstract syntactic relationships (Bloom, 1970; Schlesinger, 1971). As the child develops, word-order rules give way to more mature syntactic devices. Possession, originally signalled by word order, as in "Doggie bed," is later marked by the more mature possessive 's. Thus, content or meaning precedes language form developmentally. When the child acquires syntactic forms, they are used to express older semantic functions (Slobin, 1973).

According to this semantic hypothesis, meaning or semantics is a method of representing experience. It follows, then, that experience must be the basis for early language. Cross-cultural studies suggest that the early semantic rules are universal (Bowerman, 1973; Brown, 1973; Slobin, 1973). The common rules may represent a general pattern of cognitive development. Children learn basic relationships between entities within the environment, and these relationships are reflected in their semantic structures. Children begin to use language to talk about the things that they know. In other words, thought precedes language. Language is grafted onto existing knowledge about the world, and serves as a means of representing the world (Roberts & Horowitz, 1986).

At higher language levels, cognitive development also generally precedes linguistic (Rice, 1980). For example, children gain concepts of time and place before they begin to use the prepositions that mark these concepts. Likewise, knowledge of time sequences and increased memory are required for a child to use the linguistic relationships of "before" and "after." In the semantic/cognitive hypothesis, the child must abstract basic relationships from the physical environment and rules from the linguistic environment. Language input is interpreted using linguistic rules that reflect the cognitive relationships. Thus, language development is a product of the strategies and processes for general cognitive development.

## Pragmatics

Appropriate language use in context is another aspect of linguistic competence. To communicate successfully, the child must have knowledge of social appropriateness, as well as the knowledge of form and content (Rice, 1984). Since language is primarily used in conversations, a study of language use is also a study of discourse or conversational skills. It is the context of conversation that determines how and what the speaker chooses to say.

Bloom and Lahey (1978) have identified two aspects of use: (a) language functions and (b) linguistic selection, or the choice of words to be used. Linguistic functions or language uses may include, but are not limited to, interaction, regulation, and control (Halliday, 1975a, 1975b). The choice of codes to fulfill these functions is determined primarily by the speaker's intent (Schlesinger, 1971), but also by his perceptions of the listener, the shared

**43**

cognitive and linguistic information, and the situation. Listener characteristics that influence speaker behaviors are sex, age, race, style, dialect, social status, and role.

*Pragmatic rules* govern sequential organization and coherence of conversions, repair of errors, role, and speech acts (Rees & Wollner, 1981). Organization and coherence of conversations include turn-taking; opening, maintaining, and closing a conversation; establishing and maintaining topic; and making relevant contributions to the conversation. Repair includes giving and receiving feedback. Role skills include establishing and maintaining role, and switching linguistic codes for each role. Finally, speech acts include coding of intentions relative to the communicative context.

*A speech act is a unit of linguistic communication that contains not only the form of the utterance, but the meaning and the intention of the speaker.*

To ignore pragmatics is to concentrate on language structure and to remove language from its communicative context. The primary purpose of language is communication. **Sociolinguistic** theory considers language as it is used in communication rather than as an isolated phenomenon. Theorists who adhere to a sociolinguistic model concentrate on the social/communicative uses of language. Language use is central to the linguistic process. The motivation for language use and language acquisition is effective communication. The speaker chooses the form and content that will best fulfill her intentions based on her perception of the communication situation. In this view, language is not an abstract code but an interactive tool.

From a developmental perspective, the role of the child's communication partners is crucial. Language development is "made possible by the presence of an interpreting adult who operates as a provider, and expander and idealizer of utterances while interacting with the child" (Bruner, 1975, p. 17). Initially, the child learns to understand the rules of dialogue, not of syntax or semantics (Bruner, 1977). A communication base is established first, then language is mapped onto this base to express the intentions the child previously expressed nonverbally.

## Summary

Language is a complex system of symbols and rules for symbol use. Native speakers must be knowledgeable of the symbols employed and of the acceptable rules for use of these symbols. These rules include concept, word, morpheme, and phoneme combinations, and the use of these combinations in communication. The five aspects of language that have been described in this section are interrelated, and can help us understand both the communication process and language development.

## Language Development

Within each of the five aspects of language, development is rarely linear. At times, one aspect or a combination may be the major focus of development, as in the early stage when semantics and pragmatics appear to be the organizing principle of child language. Rates of growth within each aspect also vary. During preschool years, the child learns numerous syntactic structures. This growth slows in the school-age years.

In the following sections, we shall explore language development within generally recognized periods of development: toddler, preschool, and school-age/adult. In the toddler period, the child concentrates on vocabulary growth based on the meanings he already possesses. These referent words are used to express the intentions that the child previously expressed through gestures. During the preschool period, the child concentrates on development of language form. Although this process continues during school years at a slower rate, the content and use aspects of language development become more prominent.

## Toddler Language Development

Initial language development is characterized by single-word utterances and by early multiword combinations. It is important to remember that the child's multiword utterances are rule-based and appropriate for her level of development. While *Mommy eat* is not an acceptable adult utterance, it is fine for a 2-year-old. The adult and child rule systems are different.

Language fulfills the pragmatic functions of the child's early nonlinguistic communication. First words fill the intentions or illocutionary functions previously served by gestures and/or vocalizations. These intentions, called Primitive Speech Acts (PSA's) by Dore (1974), are presented in Table 2.l.

Phonologically, the child's first words are simple. Most contain one or two syllables; syllabic constructions usually consist of VC (vowel-consonant) (*eat*), CV (*key*), CVCV-reduplicated (*mamma*), or CVCV (*baby*). Front consonants, such as /p/, /b/, and /m/, predominate. The child's words are phonetic approximations of adult words used by the child to refer consistently to particular entities or events. Initially, the word meaning may have little in common with the meanings of more mature language users.

The child's exact word meaning is unknown. His communication partner interprets his utterance with reference to the ongoing activity and to the child's nonlinguistic behavior. Adults usually paraphrase the child's utterance as a full sentence, implying that the child encoded the full thought, although this assumption is probably false.

The toddler operates with several constraints of attention, memory, and knowledge. In particular, she has difficulty with the organization of information for storage and later retrieval (Ervin-Tripp, 1973; Olson, 1973; Slobin, 1973). Thus, the child's meanings of individual words may not even overlap with the generally accepted meaning. More frequently, however, the child's meaning encompasses a small portion of the fuller adult definition. For

**Table 2.1**   Dore's Primitive Speech Acts

| Primitive Speech Act | Child's Behavior |
|---|---|
| Labeling | Attends to object or event, does not address adult, does not await response. |
| Repeating | Attends to preceding adult utterance, may not address adult, does not await response. |
| Answering | Attends to preceding adult utterance before her utterance, addresses adult who awaits child's response and usually acknowledges response. |
| Requesting (action) | Attends to object or event, addresses adult and/or gestures, awaits response from adult who performs action. |
| Primitive Speech Act | Child's Behavior |
| Requesting (answer) | Addresses adult, awaits response. |
| Calling | Addresses adult by uttering adult's name loudly, awaits response from adult who attends or answers. |
| Greeting | Attends to adult or object to imitate or end speech event, adult returns a greeting utterance. |
| Protesting | Adult initiates speech event by performing an action the child does not like, child addresses adult, resists or denies adult's action. |
| Practicing | Attends to no specific object or event, does not address adult, does not await response. |

*Note:* Adapted from "Holophrases, Speech Acts and Language Universals" by
J. Dore, 1975, *Journal of Child Language, 2*(1), p. 33.

example, the child might hear an adult say, "Won't fit," when the child tries to pull her wagon through the door. She may later use the word *fit* to mean "too big," "I can't do it," or as a general negation of an action. The child's sources of information are the adult's naming in the presence of the referent, and the feedback received for her own utterances.

In the process of refining meanings, the child forms hypotheses about underlying concepts, and extends his current meanings to include new examples (Brown, 1965). Through this process, he gains knowledge from examples and nonexamples of the concept. Some of his concepts are restricted, while others are extended widely. Overly restricted meanings that contain fewer examples than the adult meaning are called *underextensions.* In contrast, *overextensions* are meanings that are too broad, containing more examples than the adult meaning. Calling all men *daddy* is an example of overextension.

Several linguists have suggested that children organize their early words by semantic categories. Such categorization seems basic to language learning (Nelson, 1973). At the two-word stage, children follow simple linear patterns of construction that indicate underlying semantic categories (Table 2.2). These categories are probably present before the appearance of

**Table 2.2**  Two-word Semantic Rules of Toddler Language

| Rule | Example |
|---|---|
| Agent + action | Daddy eat. Mommy throw. |
| Action + object | Eat cookie. Throw hat. |
| Agent + object | Daddy cookie. Mommy hat. |
| Modifier + head | |
| Attributive | Big doggie. |
| Possessive | Daddy shoe. |
| Recurrent | More juice. Nuther cookie. |
| Negative + X | No bed. Allgone juice. |
| Introducer + X | This cup. That doggie. |
| X + location | Doggie bed. Throw me. |

*Note:* Constructed from the work of Bloom (1970, 1973), Brown (1973), and Schlesinger (1971).

two-word utterances, suggesting a continuity from single-word to multiword structures (Greenfield & Smith, 1976; Rodgon, Jankowski, & Alenskas, 1977; Starr, 1975).

Within early two-word combinations, meaning is signalled by word order, and specific word orders fulfill specific functions. For example, the possessive function is marked by the possessor plus the possessed object. Other relationships depend primarily on one or two words that signal the semantic function. For example, the recurrence function is marked by a recurrent word, usually *more* or *nuther,* as in *more milk.* Approximately 70% of the two-word utterances of children learning language can be described by a few simple word-order rules (Table 2.2).

The child's initial two-word combinations probably reflect her rules for each individual word involved. Before long, these rules become overburdensome. Simple word-order rules relative to the child's semantic categories provide a more adequate system for elaborating her meanings and for interpreting adult utterances. Bloom and Lahey (1978) described the early combination rules as "semantic-syntactic"—semantic because the bases for combination are meaning relations, and syntactic because word-order rules and relationships are involved.

With increasing memory and processing skills, the child is able to produce longer utterances by recombining the semantic patterns. Individual differences in development may reflect different strategies for individual word and/or word class combinations (Brown & Leonard, 1986). When approximately half of the child's utterances contain two words, he begins to use three-word combinations. These consist of recombinations and expansions of the two-word semantic rules (Brown, 1973). Four-word utterances are expanded in the same way. No new relations are learned while the child develops skill with longer word combinations. The average child will be producing some four-word utterances by age 2.

Theoretically, the developmental order of semantic relationships reflects the order of development of cognitive structures. This concept has been termed *cognitive determinism*. For example, children demonstrate a concept of object permanence, or of the existence of an object that cannot be seen, before they express relationships such as appearance, disappearance, and nonexistence in their speech (Bloom, 1973; Brown, 1973; Clark, 1973; Kahn, 1975; Nelson, 1974). Children learn relationships and express that knowledge in the language that they learn subsequently.

Several cognitive abilities may need to be present for a child to use symbols (Bowerman, 1974). These include:

1. Ability to represent objects and events not perceptually present

2. Development of basic cognitive structures and operations related to space and time; ability to classify types of actions, embed action patterns within each other, establish object permanence and constancy and relationships between objects and action, and construct a model of one's own perceptual space

3. Ability to derive linguistic-processing strategies from general cognitive structures and processes

4. Ability to formulate concepts and strategies to serve as structural components for the linguistic rules

Several language development specialists consider symbolic functioning to be rooted in imitation (Bates, Benigni, Bretherton, Camaioni, & Volterra, 1979; Piaget, 1952; Sinclair-DeZwart, 1973). The child learns to imitate or represent (represent) her own motor behaviors and those of others. With language, the child is able to represent the referent with an arbitrary symbol or word. The child also manipulates objects and explores their functions. The child groups these functional features into classes to form the basis for early definitions (Nelson, 1974). Finally, development of the concept of object permanence enables the child to represent entities that are not present in the immediate context. If an object still exists even though removed from the child's immediate perception, the child can cause it to recur by evoking the symbol for it.

Other early cognitive relationships can also be seen in the presymbolic behavior of children. For example, 5-month-old children can attend to location (Robertson, 1975). By 9 months, children can discriminate between different agents. Children can discriminate between different actions by 1 year of age.

Parents respond to early child utterances by expanding the form or extending the meaning of the utterance, imitating, or giving feedback. In addition, parents continue to provide a simplified model of adult speech

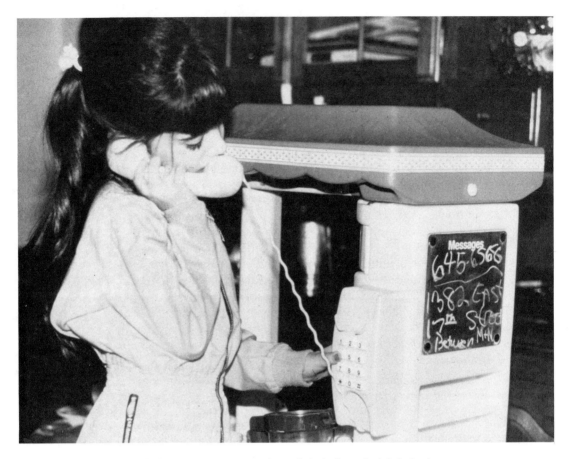

Children learn to use symbolic expression in part through imitation of adult behaviors.

(Broen, 1972; Garnica, 1977; Snow, 1972). As children begin using new structures, parents systematically modify their own language model. Children learn those structures that most effectively encode their intentions.

## Preschool Language Development

Within the preschool period, major developmental emphasis centers on language form. Preschool language development may be divided into stages characterized by the average length of the child's utterances. This average length is called *mean length of utterance* (MLU). Throughout most of the preschool period, increases in MLU correspond to increases in utterance complexity (Brown, 1973). This correlation is not as strong beyond an MLU of 4.0. There is a strong correlation between age and MLU (Miller & Chapman, 1981). From age 1.5 to 5.0 years, MLU increases approximately 1.2 morphemes per year.

Since there are qualitative differences in language development with increased MLU, we can describe several stages of language development based on MLU. These stages and the general characteristics of each are listed in Table 2.3. In the remainder of this section, we shall explore the major developments of each stage.

*Stage I* development, characterized by single-word and early multiword utterances, has been discussed under toddler language development. The relationships expressed by toddlers in simple word-order rules form the basis for later grammatical marking of these same relationships.

*Stage II* (MLU 2.0–2.5 morphemes) can be described by the appearance of morphemes that mark many of the relations marked earlier by word order. Fourteen morphemes studied by Brown (1973) are presented in Table 2.4. Each appears in Stage II (27–30 months), but many are not fully mastered (used correctly 90% of the time) until after Stage V (46+ months). The order presented reflects the order of mastery. Other early morphemes that appear in Stage II include the pronouns *I, you, them, he, she,* and *we;* auxiliary verbs *do* and *have* used as main verbs; and verb forms, such as *hafta* and *wanna.* The 2-year-old child may also exhibit the ability to use more than one function within a single utterance (Halliday, 1975b). For example, the child who doesn't own a puppy but says "I love doggie," may have more in mind than just making a statement.

**Table 2.3**  Brown's (1973) Stages of Development

| Stage | MLU | Approximate Age | Characteristics | Examples |
|---|---|---|---|---|
| I | 1.0–2.0 | 12–26 months | Semantic-syntactic rules | Daddy throw (Agent + Action)<br>Throw ball me (Action + Object + Location) |
| II | 2.0–2.5 | 27–30 months | Morphological development | Doggie *in* daddy's chair (Possessive *s*) (Preposition *in*)<br>Mommy eat*ing* cookie (Present progressive *ing*) |
| III | 2.5–3.0 | 31–34 months | Modification of basic sentence types | What man doing?<br>Where mommy will go?<br>I not eat yukky peas.<br>I don't like you. |
| IV | 3.0–3.75 | 35–40 months | Embedding | I know *what you want.* (Embedded clause in object position) |
| V | 3.75–4.5 | 41–46 months | Conjoining | I went to the party *and* I ate ice cream.<br>I hit Judy *'cause* she hitted me. |

**Table 2.4**  Brown's 14 Morphemes

| Morpheme | Example |
| --- | --- |
| Present progressive -*ing* (no auxiliary verb) | Mommy driv*ing*. |
| *In* | Ball *in* cup. |
| *On* | Doggie *on* sofa. |
| Regular plural -*s* | Kitties eat my ice cream. |
| Irregular past | *Came, fell, broke, sat, went* |
| Possessive *s* | Mommy's balloon broke. |
| Uncontractible verb *to be* as main verb | Who's sick? Response: He *is*. |
| Articles *the* and *a* | I see *a* kittie.<br>I throw *the* ball to daddy. |
| Regular past *ed* | Mommy pull*ed* the wagon. |
| Regular third person -*s* | Kathy hit*s*. |
| Irregular third person | *Does, has* |
| Uncontractible auxiliary or helping verb *to be* | Who's wearing your hat? Response: He *is*. |
| Contractible verb *to be* as main verb | Man *is* big.<br>Man's big. |
| Contractible auxiliary or helping verb *to be* | Daddy *is* drinking juice.<br>Daddy's drinking juice. |

*Note:* From *Language Development: An Introduction* (2nd ed.) by R. E. Owens,
Jr., 1988, Columbus, OH: Merrill. Copyright 1988 by Merrill Publishing Company.
Reprinted by permission.

*Stages III, IV,* and *V* can be discussed together. By Stage III (31–34 months), the language-learning child has the basic subject-verb-object sentence format, although she may omit portions in actual use. Within the last three stages, she concentrates on internal sentence development and on structural variations. In addition, she learns the phonological rules that govern use of the speech sounds she is acquiring.

The child uses both the noun and verb of simple adult declarative sentences by the last part of Stage III or early Stage IV. Once these elements are acquired, the child begins to experiment with this basic pattern. The result is the internal development of noun and verb phrases and the development of negative, interrogative, and imperative sentence forms. This process begins within Stage III.

Noun phrase elaboration in Stage III includes use of *this, that, these, those, a,* and *the* (Brown & Bellugi, 1964). Modifiers include quantifiers, such as *some, a lot* and *two*; possessives, such as *my* and *your*; and adjectives. Auxiliary or "helping" verbs, including *can, be,* and *will,* appear in late Stage III. In addition, the Stage III child will usually begin to overextend the regular past -*ed* marker to irregular verbs, thus producing *eated, goed,* and so on.

Within Stage III, the child begins to use more adult forms of both the negative sentence and the interrogative (see Table 2.5). Both forms require development of the auxiliary verb and transformations of the basic declarative sentence form. Previously, the child used forms such as *No daddy go bye-bye* to express the negative, and relied on intonation or on a *wh-*question word before a statement to express the interrogative, as in *What mommy eating?*. Within Stage III, the negative begins to appear between the subject and predicate in forms such as *don't, can't, and won't.* Auxiliary verbs also begin to appear in interrogatives. As noted in Table 2.5, it is not until the end of Stage IV that the child attains the basic adult question form.

Brown found phrasal and sentential embedding to be one of the primary characteristics of Stage IV. Embedding results when a phrase or a clause is placed within another clause. A *phrase* is a group of related words, such as *in the attic,* that does not contain a subject or a predicate. Phrases are used as modifiers or as noun substitutes. In contrast, a *clause* contains both a subject and a predicate. A clause that can stand alone as grammatically complete is independent—a *simple sentence.* Thus, *I danced* is a simple sentence. Clauses that cannot stand alone, such as *that you want,* are called *dependent* or *subordinate.* They must be joined with an independent clause to form a complex sentence, such as *Is this the toy that you want?* Most children use some form of embedding within Stage IV (Miller, 1981). Sentence embedding first appears in Stage IV (Brown, 1973; Limber, 1973). In general, these subordinate clauses have the form of simple sentences, but act as object of the sentence:

I know *you ate the candy.*
I think *I like chocolate.*
I saw *where the kitty went.*

The subordinate clause usually fills an object role for verbs such as *think, guess, wish, know, hope,* and *show.* The child initially places the newly acquired structure at the end of the sentence. It is common for new structures to appear first at the beginning or at the end of an older structure. Later, the new structure may move to a more central position within the sentence.

Relative subordinate clauses attached to the main clause appear somewhat later within Stage V (Brown, 1973; Limber, 1973; Miller, 1981). Attached to a noun with relative pronouns, such as *who, which,* and *that,* these subordinate clauses modify the noun. As before, expansion begins in the object position:

This is the kind *that I like.*

Relative clauses attached to the subject do not develop until 5 years of age, and are still rare by age 7 (Menyuk, 1977). Some examples of relative clauses attached to the subject include:

**Table 2.5**  Acquisition of Sentence Forms within Brown's Stage of Development

| Stage | Approximate Age | Negative |
|---|---|---|
| Early I (MLU: 1–1.5) | 12–22 months | Single word *no, all gone, gone.* Negative + X. ("No eat.") |
| Late I (MLU: 1.5–2.0) | 22–26 months | *No* and *not* used interchangeably. |
| Early II (MLU: 2.0–2.25) | 27–28 months | |
| Late II (MLU: 2.25–2.5) | 29–30 months | *No, not, don't,* and *can't* used interchangeably. Negative element placed between subject and predicate. |
| Early III (MLU: 2.5–2.75) | 31–32 months | |
| Late III (MLU: 2.75–3.0) | 33–34 months | *Won't* appears. Develops auxiliary forms *can, do, does, did, will,* and *be.* |
| Early IV (MLU: 3.0–3.5) | 35–37 months | |
| Late IV (MLU: 3.5–3.75) | 38–40 months | Adds *isn't, aren't doesn't,* and *didn't.* |
| Stage V (MLU: 3.75–4.5) | 41–46 months | Adds *wasn't, wouldn't, couldn't* and *shouldn't.* |
| Post V (MLU: 4.5+) | 47+ months | Adds *nobody, no one, none,* and *nothing.* Difficulty with double negatives. ("Nobody don't . . .") |

> The one *that you want* is yukky.
> The lady *who lives in that house* is nice.

By late Stage V, most children can embed phrases and clauses within a single sentence (Miller, 1981). For example, a child may place an infinitive such as "to go" within a subordinate clause such as "that we are going . . ." to produce

> I think that *we are going to the zoo.*

| Interrogative | Embedding | Conjoining |
|---|---|---|
| Yes/no asked with rising intonation on single word. *What* and *where*. | | Serial naming without *and*. ("Coat, hat.") |
| *That* + X. *What* + noun phrase + (doing)? *Where* + noun phrase + (going)? | Prepositions *in* and *on* appear. | *And* appears. ("Coat and hat.") |
| *What* or *where* + subject + predicate. | *Gonna, wanna, gotta*, etc., appear. | *But, so, or,* and *if* appear. |
| Begins to use auxiliary verbs in questions (*be, can, will, do*). ("You are going?") | Subordinate clauses appear after verbs *like, think, guess, show*. ("I know what you like.") | *Because* appears. Clauses joined with *and* appear (not until late V that most children can produce this form). |
| Begins to invert auxiliary verb and subject ("Are you going?"). Adds *when, how,* and *why*. | | |
| Adds modal auxiliary verbs (*would, could, should,* etc.). Stabilizes inverted auxiliary. | Infinitive phrases appear (to + verb) at the end of sentences. Subordinate clauses appear in object position. Multiple embeddings by late V. | Clauses joined with *if* appear. |
| | Subordinate clauses attached to the subject. Embedding and conjoining appear within same sentence beyond MLU of 5.0. | *When, because, but,* and *so* appear in clause joining beyond MLU of 5.0. |

Later forms also include more than one clause joined together in a sentence.

*Conjoining* characterizes Stage V. Conjoining occurs when two independent clauses are joined as equals, as in:

> *Mother went home,* but *she could not sleep.*

Generally, independent clauses are joined by conjunctions, such as *and, but,* and *because*.

The first clausal conjoining occurs with the conjunction *and* in Stage IV (Table 2.5). It is not until late Stage V, however, that most children can use this form (Lust & Mervis, 1980; Miller, 1981). Initially, *and* is used as an all-purpose conjunction (Bloom, Lahey, Hood, Lifter, & Fiess, 1980). Other conjunctions are used for clausal conjoining later. Even among 5-year-olds, however, *and* is the predominant conjunction (Bennett-Kaster, 1986).

Above an MLU of 5.0 most children also exhibit conjoining and embedding within the same sentence. For example, the child might produce the following:

The man who lives there is mean, and he has a big dog that bites.

These forms are rare in the speech of the typical 4-year-old, but they do occur occasionally.

Within each clause, internal changes are occurring also. By Stage IV, a noun or pronoun subject is obligatory (Ingram, 1974b). Additional modifiers, such as *some, something, other, more,* and *another* also appear. Still, the most frequent noun phrase elaborations involve only one element preceding the noun. Only gradually does the child learn multiple elements and the rules for their order in the noun phrase. Post-noun modifiers appear when the child begins to use relative clauses. An example is:

The puppy *in the window* is cute.

In this example, *in the window* modifies *puppy* to identify which puppy the speaker is discussing. This type of embedding is not widely used, however, until after Stage V. Between ages 4 and 5, the child learns quickly the use of several noun phrases in succession and, as a consequence, her storytelling abilities improve markedly.

Within the verb phrase, the auxiliary or helping verb *do* appears in negatives and questions by late Stage III or early IV. Thus, a sentence such as *She likes candy* would become the negative *She does not like candy* or the interrogative *Does she like candy?*. The modal auxiliaries *could, would, should, must,* and *might* also appear (de Villiers & de Villiers, 1973). Modal auxiliaries express moods or attitudes such as ability (*can*), permission (*may*), intent (*will*), possibility (*might*), and obligation (*must*).

By Stage V, the child has mastered both the regular and irregular past tense (*talked* and *ate,* respectively) in most contexts, the third person singular ("she talks"), and the verb "to be" ("*is* eating," "*am* happy") (Miller, 1981). Auxiliary verbs are inverted appropriately in questions and the *do* inserted when no auxiliary is present. Many verb forms are still to be mastered in poststage V. These include forms of the verb *be*, past tense modals and auxiliaries, and the passive voice.

Semantic notions, such as time and location, also affect the syntax the child uses. For example, the child must have a concept of temporal order to respond to and to use *when* and *why* questions. Causal questions such as *why* require reversibility in the response. For example, *Why did the milk spill?* requires a response explaining the events before the spill. Piaget has demonstrated the difficulty of such mental operations for the young pre-school child. When the child does not know the meaning of a temporal term, he seems to rely on the order of mention. The child has no difficulty interpreting sequences that preserve the actual order of events (Clark, 1971; French & Brown, 1977; Hatch, 1971; Johnson, 1975).

Spatial terms such as *next to* or *in front of* offer special problems. For example, *next to* includes but is not limited to the meanings "in front of," "behind," and so on. In addition, these terms differ in their meaning, depending on the locations to which they refer. With fronted objects, such as a television set, locational terms take their reference from the object, for example, the television set has its own front. With nonfronted objects, such as a ball, the term takes its location from the speaker's perspective, for example, the front of the ball is the side closest to the speaker. Thus, the listener must be able to adopt the perspective of the speaker.

Many morphological and syntactic changes are related to phonological rule development. In addition to acquiring a phonetic inventory, the pre-school child is developing rules that govern sound distribution and sequencing. As in the other aspects of language, the child developing phonological rules progresses through a long period of language decoding and hypothesis building. Many of the phonological rules used by children are listed in Table 2.6. These rules reflect *natural processes* (Oller, 1974) that act to simplify the speech stream for language-learning children; most are discarded or modified by age 4. Much of the child's morphological production will reflect his perception and production of phonological units. During the preschool years, he also "develops the ability to determine which speech sounds are used to signal differences in meaning" (Ingram, 1976, p. 22).

Once the child begins babbling, the basic speech unit she uses is the consonant-vowel (CV) syllable. The child frequently attempts to simplify production by reducing words to this form or to CVCV. The final consonant may be deleted, producing a CV structure from a CVC—*ba* (/bɔ/) for *ball*—or followed by a vowel to produce a CVCV structure—*cake-a* (/kelkʌ/) for *cake*. This process generally disappears by age 3 (Ingram, 1976; Oller, 1974; Templin, 1957). In addition, the child may delete unstressed syllables. For example, *away* becomes *way* (Oller, 1974). This deletion process continues until age 4. Reduplication is a third process for simplifying syllable structure. One syllable becomes similar to another in the word, resulting in the reduplicated structure. Thus, *mommie* becomes *mama* and *water* becomes *wawa*. Finally, the preschooler reduces or simplifies consonant clusters, usually by deleting one consonant. As she progresses, the child substitutes another consonant for the previously deleted one (Greenlee, 1974).

Assimilatory processes simplify production by permitting different sounds to be produced similarly. In general, one sound becomes similar to

**Table 2.6**  Common Phonological Processes of Preschool Children

| Processes | Examples |
|---|---|
| I. Syllable structure | |
|     Deletion of final consonants | *cu*(/kʌ/) for *cup* |
|     Deletion of unstressed syllables | *nana* for *banana* |
|     Reduplication | *mama, dada, wawa* (water) |
|     Reduction of clusters | /s/ + consonant (*stop*) = delete /s/ (*top*)Processes |
| II. Assimilatory | *beds* (/bɛdz̠/), *bets* (/bɛts̠/), *dog* becomes *gog* |
| III. Substitution processes | |
|     A. Stopping: replace sound with a plosive | *this* becomes *dis* |
|     B. Fronting | *Kenny* becomes *Tenny* |
|        1. Replace palatals and velars with alveolars (/k/ and /g/ replaced with /t/ and /d/) | *go* becomes *do* |
|        2. Nasals (/ŋ/ becomes /n/) | *something* becomes *somethin* |
|     C. Liquids | |
|        1. Gliding | *rabbit* becomes *wabbit* |
|        2. Another liquid substituted | *girl* becomes *gau* (/gɔ/) |
| IV. Deletion of sounds | *balloon* becomes *ba-oon* |

*Note:* Adapted from *Phonological Disability in Children* by D. Ingram, 1976, London: Edward Arnold.

another in the same word. For example, children produce two varieties of *doggie,* one with /d/ consonants, *doddie,* the other, *goggie,* using /g/s.

Many preschoolers substitute sounds in their speech, but these substitutions are not random. In general, substitutions can be described according to the manner of production. The two most common phonological substitution rules are *stopping* and *fronting.* In stopping, a plosive phoneme is substituted for another sound. This process is most common in the initial position in words (Oller, 1974). For example, "*show*" might become "*tow*," "*face*" becomes "*pace*," and "*valentine*" becomes "*balentine*." Fronting is a tendency to replace phonemes with other phonemes produced further forward in the mouth. Thus, /t/ and /d/ are substituted for /k/ and /g/, producing *dum* for *gum.* In conversation, it may be difficult to decipher the phonological rules a young child is using. Often, several processes in different aspects of language will be functioning simultaneously.

In his development of pragmatics, the Stage III child has not mastered adult conversational skills. He shifts topics rapidly, with only a few conversational turns devoted to each. He can revise some communication errors or mistakes, however, based on requests for clarification addressed to him by his conversational partner (Gallagher, 1977). His most frequent strategy is to simply repeat an utterance that his listener did not understand. Requests for clarification or restatement include terms such as *Huh?, What?,* and *Pardon me?.*

Within her conversation the 4-year-old child can sustain several turns, often maintaining a single topic. As she becomes more aware of the pragmatic aspects of conversation, the child acknowledges her partner's turn more through the use of fillers such as *yeah* and *uh-huh*. As she becomes more aware of her listener's shared assumptions, she deletes more shared information. For example, in response to "Who's running?" she replies, "I am." In addition, the child makes more productive use of clarification requests (*Huh?*) to maintain the conversation and attain missed information (Garvey, 1975). She is able to role play, thus taking another person's perspective to systematically change her speech (Anderson, 1977; Gleason, 1973; Sachs & Devin, 1976; Shatz & Gelman, 1973). For example, she uses words based on the speaker's perspective such as *here, there, this,* and *that.*

With maturity, the child becomes more aware of her listener's point of view and role, so that by age 4 she can adjust the form of requests and the level of politeness (Gordon & Ervin-Tripp, 1984). When the listener is an authority figure or the child is uncertain of the outcome, she is more likely to use a polite indirect form (*Can I have a cookie, please?*) rather than direct (*I want a cookie.*). At about 4½, there is a sharp increase in the number of indirect requests (James & Seebach, 1982; Wilkinson et al., 1982).

By kindergarten, the child is able to be more subtle in his language use and to disguise his intentions in indirect requests and hints (Ervin-Tripp & Mitchell-Kernan, 1977). For example, the child desiring juice might inquire, "Do we have any juice left?".

To summarize the language development of the preschool child, we can say that by age 5, the child uses most of the major varieties of the English sentence. However, there are still important syntactic advances to be made during the school-age years, a period of coordination of messages and situations (Muma, 1978). Knowledge of language use will increase. Having acquired much of the "what" of language form, the child turns to the "how" of language use.

## School Age and Adult Development

The school-age, and to some extent the adult, years are characterized by growth in all aspects of language—syntax, morphology, semantics, phonology, and pragmatics. The emphasis of development differs, however, from that seen in preschool. As in the toddler, major developmental stress is placed on semantics and pragmatics of language. The child learns to use existing forms to communicate more effectively. Metalinguistic abilities that enable a language user to think about and reflect upon language also become more prominent during this period. In addition, the child learns new means of communication, reading and writing. The child's oral language knowledge forms a base for this new learning.

Adult development continues to concentrate on semantics and pragmatics, with increased vocabulary growth and versatility in use. Vocabulary growth and categorization continues throughout life. New words are added for specialized occupations, interests, and socialization. In addition, the adult becomes an even more adept user of language, able to adapt her language style to different social contexts and different communication goals.

In the realm of language form, school-age development consists of simultaneous expansion of existing forms and acquisition of new ones. The child's syntactic growth continues with internal sentence expansion by elaboration of the noun and verb phrases, expansion of conjoining and embedding, and addition of structures such as passive voice. Most first graders do not produce adult passive sentences, reflexive pronouns, "cause" clauses, and gerunds (Menyuk, 1969). Gerunds are verbs to which -*ing* has been added to produce a form that fulfills a noun function. For example, to *fish* becomes *fishing,* as in *I enjoy fishing.* A verb can also be made into a noun by adding a suffix such as -*er,* -*man,* and -*ist.* Ninety percent of the children understand these suffixes in about second grade (Carrow, 1973a). After age 7, the child masters comprehension of the adverbial -*ly;* irregular noun and verb agreement *(The sheep is eating; The fish are eating);* imperatives *(Don't cross!);* the negative, both explicit *(The girl is not swimming)* and implicit *(Find the one that is neither the ball nor the table);* several conjunctions *(if, then);* passive sentences; and several verb tenses, such as the past participle *(has eaten),* the future *(will),* and the perfect *(has been* verb -*ing).*

Although young school-age children use most elements of the noun and verb phrase, they frequently omit them. Even at age 7, they will omit some elements such as articles, while expanding others repetitively, such as double negatives *(Nobody don't...).* In addition, school-age children still have difficulty with some prepositions, verb tensing, and plurals (Menyuk, 1965). Within the noun phrase, pronoun and adjective development continue. The child learns to differentiate between subject pronouns, such as *I, he, she, we,* and *they,* and object pronouns, such as *me, him, her, us,* and *them,* and to use reflexives, such as *myself, himself, herself,* and *ourselves.* In addition, she learns to carry pronouns across sentences.

In general, comprehension of linguistic relationships improves throughout the school years (Inhelder & Piaget, 1969; Piaget & Inhelder, 1969). The comparative relationship *(bigger than)* is the easiest for first to third graders to interpret. The cognitive skills needed for comparative relationships develop during the preschool years and must await linguistic development. Other sentential relations, such as passive, temporal, spatial, and familial, are more difficult to interpret.

Passive sentences are difficult because the form varies from the predominant subject-verb-object strategy that children use. For example, using a S-V-O interpretation strategy, the child will interpret *The cat was chased by the dog* as *The cat chased the dog.* The child does not truly comprehend passive sentences until about age 5½. Prior to this age, children use extralinguistic strategies, such as relying on context, to interpret sentences (Bridges, 1980). Approximately 80% of 7½- to 8-year-olds produce full passive sentences (Baldie, 1976). Development continues, and some forms do not appear until 11 years of age (Horgan, 1978).

The child's repertoire of embedded and conjoined forms increases throughout the school years. Conjoining expands with the addition of *because, so, therefore, if, but, or, when, before, after,* and *then* used to join clauses (Menyuk, 1969). Even though *if, so,* and *because* are produced relatively early in the school years, full understanding does not develop until much later (Bates, 1976; Hood & Bloom, 1979). Forms such as *although* and *therefore* are not mastered until late elementary school or early adolescence.

Morphological and phonological development also continues beyond the preschool years. *Morphophonemic changes* are phonological or sound modifications that result when morphemes are placed together. For example, the final sound in *electric* changes when *-ity* is added to form *electricity* (Ingram, 1974a). One rule pertains to the regular plural, possessive, and third person singular endings. In general, this rule is learned by first grade (Berko, 1958; Menyuk, 1964). The /s/ is used with voiceless and /z/ with voiced ending consonants. In contrast, /ɪz/ is used on words that end with a sibilant sound, such as /s/, /z/, /ʃ/ and /ʒ/. The /ɪz/ rule is not learned until after age 6 (Berko, 1958; Menyuk, 1964).

During the school years, the child also learns the rules for vowel shifting. For example, the /aɪ/ sound in the second syllable of *divine* changes to an /ɪ/ in *divinity.* Knowledge of vowel shifting is gained only gradually, and it is not until age 17 that most children learn to apply all the rules (Myerson, 1975).

Stress or emphasis is also learned during the school years. The stress placed on certain syllables reflects the grammatical function of the word. In English, stress varies with the relationship of two words and with a word's use as a noun or verb. For example, two words may form a phrase such as *black board,* or a compound word such as *blackboard.* The speaker stresses *board* in the phrase and *black* in the compound word. Noun-verb pairs differ also. In the noun *record,* emphasis is on the first syllable, while the verb *record* is pronounced with stress on the second. By age 12, however, most children have acquired stress contrast rules.

The new communication means of reading and writing are taught to most children during the school years, although many children begin prereading and prewriting activities prior to first grade. Gradually, the child realizes that the message is contained in the orthographic or written symbols (Ferreiro & Teberosky, 1982). In his initial reading, the child concentrates on decoding of single words. Only gradually does he begin to use the text as an aid for inferring meaning. Between grades 4 and 8, reading shifts from

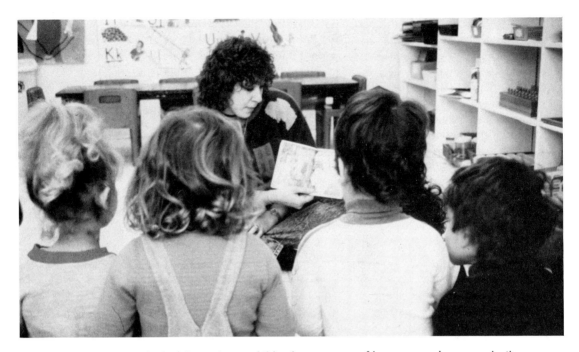

Learning to read adds a further dimension to children's awareness of language and communication.

decoding skill to comprehension with increasing rates of scanning. There is only a moderate overlap with writing. In writing, the child gradually moves from "inventive" spelling to regularity as letters are matched to speech sounds (Read, 1981). In addition, the child begins to be more aware of his reader, much as he became aware of his listener in conversations. This shift from egocentric focus to concern for the reader is evident around third to fourth grade (Bartlett, 1982). The emphasis on both reading and writing of stories requires the child to have a grasp of relational terms, such as those for time (*before, after, then, on, at*), space (*here, there, beside, between, left, right*), and comparative terms (*better than, almost, nearly, fewer, neither– nor, same*). While the basics of reading and writing are taught in the first three grades, there is a shift in fourth grade to a reliance on the skills already established.

During the school-age period and adult years, most semantic growth focuses on increases in the size of the child's vocabulary and the specificity of definition. Initial learning, in both the preschool and school-age years, seems to be receptive in nature (Dollaghan, 1985; Holdgrafer & Sorenson, 1984) and may consist of a quickly conceived tentative definition, followed by gradual refinement (Carey & Bartlett, 1978). In school-age and adult years, definitions become more dictionarylike and conventional (Wehren et al.,

1981). Gradually, the child acquires an abstract knowledge of meaning that is independent of particular contexts or individual interpretations. In this process, the individual reorganizes the semantic aspects of her language (Francis, 1972).

The school-age child begins to associate words in a different way than she has previously (Brown & Berko, 1960; Deese, 1965; Ervin, 1961, 1963; Jenkins & Palermo, 1964; McNeill, 1966). This change has been called the **syntagmatic-paradigmatic shift** (Ervin, 1961). A syntagmatic association is based on a syntactic relationship. For example, the stimulus word *girl* might elicit a child response *run*. In contrast, a paradigmatic association is based on semantic attributes. In this case, the word *girl* might elicit *boy* or *woman*. The shift represents a refinement and organization of semantic features (McNeill, 1966), and may reflect a change in general cognitive-processing strategies (Emerson & Gekoski, 1976). The period of most rapid change occurs between 5 and 9 years (Muma & Zwycewicz-Emory, 1979). It is not until the adult years, however, that paradigmatic associations become consistent and fully integrated.

One outgrowth of concept reorganization is the ability to create categories from their members and the reverse. For example, the child might say *She has a bird, two fish, a cat, a dog, and lots of other pets,* exhibiting a member-to-category process. In addition, this ability helps the child select the appropriate word when certain restrictions apply. When creating poetry, for example, the child must find a word that rhymes and also makes sense.

The school-age child also develops figurative language and uses language in a truly creative way. In **figurative language,** words are used in an imaginative sense, rather than a literal one, to create an imaginative or emotional impression. The primary types include idioms, metaphors, similes, and proverbs. *Idioms* are short expressions that have evolved through years of use and cannot be analyzed grammatically, such as *hit the roof* or *throw a party.* *Metaphors* and *similes* are figures of speech that compare actual entities with a descriptive image. In a metaphor, a resemblance or comparison is implied, as in *She had a skeletal appearance.* A simile, on the other hand, is an explicit comparison, usually introduced by *like* or *as,* such as *He ran like a gazelle.* Finally, *proverbs* are short, popular sayings that embody a generally accepted truth, useful thought, or advice. In general, proverbs are difficult for young school-age children to comprehend. Examples of proverbs are:

> Don't put all your eggs in one basket.
> You can't have your cake and eat it, too.

The 6-, 7-, or 8-year-old child interprets proverbs quite literally. Development of comprehension continues throughout adolescence and adulthood.

The area of most significant linguistic growth during the school-age and adult years is in the development of discourse or conversational skills, an area of language use or pragmatics. A preschool child does not have the skill of a junior-high student who wants something. No adult is fooled by the comment *Gee, Mom, I wonder if there's skating today.* Both parties understand the request, however indirect it may be.

During the school years, the child gains the ability to use language more subtlely. To clarify messages, she must monitor and evaluate communication and the cues regarding success or failure of the communication effort. The young school-age child has the following communication abilities or "talents" (White, 1975):

1. To gain and hold adult attention in a socially acceptable manner

2. To use others, when appropriate, as resources for assistance or information

3. To express affection or hostility and anger appropriately

4. To direct and follow peers

5. To compete with peers in storytelling and boasts

6. To express pride in herself and in her accomplishments

7. To role play

By late adolescence, the child knows not only that a communication partner's perspective and knowledge may differ from his own, but also that it is important to consider these differences. The high schooler also uses language creatively, in sarcasm, jokes, and double meanings. These begin to develop in the early school years. High schoolers make deliberate use of metaphor (Gardner, Kirchner, Winner, & Perkins, 1975) and can explain complex behavior and natural phenomena (Elkind, 1970).

One verbal strategy used widely by adults is the indirect request, an unmarked statement that refers only indirectly to what the speaker wants. For example, in the proper context the statement *The heater sure is working overtime* may be an indirect request for the heat to be turned down. Indirect requests represent a growing awareness of the importance of socially appropriate requests and of the communication context. In general, the 5-year-old is successful at directly asking, commanding, and forbidding. By age 7, she has greater facility with indirect forms (Garvey, 1975; Grimm, 1975). There is increased flexibility in indirect request forms, and the proportion of hints increases from childhood through adulthood (Ervin-Tripp, 1980).

The school-age child is able to introduce a topic into the conversation, sustain it through several turns, and close or switch the topic. These discourse skills develop only gradually through elementary school. In contrast, the 3-year-old sustains the topic only 20% of the time if her partner's preceding utterance was a topic-sharing response to one of the child's prior utterances (Bloom, Rocissano, & Hood, 1976). In other words, topics change rapidly when the conversational partner is a 3-year-old. The school-age child learns to *shadow* or to "slide" from one topic to a related one, rather than make abrupt topic changes. It is not until age 11 that the child can sustain abstract discussions.

As early as elementary school, the language of boys and girls also begins to reflect the gender differences of older children and adults (Haas, 1979). These differences can be noted in both vocabulary use and conversational style. In general, women avoid swearing and coarse language in conversation, and tend to use more polite words. Women tend to use expressions such as *oh dear, goodness,* and *gracious me,* while men use interjections like *damn it* (Farb, 1973; Lakoff, 1973). The communication experiences and needs of adults result in language systems characterized by many different language styles. Specific styles, often with their own vocabulary, are used in the workplace and with groups with particular interests. Discourse abilities continue to diversify and become more elaborate with age (Obler, 1985).

Older children and adults have the linguistic skills to select from several available communication strategies that best suit a specific context. Mature language is efficient and appropriate (Muma, 1978): efficient in that words are more specifically defined and forms do not need repetition or paraphrasing to be understood; appropriate in that utterances are selected for the psychosocial dynamics of the communication situation. The less mature language user has difficulty selecting the appropriate code because she has a limited repertoire of language forms.

# SPEECH

**Speech** is a verbal means of communicating or conveying meaning. The result of specific motor behaviors, speech requires precise neuromuscular coordination. The speech mechanism and its neuromuscular control are explained in chapter 3. Speech consists of speech sound combinations, voice quality, intonation, and rate. Each of these components is used to modify the speech message. In face-to-face conversation, much of the message is also carried by nonspeech means, such as facial expression.

The smallest unit of speech is the *phoneme,* a family of sounds that are close enough in perceptual qualities to be distinguished from other phonemes. Members of these families of sounds are called **allophones.** The allophones within a phoneme family differ from one another because of phonemic constraints, such as the effects of other phonemes on the sound, and production constraints, such as fatigue. Though phonemes are meaningless in and of themselves, they make semantic difference in use. For example, the final sounds in *cat* and *cash* are perceptually different enough to signal differences of meaning. They represent two different phonemes.

Phonemes are written between slashes to distinguish them from the alphabet. The International Phonetic Alphabet (IPA) is used rather than the English alphabet in transcribing sounds for two reasons. First, a sound may be spelled several ways, as in *day, obey,* and *weight.* Likewise, some letters, such as *c*, can be pronounced more than one way (as an *s* or *k*). This is especially true of vowels, such as the *e* in *be* and *bed*. Second, the pronunciation of the English alphabet cannot be applied to other languages, especially those that use a different alphabet system.

In English, phonemes are classified as vowels or consonants. *Vowels* are produced with a relatively unrestricted air flow in the vocal tract. *Consonants* require a closed or narrowly constricted passage that results in friction and air turbulence. The number of phonemes attributed to American English differs with the classification system used and the dialect of the speaker.

Phonemes can be described as being voiced or voiceless. *Voiced* phonemes are produced by phonation (vibration of the vocal cords); *voiceless* phonemes are not. All vowels in English are voiced, but consonants may be either voiced or voiceless.

Two classification systems are currently used for English phonemes. The more *traditional approach* emphasizes the phoneme, and classifies each according to place and manner of articulation. In contrast, the second, called the *distinctive feature approach,* emphasizes the characteristics each phoneme possesses. We will explain briefly both of these systems.

*Traditional phonemic classification* is based on the place of articulation and, for consonants, on the manner of articulation, usually the type of air release. In this system, vowels are described by the highest portion of the tongue, front-to-back positioning of the tongue, and lip rounding. Heights can be characterized as high, mid, or low, based on the position of the highest part of the tongue. The location of this highest position can be described as front, central, or back. For example, a vowel can be described as high front, or low back. The English vowels are displayed graphically in Figure 2.3. Words using each sound are printed next to each phoneme.

Lip rounding is an additional description used for vowel classification. In rounding, the lips protrude slightly, forming an "O" shape. Rounding is characteristic of some back vowels, such as the last sound in *construe*. In contrast, there is no lip rounding in *construct*.

One group of vowel-like sounds is more complex. These sounds are called **diphthongs.** A diphthong is a blend of two vowels within the same syllable. The sound begins with one vowel and glides smoothly toward another. When the word *day* is repeated slowly, the speaker can feel and hear the shift from one vowel to another at the end. The diphthongs are also presented in Figure 2.3.

Consonant descriptions are more complex than those for vowels and include manner of articulation, place of articulation, and voicing. *Manner* refers to the type of production, generally with respect to the release of air. The six generally recognized categories of manner are:

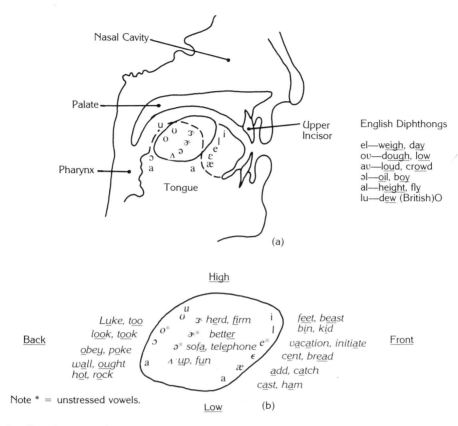

**Figure 2.3** Classification of English vowels by tongue position. *(Note: From Language Development: An Introduction (2nd ed.) by R. E. Owens, Jr., 1988, Columbus, OH: Merrill. Copyright 1988 by Merrill Publishing Company. Reprinted by permission.)*

1. *Plosive* (/p, b, t, d, k, g/)—complete obstruction of the airstream with quick release similar to an explosion.
2. *Fricative* (/f, v, θ, ð, s, z, ʃ, ʒ, h/)—narrow constriction for air to pass, creating a hissing noise.
3. *Affricate* (/tʃ, dʒ/)—a combination of a plosive followed by a fricative.
4. *Liquid* (/l, r/)—consonants with the vowel-like quality of little air turbulence. The /l/ is produced by allowing air to pass around the sides of the tongue. In contrast, the /r/ is produced by raising either the tip or back of the tongue and allowing air to pass over the tongue.
5. *Glide* (/w, j/)—produced while gliding from one vowel position to another; vowel-like qualities.

6. *Nasal* (/m, n, ŋ/)—oral cavity blocks exiting air but velum lowered to allow breath to exit via the nasal cavity.

Variations result from constriction within the oral cavity.

The place of articulation varies across the six manner categories and describes the position where the maximum constriction, either partial or complete, occurs. The seven locations are:

1. *Bilabial* (/p, b, w, m/)—lips together
2. *Labiodental* (/f, v/)—lower lip to upper incisors
3. *Linguadental* (/θ, ð/)—tongue tip to upper incisors
4. *Lingua-alveolar* (/t, d, s, z, l, r, n/)—front of tongue to upper alveolar (gum) ridge
5. *Linguapalatal* (/ʃ, ʒ, tʃ, dʒ, j/)—tongue to hard palate
6. *Linguavelar* (/k, g, ŋ/)—back of tongue to soft palate or velum
7. *Glottal* (/h/)—restriction at glottis

Many English consonant sounds differ only in voicing. When two phonemes have the same manner and place of articulation but differ in voicing, they are called *cognates.* For example, /s/ and /z/ are cognates. If you repeat the words *seal* and *zeal,* you can feel the difference at the larynx. Place and manner of articulation do not differ.

Theoretically, phonemes could be produced in almost any configuration of manner, place, and voicing. Other languages use some of the phonemes used in English, plus additional speech sounds. Some English distinctions are not present in other languages. In Spanish, for example, there is no distinction between /s/ and /z/; they are not separate phonemes. Other languages make finer distinctions that are not relevant to speakers of English (and that are therefore difficult for us to distinguish).

The other current approach to classifying speech sounds is called *distinctive feature classification.* The distinctive feature approach to speech sounds uses subphoneme units of analysis. There are several theoretical classification systems based on acoustic (Jakobson, Fant, & Halle, 1951), articulatory (Chomsky & Halle, 1968), and perceptual (Singh, Woods, & Becker, 1972) characteristics. In general, the greater the number of distinctive features that two phonemes have in common, the more alike the phonemes. Thus, common features describe the relationship between two phonemes.

Both of the approaches just discussed are ways of describing speech sounds in isolation. Although we can do this, sounds rarely occur alone in speech. Speech is a dynamic process, and movement patterns for more than one sound may occur simultaneously (MacNeilage, 1970). This co-occurrence of production characteristics of two or more phonemes is called

**coarticulation.** Coarticulation is the result of motor commands from the brain and the mechanical response of the speech muscles. Movement may occur several phonemes prior to the appearance of the phoneme associated with this movement (Daniloff & Moll, 1968). For example, in the word *construe,* lip rounding begins well before the /u/ sound. These anticipatory-movements are a clear indication that the brain is not functioning on a phoneme level.

In a mechanical system, such as the speech mechanism, there is also built-in inertia or drag. Muscle movements lag behind brain commands, thus continuing after the commands have ceased. The result is that the production characteristics of one phoneme may persist during production of another. For example, there is a nasalization of the /z/ in *runs* (/rʌnz/), caused by the insufficient time available for the velum to return to its upward position after /n/ (Daniloff, 1973).

# DEVELOPMENT OF SPEECH

As he matures, the child gains increasing control of the speech mechanism and is able to produce or articulate sounds more effectively. Although he gains much motor control within the first year, the child does not achieve-adultlike stability until mid-childhood. In this section, we shall explore the major developmental speech changes. These and other developmental changes are presented in Table 2.7.

## The Newborn

Much of the behavior of the newborn is reflexive, or beyond her immediate volitional control. The reflex of most interest for speech development is the rhythmic suck-swallow pattern, first established at 3 months prior to birth. As with other reflexes, sucking involves the midbrain and brainstem only. At birth, sucking is primarily accompanied by up-and-down jaw action. To swallow, the neonate opens her mouth slightly and protrudes and then retracts her tongue. To complete her swallow, the neonate must also close or abduct her vocal folds to protect the lungs.

The most common sounds made by the newborn are cries and partial vowel sounds (Laufer & Horii, 1977; Stark, 1978). By the end of the first month, the cries become differentiated, and mothers can usually tell the type of cry by its pattern. The noncrying sounds of the newborn include normal phonation, but lack full resonance in the oral cavity. Considerable air is emitted via the nasal cavity and the resultant sounds are nasalized.

The newborn can discriminate different phonemes and different intonational and stress patterns (Eisenberg, 1976; Hirschman & Katkin, 1974; Kearsley, 1973). This discrimination is not the same as linguistic perception, however, and does not involve sound-meaning relationships.

**Table 2.7**  Speech Development

| Age | Stage | Speech | Other Development |
|---|---|---|---|
| 0–1 month | Newborn | Reflexive behavior<br>Suck-swallow pattern<br>Non-differentiated crying<br>Vegetative sounds with phonation but incomplete resonance | 6–8 lbs., 17–21 inches<br>Can't raise head when on stomach<br>Visual and auditory preferences, best vision at 7½"<br>Sensitive to volume, pitch, and duration of sound<br>Sleeps about 70% of time |
| 2–3 months | Cooing | Definite stop and start to oral movement<br>Velar to uvular closure or near closure<br>Back consonants and back and middle vowels with incomplete resonance | Holds head up briefly while on stomach or sitting supported<br>Repeats own actions<br>Visually searches<br>Begins exploratory play<br>Excited by people<br>Social smile |
| 4–6 months | Babbling | Greater independent control of tongue<br>Prolonged strings of sounds<br>More lip or labial sounds<br>Experiments with sounds | 12–16 lbs., 23–24 inches<br>Turns head to localize sound<br>Mouths objects<br>Sits supported for half hour<br>Selective attention to faces<br>Anticipates actions<br>Excites with game play |
| 6–10 months | Reduplication babbling | Repetitive syllable production<br>Increased lip control<br>Labial and alveolar plosives (/p, b, t, d/), nasals, /j/, but not fully formed | Self-feeding<br>Progresses from creeping through crawling to standing<br>Explores objects through manipulation<br>Imitates others physically<br>Gestures |
| 11–14 months | Vocables and first words | Elevates tongue tip<br>Variegated babbling<br>Intonational patterns<br>Vocables—sound-meaning relationships<br>Predominance of /m, w, b, p/<br>First words primarily CV, VC, CVCV reduplicated, and CVCV | 26–30 lbs., 28–30 inches<br>Stands alone<br>Feeds self with spoon<br>First steps<br>Uses trial and error problem solving<br>Deferred imitation |
| 2 years | | Has acquired /p, h, w, m, n, b, k, g/ | 31–35 lbs., 32–34 inches<br>Walks without watching feet<br>Limited role playing<br>Parallel play |

close her lips when swallowing liquids. Speech is characterized by variegated babbling (Oller, 1978), in which adjacent and successive syllables are not identical. Frequently, the babbling occurs in long strings with intonational patterns that approximate adult speech. The result, an unintelligible gibberish called *jargon,* may sound like adult statements or questions.

Many speech sounds at this stage have sound-meaning relationships. These sounds, called **vocables,** function as words, even though they are not based on adult words. The child may develop a dozen such vocables before he speaks his first words. Vocables are more limited than babbling, but not as structured as adult speech. The child does not use vocables because of the difficulty of the adult models, but rather as a sound-meaning relationship. Thus, he demonstrates a recognition of linguistic regularities.

## First Words and Phoneme Acquisition

With the acquisition of words, the child's sound production becomes more constrained by the words themselves. "Emergence of the first words ... is determined as much by the child's control of articulation as by his ability to associate labels with objects" (de Villiers & de Villiers, 1979, pp. 23–24).

Children's speech is a complex interaction of the ease of both production and perception of the target syllable. The success of both processes is related to the particular phonemes involved, and to syllable stress and sound position within words (Klein, 1978). The order of appearance of the first sounds children acquire (/m, w, b, p/, Sander, 1972) cannot be explained by the frequency of appearance in English (Fourcin, 1978). The /b/, /m/, and /w/ are the simplest consonants to produce and the easiest to perceive, so they appear first.

The relationship of speech-sound perception and production in meaningful speech is complex. The lack of agreement between studies of the child's perception and production is due primarily to the child's inadequate neuromuscular control, which affects her production. Children simplify their speech in systematic ways that reflect this and other processing inadequacies and the phonological rules mentioned previously.

Several studies have attempted to establish an order of acquisition of phoneme production (Poole, 1934; Prather, Hedrick, & Kern, 1975; Templin, 1957; Wellman, Case, Mengert, & Bradbury, 1931). This order reflects the increasing speed and precision of the speech mechanism. Higher levels of cortical control and integration result in complex, integrated movements by the speech mechanism. Comparing the results of three studies (Olmsted, 1971; Templin, 1957; Wellman et al., 1931), we can make the following statements:

1. As a group, vowels are acquired before consonants. English vowels are acquired by age 3.

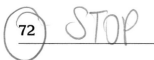

2. As a group, the nasals are acquired first, followed by the glides, plosives, liquids, fricatives, and affricatives.

3. As a group, the glottals are acquired first, followed by the labials, velars, alveolars, dentals, and palatals.

4. Sounds are first acquired in the initial position in words.

5. Consonant clusters and blends are not acquired until age 7 or 8, though some clusters appear as early as age 4. These early clusters include /s/ + nasal, /s/ + liquid, /s/ + stop, and stop + liquid in the initial position, and nasal + stop in the final.

6. There are great individual differences, and the age of acquisition for some sounds may vary by as much as 3 years.

## Summary

During the first year, the infant gains sufficient neuromuscular control of the speech mechanism to enable him to produce simple words or sound patterns. In turn, his repertoire of initial words may reflect his sound production abilities. Not all speech sounds of the parent language arereflected in these initial words, and the child may take several years to perfect his sound production. In conversational use, this speech-sound production reflects a complex interplay of language rule use.

## CONCLUSION

The terms *communication, language,* and *speech* describe different but related aspects of human behavior. The potential speech-language pathologist needs to be aware of the differences among these terms and of their interrelatedness. Not all children develop communication, language, and speech in the manner described in this chapter. The remainder of this text is devoted to disorders. As you proceed, you should keep the distinctions discussed in this chapter in mind, and be alert to the effects of any disorder on speech, language, and communcation. No doubt, as a practicing speech-language pathologist, you will someday be faced with the need to explain these terms to some unknowing soul. I hope that this chapter can provide a basis for your response. I hope that I have stirred some interest in the topic of development because it is the basis for much of the therapy that you will later provide.

## STUDY QUESTIONS

1. What are the differences among communication, language, and speech?

2. What is the significance of early communication development for later language development?

3. What are the characteristics of the five related aspects of language?

4. How does the overall emphasis of language development change during toddler, preschool, and school years?

5. How can we divide preschool language development? What are the changes that characterize each stage?

6. What are the discourse skills that develop during the school-age period?

7. What is the relationship between early speech mechanism development and early speech development?

## SELECTED READINGS

Berko Gleason, J. (1985). *The development of language.* Columbus, OH: Merrill.

Bullowa, M. (1979). *Before speech.* New York: Cambridge University Press.

DeHart, G., & Maratsos, M. (1984). Children's acquisition of presuppositional usages. In R. Schiefelbusch & J. Pickar (Eds.). *The acquisition of communication process.* Baltimore, MD: University Park Press.

de Villiers, J., & de Villiers, P. (1979). *Early language.* Cambridge, MA: Harvard University Press.

Owens, R. (1988). *Language development: An introduction* (2nd ed.). Columbus, OH: Merrill.

Rice, M. (1983). Contemporary accounts of the cognition/language relationship: Implications for speech-language clinicians. *Journal of Speech and Hearing Disorders, 48,* 347–359.

# Anatomy and Physiology of Speech

## W I L L A R D   R.   Z E M L I N

### MYTHS AND REALITIES

- *Myth:* Some people's voice problems stem from the fact that they are speaking on residual air.
- *Reality:* Residual air is air remaining in the lungs after maximum expiratory effort. It is physically impossible to speak on residual air.
- *Myth:* If an oral examination reveals no abnormal findings, an articulation problem should be classified as functional and not organic.
- *Reality:* An oral examination involves teeth and mucous membrane, and tells us nothing about the underlying neuromuscular structures. The most reasonable classification of a problem for which an organic basis cannot be readily found is "idiopathic," which simply means, we don't know.
- *Myth:* You can evaluate velopharyngeal competence by an oral examination.
- *Reality:* The only condition an oral examination will reveal is complete or partial paralysis of the soft palate. The area of contact between the palate and the pharyngeal wall is hidden from view.

- *Myth:* Anatomy has been thoroughly explored and there is nothing new to be learned about the structure of the human body.

- *Reality:* Anatomy is far from a dead branch on the tree of learning. Much has yet to be learned about individual variability, and examination at the cellular level has just begun.

- *Myth:* It is helpful during voice therapy to have clients place one or both of their hands on their diaphragm.

- *Reality:* The diaphragm is the musculotendinous partition between the thorax and abdomen. The only way a hand can be placed upon it is through surgery. Unfortunately, the epigastric region of the abdominal wall is incorrectly referred to as the diaphragm by some voice therapists and singing teachers.

- *Myth:* Some people have difficulty with their voice because they are not supporting their tone with their diaphragm.

- *Reality:* Supporting tone or voice with the diaphragm is a meaningless cliche. If tone can be supported at all, it is by virtue of the contributions of the abdominal musculature and not the diaphragm. The diaphragm can only contract during inspiration, and relax during expiration. It cannot actively contribute to the expiratory phase of breathing.

- *Myth:* People are all the same on the inside.

- *Reality:* There is a considerable degree of individual variability of structure beneath the skin, but variability is a subject still being explored.

- *Myth:* Whispering can damage your vocal cords.

- *Reality:* Nonsense. The vocal cords (folds) fail to meet at the midline during whisper, and even during forced whisper. Whisper is not abusive, but may require considerable effort on the part of the respiratory system, which may make people think their vocal folds are overworking.

- *Myth:* Baby teeth need not be cared for because they are just going to fall out anyway.

- *Reality:* Proper spacing of the deciduous (baby) teeth is extremely important because of their influence on the proper spacing of the permanent teeth.

- *Myth:* If you kiss the frog in your throat it will turn into a handsome prince.

- *Reality:* Catch the frog.


WE shall first look at the typical characteristics of speech and speech production. The structures, mechanisms, and processes of respiration will then be featured. We shall then look at phonation, and consider the anatomy and physiology of the production of voice for speech. The next section will deal with the mechanisms and processes of articulation. The last section will feature the nervous system and its role in the production of speech and language.

The phone rings, you pick it up, and say "Hello!" Between hearing the ring and the spoken message lies an intricate chain of events. To produce the word /hɛlo/, you use a complex series of nerves, muscles, and body organs.

Our task in this chapter is to explore how humans speak. We will examine the processes by which dormant air in the lungs is transformed into the meaningful sequence of sounds we call *speech.* This information about the anatomy and physiology of normal speech will serve as a foundation for the evaluation of people with disordered speech. In many cases, a speech-language pathologist must determine whether a speech problem has a physical basis or not. In other cases, the professional must predict to what extent a child or adult can overcome a physical problem, or whether a different set of skills for coping with the resultant language problem is in order. In dealing with victims of strokes, children with articulation problems, infants born with cleft palate, students with cerebral palsy (the list goes on), you will need to understand the normal processes by which we speak.

But one note of caution: in the human vocal organs, as in most human characteristics, there is a broad range of "normal." We will look at "typical" characteristics, but in practice you may see a wide span, just as adults from 5 feet to over 6 feet tall may be thought of as "normal" in height.

The highly integrated and complex structures of speech production are confined primarily to the head, neck, and trunk. The trunk is by definition the body, except for its free extremities (arms, legs, and head). It is divided into an upper thorax and a lower portion, the abdomen, which are separated by an important partition called the diaphragm (the principal muscle of inhalation). The structures illustrated in Figure 3.1 constitute the human vocal organs. They include the lungs-diaphragm-thorax complex, the larynx, and the vocal tract. The vocal tract consists of the throat or pharynx, the mouth or oral cavity, and the nasal cavities.

Air, which is drawn into the lungs during inspiration, is placed under a modest amount of pressure in the expiratory phase of respiration. Appropriate adjustments of the internal larynx result in vibration of the vocal folds, and that vibration transforms the dormant pressurized air in the lungs into a fairly regular series of air pulses during **phonation.** These pulses, in turn, excite the air column within the vocal tract. The air column resonates for a very short time with each pulse of the larynx to produce a glottal or laryngeal tone. The

Phonation *is the production of sound by vibration of the vocal folds.*

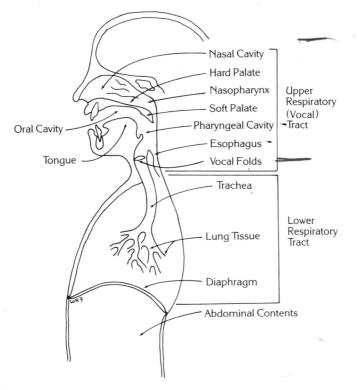

**Figure 3.1**   Human vocal organs

process is somewhat like generating a short tone in a long-necked bottle by rapping the palm of your hand over its mouth. The difference is that the larynx generates such a rapidly occurring series of short-duration tones that each successive excitation begins before its predecessor dies away. Changes in the shape and length of the vocal tract are mediated primarily by tongue, jaw, and lip movement in the process of articulation. These changes affect the resonance properties of the vocal tract, and we perceive the acoustical results as various meaningful sounds, in particular the vowels. Constrictions along the vocal tract may cause turbulent sounds to be generated, or the outward air flow may even be momentarily halted, with a mild explosive release of impounded air, to produce an entire category of sounds classified as consonants. The vocal folds may or may not be vibrating during consonant production, and so we recognize voice and unvoiced consonants. Vowels, of course, must always be voiced (except in a whisper).

Because we talk, the respiratory, phonatory, and articulatory structures shown in our model play dual roles for us—biological and nonbiological. From a purely biological viewpoint, the body is little more than a complex array of pumps, valves, and levers that function quite automatically to sustain life. One

*Resonance is the selective absorption and radiation of acoustic energy at specific wavelengths or frequencies.*

of the remarkable features of speech production is that many of the biological roles of the respiratory, pharyngeal, and articulatory structures can be at least temporarily relinquished and reassigned biosocial roles. For example, highly specialized chemoreceptors located in the large arteries of the thorax and neck are sensitive to the relative concentrations of carbon dioxide and oxygen in the blood, and they automatically trigger the respiratory muscles to become active whenever an imbalance occurs. This accounts for our regular and rhythmic breathing patterns when we are sleeping or quietly reading. Speech, however, is a conscious act. When the occasion arises, the roles of the respiratory, phonatory, and articulatory structures are suddenly transformed into elaborate and effective voluntary sequences of motor acts, and the biological functions, in a real sense, assume a secondary role.

We must acknowledge, then, the contributions of the nervous system, especially as they relate to voluntary motor acts that result in speech. We can construct a model of the act of speaking, incorporating the nervous system. Of paramount importance in this model is the role of various feedback avenues that permit an ongoing monitoring of muscle contractions and the sounds produced as a consequence of muscle activity. One almost obvious feedback channel is provided by our sense of *hearing*. It is very difficult to say something the way you intend it to be said without hearing what is being said, while it is being said.

*The communication problems of people with hearing disorders are covered in chapter 10.*

Our tasks for the remainder of the chapter are clear-cut: to examine the anatomy of the vocal and related organs, to learn under what circumstances they become active, and to specify the acoustical consequences of their activity. Bear in mind that our descriptions are highly idealized ones and that the delicate chain in our model can be broken at any link, and sometimes at more than one.

## RESPIRATION

*See chapters 13 and 14 for discussions of problems resulting from faulty respiration.*

Aside from having something to say, the first requisite for speaking is a supply of pressurized air. The **respiratory tract** begins at the mouth and nose openings and terminates deep within the lungs. As illustrated in Figure 3.1, the larynx, pharynx, and oral and nasal cavities comprise the upper respiratory tract. These same structures are associated with phonation and articulation, so we will begin with the lower respiratory tract, the skeletal framework for which is shown in Figure 3.2. Its major components include the vertebral column, ribs, sternum or breastbone, and the bony components of the pelvis.

### The Bronchial Tree and Lungs

*Remember, the thorax is the part of the trunk above the diaphragm.*

The thorax is occupied mostly by the cone-shaped lungs. Between them lie the heart, esophagus, and great blood vessels. The larynx and part of the bronchial tree are shown in Figure 3.3a, and the bronchial tree in relation to the lungs is shown in Figure 3.3b. The trachea or windpipe is composed of

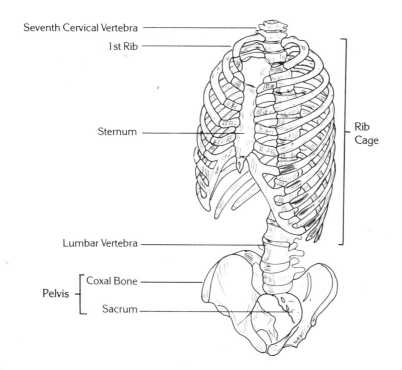

Seventh Cervical Vertebra

1st Rib

Sternum

Rib Cage

Lumbar Vertebra

Coxal Bone

Pelvis

Sacrum

**Figure 3.2**   Skeletal framework of the lower respiratory tract and of the torso

about 16 to 20 incomplete rings of cartilage that divide, giving rise to two main-stem bronchi. They in turn divide repeatedly into smaller and smaller tubes, until finally the passageway verges on the microscopic. These tubules open into about 300,000,000 minute pits (in each lung!) called **alveoli.** It is here that the gas exchange takes place between the blood and oxygen-rich air in the lungs. The combined surface area of the alveoli amounts to about 70 $m^2$, an area equal to that of a tennis court. Lung tissue is spongy and highly elastic, due to a framework of fibroelastic tissue that supports the respiratory structures.

Each lung is closely invested by a **pleural membrane,** while the thorax is lined by a similar membrane. It is tightly adherent to the inner walls of the thoracic cavity and to the surface of the diaphragm. The membranes are moist, which means the lungs can move freely in the thorax, and a rich network of pleural blood vessels tends to absorb gases and fluids. This results in a powerful negative pressure between the two pleural membranes. This pressure links the pleural membranes together with a force so great that the lungs cannot pull away from the thoracic walls, no matter how deeply we might inhale. Thus, when the diaphragm descends, and the dimensions of the rib cage increase, the lungs are literally forced into expanding.

When we are not talking, we breathe quietly about 12 times a minute. The mechanics of air exchange during quiet breathing can be stated quite

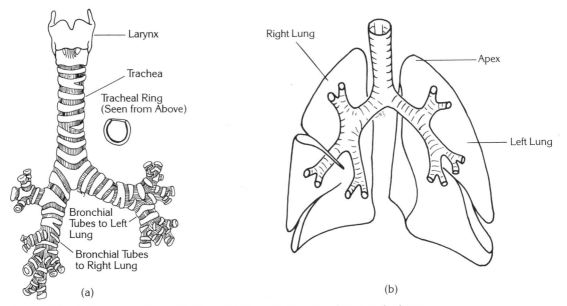

**Figure 3.3**   (a) Larynx and bronchial tree. (b) Bronchial tree in relation to the lungs.

simply. Through contraction of the thoracic muscles, the depth, width, and height of the chest cavity are increased. Since the lungs are bound to the thoracic confines by the pleural membranes, they too must expand. An increase in the size of the lungs creates a slight negative pressure (partial vacuum) within the pulmonary alveoli, and with the airway open, about 500 to 750 cm³ of air rushes into the lungs, until the alveolar pressure is the same as atmospheric. At the same time, the abdominal organs are compressed by the descending diaphragm, 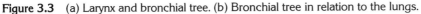 intra-abdominal pressure is elevated, and the anterior abdominal walls distend slightly. The muscles of inhalation then cease to contract somewhat gradually; the expanded thorax-lung complex rebounds, usually without the assistance of any expiratory muscles, to create a slight positive pressure within the lungs. Out goes the air.

*Atmospheric pressure is the pressure of the atmosphere, approximately 14.7 lbs/sq in. at sea level.*

Quiet breathing requires muscle activity during inspiration, but the expiratory forces are purely passive. As expiration begins, the highly elastic lungs contract as rapidly as the rebounding chest and abdominal cavities permit them to do so, and so the air within the lungs is subjected to a slight compression. Air rushes out of the lungs until once again alveolar pressure becomes the same as atmospheric.

The biomechanics of breathing for speech production or for singing are radically different from quiet or vegetative breathing, and they are not completely understood. One difference is that in quiet breathing the inspiratory and expiratory phases each last about 2.5 seconds, but when breathing for speech, a short 2- or 3-second inspiration may be followed by as much as a 15-second expiration phase (while we are talking). Another difference is that when breathing for life purposes, the entire respiratory tract is open and air flow in relatively resistance-free, but when breathing for speech production, the expiratory air flow is met with resistance by the vocal folds located within the larynx, by the articulators, or both. The pressurized air requirements for speech production place complex demands on the lower respiratory tract and its associated muscles, but for most of us, it all happens unconsciously.

Before we proceed to the process of breathing for speech, we should briefly examine the muscles responsible for air exchange.

## The Respiratory Muscles

The muscles responsible for increasing and decreasing thoracic dimensions are shown in Figure 3.4. The most important of the inspiratory muscles is the diaphragm. It alone can account for most of the thoracic expansion necessary for quiet breathing, and yet complete paralysis of the diaphragm does not handicap a person much, so great is the compensatory potential of muscles that otherwise place a minor role in breathing. The peripherally located muscular portion of the diaphragm arises from the lower margin of the rib cage and from the lower part of the vertebral column. These muscle fibers course upward and inward to insert into a tough broad sheet of central tendon. When the muscular portion contracts, the entire diaphragm moves downward and somewhat forward, compressing the abdominal organs, and at the same time expanding the lungs vertically.

Other muscles of the rib cage include the internal and external intercostals. As the name implies, they are located between the ribs. Contraction of the intercostal musculature will exert an upward force on the ribs. Because of the complex geometry of the ribs, however, upward rotation not only increases the side-to-side diameter of the rib cage, but its front-to-back diameter as well.

Twelve stout slips of muscle, the costal elevators, arise from the vertebral column, course down and outward, and attach to the ribs. As their name implies, these muscles elevate the ribs, complementing the intercostal muscles.

We have seen that quiet breathing requires muscle activity during inspiration and that the expiratory forces are purely passive. Air pressure requirements during speech production frequently necessitate active expiratory forces to augment the passive forces. This type of force is provided by the muscles of the anterior abdominal wall, which are shown in Figure 3.4. As a group these muscles compress the abdominal contents (which raises the diaphragm), depress the lower ribs, and thus pull down on the anterior part of the lower chest wall. These muscles also play an important role in coughing, bowel and bladder evacuation, or any activity requiring elevated abdominal pressure.

Muscles normally associated with the upper limbs and with the neck may produce movements of the chest wall under certain pathologic or extreme

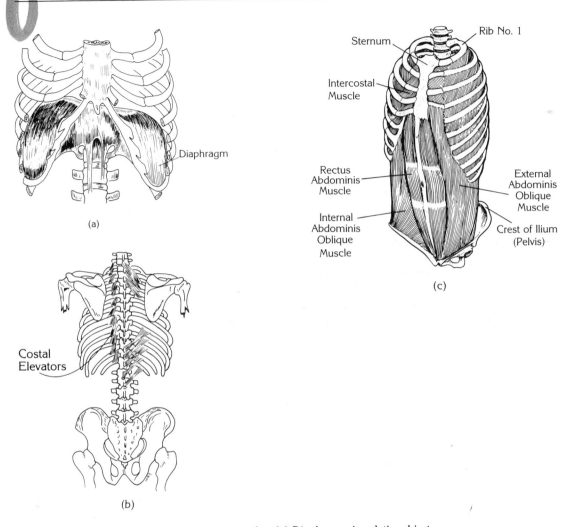

**Figure 3.4**  Schematic of the respiratory muscles. (a) Diaphragm in relationship to the rib cage and the vertebral column. (b) Costal elevators. (c) Intercostal muscles of the rib cage and the superficial-most abdominal muscles.

conditions. Severe asthma, emphysema, and other disorders that obstruct the flow of air into the lungs may require supplemental muscle activity.

## Basic Respiratory Physiology

A person breathing quietly exchanges about 500 to 750 cm$^3$ of air with each respiratory cycle. This air is called *tidal air,* and the quantity is **tidal volume.** Other lung volumes and capacities are recognized, and most of them can be measured with a **spirometer.** As a person breathes through a mouthpiece,

*See Figure 3.5.*

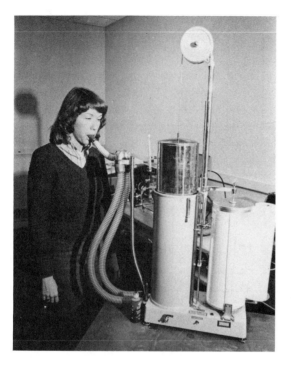

**Figure 3.5**  Subject breathing into a spirometer

air is withdrawn from and returned to a floating drum, which is coupled to a recording pen. The graphic recording is called a spirogram—the example in Figure 3.6 is self-explanatory. One important measurement is **vital capacity,** which ranges from about 3500 to 5000 cm$^3$ in young adult males, and about 1000 cm$^3$ less in adult females. Another measure, called **residual volume,** cannot be made directly, but must be computed. It is the *air remaining in the lungs after a maximum expiration,* and it amounts to about 1000 to 1500 cm$^3$ in young healthy lungs. One of the consequences of advanced age is excessive compliance of lung tissue (i.e., loss of elasticity), and in some instances residual volume can double. As a consequence, ordinary breathing requires abnormal efforts to take air in, and because of a lack of normal passive expiratory forces (which expel air without muscular effort), active expiration must accompany each breath. This shortness of breath can profoundly affect speech production in the elderly.

*Vital capacity is simply the maximum quantity of air exhaled after a maximum inhalation.*

## Speech Breathing

The amount of air remaining in the lungs after a passive exhalation amounts to about 38% of vital capacity. If we contract our abdominal muscles, our

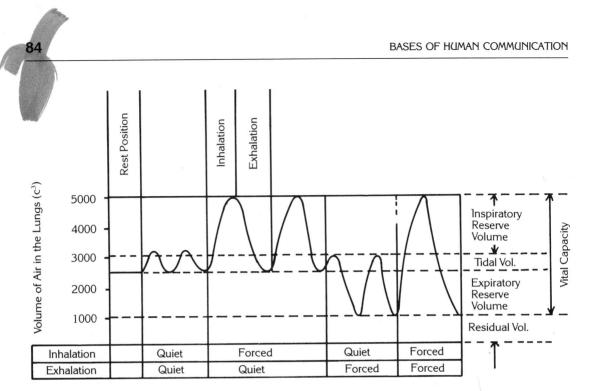

**Figure 3.6** Schematic spirogram

expiratory reserve can be completely exhaled, until only residual air remains in the lungs. A simple experiment will illustrate the significance of passive lung-thorax recoil. A water manometer can be constructed from a U-shaped glass tube with water in it, connected at the top to a length of rubber tubing. If a person inhales maximally (100% vital capacity) and then completely relaxes while exhaling into the tubing, the elastic recoil of the lung-thorax complex will generate enough air pressure to raise the column of water over 50 cm. At 80% vital capacity, the elastic recoil will raise the column about 30 cm; at 38% nothing happens; and at 0% vital capacity, about 30 cm of negative pressure is generated and the water backs up the tube.

Usually we inhale about 70% of our vital capacity prior to speaking. The "relaxation pressure" amounts to about 20 cm of water pressure. The pressure requirements for speech production, it turns out, are modest—only 5 to 10 cm of water pressure. This means that, after taking a moderately deep breath, even without any expiratory muscle activity, the relaxation pressure *exceeds* the speech requirements by 10 to 15 cm of water pressure. In other words, there is easily enough outward pressure to produce speech, without generating active expiratory forces. Normally the excessive relaxation pressure is defeated by the partial sustained contraction of the inspiratory muscles during the speech act, which simply prevents the thorax from recoiling too rapidly and with too much force. If upon prolonged phonation, we are to maintain adequate breath pressure, the expiratory muscles will be called into play, with a gradual increase in their activity as we encroach upon the expiratory reserve volume. The result of all this is that we can maintain a constant breath pressure throughout much of the lung volume range. During loud speech or in singing, the breath pressure requirements may be as high as 20 cm of water pressure and in that event, the inspiratory muscles need not counteract excessive relaxation pressure.

From all of this we begin to see a picture of complex interaction between the vocal tract and the breathing mechanism. For most of us, breath control takes place with little or no thought. In the event of certain neurological disorders (cerebral palsy), obstructive airway conditions (asthma), or lung tissue pathology (emphysema), breathing for speech can be a tormenting task.

## Summary

When one is at rest and the airway open, the pressure within the lungs (alveolar pressure) is the same as atmospheric. When we begin to inhale, contraction of the diaphragm increases the vertical dimension of the thorax and at the same time compresses the abdominal contents to elevate intra-abdominal pressure. The action of the diaphragm is complemented by the intercostal and the costal elevator muscles, which rotate the ribs outward, stiffen the intercostal spaces, and enlarge the front-to-back and lateral dimensions of the thorax. Because of powerful pleural membranes linking both, the lungs are increasingly stretched as the thorax expands. With the airway open, this expansion produces a slightly negative alveolar pressure, and air flows into the lungs until alveolar and atmospheric pressures are equalized. With increasing lung inflation, the activity of the inspiratory muscles gradually diminishes, and the passive forces of exhalation assume their role. Ribs untwist, the elevated abdominal pressure restores the position of the diaphragm, and the elasticity of the lung tissue begins to assert itself (insofar as the rebounding thorax permits it to do so). Alveolar pressure is elevated slightly and air flows outward until, once again, alveolar and atmospheric pressures are equalized. The muscles of inhalation begin to contract and a new cycle of respiration begins.

This sequence of events takes place about 12 times per minute, with about 500 ml of air exchanged each time. With increased inspiratory muscle effort, however, as much as 3 liters of air can be inhaled, starting at resting level. The magnitude of the passive forces of exhalation increases as a function of depth of inhalation. If, during exhalation, airway resistance is introduced, highly elevated alveolar pressures can be generated by the rebounding lung-thorax complex. Resistance may be introduced by the tongue, the lips, or the teeth, or resistance may be the result of the approximated vocal folds within the larynx. To further complicate matters, resistance to outward air flow may be introduced at more than one place (at the same time) along the vocal tract. For example, during the production of the voiced consonant /z/, both the teeth and the vibrating vocal folds provide resistance to air flow. The demands placed on the respiratory system for the production of /z/ are quite different from those involved in the production of the unvoiced cognate /s/.

After a deep inhalation, the passive restoration forces generated by the rebounding lung-thorax unit may produce alveolar pressures that far exceed the demands for speech production. In that event, the checking action provided by the inspiratory musculature can counteract the excessive thoracic rebound to regulate alveolar pressure.

Clearly, the demands placed on the respiratory system are complex and dynamic, but for most of us breath control takes place unconsciously.

## A Brief Clinical Note

The most common causes of respiratory disorders are diseases of the lung tissue and neurogenic respiratory disorders. Excessive lung compliance (loss of elasticity) or a lack of lung compliance (excessive stiffness of lung tissue) can result in weak speech, frequent and inappropriate inhalation, short phrases, and an inability to inject proper inflections and emphases into speech. A common finding in neurogenic respiratory disorders (in some cases of cerebral palsy, for example) is a lack of control of inhalation and inappropriate active exhalation. Such disorders may cause shallow, jerky, and frequent inspiratory gestures, and an inability to switch voluntarily from vegetative to speech breathing.

The fact that a person is poorly positioned in a wheelchair may explain difficulty in breathing. Posture can influence breathing. Try to take a deep breath, for example, while you are slumping in a chair. You can feel your torso begin to straighten out with increased depth of breath.

## THE LARYNX AND PHONATION

*Anterior means toward the front, as contrasted with* **posterior,** *toward the back.*

*That is, if you start to inhale food, you cough.*

*Dealing with people who have had their larynx removed is covered in chapter 8.*

The highly vulnerable lower respiratory tract is well protected by the larynx, a complex structure located in the **anterior** neck. The larynx is extremely sensitive to irritation. The vocal folds contained within it close, by a powerful **reflex,** to prevent the intrusion of foreign substances that might otherwise be accidently inhaled (while eating, for instance). This is usually accompanied by a reflexive contraction of the expiratory muscles to forcefully expel the invading material.

Besides its vitally important biological functions, the larynx also serves as the principal source of sound for speech. Approximated vocal folds offer resistance to the outward flow of air, and because of the elastic recoil of the lung-thorax complex, air in the lungs is placed under pressure. When the pressure is sufficient, the resistance offered by the vocal folds is overcome, and they are literally blown apart to release a strong puff of air into the vocal tract. The vocal folds quickly snap together, only to be blown apart once more. This series of events occurs about 250 times each second when an adult female is phonating, and about 130 times per second for an adult male. The vibration rate determines the fundamental frequency or what we perceive as the **pitch** of the voice. The vocal folds must comply with basic laws of physics, and depending upon their structural size, length, and muscular tension, have a particular range of natural frequency of vibration. The loudness and pitch of the voice can be varied over a wide range, depending upon the force with which the vocal folds are approximated (which influences the air pressure requirements by the larynx) and the degree to which they are stretched, the two principal adjustments of the internal larynx.

*Chapter 8 also discusses problems people have in controlling loudness, pitch, and other voice characteristics.*

No matter how we view the larynx—as a magnificently versatile musical instrument or as an effective source of sound for speech production—from a mechanical standpoint, it is not much more than a variable resistance to air flow. Perhaps we can liberate the larynx from this unglamorous description by becoming better acquainted with it.

## Anatomy of the Larynx

The human larynx is an extremely variable structure from person to person, so much so that only a generalized picture can be presented here. Descriptions of the skeletal framework of the larynx often begin with the hyoid bone, even though it is not a laryngeal structure. It forms the point of attachment for a number of muscles of the tongue and neck and is instrumental in maintaining the larynx in its proper position.

*See Figure 3.7.*

The laryngeal skeleton per se is composed of cartilage that does, however, become bonelike with age. The major cartilages are the ringlike cricoid, the shieldlike thyroid, the flexible Delphian epiglottis, and the paired arytenoids.

The thyroid is the largest of the laryngeal cartilages. It consists of two plates, joined in front at about a 90° angle. Behind, the plates are widely separated. Superior and inferior horns provide attachments to the hyoid bone and cricoid cartilages, respectively.

The cricoid cartilage surmounts the uppermost tracheal ring and is securely fastened to it. This almost circular cartilage has the shape of a truncated cylinder, with a narrow arch in front and a rectangular plate behind. The arytenoid cartilages are tetrahedral in shape. Each cartilage has a vocal process that projects into the larynx and a muscular process laterally, the underside of which has a concave articular facet. It fits onto a convex elliptical facet on the cricoid, and the architecture of this cricoarytenoid joint has an important bearing on the movements of the arytenoid cartilages and of the vocal folds that attach to them.

Even a basic appreciation of laryngeal physiology and voice production demands an understanding of the cricoarytenoid joint and its movements.

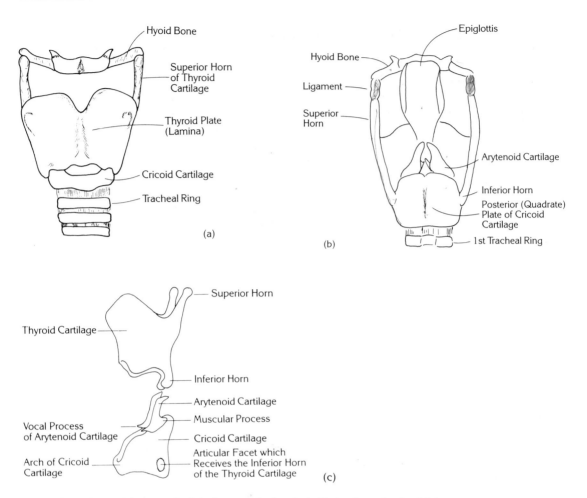

**Figure 3.7** Skeletal framework of the larynx—An "exploded" view from the front (a), from behind (b), and from the side (c).

When the cricoid cartilage is viewed from above, as in Figure 3.8, the long axis of the cricoid articular facet is directed outward, forward, and downward. This facet is sharply convex, and it accommodates a sharply concave facet on the underside of the muscular process of the arytenoid cartilage in much the same way matching cylindrical sections would fit together. Because of the outward, forward, and downward orientation of this complex joint, rocking or rotating movements result in either an upward and outward, or a downward and inward, swinging motion of the vocal processes, to which the vocal ligaments and vocal folds are attached.

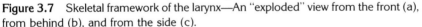

A single muscle, the posterior cricoarytenoid acts to separate or abduct the vocal folds. (See Figure 3.9.) A fairly substantial muscle, it pulls down-

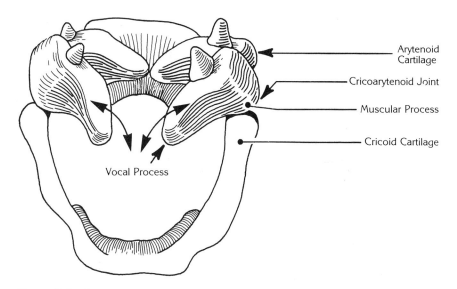

**Figure 3.8** Cricoarytenoid joint. A forward directed force on the muscular process of the arytenoid cartilage causes the vocal process and vocal folds to swing downward and toward the midline (adduction), while a backward directed force swings the vocal processes and folds upward and away from the midline (abduction).

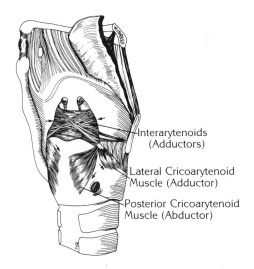

**Figure 3.9** Abductor and adductor muscles of the larynx. *(Note: From* Study Guide/Workbook to accompany *Speech and Hearing Science—Anatomy and Physiology, 3rd Ed. (W. R. Zemlin) by E. Zemlin, 1988, Champaign, Ill.: Stipes Publishing Co. Reprinted by permission.)*

ward and back on the muscular process of the arytenoid cartilage. This swings the vocal ligament and vocal folds upward and away from the midline. Two muscles, the lateral cricoarytenoid and the arytenoids, act in opposition to the posterior cricoarytenoid muscle. They swing the vocal process (and vocal folds) downward and toward the midline, and depending on the extent of this activity, the vocal folds are compressed at the midline (medial compression) with varying degrees of force. This important laryngeal adjustment causes varying degrees of resistance to the outward flow of air, thus regulating the loudness of the voice. We should realize, however, that any changes in laryngeal airflow resistance must be met with appropriate compensatory action by the respiratory system if phonation is to take place.

The vocal ligaments and vocal folds attach to the thyroid cartilage on either side of the midline in front. When rotation occurs at the cricothyroid joint, they are subjected to varying degrees of longitudinal tension, the principal mechanism by which voice pitch is regulated. A single muscle, the cricothyroid, acts on the cricothyroid joint. Its action, illustrated in Figures 3.10 and 3.11, is to reduce the distance in front between the cricoid and thyroid cartilages. This increases the distance between the vocal processes of the arytenoids behind and the thyroid angle in front—action that increases the *tension* of the vocal folds and raises the pitch of the voice. The action of the cricothyroid muscle is opposed by the thyroarytenoidmuscle, which is the vibrating part of the vocal folds we can see when the larynx is examined by a mirror placed in the back of the throat (indirect laryngoscopy—see Figure 3.12).

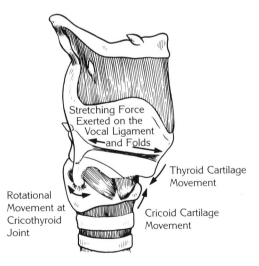

Stretching Force Exerted on the Vocal Ligament and Folds

Thyroid Cartilage Movement

Rotational Movement at Cricothyroid Joint

Cricoid Cartilage Movement

**Figure 3.10**    Rotational movement at the cricothyroid joint.

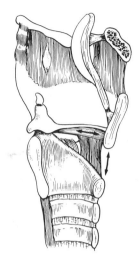

**Figure 3.11** Action of the cricothyroid and thyroarytenoid muscles

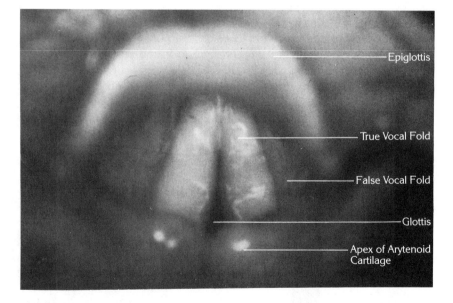

**Figure 3.12** Larynx as seen in indirect laryngoscopy

## Laryngeal Physiology

From our description of the larynx, we have learned that the vocal folds can be brought together at the midline with varying degrees of force and can be placed under varying degrees of tension. Approximation of the vocal folds is called medial compression, while the stretching force (which may or may not

92  BASES OF HUMAN COMMUNICATION

*See Figure 3.13a.*

*See Figure 3.13b.*

elongate the folds) is called longitudinal tension. Various combinations of the two, plus a variable pressurized air supply, account for the incredible versatility of the voice.

During quiet breathing, the vocal folds are relatively motionless and a triangular chink is formed by their leading edges. This opening between the free margins of the vocal folds is called the rima glottidis, or simply the **glottis.** The glottis is extremely variable in its configuration and dimensions, and as a consequence is capable of offering varying degrees of resistance to the outward flow of pressurized air from the lungs.

During forced inhalation, something we often do just prior to speaking, the vocal folds are widely separated, and so the larynx offers little resistance to the inward flow of air. As phonation begins, however, the vocal folds are brought quickly toward the midline, so they offer a certain degree of resistance to the outward flow of pressurized air, when the forces of exhalation are released. The extent of resistance is highly variable, of course, depending on the degree of medial compression and longitudinal tension. As air pressure builds up beneath the vocal folds (subglottal pressure), it quickly overcomes the laryngeal resistance. The folds are blown apart to release a puff of compressed air into the (supraglottal) vocal tract. The quantity of compressed air that is released amounts to only 1 or 2 cm$^3$; nevertheless, it results in a momentary drop in the pressure beneath the vocal folds and they snap back together. The process of phonation, then, is primarily an aerodynamic phenomenon. This building up of subglottal air pressure and the blowing apart and snapping together of the vocal folds constitute one complete cycle of vocal fold vibration. As stated earlier, in adult

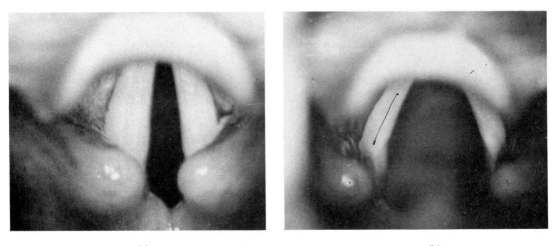

(a)                                    (b)

**Figure 3.13**  Glottal configurations during quiet breathing (a) and forced inhalation (b).

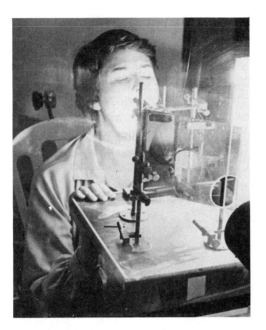

**Figure 3.14** A laryngeal physiology laboratory. This photograph was taken through the window of a sound-insulated booth that houses the (noisy) camera.

females this occurs about 200 to 260 times/sec; in adult males, who tend to have larger larynxes and longer vocal folds, the vibration rate is about 120 to 145 times/sec. During colloquial speech, however, when we might express surprise or delight or emphasize a point, the vibration rate (fundamental frequency of the voice) may encompass a range of two octaves for any given person. The fundamental frequency is the principal determinant of the pitch of the voice.

*Adult female vocal folds are about 13 to 14 mm long; male vocal folds about 21 to 22 mm.*

Ultrahigh-speed motion pictures (4,000 frames/sec) have proven to be a valuable research technique in the study of the internal larynx during phonation. When the film is projected at the standard 16 frames/sec, we see a super slow motion view of vocal fold vibration. A typical single cycle of vibration is described in terms of an opening phase, when the folds are blown apart; a closing phase, when they snap back together again; and a closed phase, when the folds are fully approximated (or nearly so) and air pressure beneath them is once again building up. The relative durations of these three phases, and the magnitude of glottal area under various phonatory conditions, provide valuable insight into the mechanics of voice production. A single cycle of vocal fold vibration (extracted from a high-speed film) is shown in Figure 3.15, and a graph of glottal area as a function of time is shown in Figure 3.16.

*Figure 3.14 shows a subject in position for such a film.*

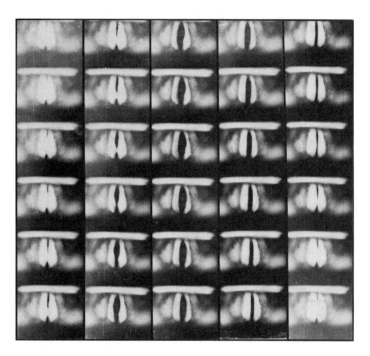

**Figure 3.15** A single cycle of vocal fold vibration, photographed at 4,000 frames/sec. The vocal folds are together in the upper left frame, which represents the beginning of the cycle. They are maximally separated in the middle row of frames, and then begin to close, until they are nearly completely approximated in the frame in the lower right. The entire event, from closed to open and closed again, represents one complete cycle of vocal fold vibration and took about 1/140 sec.

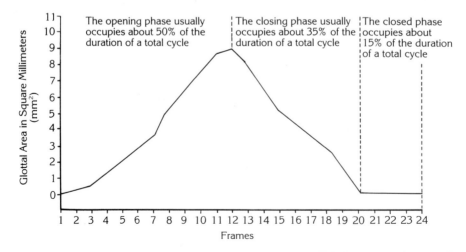

**Figure 3.16** Fairly representative graph of glottal area as a function of time

## The Pitch-Changing Mechanism

We learned earlier that action of the cricothyroid muscle tends to elongate the vocal folds and to increase their longitudinal tension. Two principal factors account for the resistance to tension that is offered by the vocal folds. One is the inherent elasticity of the vocal ligament and the vocal fold musculature. The second is the result of contraction of the muscles of the vocal folds. An additional factor that influences the frequency of vocal fold vibration is their thickness, or mass, which decreases with increases in length.

When the vocal folds are placed under stretching force, they are subjected to a certain increase in longitudinal tension, and the frequency of vibration (pitch) is raised. Active resistance due to contraction of the vocal fold muscles further increases the longitudinal tension. When the stretching force is removed from the vocal folds, their inherent elasticity tends to restore them to their original condition, and the pitch of the voice decreases. In addition, when the muscles of the vocal folds contract without opposition (by the cricothyroid), they become shorter, somewhat flaccid, and the pitch drops further. The delicate interaction between the stretching force and the resistance offered by the vocal fold tissue (active and passive) accounts in large part for the versatility of the human voice.

## The Loudness Mechanism

The loudness of everyday speech is continuously changing, just as pitch is continuously changing. If we examine ultrahigh-speed films at high intensity (loud) phonation when compared to conversational intensity, the single difference is an increase in the duration of the closed phase. The glottis opens *See Figure 3.17.* quickly, closes quickly, and then remains closed for a longer time than during phonation at conversational levels. In fact, the closed phase may occupy as much as one-half the total duration of an individual vibratory cycle. The mechanism responsible for the increase is heightened medial compression of the vocal folds, and this is regulated by activity of the lateral cricoarytenoid and arytenoid muscles (adductor muscles). Increases in medial compression produce an increase in laryngeal resistance to air flow, and so once again the lung-thorax complex must compensate. We have seen that, during phonation at conversational levels, subglottal pressure requirements are modest, amounting to 2 to 4 (or so) cm of water pressure, while loud speech requires 10 to 15 cm of pressure. Each puff of air released by the vibrating vocal folds results in an increase in the excitation of vibration of the air column of the vocal tract (pharynx, oral, and at times, the nasal cavities).

To summarize, we have seen that three factors influence the normal mode of vibration of the vocal folds. They are medial compression, longitudinal tension of the vocal folds, and subglottal air pressure. A number of additional factors can influence the behavior of the internal larynx. Many of

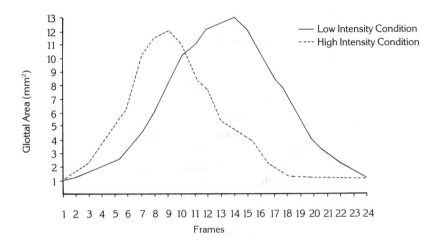

**Figure 3.17**  Graph of glottal area as a function of time, comparing conversational to loud phonation. Note the substantial increase in the duration of the closed phase for loud phonation, an indication of the increase of the resistance to air flow at the laryngeal level.

them contribute to problems with the quality and pleasantness of the voice. The mass of one or both of the vocal folds may be modified by inflammation (laryngitis) or by growths on the folds (neoplasms); as a consequence the folds may vibrate irregularly (aperiodically), which imparts an unpleasant and rough quality to the voice. A loss of mobility at the joints of the laryngeal cartilages or loss of muscular strength may impose constraints on medial compression and longitudinal tension, so the pitch range is adversely affected. If the vocal folds fail to meet at the midline with sufficient force, they will offer inadequate resistance to air flow. A weak, breathy voice may result. A great many of these negative factors can be attributed to vocal abuse. Smoking, alcohol, polluted air, and yelling in noisy environments are but a few of the abuses to which the larynx may be subjected. And finally, the aging of the tissues of the speech mechanism will ultimately impose constraints on the ability of the elderly to communicate verbally as they once did. Proper care of our bodies, however, will often defer the aging effects for a long time.

## ARTICULATION

As puffs of air are released into the vocal tract by the vibrating vocal folds, the dormant air column above the larynx is driven to produce a complex sound called the **glottal** or **laryngeal tone.** The lowest frequency component in this tone is numerically the same as the vibratory rate of the vocal folds. All of the remaining components have frequencies that are integral multiples of this lowest or fundamental frequency. The intensities of the higher frequency components fall off rather sharply, so that not much acoustic energy exists at frequencies above 3,000 Hz. This harmonically rich glottal tone is the raw material from which all of our vowels and many of our consonants are formed.

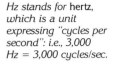

*Hz stands for* hertz, *which is a unit expressing "cycles per second": i.e., 3,000 Hz = 3,000 cycles/sec.*

With the articulators and the vocal tract in a neutral configuration (for the vowel /ʌ/, the cross-sectional area of this acoustic tube is fairly constant throughout its length. The vocal tract behaves acoustically like a tube closed at one end and open at the other. When excited, the air column in closed-open tubes oscillates or vibrates at a frequency that has a wavelength four times the length of the tube, and at odd-numbered multiples of this first frequency. For example, an adult male vocal tract is about 17.5 cm in length, so the first resonant frequency is one that has a wavelength (λ) four times the length, or 70 cm (or .70 m). From basic physics we learn that

$$f = \frac{\upsilon}{\lambda} = \frac{340 \text{ m/sec}}{.70 \text{ m}} = 485.7 \text{ Hz}$$

where $f$ = frequency in Hz, $\upsilon$ = velocity of sound in air in meters per second. The first resonant frequency of our male vocal tract is 485.7 Hz. The resonances in the vocal tract are commonly called **formants,** and their frequencies are called *format frequencies.* The second formant frequency (an odd-numbered multiple of the first) is about 1,457 Hz, while the third formant frequency is about 2,428 Hz.

When the harmonically rich glottal tone is fed into the frequency-selective vocal tract, frequency components that correspond to, or nearly correspond to, the formant frequencies are reinforced while the other frequencies tend to dissipate. Sounds that emerge from the lips will have frequency regions reinforced by the natural formant frequencies of the vocal tract.

*See Figure 3.18.*

Changes in the length or in the cross-sectional area along the vocal tract result in changes in the frequencies of the various formants. Lip rounding, lowering or raising of the larynx, changes in tongue and jaw position, or any combination of these gestures will influence the formant frequencies of the vocal tract and we hear different vowel sounds.

Our task now is to examine the mechanisms responsible for changing the acoustical properties of the vocal tract.

## The Skeletal Framework of the Vocal Tract

The skull, which forms the skeletal framework for much of the vocal tract, is composed of 22 individual bones, all rigidly joined together except for the **mandible.** It articulates with the temporal bones on either side by means of a complex double joint that permits rotation, gliding, side-to-side movements, or various combinations of the three. The skull can be divided into two major parts: (a) the cranium (braincase), which houses and protects the brain, and (b) the facial skeleton, which forms the framework for the organs

*The* mandible *is the lower jaw.*

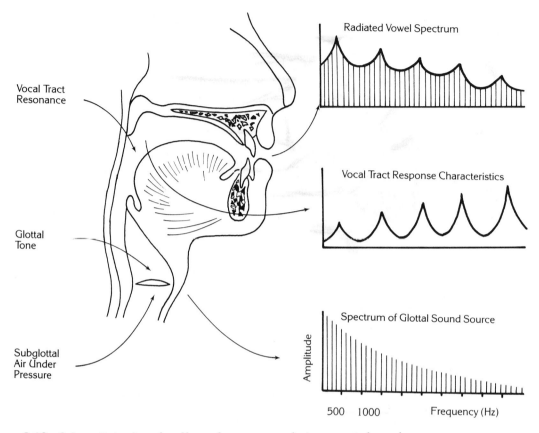

**Figure 3.18** Schematic tracing of an X-ray of a person producing a neutral vowel, vocal tract response characteristics, and spectrum of glottal sound. The radiated vowel spectrum is shown at the top of the figure.

*The results of these differential cranial and facial skeleton growth patterns can be seen in Figure 3.19.*

of mastication (teeth, jaws, and tongue), speech production (the articulators), and special senses (small, vision, taste), and the muscles of facial expression. These two parts of the skull have entirely different growth patterns. The braincase triples in volume during the first 2 years and reaches 90% of its full size by the 10th year. The facial skeleton shows bursts of growth that are related to the times of eruption of the teeth, and it continues to grow until the middle or late teens. The skull rests on the first cervical vertebra (the atlas), which together with the second (axis) vertebra forms a complex joint that is largely responsible for the mobility of the head.

## The Cavities and Associated Structures of the Vocal Tract

The cavities of the vocal tract form the resonant acoustic tube that is responsible for shaping the laryngeal tone into recognizable vowel sounds. In

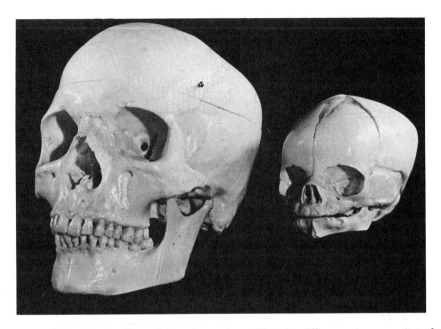

**Figure 3.19** Skulls of an adult and a newborn. Note the difference in proportion of facial height and the braincase.

addition, when constrictions along its length cause air turbulence or momentarily halt air flow, consonants can be generated.

The small but variable space between the gums and teeth is called the *buccal cavity.* Its dimensions change when, for example, we round our lips for the production of the word *who.* A circular muscle, the orbicularis oris, surrounds the mouth opening and is largely responsible for the pursing of our lips. Additional muscles (of facial expression) that insert into the corners of the mouth influence the lips.

*See Figure 3.20.*

## Dentition

The **deciduous** or temporary (baby) teeth develop very early in the embryo, and 20 of them (10 in each jaw) ultimately appear. Children begin to shed their deciduous teeth in their sixth year, and they are slowly replaced by permanent teeth. The shedding and eruption processes may continue into the early twenties, until each fully equipped permanent dental arch has 16 teeth. Aside from their obvious biological functions, the teeth play an important role in articulation. The dentition also strongly influences facial growth throughout the developing years and facial balance throughout life. The deciduous teeth are particularly important in contributing to the proper spacial relationships

*The set of teeth on one jaw is called the* **dental arch.**

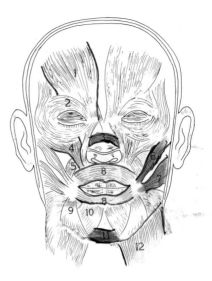

**Figure 3.20**  Some muscles of facial expression. The functions of muscles 1–12 are, briefly:
1. Frontalis wrinkles the forehead.
2. Orbicularis oculi assists in closing the eye and in winking.
3. Nasalis constricts the nostrils (twitches the nose).
4. Levator labii superior elevates and everts the upper lip.
5. Levator anguli oris elevates the corner of the mouth, as when sneering.
6. Zygomatic major assists in elevating the corner of the mouth.
7. Risorius retracts the angle of the mouth, and helps compress the lips.
8. Orbicularis oris purses the lips in a sphincterlike action (puckers).
9. Depressor anguli oris draws the corner of the mouth downward, as in pouting.
10. Depressor labii inferior draws the lower lip directly downward.
11. Mentalis wrinkles the chin, as in pouting.
12. Platysma helps retract the lips and compress them.

*Figure 3.21 shows the parts of the oral cavity.*

of the permanent teeth. Premature loss of the deciduous teeth can have profound adverse effects on the spacing of the permanent teeth.

The configuration of the oral cavity is highly variable, more so than any other of the cavities of the vocal tract. Its ability to quickly and dramatically adjust for speech sound production can be largely attributed to the mobility of the tongue and jaw.

A tongue as seen from above is shown in Figure 3.22. Anatomically it is divided into a blade and root. A shallow midline groove runs the length of the blade, and the perimeter of the blade has numerous taste buds.

## Tongue Musculature

Changes in the shape of the tongue (and acoustic properties of the oral cavity) are often attributed to muscles confined entirely to it (intrinsic muscles), while changes in tongue position are attributed to muscles that arise from structures other than the tongue and insert into it (extrinsic muscles). The muscle distribution in the tongue is extremely complex, as can be seen in Figure 3.23. Muscles course through the tongue longitudinally, transversely, and vertically, and they are interwoven like fabric. When these

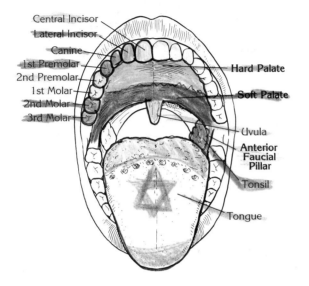

**Figure 3.21**   Schematic of an oral cavity

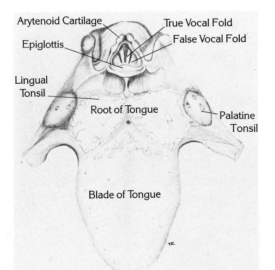

**Figure 3.22**   The tongue as seen from above, showing its relationship to some adjacent structures. (*Note: Drawing courtesy of Therese Zemlin.*)

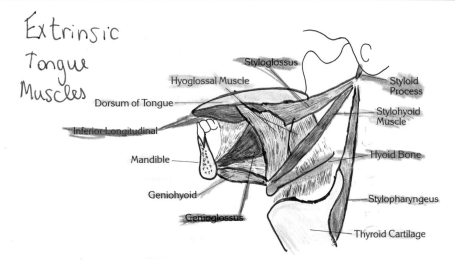

Extrinsic Tongue Muscles

**Figure 3.23**   Schematic of extrinsic tongue muscles

muscles work with or against one another, many shapes, positions, and tensions can be produced, and at an amazing rate. An important extrinsic muscle, the genioglossus, arises from the inner surface of the mandible and radiates fanlike throughout the tongue, with some of its fibers ultimately converging toward the tip. This muscle comprises the bulk of the muscular core of the tongue. Probably its most important function is to protract the body of the tongue to produce alveolar and dental consonants (and to wipe peanut butter from the roof of the mouth). Other muscles enter the tongue from beneath, above, and behind. They are instrumental in depressing, elevating, and retracting the body of the tongue, gestures that are important for vowel and consonant production.

## Mandibular Movement

The lips, teeth, tongue, and mandible are all structures associated with eating, yet they serve us well for the subtle adjustments of the vocal tract required for speech production. The musculature responsible for mandibular movement can be grouped functionally into elevators, depressors, and a single protractor. The elevators and protractor, shown in Figure 3.24, are powerful muscles used in chewing, and they contract forcefully every time we swallow. Mandibular depression requires little power, but for speech production *speed and timing are important.* The jaw must also be stabilized during the production of sounds that require the force of the tongue against the roof of the mouth, as in /t/ and /d/. This is a job for the mandibular elevators.

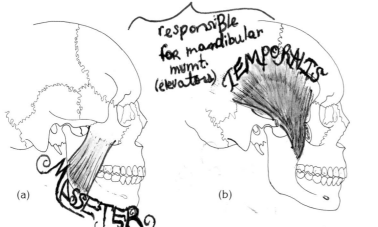

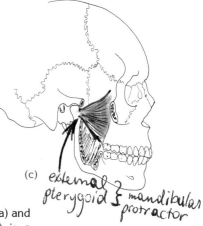

**Figure 3.24** Muscles responsible for mandibular movement: the masseter (a) and temporalis (b) are mandibular elevators, while the external pterygoid (c) is a mandibular protractor.

## The Soft Palate

The roof of the oral cavity (hard palate) is formed primarily by the bony horizontal shelves of the maxillae (upper jaw). Behind that, the hard palate is continuous with the soft palate, or **velum.**

The soft palate couples or uncouples the nasal and pharyngeal cavities. When elevated, the soft palate acts as a valve and simply closes off the nasal cavity. This is essential for the production of any consonant sound, but especially for such plosives as /p/, /b/, /t/, /d/, and /k/. The soft palate can also be actively depressed for the /m/, /n/, and /ŋ/ sounds. When that happens the complex nasal cavities act as a secondary resonator and impart to speech that quality we perceive as nasality.

From an examination of Figure 3.25, we see that the tensor and elevator (levator) muscles act to elevate the soft palate, thus sealing the opening into the nasal cavity. An inadequate seal results in excessive nasality in speech and an inability to generate pressure in the oral cavity. Two muscles, the palatoglossus (from the soft palate to the tongue) and the palatopharyngeus (from the soft palate to the pharynx), depress the soft palate.

## The Pharynx

*See Figure 3.26.*

The pharynx is essentially a muscular tube suspended from the base of the skull. Based on the relationship of its cavity to the remainder of the vocal tract, the pharynx is divided into a nasopharynx, oropharynx, and laryngopharynx. It is largely connective tissue above, becoming increasingly muscular below,

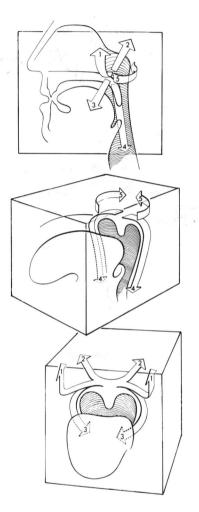

**Figure 3.25**  Schematic representation of the function of the soft palate (velopharyngeal) musculature. The arrows indicate the approximate direction of their action and influence on the soft palate.

1. Tensor palatini
2. Levator palatini
3. Palatoglossus
4. Palatopharyngeus
5. Superior pharyngeal constrictor

*(Note: From "The Velopharyngeal Muscles in Speech" by B. Fritzell, 1969.* Acta Oto- Laryngologica Supp., *No. 250. Reprinted by permission.)*

Start Here

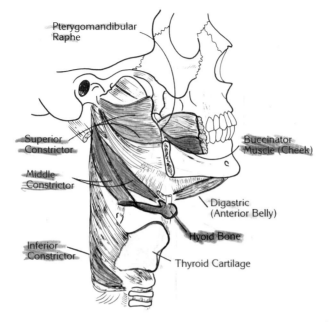

**Figure 3.26**  Schematic of the pharynx as seen from the side. Note that the cervical vertebrae and associated muscles are not shown.

where its cavity is continuous with the larynx in front and the esophagus behind. Its lowest fibers (the inferior pharyngeal constrictor) arise from the cricoid and thyroid cartilages and fan out somewhat as they course obliquely upward and toward the midline. The middle constrictor arises from the hyoid bone, while the superior constrictor fibers have a complex origin from the sides of the tongue, from the soft palate, and from the base of the skull.

The principal contribution of the pharynx to speech production is as a resonator. It is not dynamic as an articulator, and the changes that do take place in the configuration of its cavity are mediated by tongue and jaw movements, and by elevation and depression of the larynx.

The least dynamic of the resonators are the nasal cavities, which are two narrow, somewhat symmetrical chambers separated (in front) by a bony and cartilaginous nasal septum. The cavities communicate with the exterior by way of the nostrils (or nares) and with the nasopharynx by way of the choanae. The cavities are extremely complex in their overall configuration, which is attributable to the almost labyrinthine lateral walls. Its function is to filter inhaled air and bring it to body temperature on its way to the lungs, and it also functions as a complex addition to the resonator system when the soft palate is lowered.

*Look again at Figure 3.1 to see how the pharynx relates to the rest of the vocal tract.*

## Articulatory Physiology

It is now time to put our anatomy and physiology lessons together and look at the overall picture. First, let us review a bit. We have seen that a subglottal air supply can be placed under pressure by introducing air flow resistance when the forces of exhalation are released. We have also seen how resistance to outward air flow takes place at the laryngeal level to generate a glottal tone. Remember that the vibrations of the vocal folds are not the source of those sounds we ultimately hear as speech; that is, whenever the vocal folds are blown apart by the elevated subglottal pressure, a short burst of pressurized air is released into the vocal tract. With the vocal folds vibrating at a rate of 150 times/sec, for example, a discrete burst of air is released into the vocal tract each 1/150th of a second. The effect of these transient bursts of energy is to excite the dormant column of air above the larynx, and it vibrates for a short time. Although the amplitude of each vibration dies away quickly, the rapid succession of energy bursts serves to keep the air column vibrating. These short-duration vibrations generated within the supraglottal air column constitute the glottal tone, and it is rich in partials that are harmonically related to the fundamental frequency. The vocal tract, depending on its configuration, is capable of resonating to or reinforcing some of the partials in the glottal tone. We might say that the glottal tone is "shaped" by the configuration, and therefore the acoustical properties of the vocal tract, to produce our voiced speech sounds. There are just three dimensions of the vocal tract that can be modified by the articulators: the overall length, the location of a constriction, and the degree of constriction. Lip rounding, another variable, tends to increase the length of the vocal tract and at the same time impose a constriction on it. Elevation and depression of the larynx has the effect of decreasing or increasing the length of the vocal tract, and the acoustic result is to lower or raise the formant frequencies accordingly.

*A harmonic is a whole numbered multiple of the fundamental or lowest frequency.*

The location and extent of constrictions in the vocal tract often determine whether the sound radiated at the mouth will be vowel-like or consonantal (turbulent or explosive).

### Vowel Production

Each vowel in our language system is characterized by a unique energy distribution that is a consequence of a specific cross-sectional area and length of the vocal tract. For vowel production, changes are mediated by the tongue, jaw, and lips. A tracing of an X-ray of a person producing a vowel with the vocal tract in a neutral configuration is shown in Figures 3.18 and 3.27. Figure 3.18 also shows spectrum of an idealized glottal tone and the same tone after it has been shaped by the resonant characteristics of the vocal tract. The shape of the vocal tract during the production of an /i/ vowel is shown in Figure 3.28, along with the radiated vowel after shaping.

X-ray studies of speakers show that fairly predictable tongue positions can beassociated with the individual vowel sounds. For example, a vowel produced with the tongue high up and in front will be recognized as an /i/. If the tongue is moved to the opposite extreme of the oral cavity (low and back), it will probably be recognized as an /a/. See Figure 3.29.

Eight vowel configurations that describe the extremes of tongue positions for their production have been recognized. All of the vowels we produce

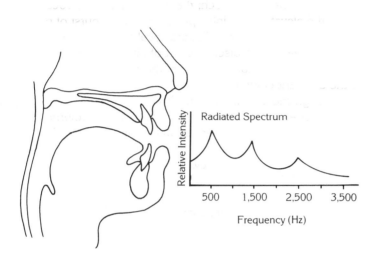

**Figure 3.27** Vocal tract in a neutral configuration and the spectrum of the sound radiated at the lips

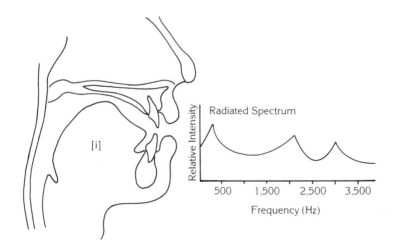

**Figure 3.28** Vocal tract in configuration for production of /i/ and the spectrum of the sound radiated at the lips.

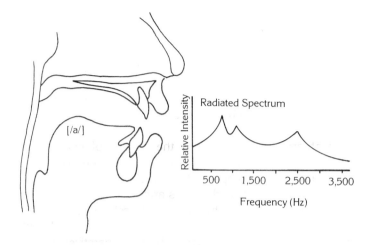

**Figure 3.29**  Vocal tract in configuration for production of /a/ and the spectrum of the sound radiated at the lips.

fall within the boundaries of these configurations. Vowels can also be classified according to tongue positions relative to the palate. When the hump of the tongue is high and near the palate, the vowel is called a *close vowel*; when the hump of the tongue is low, toward the bottom of the mouth, the vowel is called *open*. Vowels produced with the tongue in intermediate positions are called *central* or *neutral*. To round out our descriptive scheme, we also describe articulatory positions of the tongue as being either toward the front or toward the back of the oral cavity. The /i/ in *need*, for example, is a *close-front* vowel, while /u/ in *who* is a *close-back* vowel. The degree of lip rounding and relative muscle tension in articulation are also used to classify certain vowels.

A group of speech sounds similar to vowels is called **diphthongs.** They are often described as blends of two separate vowels, spoken within the same syllable. Say the word *boy* and listen to the changes in the vowel. The transition may bridge two, three, or more vowels in our everyday running speech. An example is the complex vowel in *boyandgirl,* with no break between *boyand.*

Our language system is extremely tolerant of a wide range of variability in vowel production, especially during contextual speech. Evidence of this is seen in our ability to understand speech in spite of strong foreign accents or regional dialects. Consonant production, on the other hand, demands relatively precise articulation and even minor alterations of placement can produce unwanted phonemic differences.

## Consonant Production

Consonants, which are characterized by constrictions or momentary occlusions of the vocal tract, are often described by place and manner of articulation and whether they are **voiced** or **unvoiced.** They are said to be the constrictive gestures of speech. Consonants often initiate and terminate syllables, and they comprise about 62% of all English speech sounds. They are not only more constrictive than vowels, they are more rapid and account for a large part of the transitory nature of speech. As we saw in chapter 2, places of articulation include the lips (bilabial), the teeth and lips (labiodental), the gums (alveolar), the hard palate (palatal), the soft palate (velar), and the glottis (glottal).

Manner of articulation describes the degree of constriction as the consonants initiate or terminate a syllable. If closure is complete, the consonant is a **stop;** if incomplete, it is a **fricative.** Some voiceless consonants are produced as sustained sounds and are called **continuants.** When complete closure is followed by an audible release of the impounded pressurized air, the consonant is called a **stop-plosive,** or simply a **plosive.** At other times, complete closure is followed by a comparatively slow release of the impounded air, as the tongue sweeps along the palate backward, to produce an **affricate.** Other sounds, called **glides,** are generated by rapid articulatory movement, and the noise or turbulent element is not as prominent as in plosives and fricatives. Some examples are /r/, /w/ and /j/. A small family of sounds, the **semivowels,** seem to qualify as vowel-like or consonantlike. They may be syllabic in certain contexts and so serve as vowels, while in other contexts these same sounds either initiate or terminate syllables and so serve as consonants. The semivowel /r/ serves as a consonant in the word *red*, while in the word *mother*, this same sound serves as the vowel in the second syllable. In the word *little*, the semivowel /l/ serves as the consonant in the first syllable and as a vowel in the second syllable. Three other consonant sounds /m/, n, ŋ/, classified as **nasal consonants** (when they serve as consonants) because of their quality, are also considered semivowels in some classification systems.

*Liquids* are special semivowels because of the unique manner in which they are articulated. The liquid /l/ is produced with the tongue against the alveolar ridge so the breath stream flows somewhat freely around the sides of the tongue. Sometimes a certain articulated gesture is associated with two consonants that differ only in the voiced-voiceless category. The voiced /b/ and unvoiced /p/ constitute a cognate pair. Others are the /s/ (voiceless) and /z/ (voiced) and /f/ (voiceless) and /v/ (voiced) cognates.

*Recall that these physiologically related consonants are called* **cognates.**

Consonant production is dependent on the integrity of the speech mechanism, and little leeway is allowed in their production. We seem to be far more tolerant of vowel coloration in regional and foreign dialects than we are of consonant variations.

Stop consonants are dependent on *complete closure* at some point along the vocal tract. With the release of the forces of exhalation, pressure builds up behind the occlusion until the air is released suddenly by the articulatory gesture. Closure for stop consonants occurs at the lips for the production of /b/ and its voiceless cognate /p/, with the tongue against the alveolar ridge for the

/d/ and /t/ cognate pair, and with the tongue against the soft palate for the cognates /g/ and /k/. Elevated intraoral pressures are dependent on an adequate velopharyngeal seal.

Fricative consonants are the result of a noise excitation due to a constriction somewhere along the vocal tract. Five common regions of constriction for the production of fricative consonants are used in the English language. Except for the /h/ consonant, which is generated at the glottis, all voiced fricatives have voiceless cognates.

The three nasal consonants /m/, /n/, and /ŋ/ are voiced, of course, but at the same time the vocal tract is completely constricted by the lips in /m/, by the tongue at the alveolar ridge in /n/, or by the dorsum of the tongue against the hard and/or soft palate in /ŋ/. The lowered velum results in two resonant systems, with substantially different acoustical properties, placed side by side. The effective overall length of the vocal tract is increased, which lowers the frequencies of all the formant frequencies, and because of the tortuous acoustic pathway through the nasal cavities, the amplitudes of the resonances are somewhat reduced. During normal vowel and consonant production (except for the nasals), the nasal cavities are sealed off by the soft palate. In instances of tissue deficiency (a cleft palate, for example), or an immobile soft palate (paralysis), the nasal cavity coupling is inappropriate. Thus, the person may be unable to impound pressurized air in the oral cavity for consonant production, and the vowels will be characteristically nasal. The delicate balance and subtle interplay between the respiratory, phonatory, and articulatory mechanisms during the production of ordinary everyday speech is complex, yet it seems such a simple task for most of us.

*This happens with cleft palates and related disorders; see chapter 11.*

## THE NERVOUS SYSTEM AND SPEECH PRODUCTION

The ultimate mediator of most of our voluntary behavior—as well as our adjustments to changes in our immediate environment—is the nervous system. Composed of billions of individual cells called neurons and their supportive tissues, the nervous system instigates and transmits neural impulses that stimulate our muscles to contract. At the same time, muscle contraction and movements about the joints initiate neural impulses, and they in turn travel back to the coordinating centers of the brain to "tell it" what is happening and if things are going as planned.

*One communication disorder caused by failure of the brain and nervous system is aphasia, discussed in Chapter 12.*

Except for the extensions of its cellular substance, neurons are quite similar to all other cells in the body. As shown in Figure 3.30, a neuron consists of a cell body and its extensions. The neurons that supply muscles typically have a single relatively long extension called an axon, and numerous shorter extensions clustered about the cell body, called dendrites. The terminal ending of an axon is characterized by numerous collaterals or branches (the end brush) that have little swellings or buttons at their tips. Depending on their location, end brushes terminate either on the dendrites, on the cell bodies of other neurons, or on muscle fibers.

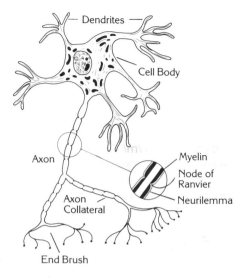

**Figure 3.30** Schematic of a neuron

Whenever a neuron is stimulated, a chemoelectrical impulse is transmitted over the entire cell and its extensions or processes. As the impulse reaches the limits of the cell processes, a transmitter agent, which is manufactured by the neuron, is released by the end brush of the axon. This transmitter agent facilitates the transmission of the impulse to the next cell body, its dendrite, or to muscle tissue.

The nervous system is divided into a **central nervous system (CNS),** which is that part enclosed and protected by the skull and vertebral column, and a **peripheral nervous system (PNS),** which is that part lying outside the bony confines of the skull and vertebral column. The central nervous system is in turn divided into the brain and spinal cord, while the peripheral nervous system is divided into a voluntary part (cranial and spinal nerves) and an involuntary part (the autonomic nervous system). A schematic nervous system is shown in Figure 3.31. Our immediate topic of interest is the central nervous system and the voluntary part of the peripheral nervous system. Neurons and chains of neurons that conduct impulses away from the central nervous system, usually to muscles, are called efferent or motor-neurons, and those that conduct toward the central nervous system are called afferent or sensory. A nerve can be thought of as a bundle of axons from a number of individual neurons. Nerves may be composed exclusively of axons that are sensory; they may be essentially motor, or they may be both motor and sensory (mixed nerves).

## The Brain

The brain is probably best studied through its embryological development. In its earliest stages, the brain consists of three hollow brain vesicles—the

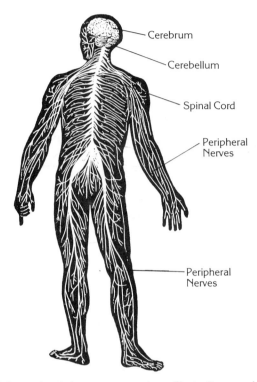

Cerebrum

Cerebellum

Spinal Cord

Peripheral
Nerves

Peripheral
Nerves

**Figure 3.31**   Schematic of the nervous system. Illustrations such as this one are based on a woodcut by Andreas Vesalius, an early 16th century anatomist (and artist) said to be the founder of modern anatomy.

forebrain, midbrain, and hindbrain. With continued growth, the structures of the brain become increasingly elaborate, and the three primary brain vesicles are divided further, as shown in Figure 3.32.

## Forebrain and Its Function

The forebrain (cerebrum) is by far the largest part of the human brain, consisting of two fairly symmetrical cerebral hemispheres, the basal nuclei, and the center for olfaction. The outermost few millimeters of each hemisphere (the cortex) are characterized by cell bodies that appear dark in color and are called gray matter. Deep within the substance of each hemisphere are aggregates or clusters of nerve cell bodies (also gray matter) that collectively are called the basal nuclei (or ganglia). These structures play an important role in coordination of motor functions. The remainder of each hemisphere consists mostly of nerve tracts, which are extensions of the cortical gray matter. These tracts appear light in color, because of a fatty deposit around them, and are called collectively white matter. Some of these

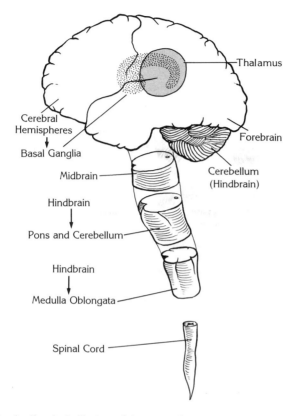

**Figure 3.32** An "exploded" view of the central nervous system showing its major divisions, which are derivatives of the three primary brain vesicles.

fibers course (a) from the cortex downward (projection fibers), connecting the cerebrum with other parts of the brain and spinal cord; (b) from the front backward (association fibers, connecting the various parts of the cerebrum on the same side; and (c) from one side of the brain to the other (commissural fibers), connecting one cerebral hemisphere with the other. The surfaces of the cerebrum have numerous ridges and furrows of varying depth. Deep furrows are called fissures, the shallow ones sulci; the ridges between them are called gyri (gyrus, singular), or convolutions. Each hemisphere is divided into lobes named after the bones of the skull that cover them. Two important landmarks, the central sulcus and lateral sulcus (or fissure) facilitate the division (see Figure 3.33).

Vertebrate nervous systems are hollow and expand into ventricles in each cerebral hemisphere. Cerebrospinal fluid, a clear liquid, circulates through the cavity system of the central nervous system, and obstructions to its circulation (hydrocephaly) can lead to brain damage, mental retardation, and death.

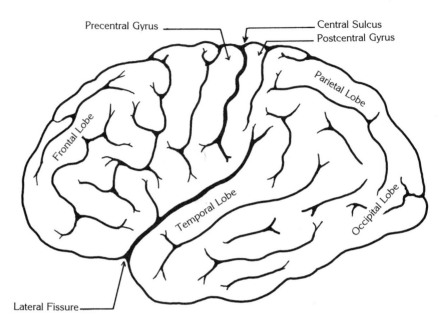

**Figure 3.33** A schematic of a left cerebral hemisphere showing the major landmarks and lobes

The cerebral functions, shown in Figure 3.34, are in part speculative, but some, such as sensory and motor, are well documented. It is mostly by virtue of the development of the cerebral cortex and association, projection, and commissural tracts that we are capable of that higher-order behavior—reason, intelligence, memory, interpretation of sensation (correlation), and the important speech and language—that makes us human. In addition to integrating and instigating voluntary motor behavior, the cerebrum places us in strong control of a lot of behavior that might otherwise be automatic or reflexive. Breathing behavior during speech is an example. Consciousness and the ability to profit or learn from experiences (memory) are attributed largely to the cerebrum. The exact changes in the incomprehensibly complex chain of neural events that might occur for the most simple speech act (saying hello) are largely unknown, however, and to even speculate staggers the imagination.

One important region, just in front of the central sulcus, is the somatic motor area. Here, the motor gestures that account for all of our voluntary movements arise. Notice in Figure 3.34 that the body is represented in an inverted manner so the region that controls the speech mechanism is at the lower limits of the motor area. The motor cortex is a highly specialized region of the brain—every site can be associated with some specific part of the

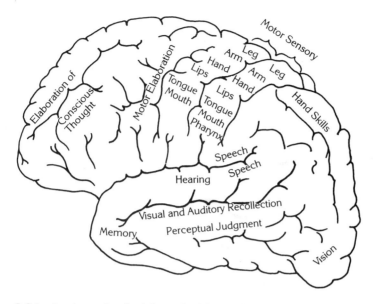

**Figure 3.34** A schematic of a left cerebral hemisphere showing areas associated with cerebral functions

body. The right motor cortex supplies motor nerve impulses to the left half of the body. Just behind the central sulcus lies the primary somatic (body) sensory area, and its "map" is similar to that for the motor cortex. The left somatic sensory area receives sensations from the right side of the body.

The motor impulses generated at the cortical level are relatively crude, but they become integrated and coordinated as they pass through the depths of the brain over the motor pathways. The principal structures for motor integration, responsible for smooth, coordinated movements, are the basal ganglia (structures deep within the cerebrum) and the cerebellum (little brain). Disorders of the basal ganglia result in rigidity; jerky and purposeless movements (chorea); slow, writhing, snakelike movements (athetosis); and sudden flailing of one (usually) arm. Cerebellar disorders result in awkwardness in gait, tendency to fall over, poor coordination of intentional movements (ataxia), a loss of tendon reflex, muscular weakness, intention tremors, and jerky eye movements (nystagmus).

In the mid-1800s, Paul Broca discovered that damage to a well-defined area of the cerebral cortex leads to a speech disorder called **aphasia.** This region, shown in Figure 3.35, is located on the side of the frontal lobe, adjacent to the part of the motor cortex that supplies the structures responsible for speech production. As a consequence, damage (stroke) to Broca's area often is accompanied by a partial (or total) paralysis of the tongue, face, jaw, and larynx. Broca made a second major discovery—

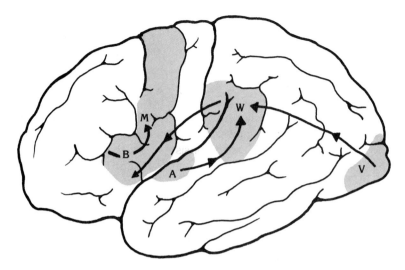

**Figure 3.35** The left cerebral hemisphere showing areas of specialization for speech production. They include the auditory area (A), Broca's area (B), the motor cortex (M), the visual cortex (V), and Wernicke's area (W). For verbal responses to visual or auditory stimuli, some representation of the response is thought to be transmitted from Wernicke's area (where speech and visual perception are integrated) to Broca's area. From Broca's area a sequential program is transmitted to the motor cortex, where commands to the speech musculature are initiated. Any interruption in this chain can lead to some form of aphasia.

damage to Broca's area on the left side (in 90% of the people) leads to aphasia, while damage to the same area on the right side of the brain does not. This has led to the concept of cerebral dominance.

During this same period, Karl Wernicke found that damage to a region in the temporal lobe and also on the left side leads to a disruption of speech, but of a different nature than Broca's aphasia. In Broca's aphasia, speech is labored and slow, and articulation is imprecise, similar to the speech of someone who has had too much to drink. The speech may make sense to a listener, but it may be grammatically incorrect. In Wernicke's aphasia, the speech may sound normal but suffers in its semantics (in other words, it may not make sense). In addition, Wernicke's aphasia may disrupt one's ability to comprehend a spoken word, and it impairs reading and writing ability.

Aphasia, one of the consequences of a stroke, is an extremely complex disorder. Neural tissue, once destroyed by a lack of oxygen, cannot regenerate, but the functions of the damaged areas of the brain can sometimes be at least partially assumed by other areas. To a certain extent, the consequences of a stroke are selective. Children under 8, for example, often make excellent recoveries, as do left-handed individuals.

The right and left primary motor and sensory areas have almost identical functions. The right hemisphere serves the left side of the body, and the left hemisphere serves the right side. Linguistic competence depends primarily on the integrity of the left hemisphere. The contributions of the right hemisphere are associated with more abstract competencies, such as perception of musical melodies, the perception and analysis of nonverbal visual patterns, and abstractions. The right hemisphere does have some rudimentary linguistic ability, however.

The remainder of the forebrain consists of the **thalamus,** a walnut-size structure located just above the midbrain. Although it is not completely understood, we do know that the thalamus receives sensory impulses from all parts of the body (except for olfactory stimuli). It also receives impulses from the cerebellum, cerebral cortex, and structures such as the basal nuclei, which are located adjacent to it. The thalamus functions in an association role, as a synthesizer and relay center and as a sensory integrating center. It regulates water balance in the body, sleep and consciousness, body temperature, and food intake.

*The* thalamus *is supposed to tell us when we have had enough to eat, a reflexive function that we seem to have little difficulty overriding at the cortical level.*

## Midbrain

The midbrain (often called the mesencephalon) consists of paired, short thick stalks (cerebral peduncles) made up of descending and ascending fiber tracts. They connect the cerebrum with the hindbrain and with the spinal cord. The midbrain also contains (in the dorsal region) important visual and auditory correlation centers, in addition to centers for motor coordination. Nerves that supply the eyes and face also originate in the midbrain.

## Hindbrain

The hindbrain consists of the cerebellum, the pons, and the medulla oblongata. The cerebellum (little brain) consists of two richly furrowed hemispheres that are joined together by a central portion, the vermis. Three pairs of cerebellar stalks connect the cerebellum with other parts of the brain. The cerebellum can be thought of as an elaborate integrating and coordinating center. Impulses from the motor center in the cerebrum, from the vestibular apparatus, and from our voluntary muscles enter the cerebellum, while outgoing impulses are relayed to the motor centers of the cerebrum, down the spinal cord, and finally to our muscles. The cerebellum helps maintain muscle tone, posture, and equilibrium, as well as muscle coordination. Injury may result in difficulty in walking, producing coordinated voluntary movements, and speaking due to a lack of coordination of the muscles of the articulators. In spite of its importance, the activities and contributions of the cerebellum never enter into our consciousness.

*The* vestibular apparatus *are organs in the inner ear which produce the sense of equilibrium, movement, and body position. See chapter 10.*

*Injury to the cerebellum can be caused by strokes; for the effects on speech, see chapter 14.*

The pons is located in front of the cerebellum, between the midbrain and the medulla oblongata. It consists of large numbers of transverse white fibers, which join the two halves of the cerebellum, and longitudinal white fibers, which link the medulla oblongata with the cerebrum. Interspersed between the white fibers is gray matter. As its name implies, the pons functions as a bridge, but it also contains the nuclei of some important cranial nerves, as well as a center for regulating breathing.

The medulla oblongata is continuous with the spinal cord, and all the ascending and descending nerve tracts of the spinal cord are found in it. Many of these tracts cross from one side to the other in the medulla. Descending motor tracts, for example, cross at the medulla, so that impulses generated on the left side of the cerebrum stimulate muscles on the right side of the body. A number of nuclei for cranial nerves are contained in the medulla, many of them important for speech production. The medulla oblongata serves as a conduction pathway between the spinal cord and the brain. It also contains centers for regulating heartbeat, dilatation and contraction of the blood vessels, and respiration, as well as reflexive centers.

## Cranial Nerves

*See Figure 3.36.*    Twelve pairs of cranial nerves emerge from the base of the brain. They are numbered according to the order in which they emerge from the brain, and are named primarily according to distribution and function. The cranial nerves important for control of the speech mechanism have their nuclei (of origin for motor nerves, of termination for sensory nerves) in the midbrain and hindbrain. Thus, damage to the structures of the midbrain and to the pons and medulla oblongata can result in specific disorders of function of the speech mechanism. Some cranial nerves are sensory, some motor, and some are mixed. Cranial nerve II, the optic, carries visual information to the occipital lobe of the cerebrum, while nerves III, IV, and VI are motor nerves that supply the muscles of the eye. Cranial nerve V is primarily the sensory nerve for the entire face, including the teeth and the eyes. This same nerve also carries motor fibers, however, that supply the muscles of the mandible and the soft palate. Nerve VII, the facial, is a mixed nerve, and its sensory fibers serve the soft palate and part of the tongue. The motor fibers supply the side of the face and the muscles of facial expression.

The important cranial nerve VIII, the acoustic nerve, is sensory and is responsible for hearing and our sense of balance. Cranial nerve IX, the glossopharyngeal, carries motor and sensory fibers that serve the tongue and pharynx. The vagus nerve, cranial nerve X, is so named because of its wandering course through the trunk of the body. It carries sensory and motor fibers that supply the larynx. The spinal accessory nerve (XI) is a motor nerve that supplies the muscles of the soft palate and muscles of the upper neck region. The hypoglossal nerve (cranial nerve XII) is an important nerve that

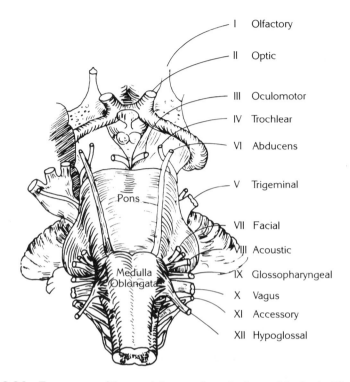

| | |
|---|---|
| I | Olfactory |
| II | Optic |
| III | Oculomotor |
| IV | Trochlear |
| VI | Abducens |
| V | Trigeminal |
| VII | Facial |
| VIII | Acoustic |
| IX | Glossopharyngeal |
| X | Vagus |
| XI | Accessory |
| XII | Hypoglossal |

**Figure 3.36**  Emergence of the cranial nerves from the base of the brain. The nerves are numbered from front to back, from I to XII, in accordance with the order in which they emerge.

supplies the musculature of the tongue. Cranial nerve functions are summarized in the illustration of Figure 3.37.

Highly specialized structures known as receptors are located in the skin and in muscle tissues and their tendons. When stimulated by touch, or by being stretched or compressed, these receptors initiate a train of neural impulses that are conveyed by sensory neurons to the central nervous system and ultimately to the cerebellum and cerebrum. It is by means of this feedback, much of it unconscious, that our nervous system learns when a muscle contraction is taking place, or when the contraction has provided us with the proper and adequate movement. Sensory feedback is a crucial link in the speech chain. Many of us have had the unpleasant experience of trying to talk with a numb face after a visit to a dentist.

## Spinal Cord and Nerves

The spinal cord extends from the medulla oblongata above to the level of the second lumbar vertebra below, and is composed of both gray and white

*See Figure 3.38.*

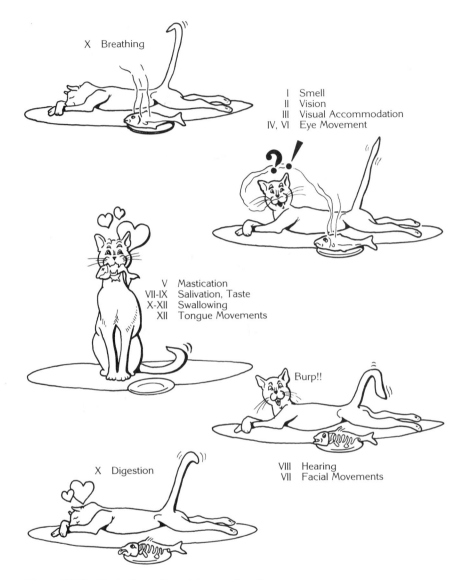

**Figure 3.37** Illustration of cranial nerve functions.

matter. The gray matter is located in the central region of the cord. When seen in cross-section, it resembles the letter H, or a butterfly. On each side of the midline, the gray matter is divided into ventral and dorsal columns or horns. The ventral column contains the cell bodies of the motor fibers of the spinal nerves, while the dorsal column contains cell bodies from which sensory fibers ascend to higher levels of the cord and to the brain. Sensory

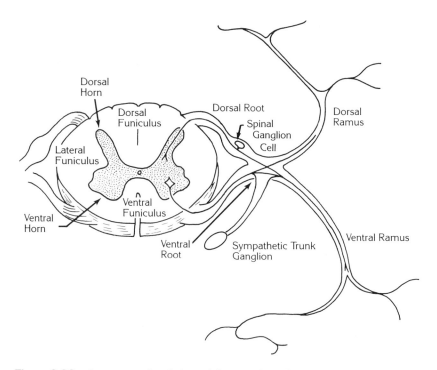

**Figure 3.38**  A cross-sectional view of the spinal cord.

fibers from the spinal ganglia enter the spinal cord and synapse with the dorsal horn neurons. Thus, any spinal nerve contains body sensory and motor fibers. Gray matter of the spinal cord also contains a large number of communicating neurons (internuncial) that transmit neural impulses up and down the cord, from one side to the other, and from the dorsal to ventral roots of the spinal nerves. The spinal cord can be thought of as a great conducting pathway to and from the brain, in addition to serving as an important reflex network for postural muscles and the limbs.

Even from this brief introduction, it becomes apparent that our language and speech production functions are utterly dependent on the integrity of the nervous system. Neural tissue is incapable of repairing itself. We are born with our full complement of an estimated 100 billion nerve cells, and although some cells die in the aging process, most cells have the same life span as their host. Damage by trauma, drug abuse, or deprivation of oxygen can result in global brain damage or comparatively selective damage. The functions normally assumed by brain tissue may or may not be compensated for by adjacent tissue. This is why the process of "reeducating" the central nervous system can be so important.

## CONCLUSION

In the process of acquiring language and the rules for grammar and syntax, a large amount of information is somehow stored in the cerebral cortex. It is information we can retrieve at will, as often as we choose, and it doesn't get used up or even wear out. Yet a tiny blood vessel can burst in the brain and the information is gone. We can automatically assemble meaningful thoughts, or we may search for words. Recall, judgment, coding, and decoding take place; almost instantly, these thoughts emerge as spoken words. And we know so little about the way in which cortical-level thought processes take place, and how they lead to sequential neural commands to the cranial and spinal nerves and then to muscles.

The phone rings, you pick it up and say hello. An in-depth explanation (on our part) of the chain of events between a sound pressure pattern entering our ear canal and a sound pressure pattern (the word *hello*) leaving our mouths, is in fact, little more than scratching the surface.

We have seen how our respiratory muscles contract and relax voluntarily to develop a reservoir of pressurized air. To say hello, the vocal folds impede outward air flow so a glottal fricative is produced. An instant later, the vocal folds move more completely toward the midline and they begin to vibrate, while simultaneously our tongue, lips, and soft palate assume the position required for production of the vowel /ɛ/. Also at the same time, the speech sounds reach our own ears as part of an integrated network of feedback channels. In the meantime, our muscles, tendons, and joints are transmitting neural impulses back to the central nervous system to help complete the feedback information. With the vocal folds still vibrating and even while the /ɛ/ is being produced, the articulators move into position for the /l/, and finally, still vibrating, they move to the position for the vowel /o/.

When stated this way, it all seems so simple to say hello—and it is for most of us. For some people, however, something in this complex chain goes wrong. A speech-language pathologist may be called on to correct the problem.

We have briefly examined the anatomical and physiological bases for speech production. But no matter how exhaustive our pursuit might be, ultimately each of us has to try to understand the whole picture. There is anatomical continuity between the tongue, hyoid bone, larynx, pharynx, soft palate, and even the lips. We can never discount what we know of the functional relationships between these structures, but we should also be aware that much has yet to be learned about the coordination of speech production.

The highly integrated and complex structures of speech production comprise a system we are just beginning to understand and fully appreciate. It is a delicately balanced, sensitive, and fragile system on one hand, resistant to disruption on the other, largely due to the human potential to compensate, a potential most of us will never put to use.

Finally, because of individual variability, our anatomical and physiological descriptions can be only representative and general in nature—it is vitally important that our constructs about structure and function never become inflexible and stereotyped.

## STUDY QUESTIONS

1. Describe the mechanisms and processes involved in one respiratory cycle (inhalation–exhalation).
2. What are the differences between quiet breathing and speech breathing?
3. Describe the laryngeal muscles and processes involved in forced inhalation before speaking.
4. Using Figures 3.15 and 3.16, describe a single cycle of vocal fold vibration as a function of time in your own words.
5. Describe how the pitch and loudness of voice are changed.
6. List the structures involved in articulation.
7. How do vowels and consonants differ?
8. List the areas of the brain involved in speech and language production and describe the primary function of each.
9. List each cranial nerve and describe its relationship to interpreting and producing speech and language.

## SELECTED READINGS

Hardcastle, W. J. (1976). *Physiology of speech production.* London: Academic Press.

Minifie, F., Hixon, T., & Williams, F. (Eds.). (1973). *Normal aspects of speech, hearing, and language.* Englewood Cliffs, NJ: Prentice-Hall.

Tarkhan, A. (1936). Ein experimenteller Beitrag zur Kenntnis der Proprioceptiven Innervation der Zunge. *Zeitschrift für Anatomie und Entwicklungsgeschichte, 105,* 349–358.

Zemlin, W. R. (1988). *Speech and hearing science: Anatomy and physiology* (3rd ed.). Englewood Cliffs, NJ: Prentice-Hall.

---

# Differences and Disorders
# of Language

# CHAPTER FOUR

# Language and Communication Differences

## ORLANDO L. TAYLOR

**MYTHS AND REALITIES**

- *Myth:* Race and culture are synonymous.

- *Reality:* Many cultures are represented within the same racial group. For example, French Cajuns in Louisiana and Irish Americans in Boston belong to the same racial group, i.e., Caucasians, but they are members of different cultural groups.

- *Myth:* A seven-year-old black male from a working class, inner city environment deletes the *-s* morpheme for plurality and possession. This indicates that he probably has a language disorder.

- *Reality:* The *-s* morpheme deletion for plurality and possession are features of Black English Vernacular. The child is probably within the realm of normalcy for his speech community.

- *Myth:* A fifteen-year-old black female from suburban Cleveland omits some final consonants and reduces final consonant clusters. She should not be considered for therapy since these are features of Black English Vernacular.

- *Reality:* After consideration of the child's speech community, it is not likely that Black English Vernacular features are a part of her middle income, highly educated environment. A possible articulation disorder or hearing loss should be considered.
- *Myth:* All dialects are nonstandard English.
- *Reality:* Several dialects of Standard English exist in the United States and are identified with regional, racial, ethnic, or language groups. Examples are Southern Standard English and Black Standard English.
- *Myth:* During classroom storytime, a ten-year-old working class black child relates the experiences of her summer vacation. The events of her story seem to have no temporal sequencing or central theme. Instead, the story is marked by loose organization that shifts across several different themes and times during the summer. Obviously, this student presents a language disorder and possible cognitive deficiency because her story is incongruent with standard discourse norms for the child's age.
- *Reality:* The student presents a topic-associating narrative style that is common among many working class black children. Narrative styles are often culture-specific. The topic-associating style is different from the topic-centered style, which is used by the middle class and is the expected narrative style within the schools. It is a difference, not a disorder of discourse.

THE above statements are examples of common dilemmas faced by speech-language pathologists in today's increasingly multicultural society. In view of the above myths and realities, what would be your decision regarding the disposition of the student described in the following clinical scenario?

*James M. is a 7-year-old working-class black male who attends a multiracial elementary school in Prince Georges County, Maryland, a suburb of Washington, D.C. James was referred for assessment by his teacher, a black female, who reported that he was inattentive, disruptive, and receiving failing grades in reading and language arts. Most of the students in James's class come from middle-class families, both black and white.*

*James was seen by the school psychologist, who administered the WISC-R test of intelligence, on which James scored in the 40th percentile. His mother reports that James is one of six children within the home.*

*James moved to Maryland from Mayfield, North Carolina, at age 5. He is reported to have had a normal childbirth and normal development. His mother, a single, working parent, reports that she has little time to read to James or to assist him with his assignments.*

*James was given the Peabody Picture Vocabulary Test and the Northwestern Syntax Screening Test. Test scores revealed that James possessed a disorder of expressive language. Many working-class black children at the school demonstrate similar language behavior.*

Communication is generally thought to be disordered when it deviates from the community standards sufficiently enough that it (a) interferes with the transmission of messages, (b) stands out as being unusually different, or (c) produces negative feelings within the communicator. Central to this is the idea that a communication disorder can only be determined in the context of a community, more specifically a **speech community.** A speech community is any group of people who routinely and frequently use a shared language to interact with each other (Gumperz & Hymes, 1972; Hymes, 1974). An accurate understanding of what constitutes a communication disorder requires an understanding of the distinction between a *communication difference* and a *communication disorder.*

In a specific geographical area or governmental jurisdiction—a city, state, or nation, for example—there might be several speech communities, although a common national language (English, for instance) is spoken. Governmental boundaries and the boundaries of speech communities need not be isomorphic. From community to community, use of one or all of the major structural or functional components of a given language—i.e., phonology, morphology, syntax, semantics, discourse, pragmatics, conversational postulates, etc.—might differ in varying degrees. These varieties of the national language are called **dialects** of that language. Despite their differences, speakers of varying dialects of a national language can generally communicate across speech communities. For example, New Englanders can obviously converse with Southerners.

Because of the intrinsic differences among the dialects of a language, speakers of certain dialects—usually ones thought by school personnel as being nonprestigious or nonstandard—are often mistakenly perceived as having a communication disorder. It is incorrect to presume that every person who speaks a dialect different from one's own, or even different from the school's educated standard, has a communication disorder, even if that dialect results in breakdowns of communication, excessive audience attention, or (because of ridicule) emotional problems for the speaker. The speech-language pathologist must know the differences between *differences* and *disorders* to accurately distinguish between individuals who need speech-language pathology services from those who may need instruction in a second dialect (or language). In determining the communication needs of an individual, several factors must be considered, including communication behavior, communication context, and the culture from which communication emanates. Moreover, a descriptive rather than a prescriptive posture should be assumed in determining these needs.

To accurately evaluate a person's communicative behavior, it is essential to understand some basic concepts pertaining to communication, language, and culture, as well as the characteristics of the dialects of American English. The same type of information can also enhance the quality of therapeutic and educational services provided to individuals with communication needs.

The American Speech-Language-Hearing Association has recognized the importance for speech-language pathologists to understand the nature of social dialects. In a 1983 position paper, ASHA asserted that no dialect of English is a disorder or a pathologic form of speech or language. ASHA supports the view that professionals must be able to distinguish between legitimate linguistic differences and speech-language disorders. Finally, ASHA suggests that two major professional competencies are needed to make these distinctions: (a) knowledge of the rules of a particular speaker's dialect, and (b) knowledge of nondiscriminatory assessment procedures.

# BASIC CONCEPTS RELATED TO CULTURE AND LANGUAGE

## Culture

**Culture** may be defined as the set of values, perceptions, beliefs, institutions, technologies, and survival systems used by members of a specified group to ensure the acquisition and perpetuation of what *they* consider to be a high quality of life. Culture is arbitrary and changeable. Cultures overlap among one another and have internal variations. In addition, culture is learned and exists at different levels of conscious awareness. Culture should not be confused with race, nationality, religion, language, or socioeconomic status, although these groups may demonstrate a common subset of identifiable cultural behaviors. The fact is that, within any one of these groups, there is enormous internal variation.

In addition to the elements of culture contained in the above definition, Saville-Troike (1978) claims that cultures tend to be characterized by modes of conduct in at least the following areas:

Family structure

Important events in life cycle

Roles of individual members

Rules of interpersonal interactions

Communication and linguistic rules

Rules for decorum and discipline

Religious beliefs

Standards for health and hygiene

Food preferences

Dress and personal appearance

History and traditions

Holidays and celebrations

Value and methods

Education

Perceptions of work and play

Perceptions of time and space

Explanation of natural phenomena

Attitudes toward pets and animals

Artistic and musical values and tastes

Life expectations and aspirations

## Culture, Language, and Communication

No matter how you define it, language is a universal human phenomenon. Some form of language is used by every group known on the planet, regardless of its race, region, education, economic, or technical development. Despite the existence of thousands of languages in the world, they all share a common set of universal rules (Greenberg, 1966). Even their patterns of acquisition are universal in some ways. It is also true that social and cultural factors universally affect the nature and use of language within human groups. The study of social and cultural influences on language structure falls within the domain of **sociolinguistics.** Similarly, the study of language use for communicative purposes, which by definition involves social and cultural considerations, falls within the domain of the **ethnography of communication.** Since the 1960s and early 1970s, with the rise of interest in sociolinguistics and ethnography of communication, authorities have increasingly recognized that disordered communication can only be defined or treated in a cultural context.

## Ethnography of Communication

The theoretical constructs and analytical procedures for examining the interplay between culture and communicative behavior are derived mostly from the field of communication ethnography. The field was defined by Dell Hymes (1966), and takes its fundamental direction from its parent field, ethnography, a branch of anthropology. Its basic orientation is descriptive, and it tends to focus on a particular type of activity, although its analytic procedures are open-ended.

Saville-Troike (1986) writes:

> The ethnography of communication provides a synthesizing focus which concentrates on *the patterning of communicative behavior* as it constitutes one of the subsystems of culture, as it functions within the holistic context of the culture of group, and as it relates to patterns in other component systems. This perspective first and foremost takes *language as a socially situated cultural form,* while at the same time recognizes the necessity to analyze the linguistic code itself and the cognitive processes of its speakers and hearers. To accept a lesser scope for the study of communication is to risk reducing it to triviality and to abandon any possibility of understanding how language actually functions in the lives of individuals and cultural groups. . . . The subject matter of the ethnography of communication is best illustrated by one of its general questions: What does a speaker need to know to communicate appropriately within a particular speech community, and how does he or she acquire this knowledge? Such knowledge, together with whatever skills are needed to make use of it, is termed *communicative competence* (Hymes, 1966). The requisite knowledge includes not only rules for communication (both linguistic and sociolinguistic) and shared rules for interaction, but also the cultural rules and knowledge that are the basis for the context and content of communicative events and interaction processes. A primary aim of this approach is to guide the collection and analysis of descriptive data about the ways in which social meaning is conveyed, constructed, and negotiated.

## Sociolinguistics

The notions of language dialects and standards are central to the understanding of sociolinguistics and its role in the study and treatment of communication disorders. A dialect is a variety of language that has developed through a complex interplay of historical, social, political, educational, and linguistic forces. In the technical sense, the term *dialect* is never used negatively, as is frequently the case with the lay public. A dialect should not be considered an inferior variety of a language, merely a variety. In this context, *all dialects are considered to be linguistically legitimate and valid.* No dialect is intrinsically a better way of speaking the language than any other dialect.

Despite the linguistic legitimacy of all dialects, the various dialects of a language tend to assume different social, economic, political, utilitarian, or educational value within a given society. Standard dialects are those spoken by politically, socially, economically, and educationally powerful and prestigious people. It is not unusual for speakers of standard dialects to have negative attitudes toward nonstandard dialects and their speakers. These standard dialects become the de facto official versions of the national language, and are used in business, education, and mass media. There may be several standard dialects within a national language.

In the United States, several dialects of Standard English do, in fact, exist. Almost all of these varieties are identified with specific regions of the country or with certain racial, ethnic, or language groups. While the dialects of Standard English (or General American English) contain differences in phonology, semantics, discourse, conversational postulates, and pragmatics (particularly in informal situations), these dialects share a common set of grammatical rules. It is, indeed, in syntax and morphology that social attitudes regarding dialect prestige are strongest (Wolfram, 1970).

Within the dialects of a language, there may be structural, stylistic, or social variations. For example, a vernacular or colloquial variation may be used in informal, casual, or intimate situations, but not in writing or in school. Variations in language use may occur as a function of the social situation in which communication occurs or the speech community of the participants. Thus, a specific linguistic structure may have various functions or values depending on the intent of the speaker. For instance, an interrogative sentence such as *Do you have the time?* is not always intended as a question, but may also be used to request the time or to command someone to provide you with the time. The selection of a specific linguistic structure, then, depends on the speaker's perception of the social situation as well as the communication intention. Finally, certain sociolinguistic variables, such as the speaker, listener, audience, topic, or setting, identify the nonlinguistic dimensions of the social context that may influence the selection of a particular language variety.

Seven major factors typically influence language behavior and acquisition:

1. Race and ethnicity
2. Social class, education, and occupation
3. Region
4. Gender
5. Situation or context
6. Peer group association or identification
7. First language community or culture

## Race and Ethnicity

Racial and ethnic influences on language and communication are neither biological nor genetic in nature. They are related to the cultural attitudes and values associated with a particular racial or ethnic group, and the group's linguistic history. Some linguistic forms and communicative behaviors are so characteristic of certain racial or ethnic groups that, when they are used, they immediately mark the speaker as either being from that group or as having had a great deal of interaction with the group.

One must be careful, however, not to assume that racial or ethnic group membership automatically predicts language behavior or prevents an individual from using language codes usually associated with other groups. To do so would be prejudicial stereotyping. In fact, many people learn the structural and functional rules of the linguistic and communicative systems of several racial and ethnic groups. Such persons are considered *bilingual* if two languages are involved, or *bidialectal* if two dialects are involved.

## Social Class, Education, and Occupation

In addition to correlating with race and ethnicity, linguistic behavior tends to reflect social class, education, and occupation. In some societies, it is considered highly inappropriate for members of the servant classes to speak the language of the aristocracy (Edwards, 1976). Even in these societies, however, it is not unusual for language behavior to be further restricted by factors such as segregation or geographical isolation. In addition to these factors, educational achievement and occupation may have a major role in determining language function (Hollingshead, 1965).

Researchers have attributed many dimensions of language variation to a number of social class influences. Chief among such factors are (a) home environment, (b) child-rearing practices, (c) family interaction patterns, and (d) travel and experience.

Bernstein (1971) has been at the forefront of those scholars who claim that social class determines a person's access to certain communication codes. He suggests that lower-class groups use a more restricted, context-dependent code with particularistic meanings and that the upper classes use a more elaborated, context-independent code with universalistic meanings. The argument against Bernstein's theory is that it has a built-in bias toward middle-class communication because it implicitly assumes that the former is the standard for determining "normalcy." This type of bias is reflected in the use of such measures as mean length of utterance (MLU), which is often used to assess language development of lower-class children using a middle-class criterion.

## Region

Regional dialects are closely tied to social dialects, but are generally defined by geographic boundaries. There are at least 10 regional dialects recognized in the contiguous United States, including Southern, Eastern New England, Western Pennsylvania, Appalachian, Central Midland, Middle Atlantic, and New York City (Nist, 1966). Figure 4.1 shows a map delineating these dialect regions. Table 4.1 on pages 142–143 contains some examples from three of

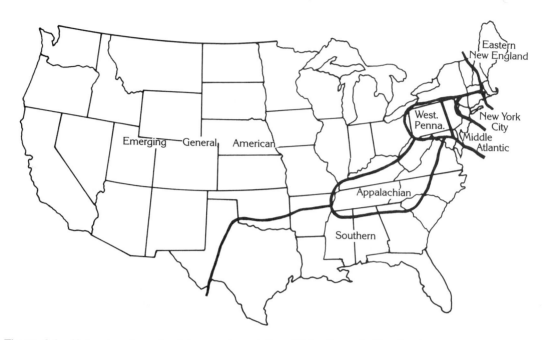

**Figure 4.1**  Major American English speech varieties. *(Note: From* A Structural History of English *(p. 371) by J. Nist, 1966, New York: St. Martin's Press. Reprinted by permission.)*

the more stigmatized regional dialects in the United States—Southern English, Southern White Nonstandard English, and Appalachian English.

The distribution of linguistic forms as a function of geography is typically related to factors such as (a) geographical features (climate, topography, water supply), (b) trade routes, (c) cultural and ethnic backgrounds of settlers, (d) religion, and (e) power relationships in the region (Wardhaugh, 1976).

In general, regional dialects are marked by specific linguistic patterns. Few native-born Americans, for example, would have difficulty recognizing a stereotyped Appalachian, New York City, or Boston dialect. The speech of people from these geographical regions is usually identifiable by a set of specific phonological features; word choices; idioms; or characteristic syntactic, prosodic, or pragmatic devices. These markings should not be confused with those associated with various registers of the language that address different styles (for example, formal or informal) of communication within a given linguistic system.

A particular speaker may choose to use a regional dialect for a variety of reasons, including local pride, local activities, or a deliberate rejection of wider affiliations. Other people may give up regionalisms because of their occupational, political, or social aspirations. Some regional dialects are viewed negatively by outsiders or by members of the upper class from the same region. Some speakers compromise by using regional dialects locally or in intimate situations, and more nonregionalized dialects when they are away from home or in formal situations. Since regional standards within a given language tend to be close to the general standard, many speakers do not find it necessary to abandon their regional dialects. Excellent discussions of several regional dialects may be found in Fasold (1984).

## Gender

Few would claim that it is difficult to distinguish between male and female speakers. We usually identify gender by pitch and intonation differences. The male voice is generally thought to be lower than the female voice because males have longer, thicker vocal cords. There may be reason to believe, however, that social programming greatly influences men to use "masculine" voices. Women are also influenced by social definitions of voice usage. Wardhaugh (1976) argues, for instance, that women typically vary their intonation patterns more extensively than men to signal endearment, excitement, "mothering," pleasure, and so on. The key point to keep in mind when discussing gender and voice usage is that culture may be at least as important as biology in determining voice use. One need only observe different voice patterns of men (or women) in various cultures around the world, even when race is kept constant.

Vocabulary and pragmatics may be even greater markers of gender than voice. For instance, in the United States there are certain taboo words (for example, profanity) and topics (such as sexually oriented jokes) that are often considered inappropriate for women to use in middle-class mixed company. These same words and topics, when used among working-class men, may be considered signs of masculinity and toughness. Trudgill (1974) even notes that men tend to use more nonstandard forms than women, as women tend to place more value on the status of standard language usage.

Wardhaugh (1976) makes the following explicit observations concerning the difference between the "characteristic language uses of men and women":

> Women tend to be more precise and "careful" in speaking: for example, they are more likely than men to pronounce the final -ing forms with a g, to say fighting rather than fightin. In general, they take more "care" in articulation. This behavior accords with other findings that women tend to be less innovative than men in their use of language and to be more conscious of preferred usages. They are also more likely than men to use "appeal tags" such as "isn't it?" or "don't you think?" ... Women use more different names for colors than men: mauve, lavender, turquoise, lilac, and beige are good examples. Men either do not use such color words, or if they

do, tend to use them with great caution. Intensifiers such as *so, such,* and *quite,* as in "He's so cute," "He's such a dear," and "We had a quite marvelous time" comprise a set of words used in a way that most men avoid; emotive adjectives such as *adorable, lovely,* and *divine* are hardly used at all by men. (p. 128)

Lakoff (1975), the author of one of the pioneer works in women's use of language in the United States, has outlined a number of gender-marked linguistic devices in semantics, syntax, and intonation. In addition to the observations already mentioned, Lakoff includes

- Greater use of "weaker" emotional particles—e.g., polite exclamations versus profane expletives
- Greater use of declarative answers with yes/no rising intonations to questions—e.g., (man) "When will dinner be ready?"; (woman) "Oh . . . around six o'clock . . . ?" (with rising intonation)
- Large stock of women's interest lexical items—e.g., *magenta, shirr, dart* (in sewing), etc.
- Greater use of hedging words of various types—e.g., *well, y'know, kinda, sorta,* etc.
- Greater use of the intensive *so*—e.g., "I like him *so* much." versus "I like him *very* much."
- Greater use of Standard English phonology and syntax
- Greater use of hyperpolite forms
- Lesser use of jokes
- Greater use of *italics* in speech, i.e., greater use of calling attention to specific words as if a failure to do so will result in their going unnoticed.

Lakoff makes the case that women—at least white, middle-class women—are taught to be "ladylike" in their speech from childhood. Therefore, such traits as nonassertiveness, uncertainty, politeness, and properness are highly stressed. Likewise, women are relegated to being authorities on the less important issues of the world, at least from the male perspective—e.g., subtleties in color differences, supercorrect grammatical forms, and empty adjectives. Lakoff concludes that women are placed in a "damned if they do and damned if they don't" position because of these gender-marker linguistic expectations. If women fail to perform in accordance with these expectations, they are considered assertive, authoritarian, and masculine. On the other hand, if they do perform in accordance with them, they are seen as being weak and trivial and behaving "just like a woman."

In the Western world, where traditional sex roles are coming under attack, it is likely we will see fewer surface differences between male and female speech in the future. Indeed, many modes of communication previously restricted to men are being used by women without penalty. In viewing male/female differences in language use in the United States, however, it is important to consider cultural and class factors. To date, most of the work on this subject has focused on gender differences among white, middle-class persons. Stanback (1985) is among a growing group of scholars who have begun to pay particular attention to the language of black women.

## Situation or Context

Language may vary according to the situation and context in which it is spoken. Several important situational and contextual variables may influence all dimensions of language behavior, the most important being

Setting

Location

Occasion

Participants

Topic

Purpose

Spatial positions of participants

Speaker's role in two-person interactions

For example, several researchers have identified a special form of address used by parents to children, often called *baby-talk* or *motherese.* They claim that parents, particularly mothers, tend to vary their pitch, intonation patterns, speed, sentence length, structure, and vocabulary to meet the needs of their children. Both Moerk (1974) and Bruner (1978) claim the mother's language gradually becomes more complex as the child's language becomes more complex.

*See Ferguson, 1964; Newport, 1976; Snow, 1972.*

Some researchers have also suggested that children, like adults, vary their speech as a function of the listener (Ervin-Tripp, 1977; Gleason, 1973; Mitchell-Kernan & Kernan, 1977; Shatz & Gelman, 1973). For instance, children may use a more restricted linguistic code when talking to strangers, especially if the strangers belong to an outside group. This point is of extreme importance for the speech-language pathologist who is attempting to obtain a valid linguistic sample from a child.

## Peer Group Association/Identification

It is widely believed that linguistic behavior, particularly during childhood, is under the control of the speech community and the parents. There is also strong research evidence to support the claim that the role of peers, including brothers and sisters, is of equal importance. Thus, a child with strong associations or identification with children from other speech communities might learn forms of language that are different from those of the home community or family. In these cases, the child may use the nonhome language or dialect only for communicating with people outside the home or home community.

Wolfram and Fasold (1974) are among several researchers who stress the importance of peer influence on language during adolescence. They report that adolescents typically learn an "in-group" dialect that is primarily used by their immediate peers. Sometimes peer pressure prevails over parental standards during this period. This point often shows up in parents' complaints that they don't understand their teenage children.

Fordham (1988) has reported that many working-class black high school students feel so strongly about their Black English Vernacular that they resist learning Standard English because they see it as "talking white." Of course, it is an error to perceive Standard English as "white English" since it is merely a way of speaking the English language by individuals within all racial groups who have had successful access to education. Taylor (1983) suggests that certain ethnic subtleties may be retained in speaking Standard English (e.g., prosodic characteristics, rhetorical styles) without losing ethnic identity. Taylor uses Black Standard English to describe ethnically identifiable educated English spoken by many black Americans, for example, Jesse Jackson.

Finally, language is often an indicator of a person's age group. Language patterns of the elderly, for instance, are different in some ways from those of younger adults (Obler & Albert, 1981), which, in turn, vary from those of teenagers, and so on. Violations of linguistic age constraints tend to draw attention to the speaker. Thus, it is not unusual to hear pronouncements like "That boy talks like a man" or "That man sounds like a teenager."

## First Language Community/Culture

People whose native language or culture is different from the official language and culture of a society typically learn the official language but retain distinct vestiges of their first language. These persons are considered bilingual, in that they presumably control parts or all of two languages. In recent years, the term *bidialectal* has been coined to refer to persons who control parts or all of two dialects.

**Code-switching** *is an individual's ability to move effectively from one language or dialect to another, as a function of the social situation. (Gleason, 1973; McCormack & Wurm, 1976).*

Bilingual and bidialectal persons typically code-switch from one language or dialect to another, depending on the social situation (Bell, 1976). In the process of code-switching, the first language may interfere with the use of linguistic structures in the second language. A person of Latino origin who speaks English, for example, might mix English and Spanish words in the same sentence: *May I have coffee con leche?* Other such speakers may make morphological errors, such as deleting the plural or possessive morphemes. Phonology and syntax in the second language may also be affected by the first language. For example, English sounds such as /v/, /ʃ/ and /ɪ/ do not occur in Spanish, and adjectives follow nouns rather than preceding them. The Spanish rules may be followed by Spanish speakers who learn English as a second language.

Social factors such as age, education, and situation influence an individual's efficiency in code-switching. The frequency with which a person hears and interacts within the second language code and the nature of instruction in it also determine a person's skill in using the second language. If a person uses a second language more than a first language, facility in the native language might be lost if it is not reinforced at home. When a whole generation of children in a given culture moves toward usage of a second language as the preferred mode of communication, "death" of the first language is inevitable. Language death is occurring rapidly, for example, for several native American and Eskimo languages in Alaska.

As you can surmise from this discussion of the social and cultural factors that influence language, no one variable operates independently of other variables. The language used during any speech event depends on the simultaneous interaction of many social, cultural, and situational factors. Therefore, no one sample of a person's speech taken from a single situation or from interaction with a single person is likely to be representative of that individual's complete linguistic repertoire. While we may be able to identify a typical speech pattern, that pattern cannot be considered the only speech variety available to that person. The speech-language pathologist must recognize an individual's potential for language variation during both assessment and training.

## DIALECTS OF AMERICAN ENGLISH

As we have mentioned, several varieties of English are spoken in the United States. These variations are caused by several factors, central among which are (a) the languages brought to the country by various cultural groups, that is, speakers of English, Polish, Chinese, Wolof, and so on; (b) the indigenous native American languages spoken in the country; (c) the mix of the various communities and regions where the cultural groups settled; (d) the political and economic power wielded by the various cultures settling in the regions; (e) the migration patterns of the cultural groups within the country; (f) geographical isolation caused by rivers, mountains, and other features, as in the dialects of the Ozark and Appalachian mountains; and (g) self-imposed social isolation or legal segregation. In particular, a cultural group that maintains a strong identity may develop a dialect of English as its children come into contact with Standard English speakers in school. An example is the dialect spoken by Puerto Ricans in New York City.

In many parts of the southern United States, for instance, the original languages spoken included a type of English brought from the southern portion of Great Britain, indigenous native American languages, and a number of languages brought from West Africa, including Wolof, Mende, and Fulani. Political and social power was usually held by the British settlers, and thus their language came to assume power in education and commerce. At the same time, English speakers were probably influenced by the languages spoken by the Africans and native Americans. As a result, a particular type of English emerged in the region, which may be loosely called Southern English. Of course, within the South, there are further regional differences.

Within each speech community, we find other linguistic variations, each of which is influenced by the social variables discussed earlier—age, gender, socioeconomic class, and so on. Again, note that these variables are *not* biological, although certain speech communities coexist with biological (racial) groups, such as the black community in the United States. Recall that the social variables are not mutually exclusive.

Many speakers are knowledgeable about and sensitive to the linguistic expectations of varying audiences and, therefore, are capable of code-switching to different dialects—even dialects that are not indigenous to their speech communities—when the situation dictates. This interaction between structure and function might be an important pragmatic consideration of sociolinguistics generally and dialectologists in particular. For example, an articulate southern black speaker might well use one dialect variety when communicating with working-class blacks **(Black English Vernacular)**, another when communicating with educated blacks **(Standard Black English)**, and still another when communicating with working-class southern whites **(Southern White Nonstandard English)**. This process can work with languages as well as dialects; a teenager might use Standard English with his employer, a vernacular English with his friends, and Chinese with his parents.

There are several excellent descriptions of dialects commonly spoken in the United States available (Fasold, 1984; Peñalosa, 1981; Smitherman, 1978; Wolfram, 1986; Wolfram & Fasold, 1974). Williams and Wolfram (1977) have prepared an excellent summary of most of the research in this area for six English dialects frequently encountered by speech-language pathologists in their professional practice—Standard English, Nonstandard English, Southern White Standard English, Southern White Nonstandard English, Black English, and Appalachian English. We will now look at some of these dialects.

## Black English

Perhaps the most controversial and most frequently written-about dialect of American English is **Black English,** variously referred to as *Black Dialect, Black English Vernacular,* and *Ebonics.* Writings on this subject began to emerge in the sociolinguistic literature in the late 1960s and early 1970s.

Loosely defined as used in much of this research, Black English may be thought of as the linguistic code used by working-class black people, especially for communication in informal situations within working-class black speech communities. Its linguistic features, like those of any other dialect, are explained on the basis of social, cultural, and historical facts, not biological differences. Speakers of Black English are presumed to be knowledgeable in other dialects of English, notably Standard English, as demonstrated by their comprehension of these other dialects.

Black English, like other dialects, is not exclusive of other dialects of English. In fact, linguistic analyses of transcripts of Black English speakers show that the overwhelming majority of their utterances conform to the rules of General American Speech (Loman, 1967).

A selected sample of the major characteristics of Black English, as described by the many writers on the subject, is presented in Table 4.1. Remember, these linguistic variations are *not* errors in the use of English. Instead they are characteristics of linguistic systems with their own rules, which are as complex and valid as those of Standard English. We can actually identify at least 29 linguistic rules of Black English that differ from Standard English (Williams & Wolfram, 1977). Careful review of these 29 linguistic rules shows considerable overlap between Black English and several other dialects, notably Southern English and Southern White Nonstandard English. Because of this overlap, we need to be careful not to assume that a particular linguistic feature used by a black speaker is a feature of Black English. Because blacks in the United States have a strong historical link with the southern states, it is not surprising that there appears to be considerable overlap between Black English and the numerous dialects spoken in the South.

Several theories have been advanced to explain the development of Black English. One of the most popular of these theories is the *creolist theory*. Briefly stated, the creolist position holds that Black English is a complex hybrid involving several African languages and four main European languages—Portuguese, Dutch, French, and English. These hybrids are believed to have developed in Africa, as well as on American plantations, in the form of pidgins and creoles.

According to DeCamp (1971), pidgin languages develop when peoples speaking different languages come in contact with each other and have a need to find a common language, usually for commerce. Typically, a pidgin is developed by speakers of a nondominant group who are in direct contact with a dominant group that speaks another language. Good examples include the pidgins still used by many Chinese and Hawaiians. At the outset of its development, a pidgin language may be informal, consisting of single words, a simplified grammar, and many gestures.

Over time, pidgin languages may become more formal, in that vocabulary items selected primarily from the dominant language are embedded into a phonological and grammatical system derived from the nondominant language. When this happens and the pidgin is accepted as a native language,

**Table 4.1** Selected Phonological and Grammatical Characteristics of Black English (B), Southern English (S), Southern White Nonstandard English (SWNS), and Appalachian English (A)

| Features | Descriptions | Examples | B | S | SWNS | A |
|---|---|---|---|---|---|---|
| Consonant cluster reduction (general) | Deletion of second of two consonants in word final position belonging to same base word | tes (test) | X | | X | |
| | Deletion of past tense (- ed) morpheme from a base word, resulting in a consonant cluster that is subsequently reduced | rub (rubbed) | X | | X | |
| | Plural formations of reduced consonant cluster assume phonetic representations of sibilants and affricatives | desses (desks) | X | | X | |
| /ϴ/ phoneme | /f/ for /ϴ/ between vowels and in word final position | nofin (nothing) Ruf (Ruth) | X | | | |
| /ð/ phoneme | /d/ for /ð/ in word initial position | dis (this) | X | | | |
| | /v/ for /ð/ between vowels and in word final positions | bavin (bathing) bave (bathe) | X | | | |
| Vowel nasalization | No contrast between vowels /I/ and /ɛ/ before nasals | pin (pin, pen) | | X | | X |
| The /r/ and /l/ phonemes | Deletion preceding a consonant | ba: game (ball game) | X | X | | |

the language is referred to as **creole.** As stated earlier, "death" of the first language often occurs at this point. Eventually, as the speakers of creole languages become more assimilated into the dominant culture, creole languages tend to move toward the standard language through an intermediate stage referred to as *decreolization.*

There are some problems with the creole theory of Black English. For instance, it tends to view the language as being European-based rather than African-based. Despite its problems, however, the creolist explanation of Black English at least provides a historical orientation for the analysis and understanding of Black American speech.

| Features | Descriptions | Examples | B | S | SWNS | A |
|---|---|---|---|---|---|---|
| Future tense forms | Use of *gonna* | She gonna go. (She is going to go.) | X | | X | |
| | *Gonna* reduced to 'ngna, 'mana, 'mon and 'ma | I'ngma go. I'mana go. I'mon go. I'ma go. (I am going to go.) | X | | | |
| Double modals | Co-occurrence of se-lected modals such as *might, could, should* | I might coulda done it. (It is possible that I could have done it.) | X | | X | X |
| Intensifying adverbs | Use of intensifiers, i.e., *right, plumb,* to refer to completeness | right large (very large) | X | | X | X |
| Negation | *Ain't* for *have/has, am/are, didn't* | He ain't go home. (He didn't go home.) | X | | | |
| Relative clauses | Deletion of relative pro-nouns | That's the dog bit me. (That's the dog that bit me.) | X | | X | X |
| Questions | Same interrogative form for direct and in-direct questions | I wonder was she walking? (I wonder if she was walking.) | X | | X | X |

*Note:* From *Social Dialects: Differences vs. Disorders* by R. Williams and W. Wolfram, 1977, Washington, D.C.: American Speech and Hearing Association. Adapted by permission.

Several researchers dispute the validity of the concept of Black English on other grounds. Some of their objections are based on the argument that it is impossible to assume that a single variety of speech accurately describes a population as culturally and geographically diverse as American blacks. Still others reject the notion of Black English on the grounds that it only describes the speech of the working class, while implicitly denying the existence of more educated forms of speech spoken by the black middle class. Finally, writers such as Smitherman (1978, 1988), Labov (1972), and Kochman (1971, 1981) argue that focus on the study of the structure of language, rather than on use of language as a communication tool, has prevented scholars from appreciating the richness of black communication behavior. For instance, oral traditions such as proverbs, rhetorical style, and verbal contests are totally ignored by the formal structured analyses of contemporary linguistics.

Taylor (1983) is among a small group of scholars who have attempted to define Black English in such a way as to account for the language and communicative behaviors of the full range of black people in the United States. He defines Black English as the speech spoken by blacks in the United States, ranging from the standard (Standard Black English) to the nonstandard (Nonstandard Black English). Taylor's model is broad enough to take the situation or context into account, as well as the rules pertaining to language structure and to language use in interpersonal interaction.

## English Influenced by Other Languages

Obviously, Black English is not the only social dialect of English used in the United States. Any cultural group's acquisition of a new language is influenced by the linguistic characteristics of that group's native language. Because there are people in the United States from so many different backgrounds, it is impossible to identify and describe all the varieties of English that have been influenced by other languages. On the other hand, these native languages typically interfere with the speaking of English when they do not contain elements that are part of English, or when the elements take a different form in the native language. A familiar example is the stereotype of the Oriental who cannot produce the English /r/ and so substitutes the /l/ instead.

Examples of language interference are commonly found in the United States among Hispanic, native American, Pan Asian, French Cajun, Gullan, Eskimo, Hawaiian, and Virgin Islands populations. In all cases, the linguistic processes underlying the variations are identical, the only differences being related to the actual languages involved, and the social, political, and economic histories of the speakers.

The largest group in the United States today with native language interference with English consists of people from Spanish-speaking backgrounds (including both Mexican Spanish and Puerto Rican Spanish). In certain regions of the nation, Asian Americans comprise a sizable portion of the population. Tables 4.2 and 4.3 present some examples of how Spanish can interfere with English phonology and syntax, respectively. Table 4.4 presents some interferences of Mandarin, Cantonese, and Vietnamese on English phonological patterns. Cheng (1987) has also provided examples of grammatical, semantic, and pragmatic interferences experienced by Asians in their speaking of English. In addition, reasonably extensive data on the influence of various languages on the speaking of English are available

**Table 4.2** Examples of Spanish Interference on English Phonology

| Features | Environments | Examples |
|---|---|---|
| /ʃ/ phoneme | /tʃ/ for /ʃ/ in all positions | chair (share); watch (watsh) |
| /z/ phoneme | /s/ for /z/ in all positions | sip (zip); racer (razor) |
| /ŋ/ phoneme | /n/ for /ŋ/ in the word final position | sin (sing) |
| /v/ phoneme | /b/ for /v/ in all positions | bat (vat); rabbel (ravel) |
| /θ/ phoneme | /t/ or /s/ for /θ/ in all positions | tin or sin (thin) |
| /ð/ phoneme | /d/ for /ð/ in all positions | den (then); ladder (lather) |
| /ɪ/ phoneme | /iy/ for /ɪ/ in all positions | cheap (chip) |

through the National Association for Bilingual Education, 1201 16th Street, N.W., Washington, DC 20036.

## Other Dimensions of Cultural Influences on Communication

Culture affects communication in its use as well as its function. For example, culture may have an impact on the conversational and discourse rules used by an individual speaker. According to Taylor (in press) these rules cover a myriad of topics:

- How to open or close a conversation
- Turn-taking during conversations
- Interruptions
- Silence as a communicative device
- Appropriate topics of conversation
- Humor and when to use it
- Nonverbal modes to accompany conversation
- Laughter as a communicative device
- Appropriate amount of speech to be used by participants
- Logical ordering of events during discourse

Narratives, the art of translating experiences into stories, are a major dimension of discourse that seem to be culture-specific. Many investigators (Heath, 1982; Michaels, 1981; Michaels & Collins, 1984; Reed, 1981) have suggested that children vary with respect to their story telling strategies as

**Table 4.3**   Examples of Spanish Interference on English Syntax

| Features | Environments | Examples |
|---|---|---|
| Forms of *to be* | Absent in present progressive | He getting hungry (He is getting hungry) |
| Pronouns | Absent as subjects of sentences when subject obvious from preceding sentence | Carol left yesterday. I think is coming back tomorrow (Carol left yesterday. I think she is coming back tomorrow) |
| Third person (*-s*) | Absent in third person verb agreements | He talk fast (He talks fast) |
| Past *(-ed)* | Absent in past tense inflections | He walk fast yesterday (He walked fast yesterday) |
| *Go* with *to* | Future markings | He go to see the game tomorrow (He is going to see the game tomorrow) |
| *No* for *don't* | Imperatives | No do that (Don't do that) |
| *The* for possessive pronoun | With body parts | I hurt the finger (I hurt my finger) |
| Present tense markings | Progressive environments | I think he come soon (I think he is coming soon) |
| Locative adverbs | Placed near verb | I think he putting down the rifle (I think he is putting the rifle down) |

they do in the surface structure features of their language. These strategies are probably related to differences in conceptualization, social interaction, and problem solving.

Tannen (1981, 1982) claims that communicative strategies vary along a cultural continuum anchored by *oral strategies* at one end and *literate strategies* at the other. Oral-based cultures are thought to place value on oral narratives and poetry, while literate-based cultures are thought to value writing and speech (Bennett, 1982; Hymes, 1981; Scollon & Scollon, 1979, 1981; Sherzer, 1983).

Of course, all individuals have a certain degree of control over both ends of this presumed continuum; however, it appears that some cultures have a

**Table 4.4**  Phonological Patterns of Interferences

|  | **Mandarin** |
|---|---|
| Substitutions: | s/θ, Z/ð, f/v |
| Confusions: | r/l and l/r |
| Omissions: | final consonants |
| Additions: | /ə/ in blends; belue/blue, gooda/good |
| Approximations: | tɕ/tʃ, ɕ/s |
| Shortening or lengthening of vowels: | seat/sit, it/eat |
|  | **Cantonese** |
| Substitutions: | s/θ, s/z, f/v, w/v, s/ʃ, l/r /e/ee |
| Omissions: | final consonants |
| Additions: | /ə/ in blends |
| Vowels: | /l/, /ʌ/, /ɔ/ are difficult for Cantonese speakers |
|  | **Vietnamese** |
| Substitutions: | s/θ, ʃ/tʃ, b/p, z/dz, d/ð, /d/dʒ/ |
| Ommissions: | final consonants and consonant blends /l/, æ/, /ʊ/, /ɔ̄/ |
| Vowels: | may be difficult at times |

*Note:* From "Cross Cultural and Linguistic Considerations in Working with Asian Populations" by L. R. L. Cheng, 1987, *Asha, 29,* p. 35. Reprinted by permission of the American Speech-Language-Hearing Association.

greater propensity for extending farther into one end or the other than other cultural groups. For example, Heather (1982) and Michaels (1981) claim that lower- and working-class children are more likely to come to school with little mastery of the literate style of communication than middle-class children. Because schools prefer the literate style, these children are often falsely perceived as having language difficulties because they do not structure their stories in a manner prescriptively perceived as normal.

In general, *topic-centered* narratives are characterized by (a) linear presentation of tightly structured discourse on a single topic or series of closely related topics with no major shifts in perspective; (b) temporal orientation or thematic focus; (c) a high degree of thematic coherence and a clear thematic progression that begins with temporal grounding, a statement of focus, introduction of key agents, and some indication of spatial grounding; and (d) an orientation that is followed by elaboration on the topic, and finishes with a punch-line resolution. The stories presume little shared knowledge between speakers and listeners, therefore requiring precise detail. They involve more telling than sharing. The topic-centered style appears to be the one most commonly used by middle-class children, possibly of all racial groups, probably because of extensive exposure to storybooks during early childhood.

*Topic-associated* stories tend to be a series of associated segments implicitly linked to a topic, event, or theme, but with no explicit theme or point. They typically begin with background statements, then shift across segments, with the shifts being marked by pitch and tempo indicators. Various segments are implicitly linked to a topical event or theme, although temporal orientation, location, and focus of segments often shift from one segment to the other. The links among the various segments are left for listener inference since there is a presumed shared knowledge between speakers and listeners. Because of this presumption, these stories tend to contain less detail than topic-centered narratives. At the same time, their focus on a number of themes results in longer presentations.

Topic-associated stories are thought to be used more often by working-class children, particularly working-class black children. They also seem to be perfectly acceptable, understandable, and frequently used by persons who come from oral cultures, regardless of racial background. Smitherman and Van Dyck (1988) have thoroughly discussed the problem of discrimination that occurs as a result of discourse differences.

## LANGUAGE DIFFERENCES AND COMMUNICATION DISORDERS

The question now is "How does a knowledge of language differences contribute to the practice of speech-language pathology?" Some possible answers to this question will be discussed.

### Attitudes

Perhaps the most important recent contribution of sociolinguistics to the field of communication disorders has to do with attitudes toward language variation. The literature clearly suggests that speech-language pathologists must view language variety as a normal phenomenon, and not necessarily as an indication of a communication problem. This is a critical prerequisite for providing clinical services that fit the language codes and expectations of clients, their parents, and their communities. ASHA's 1983 position paper on social dialects considers knowledge of the effects of attitudes on language behavior to be an essential competence for differentiating between communication differences and communication disorders.

### Definitions

Another important recent contribution of sociolinguistics to professional practice in communication disorders has to do with defining disordered communication. A sociocultural perspective toward communication disorders argues that all communication—normal or disordered—can only be defined, studied, or discussed in a cultural context. Since disordered communication is defined as a deviation from the norm, that norm has to be culturally based. In a large black community, for example, the standards against which individual communication behaviors are evaluated must obviously include rules of black communication to be valid. Of course, some black persons communicate according to the rules of some other community, usually the nonblack community that is economically, politically, or socially dominant.

There is also some evidence that societies have different values for defining minimally proficient (or normal) communication and more importantly, what to do about conditions of abnormal communication. In some societies, for example, mild deviations in communication behavior may-hardly be considered cause for alarm in the context of other priorities. Indeed, they might even be considered "cute."

Our point here is that societies may have different criteria for determining when a difference makes a difference and what to do if one exists. Some feel that little or nothing should be done about a communication disorder except to keep it hidden from the public because these disorders are perceived as acts of gods or demons. Unfortunately, there has been little research reported on what different societies, especially in Third World countries, consider disordered communication and what they think should be done about it. In the absence of data, the resourceful speech-language pathologist can, nonetheless, use imaginative interviewing techniques to determine definitions of communication disorder from clients, parents, family, or other members of the home community.

## Testing and Diagnosis

Because there are varying communication rules among different cultural groups, your examination and diagnosis of a person with a communication disorder is much more likely to be effective if you use instruments, interpersonal interaction, testing, and interpretation of findings that are consistent with the communication rules of the group from which the person comes. For this reason, effective testing and diagnostic work is directly related to sensitivity and use of culturally relevant materials and clinical orientations.

Taylor and Payne (1983) have suggested that professionals seek yes answers to a series of questions before administering any assessment instrument. Among the questions are

- Do I know the specific purpose for which this test was designed?
- Has the test been validated for this purpose?
- Do I have specific information about the group on whom the test was standardized (sociocultural, sex, age, etc.)?

■ Are the characteristics of the student being tested comparable to those in the standardization sample?

■ Does the test manual or research literature (or my own experience) indicate any differences in test performance across cultural groups?

■ Do test items take into account differences in values or adaptive behaviors?

■ Does the test use vocabulary that is cultural, regional, colloquial, or archaic?

■ Does the test rely heavily on receptive and expressive Standard English language to measure abilities other than language?

■ Am I aware of what the test demands of (or assumes about) the students in terms of (a) reading level of questions or directions, (b) style of problem solving, (c) test-taking behavior, and (d) format?

■ Has an item-by-item analysis been made of the test from the framework of the linguistic and communicative features of the group for which it is to be used?

Speech-language pathologists rely heavily on standardized tests to determine the presence or absence of communication disorders. Most tests currently used in speech-language pathology are based on Northern Midland Standard English. For this reason, many of these tests, when administered and scored according to the prescribed norms, yield results that unfairly penalize speakers of nonmainstream dialects. They give the inaccurate impression of communication disorder when, in fact, no pathology exists.

*Auditory perception is the process of identifying a sensory stimulus without necessarily attaching meaning to that stimulus.*

An excellent example of the cultural bias in communication tests may be found in many tests of auditory perception. This process is believed to be a prerequisite for the normal decoding of auditory messages. For example, a task of discrimination might require a child to tell you whether the following two nonsense syllables sound alike or different: "id" /ɪd/ and "ed" /ɛd/. The expected answer for a Standard English listener, of course, is "different." We know, however, that people tend to perceive incoming sounds according to the phonological rules of their native language. Thus, if the /ɪ/ phoneme does not exist in a particular speaker's phonological system, but the /ɛ/ does exist, he may report the word pair as "same" instead of "different." This problem is particularly apparent when speakers of nonstandard English dialects are tested for their auditory discrimination abilities in Standard English. In many cases, more errors than normal are recorded; therefore, the speech-language pathologist might inaccurately conclude that a child is 1 to 2 years behind in auditory perceptual function when, in fact, there is no delay. Several researchers (for example, Seymour & Seymour, 1977) have shown that, when cultural and sociolinguistic factors are taken into account in designing and administering language tasks, there are no statistically significant differences among cultural groups.

Taylor (1978, 1983) is among those authors who have discussed in some detail sociolinguistic dimensions in standardized tests. Drawing on his work with researchers in several related disciplines, he has discussed seven distinct sources of possible bias in tests:

1. *Social situational bias*—violation of a situation/context rule for the test taker
2. *Value bias*—mismatch between values assumed in test items and the values of the test taker
3. *Phonological bias*—mismatch between phonological rules assumed in a test item and the phonological rules of the test taker
4. *Grammatical bias*—mismatch between grammatical rules assumed in a test item and the grammatical rules of the test taker
5. *Vocabulary bias*—mismatch between words and their use between test maker and test taker (may include underlying cognitive mismatches)
6. *Pragmatic bias*—mismatch between rules of communication interaction between test maker and test taker
7. *Directions/format bias*—confusions or misunderstandings created for test taker by the use of unfamiliar or ambiguous directions and/or test formats

In addition to the above types of biases in standardized tests, Taylor and Lee (1987) suggest two additional sources of likely bias in standardized tests: communicative style and cognitive style. With respect to communicative style, they claim that test takers who prefer lengthy social greetings before getting to substantive points may be incorrectly viewed as exhibiting avoidance behaviors by testers who expect a rapid approach to the main purpose of communication. Likewise, test takers whose cultures value silence and contemplation may be viewed as lacking verbal skills by testers who expect verbosity.

Taylor and Lee also note that standardized tests tend to be based on the erroneous assumption that all individuals evidence ability through the use of similar cognitive style. Cognitive style is the manner in which individuals perceive, organize, and process experiences. Most tests presume that test takers prefer an analytical, object-oriented (field-independent) cognitive style (Goldstein & Blackman, 1978); yet research has shown that there are at least nine different preferred cognitive styles used by various cultural groups. Individuals of African and Hispanic descent tend to prefer, for example, a relational, socially oriented, field-dependent learning style in comparison to the aforementioned field-independent style, preferred by most European and Asian groups.

Test bias may also come from other culturally based differences in communicative style, in areas such as verbosity, the statement of obvious information, and preferred narrative style. Knowledge of sources of test bias can assist clinicians in interpreting test data, modifying existing tests, and constructing new scoring norms. Of course, the ultimate solution to this problem is the construction of criterion-referenced tests that assess a test taker's communication skills from the vantage point of her speech community.

The use of culturally and linguistically discriminatory assessment instruments is specifically prohibited by federal mandates such as The Education for All Handicapped Children Act of 1975 (P.L. 94-142) and its updated version (P.L. 98-199), The Bilingual Education Act of 1976 (P.L. 95-561), and Title VII of the Elementary and Secondary Education Act of 1965. In addition, several legal decisions have declared illegal the use of culturally and linguistically discriminatory assessment procedures for determining the presence of handicapping conditions; see, for example, *Dianna* v. *California State Board of Education* in 1973, *Mattie T.* v. *Halladay* in Mississippi in 1977, and *Larry P.* v. *Riles* in California in 1979.

In interpreting assessment data and diagnosing communication disorders, there is some evidence that, since different cultural communities define communication pathology differently, the speech-language pathologist must use this information. Let us take the case of stuttering to illustrate this point.

Leith and Mims (1975) note a sharp difference in stuttering patterns between blacks and whites. Whites, they report, show a strong tendency for what they call "Type I" stuttering, which is characterized by overt (audible) repetitions and prolongations with a moderate number of overt secondary characteristics, such as word phrase repetitions and accelerated speaking rates. Blacks, in contrast, show a strong tendency for "Type II" stuttering, which is characterized by more covert (nonaudible) prolongations and repetitions and a large number of relatively severe secondary characteristics, including total avoidance of speech. Black stutterers, like all Type II stutterers, often appear to have either a mild handicap or no handicap whatsoever, although they appear tense and anxious; that is, the Type II stutterer works hard to appear not to stutter.

Leith and Mims (1975) argue that blacks engage in Type II stuttering far more than whites because, as pointed out by sociolinguists such as Mitchell (1969) and Kochman (1970), the black culture in the United States places a high premium on oral proficiency and on being under control. Indeed, a substantial part of the black male self-concept is built around proficiency in oral skills like ritual insults, rapping, and verbal routines with women, and around being "cool," so as to always appear in control and never ruffled. Obviously, stuttering runs counter to these social values; therefore, the black stutterer would naturally do everything possible to mask stuttering and the way it makes him feel.

A related problem deals with the child who appears to have delayed language development. The speech-language pathologist must determine whether the child has a true language disorder/learning disability or has mastered the rules for a nonstandard dialect and is simply missing some rules for Standard English. Familiarity with the child's native speech community is the first step in the assessment process. Seymour and Miller-Jones (1981) have presented an excellent framework for assessing black children who do not speak Standard English. Erickson and Omark (1981) have provided a thorough framework for bilingual speakers. Vaughn-Cooke (1983) has made a number of suggestions for improving language assessment in minority children. Finally, Cole (1984) has developed a computer software package to assist in sociolinguistic analyses of children's language samples.

## Clinical Management

The speech-language pathologist can also apply sociocultural principles of language and communication in the delivery of therapy and education. This area is only beginning to receive attention by researchers in communication disorders. Significant changes in traditional approaches, however, have begun to appear.

First, the interpersonal dimension is a vital component of any type of effective clinical management of a communication disorder. For this reason, differences in the verbal and nonverbal rules used by the speech-language pathologist and the client can cause unintended episodes of insult, discomfort, or hypersensitivity, which could adversely affect the interpersonal dynamics needed for effective clinical work (Adler, 1973; Taylor, 1978).

Second, knowledge of developmental patterns of a particular language or dialect can help the professional determine differences between developmental variations and pathologic deviations, the appropriate time to begin speech or language therapy for pathologic features, and the course of therapy once it has started.

Seymour and Seymour (1977) have developed one of the few models for providing therapy for speech or language disorders that take language variation into account. Using Black English as their point of departure, the Seymours argue that, since many of the features of the so-called Standard English and Black English Vernacular in the United States overlap, therapy goals for Black-English-speaking children should fit with educational goals and social expectations. Therefore, their model is constructed so that particular linguistic features of both Black English Vernacular and Standard English are modified. The model recognizes the possibility of pathologic deviations from both vernacular and Standard English and the fact that true linguistic competency in the culture probably requires people to be proficient in both systems.

Miller (1984) has also presented a thorough discussion of the diagnosis and management of language disorders in bilingual populations.

## Language Education

In some professional settings, the speech-language pathologist needs to instruct speakers of nonstandard dialects in Standard English. This is in addition to the usual professional responsibility of providing therapy for people with communication disorders. In these instances, the pathologist must keep in mind that teaching a second dialect is *not* the same as correcting a disorder. In teaching a second dialect, the goal is to establish a parallel linguistic form to stand alongside an already existing, legitimate form for use in certain situations. In correcting a disorder, the goal is to eradicate unacceptable linguistic forms in favor of those that are considered "normal." It is obvious that a disorder may exist within any dialect.

ASHA's 1983 position paper on social dialects permits clinicians to provide instruction in Standard English on an *elective* basis only. To offer such instruction, however, ASHA asserts that the professional must be sensitive and competent in at least three areas: (a) linguistic features of the dialect, (b) linguistic contrastive analysis procedures, and (c) the effects of attitudes toward dialects.

Feigenbaum (1970) is one of the major writers on the subject of second-dialect instruction. Using principles from Teaching English to Speakers of Other Languages (TESOL), Feigenbaum has outlined a part "audio-lingual" or "pattern practice" approach to teaching Standard English as a second dialect. The components of the program involve the following steps:

1. Presentation of explicit examples of the two dialects, highlighting distinguishing characteristics

2. Discrimination drills between the two dialects, requiring the learner to determine sameness and difference between pairs of utterances

3. Identification drills that require the learner to properly categorize utterances as being from one dialect or the other

4. Translation drills requiring the learner to translate utterances presented in one dialect into the opposite dialect, that is, standard to nonstandard to standard

5. Response drills in which the learners respond, in quasi-spontaneous situations, to a stimulus presented in one dialect with a response consistent with that dialect or, eventually, with a response inconsistent with that dialect

Building on principles of second-language teaching and oral communication classroom techniques, Taylor (1986b) has suggested that there are eight steps through which learners must be taken if they are to acquire competence in using a particular linguistic structure of Standard English in the appropriate situations and with the correct meanings. These steps are

1. Positive attitude toward existing dialect

2. Awareness of difference between existing dialect and Standard English

3. Recognition, labeling, and contrasting of specific features of the existing dialect and Standard English

4. Recognition of different meanings coded by parallel structural forms in the two dialects

5. Recognition of situations where the existing dialect or Standard English is appropriate

6. Production of targeted features of Standard English in connected speech from a model provided by the instructor

7. Production of targeted features of Standard English in connected speech in controlled situations, for example, role playing

8. Production of targeted features of Standard English in connected speech in spontaneous situations

Taylor's program, which has been successfully field tested in several California school districts, requires instruction to focus on language structure, language use, and language as a facilitator of cognition. It emphasizes practical applications in a variety of situations, and links across the entire school curriculum, particularly in reading and writing.

Unfortunately, the decision of whether to teach English as a second language, or Standard English as a second dialect, is not always clear-cut. It is one thing to determine, for instance, that a child from a Chinese family does not have the /r/ phoneme in his phonology or that a Chicano child does not have the /i/, but it is quite another thing to determine what, if anything, should be done about these dialects educationally, who should do it, and when it should be done. Some professionals and community leaders feel that community dialects should be perceived as culturally adequate and that children should be left alone to use the language of their home speech communities (the no intervention view). Others, while respecting and preserving community dialects, feel that all children should also master the prevalent dialect, that is, Standard English, at least as a tool, so that they can use it in those situations where it is either expected or required (the bidialectal view). A few even hold the counterproductive view that community dialects have little value and should, therefore, be eradicated and replaced with Standard English (the eradication view). This rather controversial issue is not likely to be resolved in the near future. The speech-language pathologist who deals with children from any minority group—be they Blacks, Hispanics, Orientals, Hawaiians, whatever—must be sensitive to these questions and provide services to individuals in the context of the family or community expectations, the state of the art in educational linguistics, sociolinguistics, and the law.

The issue of teaching Standard English to speakers of nonstandard dialects of English, notably Black English Vernacular, has taken on legal ramifications. In 1977, a group of parents in Ann Arbor, Michigan, filed a suit in Federal Court on behalf of 15 black preschool and elementary children, charging that teachers in a local school had failed to adequately take into account the children's home dialects in the teaching of the language arts.

What are the diff. btwn these two tests?

Among their charges, the parents claimed that the teachers were not suffi-ciently knowledgeable about these dialects and, as a result, did not fully appreciate their intrinsic worth and usefulness in the educational environment. In several cases, children of the plaintiffs had been inappropriately enrolled in speech programs to "correct" their home dialects. The judge in the case concurred with the parents and ordered the Ann Arbor School Board to develop an educational plan that, among other things, would educate the teachers in the students' dialects and in how knowledge and value of the dialects can be used constructively in the language arts curriculum.

*See for instance, Taylor, 1973.*

*P.L. 94-142 also prohibits inappropriate placement into speech therapy and the use of discriminatory tests to make such placements. Because some children with language differences may, in addition, have communication disorders, the speech-language pathologist must be able to clearly distinguish between dialect and disorder.*

The Ann Arbor case places many of the issues pertaining to dialects and education into perspective. First, the fact that the parents sued to force the school to teach Standard English while preserving the home dialects corroborates data from several studies on parents' language attitudes and aspirations. Second, the arguments on behalf of the plaintiffs clearly support the bidialectal posture toward language education for nonstandard-English-speaking children. Throughout the trial, the plaintiffs' parents reiterated their belief that their right to equal protection of the laws, guaranteed by the 14th Amendment to the U.S. Constitution, requires schools to teach students Standard English, but *not* at the expense of eradicating or showing disrespect toward home and community languages and dialects. Third, the plaintiffs' lawyers attacked the inappropriate placement in speech therapy of students who demonstrate only differences, not disorders, in language and communication. Fourth, the judge's ruling in this case suggests that professionals who offer language instruction to nonstandard speakers must be properly trained in the area of language variables and in applying that training to language arts education. Training of this type may be obtained in disciplines such as sociolinguistics and bilingual education. Of course, the speech-language pathologist who assumes this role should remember that her function is that of a teacher and not of a therapist. First and foremost, the language professional must keep in mind that *different does not mean disordered.*

## CONCLUSION

At the outset of this chapter, a case history profile was presented on a seven-year-old black male child who attends a multiracial school in a suburb of Washington, D.C. At first glance, it would appear reasonable to suspect that the child has some type of a developmental language disorder. Considering the issues raised in this chapter, however, it seems quite possible that the child's classroom behavior is created by frustrations emanating from the cultural and SES differences between the child and his teacher and peers. Moreover, the child's language performance on the two assessment instruments might be attributed to a mismatch between the linguistic expectations of the instruments and the child's social/regional dialect. These suspicions are reinforced by two facts. First, many black children at the school demonstrate the same language behaviors as those demonstrated by James. Second, both of the assessment instruments contain format, lexical, and/or syntactic biases against individuals who come from speech communities like James's.

Obviously, all of these possibilities must be carefully considered by the speech-language pathologist. The guiding principle is that the entire clinical process must be culturally valid and adequate to distinguish between a language disorder and a language difference.

To achieve these objectives, the clinician must integrate ethnologic considerations into the clinical process. Taylor (in press) suggests that clinicians should:

- View each clinical encounter as a socially situated communicative event that is subject to the cultural rules governing such events by both the clinician and the client(s)

- Recognize that clients may perform differently under differing clinical conditions because of their cultural and language backgrounds

- Recognize that different modes, channels, and functions of communication events in which individuals are expected to participate in a clinical setting may result in differing levels of linguistic or communicative performance

- Utilize ethnographic techniques for evaluating communicative behavior and establish cultural norms for determining the presence or absence of communication disorders

- Recognize possible sources of conflicts in cultural assumptions and communicative norms in clients prior to clinical encounters, and take steps to prevent them from occurring during service delivery

- Recognize that learning about culture is an ongoing process that should result in a constant reassessment and revision of ideas, and greater sensitivity to cultural diversity

# STUDY QUESTIONS

1. What is a communication disorder versus a communication difference? Discuss the two from a sociocultural perspective.

2. Define Black English Vernacular. Briefly discuss its origin and the controversy surrounding the whole notion of Black English.

3. Discuss the major factors which influence language behavior and acquisition. Which of these factors do you feel could have some impact upon language differences? Defend your answer.

4. List at least five phonological and grammatical features of Black English Vernacular, Southern English, Southern White Nonstandard English, and Appalachian English. Identify specific points of overlap within your lists.

5. What are the key issues in ASHA's position statement on social dialects? Do you agree or disagree with the association's position? Defend your position.

## SELECTED READINGS

Bell, R. T. (1976). *Sociolinguistics: Goals, approaches and problems.* London: B. T. Batsford.

Fasold, R. (1984). *The Sociolinguistics of society.* London: Basil Blackwell.

Feigenbaum, I. (1970). The use of nonstandard English in teaching standard: Contrast and comparison. In R. W. Fasold & R. W. Shuy (Eds.), *Teaching standard English in the inner city.* Washington, D.C.: Center for Applied Linguistics.

Hymes, D. (1974). *Foundations of sociolinguistics: An ethnographic approach.* Philadelphia: University of Pennsylvania Press.

Saville-Troike, M. (1982). *The ethnography of communication: An introduction.* Oxford: Basil Blackwell.

Seymour, H. N., & Seymour, C. M. (1977). A therapeutic model for communicative disorders among children who speak Black English Vernacular. *Journal of Speech and Hearing Disorders, 42*(2), 247–256.

Taylor, O. L. (Ed.) (1986a). *Nature of communication disorders in culturally and linguistically diverse populations.* San Diego: College-Hill Press.

Taylor, O. L. (Ed.) (1986b). *Treatment of communication disorders in culturally and linguistically diverse populations.* San Diego: College-Hill Press.

Wolfram, W., & Fasold, R. W. (1974). *The study of social dialects in American English.* Englewood Cliffs, NJ: Prentice-Hall.

# Language Disorders in Preschool Children

## LAURENCE LEONARD

### MYTHS AND REALITIES

- *Myth:* Physically healthy children who are late talkers will catch up to their peers by kindergarten or first grade.

- *Reality:* Some children will indeed catch up, but many will not, at least not without intervention. For these children, language development can proceed slowly, and residual language problems are often present in adolescence and early adulthood.

- *Myth:* Language-disordered children with no neurological or intellectual problems must come from homes that provide poor language stimulation.

- *Reality:* There are many young language-disordered children whose home environments are not distinguishable from those of normally developing children. Often these children have siblings with age-appropriate language skills.

- *Myth:* Children's language abilities can be enhanced through intervention only to a level commensurate with their IQ.

- *Reality:* The skills assessed on IQ tests constitute only a sample of intellectual abilities. They do not represent intelligence itself. Language is also a type of intellectual ability. It is possible for a child to score low on both language and IQ tests but to score lower on the latter.

■ *Myth:* Children with language disorders are passive in conversations with other children and adults.

■ *Reality:* Some language-disordered children are generally conversationally passive, but many can be quite assertive with familiar adults and younger children.

■ *Myth:* Children whose language difficulties are limited to the production of language represent a mild case of language disorder.

■ *Reality:* Age-appropriate language comprehension ability is a positive prognostic sign; however, some children with high comprehension exhibit severe production limitations that warrant immediate clinical attention.

■ *Myth:* One cannot facilitate children's language production skills until their speech sound production abilities have been enhanced to the point where they are fairly intelligible.

■ *Reality:* Young normally developing children often attempt words that they are unable to distinguish phonologically (for example, producing *boo, spoon,* and *boot* as "boo"), and there is no justification for postponing introduction of new words until a language-disordered child can pronounce them distinctly. Furthermore, some language-disordered children use certain speech sounds only when the sounds play an important morphological role (for example, they say "bok" for *box,* but the word *ducks* is produced correctly).

Cᴸᴀʀɪꜰɪᴄᴀᴛɪᴏɴ of these erroneous assumptions is an important first step to understanding language disorders in children. Speech-language pathologists must sometimes inform parents and other health care officials that their assumptions about language-disordered children are unfounded. The picture that remains, however, is rather vague. The case study below will help to provide a clearer impression of these problems.

*Tony was first evaluated for speech and language difficulties at age 3 years, 1 month. At that time his parents reported that he produced only a few words. His most frequent communicative attempts involved gesturing, producing certain "favorite" syllables (such as* ba*), and whining. According to the parents' report, Tony seemed to understand much of what was said to him. They felt his hearing was normal, although at age 2 years he had received medication for a middle-ear infection. Tony's motor development seemed to be within normal limits.*

*The initial speech and language evaluation confirmed the parents' impressions. Tony's performance on standardized language comprehension tests was approximately 6 months below that expected for his age, and his performance on standardized language production tests suggested an ability that was more than one year below age level. This was corroborated by an analysis of a sample of his spontaneous speech, which indicated utterances limited to single words. Audiometric testing was inconclusive; however, it appeared that Tony had normal hearing in at least one ear at the frequencies most important for speech. Results from a performance scale of a standardized test of intelligence suggested a borderline level of intellectual functioning.*

*On the basis of the speech and language evaluation, it was recommended that Tony be enrolled in a daily preschool program emphasizing language-learning activities. Along with the group language stimulation activities conducted in the preschool, Tony received daily individual therapy focusing on the production of functional multiword utterances. The individual therapy sessions were 30 minutes long. Following the individual session, Tony joined the other children in the group.*

*Testing conducted 9 months after Tony was enrolled in the preschool program revealed noticeable gains in the level of his linguistic functioning. His performance on standardized language comprehension tests was age-appropriate. Tony continued to have difficulties in language production. His performance on standardized language production tests reflected a level of functioning more like that of a child one year his junior. In absolute terms, however, Tony's language production gains were significant. Utterances three to five words in length were common. In addition, he asked questions frequently (for example,* Where Josh going?*) and produced words and phrases in situations in which he had previously exhibited a pattern of whining. Tony was more cooperative during this period, making possible a more complete assessment of his hearing. Results indicated hearing within normal limits.*

*A test is* **standardized** *by administering it to a large number of children who are representative of the age levels for which the test is to be used. The results are used for comparing performances.*

Although most children seem to acquire their native language relatively easily, with no formal instruction, this critical task is difficult for some children. These children need additional assistance, which is often provided by the speech-language pathologist. It has been estimated that language-disordered children make up from 50% to 80% of the cases seen by speech-language pathologists who provide services to preschool children.

Who are these young "language-disordered" children? In general, we can say that children have a language disorder whenever their language abilities are below those expected for their age and their level of functioning. Obviously, this definition is quite broad and, we will see, allows us to consider children with widely varying characteristics as language disordered.

*This chapter focuses on preschool-age children, while the next covers the school-age language-disordered child.*

## TYPES OF LANGUAGE DISORDERS

There are at least three different ways to discuss the various types of language disorders experienced by children. As we shall see, these are not mutually exclusive. Instead, they represent three different perspectives from which the same child's problems might be described.

### Relationship to Normal Developmental Schedule and Sequence

One way of discussing a child's language disorder is to describe it in relationship to the schedule and sequence of language development usually seen in children. A number of the major characteristics of normal language development have been discussed in chapter 2. If a child is not performing like peers in language production or comprehension, there are at least five ways in which this difference might be characterized.

First, the child might be exhibiting a language delay; that is, she might be acquiring the same features of language in the same sequence as her peers but simply more slowly. Presumably, the child will eventually show the same language skills as other individuals but will not reach that point until an older age. A second possibility is that the child is slowly acquiring the same features in the same sequence as other children, but will never catch up to her peers. This resembles a language delay, but because a plateau in the child's language skills occurs, it should be distinguished from the first pattern. Both of these patterns occur, but not as frequently as one might assume.

The pattern that is observed most frequently is one in which the child is acquiring the same features of language as normal children and is generally acquiring them at a slower rate, but the features differ significantly from one another in how slowly they are developing. Although normally developing children differ from one another to some degree in the relative speed with which different features of language develop, the cases described here show greater discrepancies among features than is seen in normal development. Rather dramatic instances of this type of discrepancy can be found, but a more typical example can be seen in Table 5.1.

We can see from this table that linguistic features in general tend to be slower in emergence and development in this language-disordered child. For example, this child acquired her first words at a much later age than is seen in normal development. Similarly, two-word utterances and the use of forms such as *-ing* and *-s* were later to emerge than expected. Despite their late appearance, however, the features are not unlike those seen in a normal child's speech. The types of first words acquired are similar, and the meanings reflected in the two-word combinations are essentially the same. In addition, meanings such as recurrence (as in *more apple*) precede those such as possession (as in *Mimi purse*) in both children. Also, in both

**Table 5.1**  Pattern of Development Shown by a Language-Disordered Child and a Normally Developing Child

| Language-Disordered Child | | | Normally Developing Child | | |
|---|---|---|---|---|---|
| Age | Attainment | Example | Age | Attainment | Example |
| 27 months | First words | this, mama, bye bye, doggie | 13 months | First words | here, mama, bye bye, kitty |
| 38 months | 50-word vocabulary | | 17 months | 50-word vocabulary | |
| 40 months | First two-word combinations | this doggie more apple this mama more play | 18 months | First two-word combinations | more juice here ball more T.V. here kitty |
| 48 months | Later two-word combinations | Mimi purse Daddy coat block chair dolly table | 22 months | Later two-word combinations | Andy shoe Mommy ring cup floor keys chair |
| 52 months | Mean sentence length of 2.00 words | | 24 months | Mean sentence length of 2.00 words | |
| 55 months | First appearance of -ing | Mommy eating | | First appearance of -ing | Andy sleeping |
| 63 months | Mean sentence length of 3.10 words | | 30 months | Mean sentence length 3.10 words | |
| 66 months | First appearance of 's | The doggie's mad | | First appearance of "is" | My car's gone! |
| 73 months | Mean sentence length of 4.10 words | | 37 months | Mean sentence length 4.10 words | |
| 79 months | Mean sentence length of 4.50 words | | | First appearance of indirect requests | Can I have some cookies? |
| | First appearance of indirect requests | Can I get the ball? | 40 months | Mean sentence length of 4.50 words | |

children, suffixes such as -ing appear before function words such as is; however, the children are different in the relationships among these linguistic features in their speech. The suffix -ing shows up in the speech of the normal child at a time when her mean sentence length is 2.00 words. When the language-disordered child has achieved the same mean sentence length, she does not yet use -ing. To cite another example, the normal child shows the ability to use question forms as an indirect request at a point when her mean sentence length is 4.10 words. The language-disordered child appears to require a mean sentence length of 4.50 words before she uses indirect requests.

Another, less frequently occurring pattern is one in which the language-disordered child shows use of a feature of language also seen in normal children, but uses it with a frequency unlike that seen at any point in normal language development. The frequent use of certain types of errors is characteristic of this pattern. For example, assume a language-disordered child produces all words with word-initial [s] clusters with the [s] at the end of the syllable. Thus, *stop* is pronounced "tops," *sniff* is pronounced "niffs," *ski* is pronounced "kees," and *speeder* is produced as "peesder." This type of usage, called metathesis, is occasionally seen in young normally developing children as well. As far as I can tell, however, no normal child of any age has ever used metathesis for all words containing [s] clusters, or with such consistency.

The final pattern is also infrequent, but isolated cases do exist. This is where the language-disordered child shows use of some feature of language that has never been reported in normal children of any age. An example of this is one child who produced a voiceless ingressive alveolar fricative in place of sounds such as [s], [z], and [f] (Ingram & Terselic, 1983). This sound, produced by drawing air in rather than directing it out of the vocal tract, is not among the consonants of English, the language exposed to the child.

## Features of Language

A second way of discussing types of language disorders is to focus on the features of language giving the child the greatest difficulty. Certain aspects of the language may prove troublesome for one child, while other aspects are difficult for another child. Many children have problems with more than one aspect of language. Let's consider, then, some of the major features of language that may pose problems for a child.

Most language-disordered children are slow in acquiring their first words and in their subsequent vocabulary development. For this reason, they may be viewed as limited in their **semantic** abilities. A less obvious semantic problem is word-finding difficulties, in which the child has trouble generating a presumably known word when it is required in the situation. We have all experienced frustrating moments when we were unable to retrieve a particular name or word. Language-disordered children with word-finding difficulties experience this much more frequently.

Difficulties with **phonology** are often seen in language-disordered children. In some cases, the problem can be due to speech-motor difficulties; in others, the problem is one of phonological organization. An example of the former might be seen in the child's productions of "gup" for *cup* and "doo" for *two*. Here, the child's difficulty may be his inability to coordinate the timing of voicing so that it begins after the release of the consonant—a problem young children often experience, due presumably to their neuro-motor immaturity. An example of organizational difficulty may be seen in a child's productions of "tee" for *see* and "tack" for *sack* when the child also says "soo" for *shoe* and "sip" for *chip*. Obviously the child is capable of producing [s] but has established incorrect correspondences between the adult forms and the forms he uses.

**Syntactic** difficulties are often reflected in the reduced length of language-disordered children's utterances. For example, a 5-year-old language-disordered child might produce an utterance such as *I want to put the car on the table* as "Want put car table." A more specific form of syntactic limitation that is often reported is a problem with the auxiliary verb system of English. Even when language-impaired children can produce utterances of seven or eight words in length, they may show deletions of some elements of the auxiliary system. Thus, a child may say *My sisters like to play ball and sing,* but be unable to attempt *Daddy will have eaten.*

Problems with **morphology**—especially the use of suffixes—seem espe-cially frequent in these children. Errors on suffixes typically involve deletion. For example, errors such as "Nona like tea" and "I want Bob candy" are more likely than errors such as "We likes cake" and "I have my's dolly."

Some language-disordered children have difficulties with **pragmatics.** The following dialogue provides an illustration of this.

> **Child:** Look at that. Trees.
> **Adult:** Yeah, they're Christmas trees. See the pretty lights?
> **Child:** Trucks go fast. Them too.
> **Adult:** What else goes fast?
> **Child:** I don't know if. . . . When we take it.
> **Adult:** Oh, I see.

Of course, she didn't really see. The child's utterances did not seem to stay on the topic of conversation, and she used pronouns whose referents had not been established earlier. In short, even though this child's utterances were understandable from the standpoint of the speech sounds, words, syntax, and morphology used, little communication actually took place.

The features of semantics, phonology, syntax, morphology, and prag-matics are necessarily intertwined, so it is easy to see that if a child has problems with one, he will have some type of deficiency in one or more of the others; however, language-disordered children often have greater problems with some dimensions than with others. These children may differ from one another in their relative strengths and weaknesses.

## Distinctions Based on Presumed Etiology or Correlates

Many speech-language pathologists today would argue that the most useful ways of distinguishing among language-disordered children are the two approaches already discussed; however, these approaches were not the first to be used. The approach with the longest history is one based on the presumed cause of the child's language disorder, or, where that is difficult to determine, the correlates to the disorder. Children with language disorders attributable to different causes do sometimes differ in their language behaviors. For this reason, the etiological approach will be discussed here. Remember that language-disordered children given different etiological labels often show similar language characteristics, and children given the same label may differ significantly in their language behavior. It is often the case that the most appropriate assessment and treatment procedures for a child are unrelated to her presumed etiology.

The groups of children often distinguished using this approach include children with "specific language impairment," mentally retarded children, children with autisticlike characteristics, children with acquired language disorders, and hearing-impaired children. Some of these groups of children have been the focus of scientific investigation and discussion for many years, while others have only recently been studied. For example, the earliest scientific journals included descriptions of mentally retarded children. Descriptions of children with specific language impairment and children with acquired language disorders did not appear until the 1800s. Reports of autistic children did not seem to appear until this century. The literature on the various groups of children reveals a common trend. The earliest writings provided a general description of the disorder. Scientific articles and books soon followed, offering possible explanations for these disorders. Only in the last 25 years has there been a concerted effort to describe the language characteristics of each of these groups of children.

## Children with Specific Language Impairment

Specific language impairment *is a condition in which a child exhibits a significant deficit in linguistic functioning but shows normal hearing, motor development, and nonverbal intelligence.*

Children with **specific language impairment** have problems that seem, at least on first impression, to be confined to the area of language. (As we will see, this picture sometimes changes when more detailed testing is performed.) These children tend to perform within normal limits on tests of nonverbal intelligence. Their hearing is found to be adequate, and, except for their frustration in communicating, their emotional development seems unremarkable. Children with specific language impairment have been given various clinical labels, such as *language delayed, language deviant, language impaired, developmentally aphasic,* and *language disordered.* Some of these terms reflect a particular point of view about the nature of these children's linguistic difficulties. For instance, the label *language deviant* is sometimes used to suggest that the language of these children is somewhat different from that of younger, normally developing children. The label *developmentally aphasic* is typically used to suggest that the language problems are related to a neurological problem. But as we will see, the evidence for these points of view is not always strong. Therefore, we should not assume that children given these different clinical labels are necessarily quite different from one another.

The factors most frequently studied in relation to specific language impairment include (a) the perceptual ability of language-impaired children, (b) their symbolic abilities, (c) their interaction with other people, and (d) brain damage. Each of these factors may be linked in some way to the language difficulties of these children. It is not yet clear, however, that any of them are the cause of the language disorder. Some children with specific language impairment perform below age level on nonverbal tasks requiring symbolic ability (for example, using a pencil as if it were a spoon during pretend play); however, their performance on language tasks is even lower. To cite another example, mothers of these children are rather directive and controlling in their language use relative to mothers of normally developing children of the same age. Yet mothers of younger normally developing children show this same characteristic. Thus, mothers of children with specific language impairment may be using a pattern of language that is quite appropriate given the linguistic immaturity of their children.

A number of authors have proposed that the difficulties experienced by children with specific language impairment are a consequence of brain damage. Damage to both hemispheres of the brain is often postulated because the language development of these children is much slower than that of children suffering from acquired aphasia. Children for whom there is the most clear-cut evidence of brain damage are those whose problems involve motor and sensory as well as language deficits. For children whose difficulties seem to rest principally in language, however, the evidence for brain damage is not particularly convincing. This may change with the advent of recent technological advances that let us assess brain functioning more precisely.

The most notable feature of these children's language is that the large majority of the linguistic features reflected in their speech are slow to emerge and develop. The particular linguistic features used by these children do not seem to differ from those seen in younger, normal children. Because the linguistic features may differ from one another in their degree of delay, however, the relationship among these features in the speech of the child with specific language impairment may not always be the same as it is in normally developing children (see Table 5.1).

There has been considerable attention paid to the pragmatic abilities of children with specific language impairment. Initially, it was assumed that these children have significant deficiencies in their conversational skills. It now appears that a number of these children can serve as appropriate and active conversationalists, particularly when they are interacting with individuals whose own language skills are not fully developed and/or when the conversational adjustments required of the children do not demand much syntactic complexity (Fey, 1986).

## Mentally Retarded Children

Children described as **mentally retarded** are diagnosed according to two characteristics: (a) subaverage overall intellectual functioning and (b) personal independence and social responsibility that are below the level expected for the child's age and cultural group. Language development, too, poses a problem for these children.

In a number of children, the cause of mental retardation is suspected to be a chromosomal abnormality; for others, the suspected cause is brain injury suffered prenatally or during birth; for still others, suspicions center on genetic inheritance. Among other medical factors cited by the American Association on Mental Deficiency are infections and intoxication, disorders of metabolism, prematurity, and gestational disorders (Grossman, 1983). These biological causes are usually associated with more severe retardation. In most other cases, particularly cases of mild retardation, the exact cause is unknown; however, borderline mental retardation has often been attributed to cultural and familial patterns. The majority of these children come from "culturally deprived or different" backgrounds. They may be the victims of nutritional deficits or inadequate cultural and social stimulation. The condition may be functional and reversible with adequate stimulation, or it may be permanent. It is also possible that mild retardation has a hereditary basis.

Whatever the cause of the child's mental retardation, the fact that he is mentally retarded makes it easy to conclude that the child's linguistic deficit is caused by the retardation. Yet the matter is not so simple. Many mentally retarded children's skills in language are considerably more depressed than their skills in areas such as motor, perceptual, and even intellectual development. Therefore, the statement that a mentally retarded child's deficits can be explained by the retardation is incorrect. Unfortunately, research has not yet uncovered explanations for why mentally retarded children's linguistic skills are often so low. Early studies of children whose level of functioning was low enough to lead to institutionalization showed that these children received only limited language stimulation. There is also some evidence that parents of some subgroups of mentally retarded children do not respond to their children in quite the same way as parents of normally developing children. As with the studies of children with specific language impairment, however, the parents' behavior may simply be a reaction to the lack of responsiveness of the child.

Much of what we have said about the speech of children with specific language impairment can also be said about the speech of mentally retarded children. These children are slow to acquire most linguistic features, although the features themselves are usually the same as those seen in normal children. As with language-impaired children, mentally retarded children may show more delay with certain features than others, resulting in a somewhat different relationship among these features than is typically seen in children who have no pronounced language-learning difficulties.

In mentally retarded children, the degree of language delay may depend in part on the severity of their overall developmental disability. Some children, for example, do not begin to use words until the age of 5; others may develop only through training programs allowing them to communicate by pointing to specially designed symbols; still others may be so severely retarded as never to develop the ability to communicate. We do not yet know whether retarded children—particularly severely and profoundly retarded—learn in the same ways as normally developing children.

We do know, however, that the older a mentally retarded child is before she acquires a particular linguistic feature or ability, the less likely it is that her use of the feature or ability will resemble that of a younger, normal child. This factor of chronological age seems to be important for the study of the language of mentally retarded children. It appears that the older the child, the more likely she will acquire a linguistic feature by rote learning, and the less likely she will be to extend this feature in novel but appropriate ways. For example, children who learn the plural suffix -s at a late age may be more likely to try to learn which individual words take this suffix rather than to apply the suffix to a number of words as a general rule. Thus, when faced with a nonsense word task such as "Look, here's a meeb. Oh, here comes another meeb. Now there are two _____," an older child may not be likely to apply the plural suffix.

## Autistic Children

Language disorders are also prevalent in children described as autistic. **Autism** is a condition that we do not understand very well. It is defined according to the presence or absence of particular behaviors in the child. Among these are a failure to develop normal responsivity to other persons, a failure to use objects appropriately, and a generalized overreaction to certain sensory stimuli or a notable lack of response to other sensory stimuli. Another key ingredient in the definition of autism is the failure to develop normal verbal and nonverbal communication behaviors.

The cause of the language deficits exhibited by autistic children is also a mystery. Part of the problem is that we do not understand the root of autistic children's difficulty in relating to their environment. This question has provoked considerable controversy, and possible explanations have ranged from a reluctance to form interpersonal relationships to a malfunctioning of the child's neurophysiologic system. To complicate matters further, many autistic children meet the standard criteria of mental retardation. The most

*A diagnosis of autism is based on several factors, including a failure to develop normal responsivity and normal verbal and nonverbal communication.*

promising studies to date suggest that autisticlike children may have an impairment in functioning of the left hemisphere of the brain. Because the left hemisphere is usually thought to play a greater role in the processing of speech, this impairment may relate to these children's linguistic difficulty. At this point, however, this explanation must be regarded as sophisticated guesswork. Clearly, more research is needed.

As we have noted, autistic children are slow to acquire communicative skills. In this respect, they are similar to other language-disordered children; however, several characteristics of their linguistic functioning set them apart from mentally retarded children and children with specific language impairment. Autistic children often show a high frequency of unsolicited imitative verbal behavior, called **echolalia.** Other groups of children, including normally developing children, show spontaneous imitations of the speech of others. But in the case of children with autisticlike characteristics, the imitations sometimes seem less intentional and communicative. For example, normal children are more likely to imitate new, unfamiliar words than familiar ones. When familiar words are imitated, they sometimes serve an acknowledgment function, much as an older child or adult might use *yes.*

> **Mother:** Do you want some juice now?
> **Child:** Juice.

On the other hand, imitations like the following one are sometimes observed in autistic children.

> **Mother:** Hi, Bobby.
> **Bobby:** Hi, Bobby.

Nonetheless, it now appears that, for some autistic children, both immediate and delayed imitations may serve functions such as turn taking or affirming information in the utterance of another (see, for example, Prizant & Rydell, 1984). Other characteristics reported in these children include confusions with pronoun distinctions such as *I* and *you,* and a pronounced tendency to speak in a near-monotone. Another way autistic children's language seems different from that of other groups of children is that the articulation skills of autistic children, while not at age level, may often exceed their abilities in vocabulary, sentence structure, and social use of language. This is rarely the case with mentally retarded children or children with specific language impairment.

## Acquired Language Disorders

The language-disordered children described above have in common the fact that their language learning difficulties are apparent from an early age. Other children, however, after developing normally during the first years of life, lose some or all of their ability to function linguistically. This loss in linguistic ability can be the result of illness or cerebral trauma. The latter is often referred to as **closed head injury.** In preschool children, closed head injury is usually caused by a fall or a motor vehicle accident. Illnesses are often in the form of convulsive disorders.

Although the general cause of these children's problems is not in doubt, we have not been able to find a close correspondence between a particular type of injury and a particular type of language deficit. A major reason for this is that neither closed head injury nor convulsive disorders are selective in their damage. For example, closed head injury often causes diffuse cerebral swelling due to increased cerebral blood volume. Consequently, several areas of the brain can be affected.

The prevailing view is that, if damage is confined to a single hemisphere of the brain and occurs before the age of 9 years, the child will often regain the lost abilities and will continue to develop normally thereafter. In more serious cases, residual problems may persist. Often, though, the precise nature and extent of damage cannot be determined, and thus for many children, a timeline or even the probability of recovery cannot be specified.

The symptoms of the child's language difficulties depend somewhat on the age at which the injury took place. The child who suffers injury before 3 years of age will often become temporarily mute and will show a general unresponsiveness to the speech of others. Significant and often rapid improvement in linguistic ability then occurs, with the child seemingly proceeding through the major stages of language development seen in children acquiring language for the first time.

In children suffering from injury after the age of 3, the symptoms are usually different. Verbal output and understanding are diminished, but not absent altogether. Word-finding problems may be seen, however, where the child seems unable to retrieve and say a word that he used only moments before. For these children, recovery is somewhat slower, and residual problems are likely to be present in later years.

> Closed head injury *is a term used to refer to cerebral trauma in which one or more cognitive functions are temporarily or permanently disturbed.*

*Why have 4 different cut off points. Before three & After three Before nine + after?*

# ASSESSMENT OF CHILDREN'S LINGUISTIC SKILLS

## Identification

The identification of preschool children at risk for language disorders has long presented a challenge to speech-language pathologists. Unlike older children who attend elementary schools with organized speech-language screening programs, younger children often attend preschools with no formal arrangement for screening, or attend no school at all. Identification of these children, then, has depended on the vigilance of parents, preschool teachers, physicians, and other health professionals. Fortunately, some recent developments have facilitated this process.

Probably the most significant of these developments was passage of federal legislation requiring states to provide services to handicapped children—including children with language disorders—who are 3 to 5 years of age. This legislation, P.L. 99-457, also encourages states to offer services to children even younger, from birth to 2 years. The significance of this law rests not only with the fact that evaluation and treatment can now be given to many children for whom these services were previously unavailable, it will also serve to raise the awareness of many health care professionals about the importance of identifying young children with potential language problems. As a result, the disappearance of the myths concerning early intervention (see pp. 159–160) may be hastened.

## Testing

*A norm-referenced test allows an examiner to compare a child's performance to that of her age-level peers in the standardization sample.*

*Normative data are performance scores—raw scores, standardized scores, or percentile levels—that allow an examiner to compare a child's scores to those obtained by his age peers in the standardization sample.*

*Cutoff scores are either raw scores or percentile levels below which an individual child's performance is considered to be significantly lower than that expected for her age level.*

*Percentile levels or ranks indicate the percentage of children in the standardization sample for an age level who scored below a given raw score.*

Before we say that a child has a language disorder, we must conduct a thorough examination of the child's linguistic skills. Guiding this examination process is information provided by the child's parents. Such information includes the child's medical and developmental history, the nature of the communicative limitations experienced by the child, and the contexts in which these limitations are most notable. Usually two forms of assessment are used in the examination process. One form is the **norm-referenced standardized test.** Standardized language tests are available for both screening and diagnosis. Both types of standardized tests usually include **normative data** that indicate how children of various ages might be expected to perform on the test. Screening tests typically employ **cut-off scores.** If a child's performance falls below the cutoff for her chronological age, further testing is warranted.

Diagnostic tests usually provide **percentile scores** or **ranks** for each age level. Children who perform at a low percentile level, such as the 10th percentile, are generally suspected of having difficulties with the linguistic skills in question. Other diagnostic tests employ **standard scores.** The child's score is converted to a score that takes into account the average score and variability of scores obtained by similar age children. Children whose standard scores fall, say, two standard deviations below the mean are typically regarded as having difficulties with the types of linguistic skills assessed by the test.

Certain other tests are standardized in the sense that they include items that should be passed by children at designated age levels, according to the research findings of the test developer or others. Percentiles or standard scores are usually not available for these tests. Instead, the speech-language pathologist reports the specific items or developmental level of the items passed by the child. These tests might be called **descriptive tests.**

The tests available to speech-language pathologists for use with young children vary widely in terms of the specific dimensions of language tested, the theory behind the development of the tests, and importantly, how well they were standardized. A diagnostic test that is poorly standardized may provide relatively little useful information.

The second form of assessment used is the *nonstandardized probe.* Generally, these probes are individually selected or devised for each child. They are often **criterion-referenced** and are designed to examine some specific linguistic skill in considerable detail. Unlike the standardized test, no information is available concerning how a child of a particular age might be expected to perform on the probe. The speech-language pathologist must instead rely on his knowledge of normal language development. The major advantage of nonstandardized probes is that they provide considerably more detail concerning the consistency of a child's problem with a linguistic feature and the contexts in which the problem is most notable. Another valuable aspect of nonstandardized probes is that they permit the speech-language pathologist to assess a number of pragmatic skills (for instance, conversational turn taking and understanding indirect requests such as *Can you open the door?*) that are not included in standardized tests.

Standardized tests and nonstandardized probes use many of the same types of tasks. These tasks can be divided into receptive tasks, involving comprehension, and expressive tasks, involving production.

> Standard scores *are converted raw scores that have been weighted by accounting for the group mean and variability of scores (standard deviation) for the age level.*

> Criterion-referenced tests *probe behavioral repertories known to be acquired by the majority of children, usually 85%, at a specific age or stage of linguistic development.*

## Receptive Tasks

The most common form of receptive task involves **identification** or recognition. In this task, the examiner produces a word or sentence and the child chooses the picture (from several alternatives) that represents an appropriate match. For example, the speech-language pathologist may place several pictures depicting actions in front of the child and say, "Show me 'running.'" Some common tests that use this task are the Test for Auditory Comprehension of Language (Carrow, 1973) and the Peabody Picture Vocabulary Test (Dunn, 1965/1980). These tasks are especially useful in assessing the lexicon and morphology.

> Identification tasks *require the child to select a picture (or object) in response to the examiner's question.*

Another receptive task is **acting out.** Typically, this task uses toys or objects that the child can manipulate. The examiner produces a sentence, and the child acts with the objects in a manner consistent with the sentence. For example, the speech-language pathologist might place a doll and a toy car in front of the child and say, "Put the baby behind the car." The Vocabulary Comprehension Scale (Bangs, 1975) is an example of a test that uses an acting out task. Acting out can be used to assess vocabulary, morphology, syntax, and semantics.

> *In an* acting out task, *the child performs an action with an object in accordance with the examiner's request.*

The most difficult of the receptive tasks is the judgment task. **Judgment tasks** require the child to make a formal judgment of the suitability of a word or sentence. A sentence is produced by the examiner, and the child is asked whether it was "right" or "wrong" or "silly" or "O.K." For example, the

> *In a* judgment task, *the child indicates the suitability of the examiner's sentence by giving a "right" or "wrong" response.*

examiner might ask, "Is this silly or O.K.—The is shining sun?" This task can be seen in several items of the Bankson Language Screening Test (Bankson, 1977). Again, it can be used to assess the lexicon, morphology, syntax, and semantics.

The speech-language pathologist must be aware of the limitations of each of these tasks. In the identification task, a child may appear to comprehend when actually her identification of the appropriate picture is based on a lucky guess. A child might also make a correct response on this test not because she knows the word or sentence, but because she knows enough about the alternative pictures to rule them out as possible selections. (Many of us have used a similar strategy when faced with multiple-choice tests.) Finally, identification tasks test a relatively superficial form of comprehension, that of recognition. Probably we have all had the experience of forgetting the melody or lyrics of a song that, when played for us, we recognize as the song in question. A similar process seems to be involved in identification tasks.

The chief precaution to take when administering an acting out task is to ensure that the child is not using a strategy requiring full understanding of the material being presented. For example, young children may respond correctly to the sentence *The truck is pushing the car,* not because they fully comprehend the sentence, but because their knowledge of the real world suggests that it is more likely for a truck to push a car than vice versa.

The major limitation of the judgment task is that it often proves too difficult for children under the age of 4 years. The apparent reason is that this task requires the child to think about the form of a word or sentence independent of its meaning. For example, young children seem to attend to the fact that two sentences such as *The boy runs down the street* and *The boy run down the street* have the same meaning. Not until they reach at least age 4 do they attend to the fact that one of these sentences is not constructed as well as it might be.

## Expressive Tasks

Elicited imitation tasks *require the child to repeat the examiner's utterances.*

One of the most commonly used tasks of linguistic expression is the **elicited imitation task.** In this task, the examiner produces a sentence, and the child is asked to repeat it. The assumption behind this task is that, if a child does not use a particular linguistic feature properly, he is unlikely to use it in imitation—particularly if no undue attention is placed on the feature when it is presented by the speech-language pathologist. For example, a child who does not ordinarily use the article *the* in everyday speech is likely to imitate the sentence *Daddy put the ball on the table* as "Daddy put ball on table." The Stephens Oral Language Screening Test (Stephens, 1977) is one of several tests that employ elicited imitation. This task is helpful for assessing morphology, syntax, and semantics.

A somewhat similar procedure, used to assess the same skills, is the **delayed imitation task.** In this task, the child's response is further removed in time from the speech-language pathologist's production than is the case for the elicited imitation task. Assume, for example, that a child's use of the plural -s is in question. The examiner might pace two pictures in front of the child and say, "The man sees the boy," "The man sees the boys"; then, pointing to one of the pictures, "Which one is this?" This task is used in the Northwestern Syntax Screening Test (Lee, 1971).

*In* ta: *tu produced by the examiner, and repeats the one that matches an accompanying picture.*

The **carrier phrase task** is another task of linguistic expression. A portion of a sentence is spoken by the examiner, and the child is asked to complete it. For instance, a child's use of the pronoun *she* might be tested by presenting three pictures of a particular girl performing different activities. The speech-language pathologist might describe the first two pictures for the child, and have the child describe the third. The following sequence might set the occasion for the child's use of a response that includes *she*: "Look, here the girl is riding a bike, and here the girl is eating a cookie, and here (pointing to a picture of the girl throwing a ball) _____." This task can be seen, for example, in one of the subtests of the Test of Language Development-Primary (Newcomer & Hammill, 1977). It is especially useful in assessing morphology and syntax.

*The child completes the examiner's sentence with the appropriate word or phrase in a* carrier phrase task.

An expressive task that has certain features in common with the carrier phrase task is the **parallel sentence production task.** Typically, two pictures are placed in front of the child. The speech-language pathologist describes the first picture using a particular sentence pattern, and the child is asked to describe the second picture. It is assumed that the pattern used in the examiner's sentence will influence the type of sentence attempted by the child. For example, if a picture of a large ball and a picture of a small ball were used, the following interchange might be expected.

*In a parallel sentence production task, the examiner describes pictures (in a particular manner), and then asks the child to describe new pictures that can be described using the same sentence pattern.*

> **Examiner:** I'm going to talk about this picture (points to picture), and then you talk about that picture (points to other picture.) Ready? (Points to first picture.) This is a big ball.
> **Child:** (Points to second picture.) This is a little ball.

The parallel sentence production task is quite useful in testing morphological and syntactic features that children might not otherwise attempt frequently. An example of this task can be seen in the CID Grammatical Analysis of Elicited Language (Moog & Geers, 1979).

A child's expressive language is often assessed by examining a sample of her spontaneous speech. If the child's utterances are to be truly spontaneous, of course, nothing in the questions or instructions should dictate how the child should respond. However, to increase the likelihood that the child will provide a sufficient number of utterances, or a sufficient number of utterances of a certain type, open-ended questions or requests are often presented (for example, "Tell me about this"). Thus, the utterances the child produces during these sampling situations are evoked or influenced to some degree by the speech-language pathologist. Collecting and analyzing a sample of a child's speech are usually more time consuming than giving any one test of language. Several studies have indicated that this inconvenience is offset, however, by the fact that speech samples often yield more information about a child's linguistic skills than language tests. Speech samples are especially useful in assessing pragmatic abilities (see, for example, Prutting & Kirchner, 1987). Analysis time can be reduced considerably through use of computer-assisted programs that are now available. Each of these requires the speech-language pathologist to transcribe the tape recordings of the child's utterances and to enter these utterances on the computer. Once entered, the utterances are automatically and rapidly analyzed for a range of semantic, syntactic, and phonological features. Two examples of computer-assisted analysis programs are Systematic Analysis of Language Transcripts (Miller & Chapman, 1983) and Computerized Profiling (Long, 1987).

As with receptive tasks, there are limitations to the use of expressive tasks. One risk involved in the use of imitation is that the child may have good auditory memory skills and repeat a sentence with greater accuracy than might be expected given his spontaneous speech characteristics. Carrier phrase tasks usually require only a one- or two-word response from the child. Therefore, even if a child produces a plural or past tense ending correctly, we do not know whether he can do so in a complete sentence. The greatest limitation of a spontaneous speech sample is that it may not include a number of linguistic features that infrequently occur. For example, the child may not attempt sentences in the passive voice such as *The car was hit by the train,* or words that require the plural *-es* such as *dishes* in the speech sample. Yet the child might have difficulties with these linguistic features.

## The Assessment Process

An example might be helpful in illustrating the assessment of a child who is suspected of having linguistic difficulties. Assume that a 4-year-old child is brought to a speech-language clinic with the parental complaint that he "doesn't seem to understand when we ask him to do things." Initial contact with the child in an informal rapport-building play activity suggests that the child's productions are limited to single- and two-word utterances. Because this level of linguistic expression is markedly delayed relative to his age, attention turns to whether or not this expressive problem might be due to limitations in comprehension.

After we have determined that the child's hearing sensitivity, based on audiometric testing, is within normal limits, we might give him a standardized comprehension test that includes both word comprehension and sentence comprehension. Assume that the child is found to perform slightly below average for his age level on the word comprehension section, and well below age level on the section dealing with sentence comprehension. Noting that the sentences on which the child had the greatest difficulty were not only the most grammatically complex but also the longest, we might administer another standardized comprehension test, one that tests the child's comprehension of increasingly longer sentences that have only limited grammatical complexity. Let us assume that on this test the child performs only slightly below age level.

If these two tests used the same type of task and were both standardized on children with cultural and socioeconomic backgrounds comparable to that of the child, we might assume that the child's problems rest mainly in comprehension difficulty with relatively complex grammatical constructions. Ordinarily, we should determine whether this apparent problem is caused by difficulty the child has with the type of task used in the standardized test. In this case, however, we know that the child performed considerably better on the word comprehension section of the same test, which used the same task. Therefore, it seems reasonable to assume that the child's difficulty rests with the grammatical constructions themselves.

Some standardized tests use a variety of tasks. When a child performs better on one section of the test than another, we cannot always tell whether the child has greater ability with the linguistic features assessed in the section or greater ability with the task used as the means of assessment.

At this point, nonstandardized probes would probably be selected. The probes would help us determine the degree of difficulty the child has with some of the grammatical constructions used in the standardized test. Typically, standardized tests cover a range of abilities falling within some fairly broad area of language, such as receptive vocabulary or receptive grammar. Only a few test items are devoted to any particular type of word or grammatical construction. Without the use of probes, we would have evidence that the child is performing below age level in some area such as receptive grammar, but we would be somewhat hard pressed to select a particular grammatical construction to teach the child.

In selecting particular grammatical constructions for detailed probing, we would examine the results of the standardized test and select those constructions the child found troublesome and that are ordinarily acquired at the earliest ages. Alternatively, we might select from the test those constructions whose appearance in the everyday speech the child hears might well cause the kinds of comprehension problems noted by his parents. We might select two such grammatical constructions and design 10 probe items for each. The child's performance on these probes should provide more detailed information concerning the degree of difficulty he has with these constructions, and the appropriateness of these constructions as a focus for language intervention, than would be possible through an examination of the child's standardized test performance alone.

## Instruction in the Assessment Process

An adequate evaluation of a child's linguistic skills should not be limited to the overall assessment of linguistic functioning and the identification of one or two linguistic features that might serve as initial targets for intervention. Attempts should also be made to determine whether the child's comprehension or production of the feature seems amenable to instruction and, if so, which procedure seems most suitable. Generally, this process involves trying a sampling of plausible intervention procedures with the child until you find one or two that may be promising. These efforts usually take only a few minutes, as they are generally conducted during a diagnostic session that includes other activities important to the evaluation process—obtaining case history information, audiometric testing, the administration of language tests and probes, the assessment of the child's oral structure and functioning, and the assessment of other suspect aspects of the child's communicative functioning. The information obtained from these attempts at modifying the child's performance with these linguistic features can be invaluable to the process of designing intervention activities. Many of the procedures that might be appropriate to try during the diagnostic session are discussed in the following section on intervention procedures.

## PROCEDURES FOR TEACHING SPECIFIC LINGUISTIC FEATURES

In certain respects, language intervention is not much different from articulation training, therapy directed toward increasing vocal control, or other treatment. When approaching the task of modifying any behavior, the speech-language pathologist must keep certain principles in mind. For example, a careful specification of the desired or "terminal" behavior is needed, as well as a detailed description of the child's current or "entry" behavior. A carefully constructed sequence of steps proceeding from the entry to the terminal behavior is also crucial. In addition, the criterion for moving from one step to the next must be spelled out. Within any given step, we should specify the verbal and/or visual stimuli used to evoke the child's response and describe the characteristics of the child's response that are needed for the response to be judged as accurate. Finally, the nature of the feedback the child receives for correct and incorrect responses must be detailed.

These principles do not dictate any specific procedure that must be used; in fact, a number of language intervention procedures have been successfully employed. The particular procedures used are often based on the age and language abilities of the child and the theoretical orientation of the speech-language pathologist. Of course, trends can be seen in the language intervention procedures adopted. For example, there has been a trend toward procedures used in group settings that emphasize the social functions of language. There has also been a trend toward developing procedures for very young children. As long as children vary as widely as they do in the nature and severity of their linguistic difficulties and in the relative strengths they bring to language-learning tasks, there will always be a range of intervention procedures with which the speech-language pathologist should be familiar. We will discuss representative procedures, divided according to their major focus. These procedures can be used for work on pragmatic, morphological, syntactic, or semantic features. By introducing new words as the child masters the use of the feature, the speech-language pathologist can also help the child expand her vocabulary.

# Oral Language Production

## Procedures Involving Direct Imitation

A significant number of intervention procedures use an **imitation-based approach.** Often imitation procedures involve visual stimuli, such as pictures or enactments performed in the child's presence; verbal stimuli, such as a request or question asked of the child; and the use of an imitative prompt (see, for example, Connell, 1987). For example, a procedure designed to teach the child the use of two-word utterances such as *push truck* and *throw ball* might include the following sequence at the outset.

Imitation-based approaches *require the child to imitate the speech-language pathologist's utterance in response to a verbal prompt.*

> **Speech-language pathologist:** (Pushes a toy truck.) What am I doing? Say "push truck."
> **Child:** Push truck.

These components are used to provide the child with maximum assistance during the initial stage of training, assistance that may be necessary because the child is being asked to attempt a linguistic feature that he has not used before. As the child becomes more proficient with the feature, the imitative prompt is removed.

> **Speech-language pathologist:** (Tosses a ball.) What am I doing?
> **Child:** Throw ball.

Other procedures using imitation appear to place fewer demands on the child (see Warren & Kaiser, 1986). Some of these employ an informal play format. A close inspection of these sessions often reveals considerably more than first meets the eye. Consider the following events. The setting is a preschool play/work room containing a number of toys such as blocks, toy silverware, dolls, wind-up toys, a ball, and several toy cars. Three children attend the preschool sessions. Each produces speech limited for the most part to single-word utterances, although some two-word utterances are heard. Some of the activities of one of these children are described below.

> (Child picks up a clear plastic box containing several toy cars. The child is unable to remove the lid of the box and looks up at the speech-language pathologist.)
> **Child:** Car.
> (Speech-language pathologist looks toward child, pauses.)

**Child:** Car.
**Speech-language pathologist:** What do you want?
**Child:** Want car.
**Speech-language pathologist:** Oh, let me help (opens box and child takes out a toy car).
(A few minutes later the child joins the speech-language pathologist, who is playing with a doll. The speech-language pathologist "feeds" the doll using a toy fork.)
**Speech-language pathologist:** Here, you play with the baby (gives child doll, continues to hold the fork, spoon, and cup). Maybe she wants a drink.
(Child looks up at speech-language pathclogist.)
**Child:** Cup.
(Speech-language pathologist looks toward the child, pauses.)
**Child:** Want cup.
**Speech-language pathologist:** (Hands the cup to the child) Here's the cup.
(Several minutes later the child picks up the ball.)
**Speech-language pathologist:** Oh, roll the ball over here. Roll the ball.
(Child rolls the ball to speech-language pathologist, who then rolls it back.)
**Speech-language pathologist:** Roll it again.
(Child rolls ball to speech-language pathologist, who then pretends to attend to something else while still holding ball.)
**Child:** Ball.
(Speech-language pathologist looks toward child, pauses.)
**Child:** Ball.
**Speech-language pathologist:** Say "want ball."
**Child:** Want ball.

The speech-language pathologist's goal for this session was to increase the child's use of certain highly functional two-word constructions, such as *want* combined with the name of the object or action desired (*want cookie, want ball, want do*). The procedure adopted requires the use of the target construction in a natural and situationally appropriate context. For this reason, the speech-language pathologist carefully selected the materials to be used in the session and determined beforehand the activities involving these materials that might set the occasion for the child's use of the target construction. Thus, the speech-language pathologist had placed some presumably desirable objects (toy cars) in a clear plastic container that she knew would be difficult for the child to open. Similarly, she deliberately withheld the cup when giving the child the doll and knowingly failed to roll the ball back to the child. Each of these was designed to result in a situation where the child had to make a request that could be expressed with the target construction. The speech-language pathologist gave the desired assistance only when the child produced the request with this construction. As this was a new linguistic behavior for the child, however, "correct" requests could not be expected in each instance. Therefore, the speech-language pathologist planned the following strategy.

1. Set the occasion for a request by the child.
2. If the request is expressed in the target construction, give the child the assistance requested.
3. If not, look at the child and pause. Give assistance if the target construction is used.
4. If not, ask a question that contains one of the words the child should use in the request (*What do you want?*) Give assistance if the target construction is used.
5. If not, produce the request for, the child to imitate. Give assistance if the imitation is accurate.

As you can see, additional clues are provided only when they seem necessary. With this procedure, it is assumed that when the child gains greater control of the target construction he will use it in his initial request, since this would enable him to obtain assistance most quickly.

A major advantage of imitation procedures is their effectiveness in evoking responses from the child that at least approximate the desired behavior. The intellectual and motor skills necessary to match the behavior of another person are intact in most children, provided that the particular behavior the child is asked to imitate does not greatly exceed his current skill level.

One of the limitations of imitation procedures is that they are somewhat awkward to use when attempting to teach pragmatics, or linguistic features that are closely related to discourse. For example, children gradually develop an awareness that, when a question is asked of them, a response to the question is expected. In an imitation approach, the child must inhibit the tendency to respond to the question and instead attempt to produce the question himself.

> **Speech-language pathologist:** Say "Where am I going?"
> **Child:** Where am I going?

## Procedures Involving Modeling

Several other language intervention procedures use a **modeling approach.** In this approach, the child observes someone else, usually the speech-language pathologist or a third participant, present examples of the linguistic feature serving as the focus of intervention. The child is not asked to imitate the modeled examples. Rather, the child is instructed that the model will be talking in a "special way" and that she should listen carefully, for she will soon be given a turn to speak (see Connell, 1987). An example of a segment from a modeling session is presented below. In this session, a third participant is serving as the model. The focus of intervention is on the use of questions containing both *what* and the auxiliary verb *is.*

*Modeling approaches involve the production of examples of a sentence pattern by the speech-language pathologist or a third participant to describe pictures. The child is asked to listen to the examples and describe new pictures using the same pattern.*

**Speech-language pathologist:** I have some pictures of some people doing some things and some animals doing some things. I'm not going to show you the pictures unless you ask me about them. But you have to ask in a special way. Bobby [the child], you listen to Julie [the model] first and then it will be your turn to ask questions. Ready? (Speech-language pathologist turns to model.) Ask me about the first picture. It shows a boy eating.

**Julie:** What is the boy eating?

**Speech-language pathologist:** The boy is eating an apple. See? (Shows picture.) That was a good question. This next picture shows a dog watching.

**Julie:** What dog watching?

**Speech-language pathologist:** You didn't ask very well.

**Julie:** What *is* the dog watching?

**Speech-language pathologist:** See? (Shows picture.) The dog is watching the goldfish. That was a good question. Try another. This shows the girl throwing.

**Julie:** What is the girl throwing?

**Speech-language pathologist:** (Shows picture.) An egg. I bet that will make a mess. That was a good question. O.K., Bobby, you ask some questions now. This picture shows a man cleaning.

**Bobby:** What the man is cleaning?

As you can see, in a modeling procedure, the child does not attempt to immediately repeat the model's utterance. Instead, the child attempts to determine what form the utterance is expected to take by listening to the model and observing whether the speech-language pathologist regards the model's utterance as acceptable. Of course, this is a type of imitation, but it is a rule for combining and sequencing words that the child is imitating, not particular utterances that were spoken by the model. For example, the model had never produced the question *What is the man cleaning?* in the session described above, yet the child was asked to produce this question. (In our example, Bobby did not produce it with complete accuracy.) This approach can be helpful in working on pragmatics skills, as well as other linguistic abilities.

One language intervention approach that shares certain characteristics with this modeling approach might be called a **focused stimulation approach.** The approach of Lee, Koenigsknecht, and Mulhern (1975) seems to fall in this category. In this approach, the child is provided with concentrated exposure to particular linguistic features with which he has been found to have difficulty. In those instances where the child's expressive ability with these features is in question, he may be asked to produce the linguistic feature. Compared with the modeling approach we have already described, however, focused stimulation involves a considerably higher degree of exposure for the number of responses required of the child.

A storytelling format is frequently used in this approach. The story told to the child contains two or three linguistic features proving troublesome for the child. Several examples of each feature appear in the story. For example, assume a child shows a tendency to produce *him* and *her* when *he* and *she,*

*In a focused stimulation approach, the speech-language pathologist provides many examples of a linguistic feature, and, on occasion, may ask the child to use the feature.*

respectively, should be used (*Him flying a plane, Her sleeping*), and uses the negative form *not* when *can't* should be used. The speech-language pathologist might devise several stories that include these features. Pictures might also be used to accompany the stories, to help the child understand the story.

> Here is a girl who likes to play games. *She* likes hide-and-seek and hopscotch. *She* likes baseball too. The girl wants to learn new games. *She* wants to play football with her brothers. But the girl's father says no. "You *can't* play football," the father says. "You *can't* throw the ball far and you will get hurt if they tackle you." "Then I'll tackle them," says the girl. "But you *can't* tackle them. They're too big," the father says. The girl is sad. But then *she* finds a new game—running.

Following the story, the speech-language pathologist may ask questions such as *What did the father say?* to give the child practice in producing the target linguistic features. Through the use of several stories containing these features, the child should acquire greater understanding of these features and how and where they are used in sentences. By being given the opportunity to respond verbally after each story, the child will gain greater control over her production of these features.

Procedures involving modeling seem well suited for teaching children various linguistic features. Through the use of carefully selected examples produced by a model, the child is in a position to learn how and where the linguistic feature is to be used. In addition, modeling seems somewhat less artificial than some approaches, making the transfer from use in the teaching environment to use in the child's natural environment more likely. However, the effectiveness of modeling depends on the child's ability to pay attention. Unfortunately, a number of children do not demonstrate anything more than sporadic and fleeting attention to the speech of others. For these children, modeling procedures are probably not effective.

## Reactive Language Stimulation Approaches

The approaches described above have at least two features in common: they focus on specific linguistic forms, and the speech-language pathologist controls the activities and the topic of conversation. In contrast, some approaches have as their aim general language stimulation. An assumption behind some of these approaches, known as **reactive language stimulation approaches,** is that the best language-learning environment is one in which the child is free to control the topic and the speech-language pathologist reacts, nonpunitively, to the child's utterances. One of the techniques used in these approaches is *expansion*, as in the example below.

**Child:** (Looking at a picture.) Dolly bed.
**Speech-language pathologist:** The dolly is in her bed.

*Reactive language stimulation approaches permit the child to control the topic and activities. The speech-language pathologist reacts to the child's utterances, often using features that illustrate more accurate ways of saying the same thing.*

Often, approaches such as these are used in a classroom or group setting. Although this general approach has been in existence for some time, updated versions have been developed (see Weiss, 1981).

### Oral Language Comprehension

*In a* comprehension-based approach, *the child is taught to comprehend a feature of language before (or instead of) being taught to produce it.*

Several language intervention procedures can be characterized as **comprehension-based approaches** (see, for example, Winitz, 1973). The assumption behind some of these procedures is that the child needs to understand particular linguistic features before she can be taught to produce them. Other procedures assume that if a child learns to comprehend these features, she will begin to produce them with little or no direct instruction in expression. The two types of procedures are similar in their methodology.

For example, assume that a child does not yet comprehend the double object construction used in utterances such as *She showed the boy the car* and *Daddy gave Mommy the baby.* The speech-language pathologist may place three pictures in front of the child. One picture might depict a woman showing a boy a car, another might depict a boy showing a woman a car, and a third might depict a woman pointing to the boy while looking at the car (as if "showing" the boy to the car). The child would be asked, "Point to *She showed the boy the car.*" If the child points to the wrong picture, the speech-language pathologist would indicate which picture was correct. This method would continue, using additional sets of pictures appropriate for other possible sentences involving the double object construction. Once the child consistently indicates comprehension, a production probe might be administered. For example, the speech-language pathologist may use a parallel sentence production task, where he describes a picture using the double object construction and asks the child to describe a second picture. The extent to which the child is able to use this construction will indicate the extent to which the comprehension training facilitated the child's production abilities.

## NONSPEECH COMMUNICATION

For some children, the acquisition of spoken language is not a realistic goal. The limited degree of physical control these children have over their speech mechanisms makes it unlikely that they would acquire the ability to produce recognizable speech; however, many of these children can acquire the ability to communicate if given alternative means. In recent years, a number of communication systems have been devised for these children (see, for example, Capozzi & Mineo, 1984; Fristoe & Lloyd, 1979). These systems allow the child to transmit messages without use of spoken language.

The particular nonvocal communication system selected will depend on the motor abilities of the child and her level of intellectual functioning. The systems available cover an enormous range. For children with sufficient physical coordination, sign systems such as American Sign Language may be used. Frequently other types of systems are employed. For example, children with physical coordination and intellectual limitations may use a system where the child nods when another person points to a picture representing a desired object. Children with greater intellectual ability might use a system where the child spells messages on a grid using row-column scanning with an electronic device. Other children might use a system in which the child constructs a message on a specially designed typewriter whose output is displayed on a television monitor.

Before some of these systems can be used by the child, the optimal means of responding must be determined. This decision is based not only on the nature of physical control the child has over her body, but also on how well the communication system can be adapted to responsiveness to this type of control. Often innovative solutions have arisen from such considerations. Some children can make use of sophisticated communication systems by either direct selection or a code, such as Morse Code; with head movements; sipping and blowing through a tube; and even with movements of the big toe.

Without question, the area of nonspeech communication will continue to undergo rapid expansion. New systems will be developed and clever ways of interacting with these systems will be devised. Microcomputers, already used in some nonspeech communication systems, will play an even larger part in the years to come.

For many children unable to speak, the greatest need is to select an appropriate nonspeech communication system. These children often have adequate (or superior) intellectual skills, so the learning of the system requires primarily a familiarization phase and a great deal of practice. For other children, however, selection of a system is but a small part of the solution. These children must learn the function of the system; that is, they must learn not only how to use the system but that the system is used to communicate.

Let us look at an example of how a system of nonspeech communication might be taught to this type of child. Assume that a speech-language pathologist is working with a multiply handicapped child who is mentally retarded and has severe motor limitations that have prevented him from gaining any benefit from training in spoken language. The speech-language pathologist selects or designs a "communication board" to sit on the child's wheelchair arms. The board contains a number of pictures of common objects and activities arranged in rows and columns.

A major goal in this approach is to teach the child that his pointing at a particular picture serves as a request for the object or activity shown in that picture. He must also learn the picture that corresponds to each object or activity. The speech-language pathologist might initially place a single picture in front of the child. She would place the child's finger on the picture and then present the corresponding object (for example, a radio) or have the child perform the corresponding activity (for example, drink some juice). Eventually, the child would be required to point to the picture without assistance from the speech-language pathologist to receive the desired object or activity.

Once the child consistently points to the first object, the speech-language pathologist would introduce additional pictures corresponding to other objects and activities. Initially, the pictures would be presented singly to ensure that the child has opportunity to learn the meanings of each one. Subsequently, two pictures would be presented at the same time, then three, and so on, until the child shows the ability to point appropriately when the full complement of pictures is before him. As with other procedures, it is important to introduce new elements one at a time and to reinforce the child for gradually improving approximations of the correct response.

# GENERALIZATION

As we have seen, we cannot discuss the issue of language intervention without also discussing generalization. Teaching a child to use a new linguistic feature is only half the battle. The other half comes in ensuring that the child is able to construct her own utterances involving the new linguistic feature and that she is able to use these utterances in settings quite different from the setting in which the feature was first taught. Language consists of an infinite number of word combinations, and it is impossible to provide a child with direct training on each of them. Similarly, the professional cannot accompany the child to every situation in which she might speak to ensure that she has received training in every possible setting. Fortunately, generalization need not be left to chance. The speech-language pathologist can take active steps to increase its likelihood. We will describe some of these steps next.

## Utterance Form Generalization

Utterance form generalization *is the ability to apply a learned sentence pattern to new utterances.*

One type of generalization might be called **utterance form generalization.** This type of generalization is essential for any language intervention procedure designed to teach some type of linguistic rule or construction. For example, assume that a child is taught the use of two-word utterances reflecting the action + object construction. Let us assume that these utterances were learned in the context of describing the speech-language pathologist's actions on the objects mentioned in the utterances. For example, the child learned to say *kick truck* when watching the speech-language pathologist kick a toy truck.

There would certainly be little reason to believe that the child had acquired a linguistic rule if he did not also show untrained usage, like the examples in the second column in Table 5.2. In this column, the utterance listed involves both an action and object that were used during action + object training. During this training, however, the action was not performed on this particular object; other actions were used with the object. As this utterance represents only a recombination of trained material, it does not represent a significant extension of the trained behavior. As we move to the third and fourth columns of the table, however, the utterances reflect greater ability on the child's part to incorporate new words into the trained pattern. This usage seems to constitute evidence that the child has learned the rule. To cite an example, the child's use of *push block* reflects an ability to combine two words that were never used in action + object training. The fact that he could do this suggests that, during training, the child was learning a rule for combining words involved in an action-on-object relationship, not merely a series of particular word combinations. It is the speech-language pathologist's responsibility not only to teach the child a number of word combinations reflecting a particular construction or rule, but also to ensure, through the use of untrained probes, that the child's usage reflects the rule rather than rote learning. If the child does not show rule application, the usual strategy is to provide additional examples of the rule in training. The assumption is that additional examples may tax the child's rote memory, leading him to look for more general principles that may provide cues as to how the words should be combined.

## Position Generalization

Along with utterance form generalization, speech-language pathologists rely on **position generalization.** Several linguistic features, such as the articles *a* and *the,* adjectives, prepositions, and even certain verbs, can appear in different sentence positions. For example, *the* may appear in sentences such as *The knife is gone* as well as *Wanda saw the ghost. Was* may appear in sentences such as *Hal was a singer* as well as *Was the man here?*

*In* position generalization, *the child uses a newly taught feature in a new sentence position.*

**Table 5.2**  Some Examples of Utterance Form Generalization

| Trained Examples | Untrained Examples Observed During Probes | | |
| | New Permutation | One New Element | Two New Elements |
| --- | --- | --- | --- |
| throw ball throw truck kick truck | kick ball | roll truck | push block |

Position generalization may be promoted by providing the child with practice in using the trained linguistic feature in more than one sentence position. For example, the child might be taught the use of *the* in sentences such as *The ball rolled away* and *I took the ball from Jason*. In the initial stage of this process, it might be helpful to the child if *the* preceded the same word (*ball*) when its position in the sentence is changed. Subsequently, the words immediately following *the* could vary. Following this training, probes could be used to determine if the child is beginning to use *the* in still other sentence positions. For example, the child could be tested on sentences such as *He put it on the table.*

## Stimulus Generalization

Stimulus generalization *is the ability to use a newly taught feature when the physical setting, interactants, and/or verbal context are changed.*

One of the most exasperating experiences a speech-language pathologist can face is working with a child who shows good use of linguistic features in the clinic setting, but who shows little or no use of the features in everyday surroundings. Unfortunately, this problem is frequently encountered. The solution is to take active steps to facilitate **stimulus generalization.** A first step in promoting stimulus generalization is to note the differences between the stimulus conditions involved during language intervention activities and the conditions involved in the child's everyday speech. Minimally, these involve the physical setting in which the child's use of the trained linguistic feature may occur, the persons to whom the child may speak while using (or failing to use) the trained linguistic feature, and the particular utterances directed to the child that might lead her to respond with an utterance containing (or omitting) the trained linguistic feature. Once the child shows an ability to use the linguistic feature in one circumstance, the speech-language pathologist attempts to gradually modify the conditions surrounding this circumstance until they resemble the speaking situations in which the child ordinarily finds herself.

An example of the steps involved in facilitating stimulus generalization may be helpful. Assume that a severely retarded child has been taught to vocalize to get another person's attention, and then to make the sign for "eat" or "drink" whenever she wishes some food or beverage. The procedure involved the speech-language pathologist taking some food or beverage from a bag and preparing to eat it, without offering any to the child. All treatment sessions took placed in an assigned therapy room in the child's school. At this point, the parent could be asked to perform this same act of preparing food in the same therapy room. The next step might involve the parent using new food items that might appeal to the child. Once the child shows an ability to vocalize and sign under these circumstances, the activity could be repeated in another room in the school, and, eventually, in the home. Finally, other family members could perform the food preparation in the child's presence. Through the use of several settings, a range of foods and beverages, and several interactants, the child should learn that the behavior taught is communication itself, and not simply part of a game that is played whenever she is with the speech-language pathologist.

# COUNSELING

Like other communication disorders, language disorders constitute a family problem, not simply a problem of the child. The family considerations involved can take a number of forms. First, we must determine whether the ways in which family members interact with the child might be contributing to the child's problem. Earlier in this chapter, we noted that the interactions between language-disordered children and their parents are somewhat different from those between normally developing children and their parents; however, the reasons for this difference are unclear. Language-disordered children are sometimes not very responsive to parents' attempts to communicate. Therefore, it would be unwise to assume that parents of language-disordered children, even those who seem more directive than most parents, are the cause of their children's language problems.

At the same time, the speech-language pathologist must be on the lookout for extreme cases. For example, if a parent simply gives up and stops talking to the child, or talks to the child as if the child understood nothing that was said, the speech-language pathologist would have reason for concern. In these cases, it would be valuable to counsel the parents concerning the linguistic abilities the child does possess and the ways in which the parents might change their communications with the child. When parents of language-disordered children are encouraged to increase their verbal commentary on their activities and supplement it with occasional questions directed to their child, significant increases in the child's linguistic skills may result.

The literature on the interactions between parents and their normally developing children also offers a few suggestions concerning possible ways parents might interact with their language-disordered children. For example, parents of normal children typically produce utterances that are shorter, grammatically and semantically simpler, more fluent, and more redundant when talking with less linguistically sophisticated children than when talking with more sophisticated children and adults. Their explicit corrective feedback seems limited to semantic inaccuracies in their children's utterances; corrections of grammatical inaccuracies are less frequent, and when they occur, they are rarely accompanied by words such as *no*.

> **Child:** (Looking at picture in book.) See horsie, mom.
> **Mother:** No, that's a giraffe.
> **Child:** Waffe (looks at picture). Sheeps. Look a sheeps.
> **Mother:** Yes, sheep. They're eating some grass for dinner.

Parents might also be alerted to the influences that siblings may have on a child's linguistic development. Parents of language-disordered children often express concern that older siblings may have a detrimental effect on their child's development because the older children understand the younger child's communicative intents and do not encourage the child to use his best speech; however, research with normally developing children suggests that the age differential between older and younger child is a critical factor. When no more than 2 years separate the older and younger child, the linguistic development of the younger child actually seems to benefit, proceeding faster than that of only children and children with siblings who are considerably older.

Although parents of language-disordered children may not be the cause of their child's difficulties with language, they may often feel that they are. Certainly many parents are concerned about whether their interactions with their child promote the child's linguistic development. Other parents feel guilty—ranging from a feeling that they may have provided inadequate language stimulation for their child to acquire language properly, to a feeling of guilt for not being able to produce a normal, healthy baby. The speech-language pathologist must determine the nature and degree of the parents' concerns. For those parents whose concerns are over providing the child with the most facilitative linguistic environment possible, counseling might include discussion of methods of providing the child with the most optimal linguistic input and the types of activities and interactions that might be most beneficial.

This is not to say that these parents have no needs of their own. One of my most vivid memories is of a mother who was faced with the problem of determining what to do about her son's tendency to get up in the middle of the night and explore electrical appliances, taste food kept in the refrigerator, and bend or break small household objects. Her decision, after considering the danger that might come to her son even with added precautions, was to lock him in his room once he went to sleep. The mother needed a great deal of support once this difficult decision was made. In some cases, counseling should be principally limited to the needs of the parents. These are the parents who may feel that they have caused or contributed in some way to their child's problem. These feelings may have been aggravated by other professionals (perhaps physicians or psychologists) who explicitly blame the parents for the young child's language delay. This is a particular concern with autism, which some feel to be basically an emotional problem. For parents such as these, efforts at instructing them in optimal language stimulation activities may simply confirm in their mind that they had been doing things wrong all along. The unwarranted guilt of these parents must be allayed before the focus turns to the linguistic needs of the child.

One of the chief counseling responsibilities of the speech-language pathologist is to inform parents when he feels the child would benefit from being seen by professionals in other fields. For example, a child's lack of

motor coordination and poor attention span might justify an examination '
a pediatric neurologist. A child's slow progress during language train,
coupled with an apparent difficulty comprehending tasks whose instructions
can be conveyed without the use of language, might warrant referral for
psychological testing. It is important that the speech-language pathologist
justify the referral. For example, parents need to know that a thorough
neurological examination may result in the recommendation that the child
do particular neuromotor exercises to improve coordination or that the child
receive medication to improve his attention span. Psychological testing
might suggest the need for instruction directed at other developmental skills
in addition to language. It is not adequate to justify the economic and
emotional expense of these referrals by simply telling parents that "more
information would be helpful." The speech-language pathologist should
clearly state what information can be gained and how it might be helpful.

Finally, it is important that speech-language pathologists provide parents
with a reasonable estimate of what to expect for the future. We cannot and
should not make detailed predictions of a child's future status; however, we
can certainly provide parents with some general idea of the expected
duration of treatment. Many language-disordered children require years of
treatment for their linguistic difficulties, and most experienced speech-
language pathologists can identify these children by the initial severity of their
problems and by their slow progress during the first several months of
intervention. It would be unfair to convey a wait-and-see attitude to the
parents of these children. They may need to make financial plans for a long
period of receiving professional services, and they may need time to arrange
their lifestyle to accommodate a long-term routine of transporting the child
to the treatment facility.

The speech-language pathologist must also assume one other responsibility. A number of long-term studies of language-disordered children reveal
that these children may have residual linguistic difficulties throughout
childhood and into adolescence (Weiner, 1985). Often these difficulties make
the process of learning to read and write more problematic. Many of these
children require extra help in reading and writing and may even be assigned
to "special" classes to accomplish this end. The parents of children with
more serious language problems should probably be alerted to this possibility, and they should be informed of some of the professionals in other fields
who may provide useful guidance in this matter. The related problem of
language disorders as they affect school-age children is examined in depth
in the next chapter.

# STUDY QUESTIONS

1. Language-disordered children are often examined relative to the stages of
   development seen in normal children. Using features of normal language

development from chapter 2, replace the attainments listed in Table 5.1 with new ones. Try to construct this new table so that language-disordered children's development lags behind that of normally developing children.

2. Where possible, identify characteristics of language that distinguish the following groups of children from the others: children with specific language impairment, mental retardation, autism, acquired language disorders.

3. Design three items that exemplify each of the assessment tasks described in the chapter.

4. Select two of the teaching approaches described in the chapter and describe how you would teach three-word utterances, for example, *Mommy chase kitty,* using each approach.

5. Generalization of linguistic features is discussed on pages 186–189. Three forms are mentioned: utterance form, position, and stimulus generalization. Reflect on your own experiences in learning to read or learning math in the elementary grades, or consult elementary level texts. Identify and describe analogies to three types of generalization. You may, for example, analyze generalization in teaching math concepts, operations, and applications to verbal math problems, or to teaching the alphabet, long and short vowels, and reading of word families and sentences.

6. Select two systems of nonspeech communication and describe the motor and intellectual abilities of a child who might be appropriate for each.

## SELECTED READINGS

Bloom, L., & Lahey, M. (1978). *Language development and language disorders.* New York: John Wiley.

Fey, M. (1986). *Language intervention with young children.* San Diego: College-Hill Press.

Gallagher, T., & Prutting, C. (1983). *Pragmatic assessment and intervention issues in language.* San Diego: College-Hill Press.

McLean, J., & Snyder-McLean, L. (1978). *A transactional approach to early language training.* Columbus, Ohio: Merrill.

# Language Disabilities in School-Age Children and Youth

## E L I S A B E T H   H.   W I I G

## MYTHS AND REALITIES

- *Myth:* Children outgrow language-learning disabilities by the time they are adolescents, so why worry?
- *Reality:* Studies tell us that maturation by itself does not take care of the communication disorders associated with language-learning disabilities.
- *Myth:* Only boys have language-learning disabilities, girls do not.
- *Reality:* The ratio of boys to girls with language-learning disabilities is commonly reported to be about 4:1. Because professionals have better knowledge of the nature of language-learning disabilities, more girls are now being identified and treated for language-learning disabilities. As a result, the boy/girl ratio is changing.
- *Myth:* Everyone has some type of a learning disability if you look closely.
- *Reality:* Everyone has areas in which they perform better or more poorly than their average. This is part of the normal variation in development. The

nature, extent, and degree of a deficit must be such that it interferes with normal learning processes and causes underachievement in several areas of learning for it to be considered a learning disability. We can expect that about 5% of the population has a learning disability as defined in this chapter.

■ *Myth:* If I send my child to a competent speech-language pathologist, she can diagnose a language-learning disability.

■ *Reality:* The diagnosis of a language-learning disability should be made by a multidisciplinary team of professionals. Such a team should include professionals with expertise in, among other areas, audiology, learning disabilities, psychology, reading, regular education, and, of course, speech-language pathology.

■ *Myth:* Language is fully developed by the third grade, so there is no reason to screen or test for language-learning disabilities after that.

■ *Reality:* The majority of the basic linguistic rules and structures are acquired by about age 8; however, important abilities and aspects of how to use language effectively as a tool for communication do not mature until about ages 11 to 13.

■ *Myth:* It is too late to start language intervention after the third grade, and intervention is not effective with adolescents.

■ *Reality:* Studies of the effectiveness of language intervention with elementary school children and adolescents with language-learning disabilities show that both groups can make significant gains.

■ *Myth:* Children and youth with language-learning disabilities will never amount to anything.

■ *Reality:* A diagnosis of a learning disability, including language-learning disability, implies that the person shows areas of strength, as well as weakness, in performance. What a language-learning disabled student can achieve depends on the nature and degree of strengths in thinking and performance. Many persons with diagnosed and treated language-learning disabilities attend college, and colleges provide support services to allow them to reach their intellectual and academic potential.

IN this chapter, we shall look first at a rather typical case history of a student who grew up with a language-learning disability. Then we shall consider definitions, characteristics, and etiologies. Finally, we shall take a closer look at the language and communication problems typical of children and adolescents with a language-learning disability, and consider how to assess and treat this type of disorder. The goal is to dispel the myths, and to establish greater awareness and knowledge of the realities.

*Jim is an attractive young college man who carried a number of diagnostic labels during his preschool and school years. He was said to have articulation disorders, apraxia of speech, a dysfluency disorder, delayed language acquisition, and a language-learning disability. Jim is not atypical of the children discussed in this chapter. The combined efforts of speech-language pathologists, learning disability specialists, classroom teachers, and parents made it possible for Jim to achieve in some areas and to enter college.*

*Jim's early motor development was normal. His speech and language development did not, however, conform to the normal pattern. When he was 18 months old, he was referred to an audiologist for a hearing evaluation and to a speech-language pathologist for language evaluation because he did not yet talk. At $2\frac{1}{2}$ years, Jim still did not talk, but he understood everything said to him. His intellectual ability was evaluated and all evaluations indicated performance within normal limits. At about age 3, Jim uttered his first sentence but his speech was unintelligible to anyone outside the family. At 4, Jim entered a nursery school with a language stimulation class. His language development began to follow a normal pattern of growth, but was still delayed. At 5, Jim entered the local kindergarten. His teacher soon noticed that Jim had a poorer command of words than his classmates. He was hard to understand, and he substituted and omitted speech sounds. During the year, Jim became highly disfluent. Sometimes his speech would come to a complete halt in his effort to say a word. In the spring, Jim was referred to a speech-language pathologist for evaluation and therapy.*

*The evaluation indicated that Jim's articulation difficulty was rooted in a sensory-motor integration problem (**apraxia of speech**). Jim had problems in programming, timing, and executing sequences of speech sounds. As Jim's articulation improved, problems in finding the words to express ideas became more obvious. Jim's vocabulary was also delayed, especially for space and time terms. Speech and language therapy was continued until the end of the first grade, when Jim was dismissed.*   *See chapter 13.*

*In the spring of the second grade, Jim was referred back to the speech-language pathologist. The classroom teacher stressed that Jim had problems in spelling and oral reading. Jim was again given language therapy. Language training focused on developing his vocabulary and on teaching some strategies for finding words. After about a year and a half, Jim was again dismissed from therapy.*

*By now, Jim was diagnosed as having a language-learning disability, and his teachers were alerted to his problems. In the fifth grade, yet another language-related problem emerged: Jim was not able to perform up to expectations in language arts and English composition. Extra efforts were made in the classroom and in consultation with the speech-language pathologist and learning disabilities specialist.*

*Jim's future in junior high raised some questions in the minds of his teachers and parents. Everyone expected that he would need assistance for English and social studies. No one anticipated, however, that he would fail three foreign languages in succession. Throughout junior high, Jim was provided with study skills and language assistance. It was also decided to exempt Jim from learning a foreign language. Instead, he was allowed to substitute sign language and a computer language for this requirement. Jim was an active partner in his support service program in junior high. He alerted the special education staff to problems in academic areas as they occurred. He asked for assistance and contracted for the amount of support time needed.*

*In high school, Jim continued to emphasize sciences, in which he achieved. Jim's SAT scores showed a discrepancy of more than 300 points between the math and verbal scores, which supported the diagnosis that Jim still had a language-learning disability. Jim is now in college pursuing studies in the sciences. He is able to look back at his early years and assess the impact of his language-learning disability. He talks of his loneliness and depression in the early school years. He tells of losing motivation in the fourth and fifth grades, when the struggles seemed insurmountable and he opted to be truant. He talks about being frustrated by knowing more in his head than he was able to express with words, and about being underestimated and misjudged.*

## DEFINITIONS

In chapter 5, we looked at the kinds of difficulties some young children have as they develop language skills. Many of these children, even those who receive speech-language therapy, continue to have language problems when they enter school. Other children have language problems that become evident only when they are faced with the academic challenges of school, or are compared with their classmates in terms of speech and language skills. Their language problems are often detected after they fail to achieve as well as their peers in school. The language problems may seem to come and go, or to get better or worse, as the child advances to new academic levels. Furthermore, the changes we have all faced in growing up—particularly the stresses associated with adolescence—can be accompanied by flare-ups or aggravation of language problems.

Language and communication disorders are common among children with school and social learning problems. These children are called learning disabled, slow learners, learning handicapped, or language-disabled. Whatever the label, these children have been the subject of concern for years, partially because the ability to use language is so critical in acquiring academic skills. A child cannot learn to read and write fluently if the native language has not been learned adequately. There are few subjects a child can learn without reading (or understanding what is said in the classroom), and few tests that can be passed without writing (or expressing knowledge by using language).

Speech-language pathologists, in cooperation with other specialists in the school system, deal with students for whom language and communication are the major problems. They also deal with students for whom a language disability is only a part of an overall learning delay.

It is recognized by legislation that some school-age children and adolescents have handicaps attributable to specific learning disabilities. This group of children has been defined in The Education of All Handicapped Children Act (P.L. 94-142, 1975):

> Children with specific learning disabilities exhibit a disorder in one or more of the basic psychological processes involved in understanding or using spoken or written language. These may be manifested in writing, spelling, or arithmetic. They include conditions which have been referred to as perceptual handicaps, brain injury, brain dysfunction, dyslexia, developmental aphasia, etc. They do not include learning problems which are due primarily to visual, hearing, or motor handicaps, to mental retardation, or to environmental disadvantage (p. 42478).

While this definition had substantial impact in the field of special education, it is not completely useful. It gives a list of diagnostic labels often used for these children, but it does not describe behavioral characteristics or give precise criteria for deciding if a given child or student fits the category. Most special educators, however, seem to agree on three essential aspects of the definition (Johnson & Morasky, 1977):

*For a definition of dyslexia, see page 199. Aphasia refers to a language disorder caused by brain damage, resulting in partial or complete impairment of language comprehension, formulation, and use for communication. (See also chapter 12.)*

1. The children must have one or more significant delays or deficits in essential learning processes (perception, integration, verbal or nonverbal expression) and must require special education procedures for intervention or remediation.

2. The significance of a delay or deficit in the essential learning processes must be determined by accepted diagnostic procedures in education, special education, and psychology.

3. The child must show a discrepancy between expected performance, based on assessed intelligence, and actual achievement in one or more areas such as spoken, read, or written language; spelling; mathematics; and/or spatial orientation.

Within the definition of the law, a learning-disabled child will have problems in some but not all academic skill areas. The learning disability may be reflected in the child's oral expression, listening comprehension, written expression, basic reading skills, reading comprehension, mathematics calculation, or mathematics reasoning (Federal Register, 42:250, December 29, 1977, p. 65083). Learning disabilities are not necessarily accompanied by delays in social skills, or by emotional or behavioral problems. In contrast, as we saw in chapter 5, a child with mental retardation shows "significantly subaverage general intellectual functioning existing concurrently with deficits in adaptive behavior" (Grossman, 1983).

The definition of learning disabilities featured in P.L. 94-142 was challenged by the National Joint Committee on Learning Disabilities (NJCLD), a group consisting of representatives from professional organizations concerned with individuals with learning disabilities, among them ASHA. According to the NJCLD, the definition is often misinterpreted to refer to a homogeneous, rather than a heterogeneous, group of individuals. The definition applies only to the age range from birth to 21 years, and fails to recognize that a learning disability may continue into adulthood. Finally, it provides an "exclusion clause" that can be interpreted as though individuals with learning disabilities cannot have multiple handicapping conditions or come from minority cultural or linguistic backgrounds. As a result of these concerns, the NJCLD recommended the following definition:

> Learning disabilities is a generic term that refers to a heterogeneous group of disorders manifested by significant difficulties in the acquisition and use of listening, speaking, reading, writing, reasoning, or mathematical abilities. These disorders are intrinsic to the individual and presumed to be due to central nervous dysfunction. Even though a learning disability may occur concomitantly with other handicapping conditions (e.g., sensory impairment, mental retardation, social and emotional disturbances) or environmental influences (e.g., cultural differences, insufficient/inappropriate instruction, psychogenic factors), it is not the direct result of those conditions or influences. (Hammill, Leigh, McNutt, & Larsen, 1981, p. 336)

## Types of Learning Disabilities

Syndrome *refers to a cluster of usually co-occurring characteristics that form a pattern.*

Graphomotor *refers to the process involved in executing written language.*

Children with learning disabilities are not all alike. They differ by type, degree of involvement, and the combination of problems they show. There are at least three independent clusters of difficulties (**syndromes**) among children with learning disabilities (Denckla, 1978; Erenberg, Mattis, & French, 1976; Mattis, French, & Rapin, 1975). The most common is considered to be a *language disorder syndrome.* It is characterized by problems in language comprehension, expression and use; word finding difficulties; and sometimes by auditory processing and speech discrimination problems. This syndrome is termed *language-learning disability* in this chapter.

The second syndrome is called *articulatory and graphomotor dyscoordination syndrome.* It is characterized by articulation, writing, and drawing difficulties, and is sometimes referred to as a *"clumsy child"* syndrome or as *developmental apraxia.* It may or may not include apraxia of speech. The syndrome is related to the apraxia syndromes found in adults with **neurogenic** disorders of speech and acquired apraxias (see chapter 13).

The third syndrome is a *visuospatial perceptual deficit syndrome.* It is characterized by visual discrimination, visual memory, and spatial orientation problems. Children with this syndrome typically confuse look-alike letters, such as *b* and *d,* in reading and have problems orienting themselves in space.

Combinations of the three major syndromes also exist. The language disorder syndrome may combine with the articulatory and graphomotor dyscoordination syndrome. It may also combine with the visuospatial perceptual deficit syndrome.

## Terms Used with Language-Learning Disabilities

In the evolution of the study of children with language and learning problems, many terms have been used to refer to various aspects of the problem. Some of these are widely used; others are less common. Any of the terms may, however, turn up in case histories or evaluation reports of the children seen by speech-language pathologists.

One common diagnostic term is **dyslexia.** It refers to a specific learning disability involving failure to master reading at normal levels for age. This term is used in the absence of a major debilitating disorder, such as mental retardation, major acquired brain injury, or severe emotional disturbance.

**Dysnomia** refers to a word-finding difficulty that interferes with a child's accuracy in finding and using names for persons, animals, objects, actions, or attributes. This term covers only one aspect of the language syndrome associated with learning disabilities.

*The related disorder anomia is discussed in chapter 12.*

Lastly, the term **language-learning disability** refers to the language disorder syndrome associated with learning disabilities. Language-learning disabilities are often subtle enough to escape early detection, but severe enough to interfere with the acquisition and use of language and communication for learning and socialization. In this chapter, language-learning disabilities are differentiated from language disorders in early childhood because of differences in the scope and degree of involvement and the usual time of detection of the problem.

## Jim's Case: Syndrome Type

In Jim's case, a combination syndrome was observed. In the preschool years, the articulatory deficits (apraxia of speech) associated with an articulatory-graphomotor dyscoordination syndrome assumed the greatest importance. After treatment of the articulatory problems, an evaluation revealed that Jim also showed a language disorder syndrome. It was difficult to determine at the time of diagnosis which deficit should be considered primary and which secondary. As Jim reached the third and fourth grades, the language disorder syndrome (language-learning disability) had the greatest impact on Jim's learning. It was therefore given primary status.

# EXAMPLES AND CHARACTERISTICS

## Linguistic Transitions

In the last decade, there has been an increase in the number of investigations of the linguistic transitions in the period from the early elementary years through adolescence. It is now widely accepted that the linguistic attainments in the years from 8 to 15 or 16 may be as significant as those of the preschool years (Menyuk, 1983; Simon, 1985; Wallach & Butler, 1984; Wiig & Semel, 1984). If we observe children during this transition period, we find that there are important changes in the ways they approach problem solving. These changes are reflected in increasing ability to think about and analyze how a problem can be solved (Flavell, 1976). This ability is called *metacognition*. At the same time, we observe increasing ability to think about and use language effectively, so-called metalinguistic abilities (Menyuk, 1983). Stated differently, the transitions seem to reflect the differences between acquiring functional use of language and developing ability to think and talk about language as an object, entity, or tool and using it for thinking, learning, problem solving, and effective communication.

*In a paraphrase, words and structural forms can be changed.*

We can identify some of the attainments that contribute to the acquisition of metalinguistic ability (Menyuk, 1983). First, there is a drastic increase in the available lexicon, the awareness of the multiple meanings and uses of words, and the possible combinations of and relations among them for expressing ideas and reactions. Second, the knowledge of the structural rules and the syntactic possibilities for paraphrasing ideas and intents increases. Third, there is improved sociolinguistic awareness and knowledge of the rules of language usage. This is reflected in changes in communication style or dialect as a function of the social situation or context (*code-switching*), and in adapting to the listener's point of view (*perspective taking*) in speaker-listener interactions. Fourth, there is an increasing ability to relate spoken information to past experiences and internalized knowledge and to make inferences. Fifth, there is a growing ability to view language as an object and to analyze words, phrases, sentences, and expression of intentions, so-called speech acts. Menyuk summarizes the attainments: "In all aspects of language new categories of language knowledge are acquired and this knowledge is applied in new contextual and linguistic domains" (p. 155).

Some aspects of metalinguistic ability appear to show the greatest developmental gains during the middle childhood years. This seems to be the case for the ability to segment words into sound (*phonemes*) and meaning units (*morphemes*), and to see the relationships between spoken and written words, all important for reading (Hakes, 1980). Other aspects of metalinguistic ability seem to change the most during the period from 8 or 9 to 11 or 13 years. Among them are the ability to interpret sentences with more than one meaning due to word choices or structure (**ambiguous sentences**), figurative language, jokes and sarcasm, and the ability to plan for language production whether for discourse, narrative, or writing. By adolescence, the communicatively competent student has developed and uses all the communication repertories effectively (Allen & Brown, 1977). She can

- Present, understand, and respond to information in complex spoken or written sentences that relate to persons, objects, events, or processes not immediately visible.
- Adapt messages, spoken or written, to the needs of others based on listener age, status, and nonverbal reactions and on the setting and medium used.
- Express positive and negative feelings and reactions to others acceptably and control others politely, formally, and with perspective taking.
- Take the role of another person effectively and approach conversations and verbal interactions with expectations of what to say, how to say it, and when to say it based on prior experiences and observations of others.

As language use increases in sophistication, the curriculum also places greater and greater demands on language as a tool for thinking, learning, and problem solving. Some of these demands have been discussed by, among others, Levine (1987) and Wiig and Semel (1984). In the middle and high school years, teachers expect students to be able to express their thoughts and knowledge accurately and concisely. They are supposed to retrieve information rapidly from memory. The expressions of knowledge and information must be organized and must adhere to the rules for discourse, narrative, or composition. Students must be able to integrate, restate, and paraphrase information they have obtained from many sources through listening or reading. Students are expected to show higher-order conceptualization and to interpret and use, among others, *verbal analogies* and metaphoric expressions.

*A verbal analogy compares two relationships, as in the comparison "Apples are to pears as lemons are to _____."*

Inadequacies in the linguistic attainments during the transition to adolescence can be expected to result in underachievement. Halliday (1978) comments on the interaction between language and academic achievement:

> Suppose that [language] functions that are relatively stressed [or acquired] by one group are positive with respect to school. They are favored and extended in the educational process, while those that are relatively stressed [or acquired] by another group are largely irrelevant or even negative in the educational context. We have, then, a plausible interpretation of the role of language in educational failure. (p. 106)

## Linguistic and Metalinguistic Delays

There are comprehensive accounts of the nature of linguistic delays associated with language-learning disabilities in the elementary school years (Lord Larson & McKinley, 1987; Simon, 1985; Wallach & Butler, 1984; Wiig & Semel, 1984). These delays cut across linguistic domains and can be found at the levels of morphology and syntax, semantics, and pragmatics. We shall look at the evidence of pragmatic deficits, and then examine the evidence of deficits at the levels of content (semantics) and structure (morphology and syntax). First, however, the short speech sample that follows serves to illustrate the pragmatic deficits seen among children with language-learning disabilities. The sample is of a 9-year-old girl who was asked to tell her class how to play a game of baseball.

> "Well ... you have to pitch the ball and you have to hit it and if you ... sometimes you get four balls and you walk to first base and then you get a hit like a home run. You have to hold the ball to see if the man is on which base and the persons gonna try to run from the base will run to first, second, third, home ... and that's it." (Bashir, Wiig, & Abrams, 1987, p. 149)

Evidence of the nature of pragmatic deficits comes from studies of discourse, narrative, and descriptive communication ability, and the ability to express complex intentions. Efficiency at discourse and narrative requires ability to follow a pattern or schema for an underlying structure, as well as a set of rules for the surface structure of cohesion (Clark & Clark, 1977; Stubbs, 1983). Among the cohesive mechanisms are lexical repetitions, shared lexis through repetition of words across utterances, repeated elements or phrases, use of lexical items from a well-defined semantic field, and lexical-syntactic patterning (Stubbs, 1983). Students with language-learning disabilities have the greatest problems at the level of cohesion related to the surface structure, both in discourse and narrative. Donahue (1985) reports that the narratives of children with learning disabilities include fewer words and idea units, a smaller proportion of syntactically complex sentences, and a greater proportion of pronouns for which the referents were not previously specified when compared to those of their academically achieving peers. Similarly, adolescents with learning disabilities use fewer referent-creating features and cohesive mechanisms in their narratives than their peers do. Lack of ability to use cohesive mechanisms has been observed in discourse. One study also looked at the effects of narrative style by students with learning disabilities on their classmates' willingness to listen (Silliman, 1984). The willingness to listen was influenced more by production factors, such as dysfluencies and false starts, than by the level of complexity of the narrative.

The pragmatic difficulties extend to the levels of providing descriptions in descriptive communication tasks and expressing complex intentions. Students with learning disabilities are much less skilled than their peers at formulating descriptions that are helpful to their partners in the task. They also have problems in clarifying messages they have not understood or misunderstood. They do not seem to realize that the listener must ask for clarification when a speaker's message is not understood. There are also problems with expressing complex intentions. Teenagers with learning disabilities are unable to negotiate conflicting situations and to resist peer pressure (Donahue, 1985). This observation is interpreted to mean that these teens show deficits in the social-cognitive strategies required to carry out persuasive appeals.

All of these problems can have devastating effects on academic achievement and social adjustment. In class, students are required to talk or write about experiences and events. Without adequate control of narrative structure, they are less able to display their knowledge than their peers, and they accordingly earn lower grades. Asking others, including teachers, for clarification of messages that were not understood is a potent tool for learning and acquiring new information. Without this ability to initiate clarification of messages, students with language-learning disabilities may fall more and more behind their peers in knowledge acquisition and academic achievement. Descriptive communication is often a part of social interaction. It is part of giving directions or messages and of playing social games. When the descriptions are less than helpful to the participants, the child or adolescent with a language-learning disability may well be left out of the interaction or rejected outright. Social interaction also requires ability to get complex and sometimes negative or controversial intentions across to others. Without ability to express complex intentions, the child or adolescent with a language-learning disability is left without a tool for controlling his own destiny. We shall now take a closer look at some of the semantic and syntactic problems that are reflected in the pragmatic communications.

## Semantic Deficits

### Word Meaning

The effectiveness of a communication hinges partly on the vocabulary used to convey the content and on the relationships among elements of the message. On the surface, children and adolescents with language-learning disabilities may appear to have vocabularies that match expectations for their age and grade. When they are tested with picture vocabulary tests, such as the Peabody Picture Vocabulary Test-Revised (Dunn, 1980), this observation often seems confirmed because they may earn scores that fall within the normal limits. Nonetheless, some students with language-learning disabilities present striking and specific lags in vocabulary knowledge and use. One problem seems to be the extent to which the meaning features associated with a word or concept are acquired. In normal vocabulary acquisition, a child's appreciation of a word develops in two stages (Miller & Gildea, 1987). During the first stage, which is relatively fast, a new word is assigned to a broad semantic category, such as names of fruits if the new word is *pomegranate*. During the second stage, which is relatively slow, the distinctions among words within the semantic category are worked out. This is accomplished by comparing and contrasting shared and nonshared features of meaning (*semantic features*). Before these distinctions are worked out, a new word may be overextended in use. Observations suggest that it is at the second stage in the acquisition of new vocabulary when students with language-learning disabilities show inadequacies. Often the distinctions among members of the same semantic class are incomplete, and words are misused or substituted.

The meaning of words may change somewhat depending on the context in which they are used. Consider, for example, the meanings of the word *beautiful* in these contexts: *I saw a beautiful butterfly, I saw a beautiful house*. In the first case, we might be referring to color as the significant attribute. In the second, we may be referring to size and architecture as the significant attributes. Children and adolescents with language-learning disabilities often fail to perceive the subtle shifts in word meaning that follow from changes in context. As a result, they may show incomplete understanding of what was meant and they may be less than precise in expressing themselves.

The same word may also be used to refer to essentially different references or contexts, for example, the word *glasses*. It can be used to refer to drinking glasses or eyeglasses. Children with normal language development recognize the multiple meanings of frequently used words by age 8 or 9. In contrast, adolescents with language-learning disabilities may not perceive the multiple meanings of even the most frequently used words (Wiig, Semel, & Abele, 1981; Wiig & Secord, 1985). This may lead to misinterpretations when they listen or read because they seem to come up with a single interpretation, based on their own past experiences with the word and its preferred reference. For example, a student with language-learning disabilities who wore glasses would be most likely to interpret the statement *He wiped the glasses carefully* as a reference to eyeglasses and fail to consider other alternatives.

Adding to the complexity of word meanings are words for which there are objective references that may be used figuratively to refer to behaviors, states, or conditions. In children with normal language development, we expect the ability to interpret most figurative expressions to be developed by ages 11 to 13. This is not the case among students with language-learning disabilities. Although they may have reached adolescence, they may still interpret common metaphoric expressions literally or incompletely (Nippold, 1985; Wiig & Secord, 1985). As an example, the expression *It is still up in the air* may be taken to mean that a plane has not yet landed. Delays in the acquisition of figurative ability have a significant impact on students' performance in school and on social interaction and adjustment, especially when we consider the uses and functions of metaphors (Wiig, 1989). Metaphoric expressions can serve as important memory aids. They are often used to summarize complex events into universal images. They can be used to refer to topics that are otherwise taboo, and they can convey the inner feelings and dynamics of a person in an acceptable manner. They are also tools in teaching and problem solving because they can let us see an abstract situation or problem as if it were a simple, concrete one.

There is yet another category of words and functions that cause problems for students with language-learning disabilities: words that indicate relationships among two or more arguments in sentences or sentence sequences (transition words). This category includes conjunctions (for example, *if, before, although*) and words such as *accordingly, subsequently,* and *regardless.* Students with language-learning disabilities, even at the college level, may have difficulty interpreting and using these words. They do not seem to understand the function of transition words in relation to the arguments that constitute sentences or sentence sequences, whether in speaking or writing. As an example, the word *although* indicates that a positive argument is followed by a negative argument, or vice versa, as in the statement *Although it's not my favorite color, I'll take the jacket at that price.* The problem then seems related to the logical structure of successive and related arguments in communication. Students with language-learning disabilities often misuse transition words, or they avoid making complex sentences or relating successive arguments to each other. As a result, discourse and narrative often consist of a string of repetitive arguments, each of which modifies the overall meaning or intent only somewhat.

## Word Finding

All of us have experienced problems in recalling an intended word from the word store (**lexicon**) in our brain. Sometimes we have trouble with a proper name, or can't get at a special term to label something precisely. For most of us, word-finding problems occur every now and then, and not every time we try to get an idea or intent across.

Johnson and Myklebust (1967) first called attention to the word-finding problems of children with learning disabilities. They named these difficulties **dysnomia** and described the problem as being "a deficit primarily in reauditorization and word selection" (p. 114). They also pointed out that children with dysnomia understand and recognize the intended word, but they are unable to retrieve the intended word on command. These children may resort to gestures that can be highly descriptive and dramatic when they search for a word. In rapid conversation, the recurring search for specific words often results in dysfluencies and false starts. The speech sample in Table 6.1 illustrates these patterns.

There are two hypotheses for explaining word-finding difficulties among children and youth with language-learning disabilities. The first holds that the

**Table 6.1**  Language Sample From an 8-Year-10-Month-Old Boy in the Second Grade, Illustrating His Word-Finding Problems

Examiner: Tell me about your favorite TV show:

1. (I seen it) I seen it today.
2. It wasn't that much.
3. Well (there was) they were chasing after (them) the both.
4. (And) (and) (they) (they) and (Tom and Jerry) (Tom) he (went) ranned into a dog.
5. (And) the dog was mad.
6. (And) he ran after 'em.
7. (So he) (so Tom) (little Jerry) (he went) (he) he pushed the metal thing up on the street.
8. (And he) (and he) (and he) the dog walked like a string.
9. Well he was just walking like a string.
10. And that was it.
11. They were just jumping on a jumping beam.
12. (Then they) (then the house) (then the house) (they) (they were com . . .) they came out of the house.
13. And they were fighting.
14. (And they didn't do) and they were just funny.
15. There was a little puppy (and a) and a father dog, right?
16. (And) the father dog. "You better not hurt that dog (unless you're gonna) unless you're gonna get a beatin."
17. (And) so he got a beatin.
18. (And) he sticked his tongue out.
19. (And) he got a beating.
20. (And) (so he just) (so he just) (and he) (and his) (and) he gave the dog food.
21. (And) then that was it.
22. Like I just told you the two (some) of the same thing.
23. It's (just they) they just go on a rocket flight.
24. (And) they just go on a spooky planet.
25. (And) (then) then they get caught.
26. (And) that's it.

*Note:* From *Language Assessment and Intervention for the Learning Disabled* (2nd ed.) (pp. 182–183) by E. H. Wiig and E. M. Semel, 1984, Columbus, Ohio: Merrill Publishing Co. Copyright © 1984 by Merrill Publishing Company. Used by permission.

difficulties arise because the child has not learned the names for lexical items adequately, and therefore cannot recall them rapidly, automatically, and accurately. This hypothesis, the *storage hypothesis*, seems true for some children (Leonard et al., 1983). A second hypothesis is that the stored lexical representations or names for objects are adequately learned, but that the information is insufficiently accessible when needed. This hypothesis, the *retrieval hypothesis*, seems true for other children studied (Denckla & Rudel, 1976; Fried-Oken, 1983). The reason for considering the mechanisms associated with word-finding problems is that treatment would differ, depending on whether the problem was related primarily to storage or retrieval. In the first case, therapy would focus on strengthening the lexical representations. In the second case, therapy would focus on developing strategies for retrieval.

Studies of word-finding problems generally use picture naming, naming to description, and open-ended question tasks (Fried-Oken, 1983; German, 1982; White, 1979). One study indicates that the high frequency of **circumlocution** differentiates elementary school children with language-learning disabilities from their peers. Among adolescents, the high frequency of circumlocuting and of making word association errors also differentiates students with dyslexia from their academically achieving peers.

> *Circumlocution is a roundabout way of referring to an object, action, or event when a speaker cannot find the exact or intended word.*

The significance of a word-finding problem is that it interferes with pragmatic competence (see Table 6.1). It is hard to follow the topic of conversation or narrative when there are false starts and repairs, and when essential words are substituted. The word-finding efforts also interfere with the formulation of sentences and the organization of arguments because they occupy processing space.

## Morphologic and Syntactic Deficits

One of the attainments associated with metalinguistic ability is code-switching in response to the needs and characteristics of participants in a communicative interaction. This ability emerges with increasing sociolinguistic awareness, and with increasing ability to control the structural forms as well as the content of messages and expressions of intention (speech acts). Several studies indicate that children and adolescents with language-learning disabilities are not as capable of adapting their language and communication styles to the listener's needs, or to the interpersonal context, as their peers with normal language development (Bryan, 1978; Wiig, 1982; Wiig et al., 1983). In interpersonal communication, regardless of the status of the participants, they tend to use simple, rather than complex and elaborated, forms of messages. They tend to use the prototypical forms for getting their intents across to others, rather than the attenuated, more polite, or indirect forms. As an example, they often use imperatives to request actions (*Answer that phone*), rather than more mature forms that give reasons (*Would you please answer the phone for me? I can't leave the stove right now*). Two reasons are postulated for the immature response forms. First, the student with a language-learning disability may not have acquired the syntactic transformations needed to soften the impact of a message or a command (often by using modals and complex verb forms [attenuation] to make them more polite). Second, they may not be able to take the perspective of the listener and understand what effect the message form has on others. Generally, the two reasons coexist, and therapy needs to address both sides of the problem. If we accept that syntactic deficits may have adverse effects on message adaptation or code-switching, then we need to take a closer look at the nature of the problems in acquiring the structural rules (*syntax*).

Several studies indicate that children with language-learning disabilities do not acquire the rules for forming words (*morphology*) at the same rate, and with the same consistency and degree of sophistication, as children with normal language development (Golick, 1976; Vogel, 1977; Wiig, Semel, & Crouse, 1973). These children appear to ignore hard-to-hear parts of words (for example, word endings, unstressed words, phrases, and parts of clauses) when listening to and interpreting spoken language. As a result, they may not learn the rules for using words such as auxiliaries (*can, will*), modals (*could, would*), prepositions, conjunctions, and other grammatical markers that tend to receive low stress in speech. Instead, they tend to focus on and remember the words that stand out, either because of stress or high information content. Unfortunately, one of the means for attenuating messages and making them more polite is to adapt the verb phrase and to use modals and remote verb tenses (for example, "Would you *mind moving over one seat?*"). If the modals and complex verb forms are not acquired and their function in message adaptation is not understood, code-switching may not be possible from a planning and production perspective.

Along with difficulties in semantics and morphology, children with language-learning disabilities may have significant problems in learning and using the rules for forming sentences. The nature and extent of these problems may vary. In some instances, the greatest problem is in the process of forming ideas, thoughts, or images (**ideation**) and productivity; in others, it is primarily syntactic-pragmatic. In the majority, however, both problems seem to be present.

When the problems observed are compared across studies, we see a remarkable consistency (Donahue, 1985; Simon, 1985; Wiig & Semel, 1984). Sentences in which the usual order of the agent-action-object is either interrupted or reversed (**transformations**) are delayed in acquisition. This includes sentence transformations such as passives (*The train was hit by the car*), and sentences with relative clauses (*The boy, who lives next door, went to camp*), noun complements (*Your plans to camp out in winter don't please me*), or indirect-direct object order (*The girl showed the boy the baby*). Adolescents with language-learning disabilities also have problems coming up with alternative interpretations for sentences with ambiguities caused by structure (*Jane didn't blame Jack as much as his mother*) (Wiig, Semel, & Abele, 1981). Inadequacies in syntactic development, and lack of versatility in interpreting and formulating sentence structures can be expected to adversely affect socialization and achievement in reading, writing, and other language-based curriculum areas.

## Language After Traumatic Head Injury

It was mentioned earlier that language-learning disabilities can result from traumatic head injury. There are different views about the nature of the language disorder syndrome that follows head injury. One view holds that the language impairments are specific or categorical, and that the syndromes resemble the *aphasias* observed in adults who have suffered strokes (Heilman, Safron, & Geschwind, 1971; Sarno, 1980, 1984; Waterhouse & Fein, 1982).

*See chapter 12.*

The second view holds that language becomes disorganized as part of a global disorganization process (Bernstein-Ellis, Wertz, Dronkers, & Milton, 1985; Hagen, 1982, 1984; Holland, 1982; Wiig, Alexander, & Secord, 1987). The global disorganization has been tied to a generalized cognitive dysfunction following traumatic head injury. Language lacks variation in form and style, is no longer used with originality or creativity, and is terse and not elaborated upon. In addition, there may be problems with attention, retention, and auditory and recent memory. The language deficits are similar to those seen in students with developmental language-learning disabilities, but the problems generally cut across the areas of semantics, syntax, and pragmatics. Children and adolescents with language disorders resulting from traumatic head injury generally have marked word-finding problems. They also have problems with the more abstract levels of language interpretation and use required for figurative language, jokes, and sarcasm. The problems also involve planning and organizing language for production both at the sentence, discourse, and narrative levels. The degree and extent of the language disorders after traumatic head injury seem closely tied to the level of recovery of cognitive functioning (Wiig, Alexander, & Secord, 1987).

Children and adolescents with traumatic head injury can be expected to present with concomitant physical and perceptual-motor deficits and organically based behavior and emotional disorders (DePompei & Blosser, 1987). Among physical deficits are impairments of mobility, strength, vision, and/or hearing. Possible perceptual-motor deficits are visual neglect, visual field cuts, and motor apraxia. Behavior and emotional disorders might include impulsivity, disinhibition, denial, depression, emotionality, apathy, and lethargy. The presence of concomitant problems complicates the rehabilitation process, return to an educational setting, and need for classroom adaptations.

## The Case of Jim: Language Characteristics

Jim was observed to have language deficits in several areas. In the late pre-school and early elementary years, the delays in vocabulary development and concept formation assumed the greatest importance in therapy. His word-finding problems were, at that time, thought to reflect inadequacies in word knowledge. As Jim's vocabulary knowledge grew, the severity of his word-finding problems was reduced somewhat; however, he still experienced word-finding difficulties more often than expected for his age, and he substituted familiar words in a pattern characteristic of dysnomia. For example, he would say that a fork was missing at dinner when the knife was missing (age 8 to 9 years). He substituted antonyms consistently, and would say he was going downstairs when he was on his way upstairs (age 10 to 11 years). He could not keep words with prefixes straight: "I'll excard (for *discard*) that," "I'm going to watch the telephone (for *television*), there's a special on," (age 13 to 15 years). He had trouble in geography with directional terms, never quite knowing if the direction in question was north, south, east, or west. As a teenager, Jim's delays in acquiring control over verbal-social repertoires (pragmatics) came to the fore. He did not know the rules for telephoning and initiating conversation or leaving messages. He did not know how to complain politely, respond to complaints, or negotiate changes in appointments. The pragmatic problems emerged as the require-ments for verbal-social interactions and styles became more stringent and complex in everyday life and in academic areas, such as English literature and composition. Jim never had problems with the syntactic rules, a fact that helped him considerably.

## PREVALENCE

Estimates of the prevalence of learning disabilities among school-age children vary widely due to differences in definitions or criteria for inclusion. High estimates indicate that 15% of school-age children suffer reading or learning disabilities due to minimal brain damage (Calvin & Ojemann, 1980). Some estimates are lower because they are affected by practical constraints of finances or professional resources available. For example, several states say only from 1% to 3% of all school-age children may demonstrate a learning disability.

Not all children with learning disabilities have significant difficulties with language, but a major midwestern special school district reports that 80% of the students receiving language therapy also carry a learning disability diagnosis. The prevalence of the language-learning disability syndrome among children with diagnosed learning disabilities is estimated to range from about 40% to 60%. The prevalence of the articulatory and graphomo-tor dyscoordination syndrome among the learning disabled is estimated to range from 10% to 40%. The visuospatial perceptual deficit syndrome is estimated to occur in from 5% to 15% of the learning disabled.

Among students who receive special education for learning disabilities, 20% are estimated to have acquired brain injury caused by head trauma. The group of males between 15 and 24 years of age is especially vulnerable and appears to constitute 50% of all head injury cases. The incidence rate for head injury in that age group is 600 per 100,000. A large proportion of these cases will suffer permanent language-learning disabilities (Bigler, 1987a, 1987b).

# UNDERLYING MECHANISMS

In chapter 5, we looked at some of the possible causes and underlying mechanisms in early childhood language disorders. At this point we need take only a brief look at some additional research of the causes of learning and language-learning disabilities.

Levine and Zallan (1984) state that academic underachievement and learning problems in older children and adolescents are "the product of multiple convergent factors, including underlying often concealed disabilities, secondary affective and motivational changes, responses to extrinsic pressures, and a repertoire of learned styles and face-saving strategies" (p. 345). This view leads us to a combination of factors rather than a single factor or mechanism for language-learning disabilities. There are organic factors and underlying mechanisms that may contribute to a language-learning disability.

Several authorities consider attentional deficits to be a significant underlying factor in learning and language-learning disabilities (Calvin & Ojemann, 1980; Levine, 1984). This deficit syndrome is associated with restlessness or hyperactivity, distractibility, inconsistencies in performance, a tendency to fatigue easily, difficulty in delaying gratification, and burnout on tasks that require maintenance of attention during problem solving. The attentional deficit syndrome can be related to dysfunction of the brain's activating system, specifically the thalamus and striatum.

*Areas of the brain and their functions are discussed in chapters 3, 12, and 13.*

The primary area for auditory language processing and association in the left hemisphere (Wernicke's area) has also been implied as a brain site and underlying mechanism in language-learning disabilities. One source of evidence comes from autopsy studies of adults with lifelong histories of language and reading disorders (Galaburda & Kemper, 1979). It was found that the brains showed signs of abnormalities and distortions in the architecture of the left temporal lobe. A second source comes from studies of discrimination and sequencing of rapidly presented speech stimuli (Tallal, 1987). These studies found that children with specific developmental language disorders had a slowed rate of processing a series of auditory stimuli, both speech and nonspeech, and of producing syllables rapidly. In adults, damage to the left, but not to the right, hemisphere of the brain disturbs the rapid discrimination of changing auditory stimuli. Electrical stimulation of the temporal lobe in the left half of the brain also has been shown to change both the discrimination of speech sounds and the ability to produce oral movements in rapid sequence (Ojemann & Mateer, 1979).

Genetic and hereditary causes for language-learning disabilities must also be considered. Several studies suggest that verbal and spatial abilities are inherited (De Fries et al., 1976). Hereditary patterns observed in twins and among families of dyslexics and disabled readers suggest that certain types of specific learning disabilities may also be determined by heredity (Finucci, Guthrie, Childs, Abbey, & Childs, 1976; Hallgren, 1950; Hermann, 1959; Owen et al., 1971).

When traumatic head injury is the cause of language-learning disability, the disability is acquired. The resulting language deficit syndrome shares characteristics of the developmental language-learning disability syndrome, but varies in some dimensions. In traumatic closed head injury, the lesion to the brain is nonfocal, and a single or primary site of lesion cannot be identified.

Cortical *refers to the outer layer of the brain.* Subcortical *refers to the areas of the brain lying beneath the cerebral cortex.*

The resulting lesion generally encompasses **cortical** as well as **subcortical** structures. Attentional and memory deficits and impaired abstract reasoning ability are significant components of the syndrome (Bigler, 1987a, 1987b).

Summarizing the studies of potential causes of language-learning disabilities, we must conclude that several causes are possible and several underlying mechanisms may be involved. In addition, several of the causal factors may be present. As we saw in early childhood language disorders, it is difficult to distinguish between causes and correlates of language-learning disabilities. There is enough evidence of a connection between physical causes and language-learning disabilities to suggest, however, that the child or youth with this problem should be evaluated by medical specialists as part of an in-depth educational assessment.

## Jim's Case: Causes and Underlying Mechanisms

Several factors may have contributed to Jim's problems. One evident factor was heredity. Jim's father was found to have a language-learning disability with a developmental history that was similar to Jim's. The father's family showed a history of learning disabilities, generally affecting the males but also affecting an occasional female. Jim was diagnosed by a neurologist as having attentional deficits with distractibility and hyperactivity, and these deficits were also thought to underlie his language-learning disability.

# APPROACHES TO DIAGNOSIS

## Identification of Children at Risk

Clearly it would be helpful and cost-effective if we could identify children at risk for language-learning disabilities on the basis of their early histories and existing school records. Early language delays or histories of speech or language problems are important signals of potential language-learning disabilities (Ingram, 1970; Mason, 1976; Strominger, 1982). The implications are that speech-language pathologists should follow children with histories of early speech or language delays and be alert to emerging language-learning disabilities.

Patterns of intellectual functioning may also help identify school-age children with potential language-learning disabilities. The Wechsler Intelligence Scale for Children—Revised (Wechsler, 1974), a widely used standardized test, may provide evidence of discrepancies between verbal and performance measures of intelligence. A significant verbal-performance IQ discrepancy (12 or more IQ points) may indicate that the child is at risk for, or has, a language-learning disability. The implications are that children with this pattern of intellectual performance should be referred for language assessment.

Profiles of academic underachievement in children with normal overall potential for learning may also be used to identify those who may have or may develop language-learning disabilities. Many children with language-learning disabilities show one of two academic achievement test patterns (Rourke, 1975). In the first pattern, reading and spelling achievement are significantly below grade level (two grades or more). In the second, academic achievement in reading, spelling, and arithmetic are uniformly below grade- or intellectual-level expectations. Again, school-age children who show either of these patterns should be considered at risk and evaluated for language-learning disabilities.

## The Case of Jim: Identifiers

In Jim's case, his early articulation and language delays should have been a warning that he was at risk for language-learning disabilities. When his intelligence was tested in the early grades, his verbal IQ was about 20 points lower than his performance IQ. During the school years, Jim's academic achievement record also showed discrepancies. He achieved above average in math and sciences, significantly below average in reading and spelling, and failed foreign language requirements. His development followed typical patterns for children with language-learning disabilities.

## Language Screening

Children with language-learning disabilities can also be identified through language screening. If possible, every child who enters kindergarten or elementary school should be screened for potential language disabilities. At the very least, all children who are suspected of being at risk for language-learning disabilities; referred by teachers, parents, physicians, or other specialists; or who do not achieve to potential in reading, spelling, or arithmetic should be referred for language screening.

There are other stages in the educational process when children at risk for language disabilities should be evaluated at least briefly. Critical points in the educational process occur at the transitions from third to fourth grade, from elementary to junior high, and from junior high to senior high school.

Depending on the age and grade level, one of several language screening tests may be used to identify preschool and early elementary school children with potential language disabilities. An example is the Bankson Language Screening Test (Bankson, 1977). It probes word knowledge, morphology, syntax, and visual and auditory perception. Another example is the Merrill Language Screening Test (Mumm, Secord, & Dykstra, 1980). It uses a storytelling format to elicit retelling. Each child's story is then analyzed for structure, elaboration, and narrative style.

There are also language screening tests for older children. One example is the Clinical Evaluation of Language Fundamentals—Revised Screening Test (Semel, Wiig, & Secord, in press). It samples word knowledge, syntax, and memory for spoken language. Another example is the Screening Test of Adolescent Language (Prather, Beecher, Stafford, & Wallace, 1980).

Language screening tests take a relatively short time to administer and are easy to score. They give norm-referenced scores to allow comparison between the performance of children or adolescents and their peers. If a student's performance is judged to be significantly below that of peers, a referral is made for a language evaluation.

## Evaluation and Diagnosis

Although the term *diagnosis* is somewhat imprecise, it most often refers to the process of identifying a child's or adolescent's strengths or weaknesses in a given ability, such as language. Inherent in the definition is the concept that diagnosis involves a process. P.L. 94-142 indicates that the diagnosis of a language or learning disability must be made by a multidisciplinary team. The team must include the classroom teacher, a psychologist, a special educator, and other professional specialists. If a language-learning disability is suspected, the speech-language pathologist should be included.

The first step in the diagnostic process is to obtain a case history. This history should include information about the student's language and other development, academic achievement and existing problems in learning, home and social environment and dialectical or linguistic background, communication and interaction style and existing problems, and the student's own view of and reactions to the language and communication problems.

The next step is to obtain reliable, valid, objective, and measurable information about the student's language abilities and behaviors. P.L. 94-142 indicates that at least two independent tests must be used to diagnose a language-learning disability. It also stipulates that tests used for diagnosing language or learning disabilities must be standardized and report standard scores to allow for comparison of performances to a group of peers. No formal test of language is completely reliable, and a wider range of abilities will be sampled if different language tests are employed. The speech-language pathologist may use language probes and behavioral observation to supplement the diagnostic findings. The specific language tests, probes, and methods of behavioral observation used will depend on the diagnostician's views of the nature of the language-learning disabilities and on the current state of the art. We can identify several major approaches to the assessment of language disabilities in school-age children and adolescents. Three commonly used approaches will be discussed.

## Semantic-Syntactic Approaches

The semantic-syntactic approaches evaluate the language characteristics of a student in relation to the linguistic domains, semantics, morphology, and syntax. Tests and tasks usually focus primarily on either word knowledge, or knowledge of morphologic and syntactic rules and structures. The tests and tasks are not primarily concerned with how the student communicates in real-life interactions. As such, the language used in the tests and tasks can be considered decontextualized. The standardized tests that use a semantic-syntactic approach to assessment are generally reliable. They are valid diagnostically because they are able to differentiate students with language disabilities from those with normal language development at high levels of accuracy. When tests in this category are used, it is essential to recognize the limitations of the test in relation to real-life communication (pragmatics).

Examples of comprehensive standardized language tests in this category are the Test of Language Development (Newcomer & Hammill, 1977) and the Test of Adolescent Language (Hammill, Brown, Larsen, & Wiederholt, 1980). These tests are designed to probe receptive and expressive language abilities for morphology, syntax, and semantics. The Clinical Evaluation of Language Fundamentals—Revised (CELF—R) (Semel, Wiig, & Secord, 1987) also belongs in this category. Subtests of the CELF—R probe morphology and syntax, semantics, and recall of spoken language. Tasks and methods for extension testing to identify the language variables that either facilitate or present a barrier to accurate responding are included.

## Pragmatic Approaches

These approaches seek to assess aspects of a student's ability to communicate ideas and intentions effectively in a variety of educational and social communication contexts. The objective of assessment is to evaluate the relationships among spoken messages, the contexts in which they occur, and the interpreters of the messages. The focus is on identifying a student's existing strengths and weaknesses as a communicator and recipient of messages and intents.

The communicative competence of the child or adolescent is judged in relation to his effectiveness in following the rules for interpersonal communication, whether in discourse or narrative. It is judged by the effectiveness in controlling arguments, reasons and intentions, the forms that best express them, and the timing that is expected in interpersonal interchanges. In simpler words, it looks at the *why,* the *how,* and the *when* of communication.

Several formats can be used for pragmatic assessment. One is spontaneous language sample analysis. It has been proposed that the spontaneous language sample to be analyzed should be gathered in three separate, fifteen-minute samples (Miller, 1981). This procedure is also recommended for school-age children. The spontaneous language samples can be analyzed for length of utterances, grammar, and syntactic complexity (Miller, 1981), and discourse structure (Stubbs, 1983).

*Spontaneous language sample analysis has been discussed in chapter 5.*

The descriptive communication task is another commonly used format for pragmatic assessment (Glucksberg, Krauss, & Weisberg, 1966). In this format, the student describes objects, pictures, events, or object assemblies or designs to another person. The listener either has to identify the item described or follow directions for making designs. The effectiveness of communicating is judged by the listener's ability to identify the items or carry out the actions described.

Behavioral observation and interviewing others about a student's pragmatic behaviors are also commonly used procedures. Gallagher (1983) introduced a pragmatic pre-assessment questionnaire. It was designed to elicit descriptions of the communicative behaviors of a student, in general first, and then in relation to variations in partners, topics, activity contexts, and physical settings. This questionnaire is often used as part of gathering the background case history. Prutting and Kirchner (1983) presented a Pragmatic Protocol for observing and recording observations of communicative behaviors and interactions. This protocol provides for observation of behaviors in three broad areas: (1) the utterance acts, relating to features such as intensity and quality of voice, prosody, proximity, body posture, facial expressions, and gaze patterns; (2) the propositional acts, relating to the lexical use, word order, and stylistic variations of the messages and expressed intents; and (3) the illocutionary and perlocutionary acts, relating to the types of speech acts used, the topical focus and topic maintenance, and turn taking.

Pragmatic abilities may also be assessed in structured elicitation. There are three formal tests that use this method. One uses a game format to elicit expressions of intents and turn taking (Blagden & McConnell, 1983). The others use illustrations of interactions to elicit a variety of expressed intents, first as if to peers and then as if to authority figures (Bray & Wiig, 1987; Wiig, 1982).

## Cognitive-Linguistic Strategy Approaches

This approach seeks to identify how well a student plans for and solves problems with language either as stimuli or responses. The objective is to assess whether or not the student has acquired metalinguistic ability, can use language as a tool, and can analyze and evaluate language. The focus is on identifying strengths and weaknesses in, among others, dealing with higher level or more abstract language, such as multiple meanings or metaphoric uses; making inferences; or planning for language production, either at the sentence, paragraph, discourse, or narrative levels. The student's performances are judged against criteria for responding. The criteria vary as a function of the task and may include whether the student can come up with several meanings for words or sentences, interpret metaphoric expressions, make several inferences from spoken narrative, or plan and organize spoken presentations.

Several formats can be used for cognitive-linguistic strategy assessment. One elicits a narrative, which is analyzed to evaluate how well the rules for narrative structure are followed (Stubbs, 1983). A second format asks a person to describe something fairly complex, such as the layout of an apartment. The description can be analyzed for how well rules for description were followed (Linde & Labov, 1975).

There are two standardized tests that evaluate aspects of the emergence and maturation of metalinguistic abilities. The first, the Test of Language Competence—Expanded (Wiig & Secord, 1985, 1988), evaluates the ability to give two interpretations of ambiguous sentences, make two plausible inferences, plan for and produce spoken messages with given word choices in response to illustrated contexts, and interpret and match metaphors. This test was originally designed for preadolescents and adolescents. Its simpler version explores the same abilities in easier tasks to evaluate the emergence of metalinguistic abilities.

## LANGUAGE THERAPY

Language therapy with school-age children and youth should be broadly based and integrated with the requirements of the settings in which the child has to function and perform. As a result, therapy may take a direct as well as an indirect approach. Lord Larson and McKinley (1987) have described a broadly based prototype delivery model for speech-language pathologists. The direct component of language therapy is directed toward developing thinking, listening, speaking, and nonverbal communication skills and survival language. They suggest that referential communication, simulation and role-playing activities, narrative skill-building activities, and other approaches may be used to develop these skills.

The indirect therapy component focuses on two groups. The first consists of members of the student's educational system, and the second consists of members of the environmental system. With both groups, the model advocates modifications of the educational and environmental systems through, among others, consultation, content area tutoring, adaptation of classroom discourse and of educational materials, and counseling.

The therapy component of the delivery model is complemented by dissemination of information about available speech and language services to administrators, regular educators, special educators and other professionals, parents, and the community at large. It is also complemented by follow-up to determine the benefits of the student's program. This is accomplished by surveys in the form of interviews and questionnaires, direct testing, and research. More specifically, they suggest that language therapy should be provided in one-hour daily delivery modules, and that therapy should occur in group settings. The students, especially if they are adolescents, should be given academic credit for participating in language therapy. Finally, they suggest that language therapy should be provided under supportive labels, using terms such as *oral communication strategies* rather than *therapy*.

# COUNSELING

In recent years, there has been an increasing awareness of the interaction among language disorders, learning disabilities, and adverse social and emotional growth and development. Some of these interactions can be reflected in maladaptive behavior characteristics in kindergarten. Kindergarten children with language and learning disabilities have been described as immature, poorly adjusted socially, and impulsive. They may show aggression, lack of responsibility; poor interpersonal relationships; and disinterested, angry, and hostile reactions and behaviors (Keogh, Tchir, & Windeguth-Behn, 1974). In elementary school children with language and learning disabilities, negative communication features and postures become more obvious. These children seem to have general problems in interacting both with peers and with teachers. They come across as egocentric. As we saw, they do not switch social register, do not give sufficient details when they communicate, and are less assertive and effective in conversations than their peers. They also are less able to negotiate conflicting situations and resist peer pressures, and they do not maintain proper control of communicative interactions (Donahue, 1985).

There are also indications that children and youth with language and learning disabilities are at risk for psychiatric disorders, behavior disorders, and delinquency (Cantwell & Carlson, 1983; Thompson, 1986). It is now the accepted view that the relationships among emotional problems, delinquency, and language-learning disabilities must be understood by addressing the interactions among the primary vulnerabilities and environmental stresses (Bashir, Wiig, & Abrams, 1987). This recognition has led to the recommendation that treatment must address the acquisition of essential linguistic and basic academic skills, learning of curriculum content, and development of appropriate perspectives of the self and the environment in a functionally coordinated manner, with counseling being one component of treatment (Bashir, Wiig, & Abrams, 1987; Simon, 1985).

Experiences with counseling language-learning disabled adolescents and young adults suggest that insight into the nature and implications of the communication difficulties may have several benefits. It may improve motivation for language therapy. It may facilitate compensation for specific difficulties and result in the development of more adaptive coping strategies.

In counseling, the speech-language pathologist may use both a nondirect and a direct approach. In nondirect counseling, open and spontaneous expressions of feelings, reactions, and attitudes are encouraged. The counselor guides the student in gaining insights into the causes and dynamics of the expressed feelings in a self-discovery process. In the direct approach, the speech-language pathologist would share professional knowledge and experiences with the student to further the student's understanding of her problems and of how to cope effectively. Simon (1985) adds some practical suggestions for the speech-language pathologist: (1) beware of signs of depression and refer to psychological services if necessary, (2) determine if psychological problems are primary or secondary in nature, (3) gather descriptive information about the roots of the problems and what forces maintain them, (4) consider multidisciplinary and multimodality intervention, and (5) provide counseling as needed.

## CONCLUSION

Jim's case illustrates that language-learning disabilities can be expected to persist over the life span. It is therefore important to track and assess children with early language disorders and those who are at risk for language-learning disabilities throughout their school years. Even if an adolescent has been through a successful course of language therapy as a child, new problems may crop up as the demands for language sophistication increase. Experience shows that it is never too late to provide language and communication training for the language-learning disabled, even in adulthood. The effects of a language-learning disability on school performance and everyday life interactions can be so wide ranging that we must be prepared to intervene whenever necessary.

## STUDY QUESTIONS

1. Compare the two definitions of learning disabilities (P.L. 94-142 and NJCLD). How are they alike? How do they differ?

2. Read Jim's case history and make a developmental chart with age and grade levels and the language and learning problems he experienced.

3. What are the three major syndromes in learning disabilities? How do you think each would influence learning to read, spell, write, and do mathematics and geometry?

4. Identify six or more linguistic and pragmatic behaviors that reflect the attainment of metalinguistic ability.

5. Identify and outline the pragmatic behavior deficits described in students with language-learning disabilities.

6. Compare and contrast the two hypotheses for word-finding problems (dysnomia). When you have occasional word-finding problems, which hypothesis best describes the origin?

7. Outline the process involved in identifying and assessing students with language-learning disabilities.

8. Compare and contrast the three approaches to language assessment. Suggest one or more additional tasks or tests for each approach.

## SELECTED READINGS

Bryan, T. H., & Bryan, J. H. (1978). *Understanding learning disabilities* (2nd ed.). Sherman Oaks, Calif.: Alfred Publishing.

Mercer, C. D. (1987). *Students with learning disabilities* (3rd ed.). Columbus, Ohio: Merrill Publishing Co.

Simon, C. S. (1985). *Communication skills and classroom success.* San Diego: College-Hill Press.

Wallach, G. P., & Butler, K. G. (1984). *Language learning disabilities in school-age children.* Baltimore: Williams & Wilkins.

Wiig, E. H., & Semel, E. M. (1984). *Language assessment and intervention for the learning disabled* (2nd ed.). Columbus, Ohio: Merrill Publishing Co.

# PART FOUR

# Disorders of Articulation, Voice, and Fluency

# Articulation and Phonological Disorders

LEIJA V. McREYNOLDS

## MYTHS AND REALITIES

- *Myth:* Developmentally, children acquire sounds in the same sequence and at the same ages.

- *Reality:* Normative studies differ in the developmental information they present, so they need to be applied with caution. Longitudinal studies of phonological acquisition show that children vary a great deal from each other in the way they learn the phonology of their language.

- *Myth:* If a child learns the target sound according to criterion and produces it correctly in the clinic, it will generalize to the natural environment.

- *Reality:* Generalization does not occur as readily as expected. Carryover is a serious problem in treatment. The clinician should plan for generalization from the beginning of training by introducing variables that will facilitate carryover.

- *Myth:* All children with articulation errors have phonological problems.

- *Reality:* A phonological problem suggests that a child has a problem with the organization of his phonological system. Not all articulation problems are organizational. Some children may have motor or perceptual problems, which may not necessarily be phonological.

- *Myth:* If a client with an articulation disorder can make the discriminations required on a general test of discrimination, she does not have a discrimination problem.
- *Reality:* Research has shown that general tests of speech sound discrimination do not reveal the discrimination deficits of children with articulation disorders. Misarticulating children need to be tested on their specific error sounds if their discrimination problems are to be revealed. In fact, the best discrimination test is one in which the child evaluates his own productions of the target sound.
- *Myth:* A phonological process analysis explains a child's articulation problem.
- *Reality:* A phonological process analysis is a descriptive procedure, not an explanatory one. The analysis is used to reveal patterns in the articulation errors produced by children. The analysis does not explain the patterns or why they occur.

WITH these myths and realities as a background, we turn to some of the facts of articulation and phonological disorders. Some of the realities are illustrated in the introductory case study of a 7-year-old. Phoneme production and articulation development are then introduced, with the characteristics of articulation and phonological disorders discussed next. Approaches to the evaluation and remediation of articulation disorders are discussed and evaluated.

Bobby, a 7-year-old, was referred to the Speech and Hearing Clinic by his classroom teacher and his parents. His problem was described as a severe articulation disorder.

Bob's birth and developmental history were unremarkable except for language. The mother reported that Bobby did not start talking until he was 3½ years old. Otherwise, his physical and motor development fell within the normal range.

Bobby had suffered no unusual or prolonged illnesses or injuries. He had a number of colds and ear infections, but according to the pediatrician, these were not any more numerous or severe than most children's bouts with the same illnesses. The pediatrician rated Bobby's health as average over the 7 years under his care.

No speech disorders have been observed in the immediate family. Bobby has one sister who is 2 years older. According to his mother, the boy plays well with his peers and his relationship with the sister is quite good. Bobby participates in social and sports activities in school and at home. Although he is not a leader, he participates as an equal in these activities. Bobby had not demonstrated any inhibitions in speaking to others until first grade. At that time, he expressed annoyance when he was not understood by the teacher and some of his classmates. Until first grade, he seemed unaware that his speech was different from that of others. His performance in school is slightly below the average, but IQ tests place him within the normal range.

Bobby was given a comprehensive assessment. Normal hearing acuity was noted for each ear with pure tone and speech stimulation. Word discrimination ability could not be tested due to the presence of numerous articulation errors in repeating discrimination test words. His receptive language was tested on the Peabody Picture Vocabulary Test and the Test for Auditory Comprehension of Language. In both measures, Bobby obtained scores well within the norms for his age group. His expressive language was assessed by administering the Carrow Elicited Language Inventory and the Expressive One-Word Picture Vocabulary Test. A conversational language sample was also obtained. On both formal tests Bobby scored at the 25th percentile, indicating that his performance fell within the boundaries of the lower 25% of the standardized populations. The numerous articulation errors made evaluation of his conversational language sample difficult; however, Bob's expressive language consisted of complete sentences and phrases.

The oral-peripheral physical examination revealed no structural abnormalities in the mouth. Tongue movements on nonspeech activities were appropriate. No malocclusion was evident in the alignment of teeth. Bobby's repetition of pa-ta-ka was slow, however. The oral-peripheral examination revealed no obvious physical or organic problems.

The Templin-Darley Articulation Test and the Goldman-Fristoe Articulation Test were administered. The following results were obtained:

|  | Substitutions | Omissions |
|---|---|---|
| Initial position | d/g, t/k, t/s, d/z, p/f, b/v, t/ʃ, t/tʃ, d/dʒ, d/ʒ, w/r, w/l, t/θ, d/ð | -/r, -/l, -/dʒ |
| Medial position | n/d, d/g, d/k, t/s, n/tʃ, n/ʃ, d/z, t/dʒ | -/r, -/l, -/s, -/f, -/v, -/θ, -/ð, -/z, -/tʃ, -/ʃ |
| Final position | t/s, n/t, p/k, d/z, m/b, b/g | -/r, -/l, -/f, -/v, -/s, -/z, -/ʃ, -/dʒ, -/tʃ, -/g, -/k, -/θ, -/ð, -/t, -/d, -/p, -/b |

*According to Templin's normative data, Bobby's raw score is below the 3-year level of articulatory functioning on consonants. Stimulability was tested by requesting the child to imitate his error sounds. On this test, Bobby correctly produced the /t/, /k/, /g/, /v/, and /f/ with instructional aid. A distinctive feature analysis revealed errors on (+) stridency and (+) continuancy at 90%. A high percentage of errors also occurred on the place features (+) back, (+) high, and (+) coronal.*

*A phonological process analysis of Bobby's conversational sample revealed that cluster reduction, final consonant deletion, stopping, and assimilation were possible phonological processes present in his articulation errors. Further testing of processes was undertaken to determine whether the sounds affected by the processes were used by the child in any contexts contrastively.*

*A morphophonemic alteration procedure, used to examine the child's underlying representations for the error sounds, revealed that the adult form could be present for all error sounds except the /g/, /k/, and /s/. Position and contextual constraints for /f/, /v/, /ʃ/, /tʃ/, /dʒ/, /r/, /l/, /θ/, and /ð/ were identified. The analysis revealed least phonological knowledge for /g, k, and s/, some knowledge for /f, v, ʃ, tʃ, dʒ, r, l, θ and ə/, and most knowledge for /p, b, t, d, m, n, n, ŋ/.*

*Bobby's past history and present status indicate that physically he is performing adequately. Academically his performance is lower than average, but this may be due partially to his speech problem, since his IQ has been established to be within the normal range. Socially the child is functioning normally and enjoys interacting with his family and peers. No medical reason for his speech problem has been identified.*

*On the formal hearing tests, Bobby evidenced no hearing problem. His language scores on the expressive language tests placed him in the lower 25th percentile, but his articulatory deficit made it difficult to score the language tests. Articulation measures revealed numerous articulation errors of substitutions and omissions. These errors make his speech difficult to understand.*

*Bobby may be described as a child with a severe articulation disorder of unknown origin. The disorder could also be described as a phonological disorder. Several recommendations were made. First, it was recommended that Bobby be enrolled in direct intensive articulation training. He should be seen by the speech-language pathologist individually 5 days a week. Next, it was recommended that a structured treatment program be developed to establish correct production of sound classes through a selected sample of exemplars from two classes. Third, initially, contrast training between stops and fricatives should be administered. For example, the child can be trained to produce the /p/ and /f/ contrastively, first in nonsense-syllable contexts and then in words. The /p/ and /f/ are likely targets because Bob can and does produce /p/ appropriately, and is stimulable on the /f/. Finally, generalization to other stops and fricatives should be tested frequently and always prior to initiating training on another sound pair. The generalization testing can be used to determine progress and to select future target sounds and contexts for training.*

As we have seen, for two people to communicate successfully, the sender must use a shared language to encode a meaning that the receiver can decode. If I'm talking to you, I must use words and structures that you understand. I must pronounce those words so that you can recognize them, at least within certain limits. **Articulation** is the process of producing the speech sounds of a language, and **intelligibility** describes how readily speech can be understood by listeners. The most precise words and the clearest structures are useless if you cannot understand them because the sounds are not intelligible. Unfortunately, problems with articulation are common—in fact, they occur more often than any other type of disorder seen by most speech-language pathologists.

This chapter discusses functional articulation and phonological disorders, beginning with a short explanation of articulation and how it develops normally. A definition of *disordered articulation* follows, and later a definition of *functional articulation* and *phonological disorders* is offered. Next, we will summarize the most common explanations of the nature of functional articulation disorders and how remediation is approached within each explanation. The final sections are devoted to evaluation and treatment of articulation and phonological disorders. These sections describe the variables measured in assessing articulation disorders, with special emphasis on variables that seem to be useful in **prognosis** and in planning remediation programs. In this final section, general principles for planning remediation programs are also set forth.

*A prognosis is a prediction of how quickly and how well a person will recover from or overcome a condition with/without intervention.*

## ARTICULATION AND ARTICULATION DEVELOPMENT

*Articulation* refers to the movements of the articulators in production of the speech sounds that make up the words of our language. It is more than that, however, because production of each speech sound (phone) in each word must be related to the abstract representations (phonemes) of the language; that is, speech sounds are represented on two levels, the phonetic and the phonological level. On the phonetic level, there are many phones for one phoneme because individual speakers produce sounds differently. A child will produce a sound somewhat differently from the way an adult produces the same sound because her vocal-tract size is different from that of adults. The context (word or syllable) in which a sound is produced influences the phone as well. For example, the phoneme /p/ will be produced differently in the words *pin* and *spin*. The [p] in *pin* is accompanied by aspiration (breath), while in the word *spin* the [p] is unaspirated. Thus, the phoneme for both productions is /p/, and the two ways of producing [p] in *pin* and *spin*

*To review, a phoneme is indicated with slash marks //, and phones are enclosed in brackets [ ].*

constitute phones because the contexts in which they are produced influence their production.

On the phonological level, phonemes are linguistically important because they act as **contrastive elements** in the language—they serve to distinguish meaning, as the /p/ and /b/ do in the words *pin* and *bin*. Only the /p/ and /b/ are different in the two words; because they differ, we know that these are two words, each with a different meaning. The /p/ and /b/ thus contrast with each other. This contrast allows a differentiation of the two words with regard to meaning; therefore, the contrast is linguistic. Articulation, therefore, helps (a) to differentiate words from each other and (b) to make productions of sounds more precise. Of course, as pointed out in chapter 2, phonology describes not only contrastive elements, but also permissible sequences of sounds and combinations of sounds.

The English language consists of approximately 40 phonemes, categorized into vowels and consonants. Children learn these sounds gradually, and this gradual development has been studied to identify the sequence in which sounds are acquired (Ferguson, 1979; Ferguson & Farwell, 1975; Poole, 1934; Prather, Hedrick, & Kern, 1975; Templin, 1957; Wellman, Case, Mengert, & Bradbury, 1931). The beginning of this gradual development has been studied by linguists, child development investigators, psychologists, and speech pathologists. One issue in sound acquisition is whether there is a relationship between early infant vocalization and later sound production in words. Jakobson (1968) originally theorized a discontinuity between the two, stating that there is no relationship between early infant vocalizations and later phonetic forms in meaningful words. That position has been modified considerably, and it is now acknowledged that there is continuity between babbling and meaningful speech. In fact, the child is thought to be an active participant in the entire process of learning the phonology of the community language (Ferguson & Macken, 1983; Kiparsky & Menn, 1977; Macken & Ferguson, 1983; Vihman, Macken, Miller, Simmons, & Miller, 1985).

Thus, we now recognize that infant vocal behavior probably has relevance to the sound acquisition patterns of children as they begin to acquire language; the similarities between infant vocal behavior and early language acquisition support an interactionist-discovery theory of phonological acquisition (Kiparsky & Menn, 1977; Menn, 1976, 1983). Normative data for infant sound patterns are not yet available, but investigations continue. These studies offer important information for our understanding of how children go about acquiring the sounds of their language. The studies provide data on the patterns of sound acquisition and the strategies children use during acquisition of the first 50 words, and even on earlier vocalizations (Stoel-Gammon & Dunn, 1985; Vihman et al., 1985).

Of primary interest to speech-language pathologists is the sequence of consonant acquisition because consonants are more important to intelligibility than vowels. Normative data for ages at which particular consonants are

*Normative data result from the study of large groups of normally developing subjects to evaluate behavior at different age levels.*

usually present are reported in Table 7.1. These data are from two studies, one completed by Templin in 1957, and the other by Prather, Hedrick, and Kern in 1975. Younger children (ages 2 years to 4 years) were tested in the 1975 study; in the Templin study, the children ranged in age from 3 to 8 years. As you can see in the table, the sequence in which sounds appear in children's speech is similar in the two studies, but the Prather et al. data indicate that sounds may be acquired at younger ages than we used to think. Prather and colleagues caution, however, that they tested each consonant in just two positions in words (initial and final), while Templin tested the consonants in three positions in words (initial, medial, and final). This difference may be responsible for the different results obtained in the two studies.

*The initial position is the first sound in a word, the final is the last sound, the medial falls in the middle. A child may be able to produce a phoneme in only one or two of these positions.*

More detailed analyses of the data from normative studies and the more recent longitudinal studies of individual children have emphasized the

**Table 7.1**   Ages (in Years and Months) at Which 75% of Children Correctly Produced Consonant Sounds

| Sound | Templin (1957) 3 Positions | Prather et al. (1975) 2 Positions | Sound | Templin (1957) 3 Positions | Prather et al. (1975) 2 Positions |
|-------|---------------------------|-----------------------------------|-------|---------------------------|-----------------------------------|
| m | 3 | 2 | g | 4 | 3 |
| n | 3 | 2 | s | 4–6 | 3† |
| h | 3 | 2 | r | 4 | 3–4† |
| p | 3 | 2 | l | 6 | 3–4† |
| ŋ | 3 | 2 | ʃ | 4–6 | 3–8 |
| f | 3 | 2–4 | tʃ | 4–6 | 3–8 |
| j | 3–6 | 2–4 | ð | 7 | 4 |
| k | 4 | 2–4 | ʒ | 7 | 4 |
| d | 4 | 2–4 | dʒ | 7 | 4†* |
| w | 3 | 2–8 | θ | 6 | 4†* |
| b | 4 | 2–8 | v | 6 | 4†* |
| t | 6 | 2–8 | z | 7 | 4†* |
|   |   |   | hw | * | 4†* |

*Sound tested but not produced correctly by 75% of subjects at oldest age tested.

†Reversal: Reported at earliest age level if only one reversal occurred and percentage at 11 older age levels exceeded 75%.

*Note:* The data in this table are from *Certain Language Skills in Children* by M. C. Templin, 1957, Minneapolis: University of Minnesota Press and from "Articulation Development in Children Aged Two to Four Years" by E. M. Prather, D. L. Hedrick, and C. A. Kern, 1975, *Journal of Speech and Hearing Disorders, 40*. Used by permission.

individual variability children exhibit in the acquisition process. Partly to adjust for that variability and partly to account for the differences in the procedures used to gather the data across studies, Sander (1972) reanalyzed data presented by Templin (1957) and Wellman et al. (1931). His purpose was to present the average age of sound production rather than just upper age limits. He suggested that such an analysis would show the customary age at which a child produces the sounds. *Customary age* was defined as the age at which a child produces a sound correctly more often than incorrectly in two out of three word positions. Sander's reanalysis of the Templin and Wellman et al. data resulted in the graph shown in Figure 7.1. An age range of sound development is shown for each consonant. The range begins where 50% of the children used each sound correctly in two of three word positions, and ends where 90% of the children used the sound correctly in three word positions.

Developmental information presents a broad guideline for sound acquisition, as evidenced by the ranges in the graph. The speech-language pathologist should keep in mind that the guidelines are indeed broad; specific children vary a great deal within the guidelines. It has been pointed out in many sources (Bernthal & Bankson, 1988; Hanson, 1983; Weiss, Lillywhite, & Gordon, 1980) that it is difficult to compare data across studies because of methodological and criterion level differences. A review by Smit (1986) of several normative studies examined differences in methodology and results. She wished to explore the validity of data sets that clinicians use. Smit found large discrepancies in sampling sets, ages studied, experience of the examiners, reliability of scoring, elicitation methods, and cut-off criteria. Smit concluded that these discrepancies seriously limit how much reliance clinicians can place on the norms reported in the studies. Her suggestion was that all normative data should be used with caution when determining if a child has an articulation disorder, and when selecting a target sound for training. Thus, norms can be used by speech-language pathologists as long as two important facts are considered when applying them to specific children: (a) there is a discrepancy among the ages in the different sets of normative data due to the manner in which the norms were developed, and (b) longitudinal data on individual children are beginning to suggest that each child uses his own strategies during acquisition—no two develop in exactly the same way (Ferguson, 1979; Ferguson & Farwell, 1975; Vihman et al., 1985). For example, a young child may produce words with a sound that is considered to be later developing, such as /f/, if the word *fish* is important to him.

## DEFINITION OF DISORDERED ARTICULATION

When an articulation error occurs, production of a phoneme is imprecise in one of several ways. Sometimes the intended phoneme is replaced by

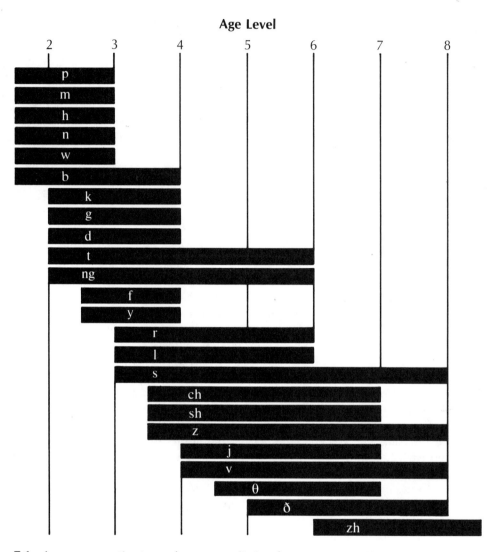

**Figure 7.1** <u>Average</u> age estimates and upper age limits of customary consonant production. The solid bar corresponding to each sound starts at the median age of customary articulation; it stops at an age level at which 90% of all children are customarily producing the sound. (*Note: From "When Are Speech Sounds Learned?" by E. K. Sander, 1972,* Journal of Speech and Hearing Disorders, *37(1), p. 62. Reprinted by permission.*)

another phoneme. In that case, the error is one of **substitution;** the appropriate phoneme is replaced by an inappropriate phoneme. If a person says, "Don't *wet* me" when she means "Don't *let* me," she is substituting a /w/ for an /l/, and the substitution results in a shift from the word *let* to *wet*.

This misproduction is likely to cause a misunderstanding of the intended word because the /l/ and /w/ function contrastively in the two words to differentiate them and their two meanings.

In other instances, a misproduction makes a phoneme sound different, but not different enough to shift the production into another phoneme. For example, a person might use aspiration in producing the [p] in *spin* when it should have been produced without aspiration. The aspirated [ph] in *spin* sounds funny, but the listener recognizes it as a /p/, not some other phoneme. The word is understood, although the [p] is distorted. This kind of production is referred to as a **distortion** because the sound has not been produced in the standard manner, but the production is perceived as the appropriate phoneme.

In disordered articulation, sounds within words are sometimes omitted entirely. When this happens, it is not always possible to determine what the phoneme should have been; and of course, since nothing is produced, it isn't possible to determine if the phone was produced in a standard manner. If a child says, "My ca ____ is lost," you wouldn't know if the word was supposed to be *cat* or *cap* because, in this case, the final sound in the word identifies what the word is and that sound is missing. These errors are called **omission** errors. The error types with examples are summarized in Table 7.2.

Thus, an articulation error may consist of a substitution, distortion, or omission of sounds (and, infrequently, addition of extra sounds). At times, a word is changed to another word because the error is a substitution that changes the intended phoneme. An articulation error may also result in distorting a sound without changing the intended phoneme, thus leaving the intended word unchanged, although strange. Finally, sounds may be omitted entirely from words, and the omission is an articulation error.

But of course, it takes more than just one substitution, distortion, or omission to diagnose articulation errors as articulation disorders. We do not have standard criteria for determining how many or what kinds of errors

**Table 7.2** Kinds of Articulation Errors

| Error Type | Definition | Example |
|---|---|---|
| Substitution | Replace one sound with another sound | Standard: The ball is red Substitution: The ball is wed |
| Distortion | A sound is produced in an unfamiliar manner | Standard: Give the pencil to Sally Distortion: Give the pencil to Sally (the /p/ is nasalized) |
| Omission | A sound is omitted in a word | Standard: Play the piano Omission: P_ay the piano |
| Addition | An extra sound is inserted within a word | Standard: I have a black horse Addition: I have a balack horse |

comprise a disorder, but several variables are considered by speech-language pathologists in arriving at the conclusion that a child or adult has an articulation problem. Foremost in arriving at a decision is a judgment about how severely intelligibility is affected. This judgment depends on a number of variables, such as number of errors, type of error, and consistency of errors.

*These variables will be discussed in more detail in the evaluation section of this chapter.*

Frequently, however, the decision that a person has an articulation disorder is also influenced by the speech-language pathologist's own views concerning articulation and phonological disorders; that is, individual professionals have personal opinions about what constitutes an articulation disorder. These biases help determine the variables to be measured in evaluation and the weight given to each measured factor.

## Definition of Functional Articulation Disorders

Sometimes articulation errors are accompanied by physical abnormalities such as that seen in cleft palate, or by neurological deficits as in cerebral palsy and apraxia. It is generally accepted in these instances that the structural or neurologic deficit is at least partially responsible for the articulation defect. Although articulation is affected in special populations such as children with cleft palate or cerebral palsy, articulation is not always the first concern in these disorders. For example, in cerebral palsy, not only is muscle movement abnormal, often the neuromotor problem is accompanied by sensory, behavioral, and cognitive disabilities. As suggested in chapter 14, these individuals need much more than articulation training. Similarly, in cleft palate children, repair of the cleft may take precedence (see chapter 11). Some children with articulation errors are diagnosed as apraxic, indicating that a neurologic component is present, which requires a different kind of treatment from children without neurologic involvement (for a discussion of apraxia, see chapter 13). Articulation problems are prevalent in the hearing-impaired population, and treatment needs to be planned to take into consideration the sensory deficit (chapter 10). The exact relationship between the physical condition and the defective articulation may not be easy to establish; nevertheless, there appears to be some evidence that the two are related.

A large group of articulation problems, however, have no known or obvious organic, neurologic, or physical correlates. Since the cause or causes for these problems are unknown, they have been relegated to a category labeled **functional** articulation disorders. *Functional* may mean any number of things; mostly, it serves as a wastebasket label denoting only that

*The etiology of a condition is its cause or causes.*

the **etiology** for the disorder is unclear and no causal components can be identified (Shelton, 1978). It isn't that investigators have not attempted to identify causes; as a matter of fact, many variables have been explored with the expectation that one or more would be found to be responsible for articulation problems, or at least closely related to them. Variables such as intelligence, motor skills, auditory discrimination, auditory memory, socio-economic status, sex, personality, academic performance, dentition, and many others have all been explored in the hope that one or more would reveal a causal link (Winitz, 1969). Unfortunately, few of the variables were found to be related to disordered articulation, at least to the extent that they could be causing the articulation problem. The variable showing the strongest relationship was *auditory discrimination*, the ability to discriminate between speech sounds. This factor has *not* been shown to cause disordered articulation, but there is a correlation.

*doesn't cause but there is a correlation*

The lack of a relationship between articulation disorders and the numerous variables studied has led most experts to assume that articulation disorders have multiple causes, and attempts to find causes have received less emphasis. Attention has shifted to describing articulatory behavior itself, seeking ways in which the variables could contribute to evaluation for determining the presence of the disorder, making statements about prognosis, and developing efficient treatment programs.

The omissions, substitutions, and distortions described earlier have been analyzed to reflect patterns of errors or categories of errors (Hodson, 1986; Ingram, 1981; Shriberg & Kwiatkowski, 1980; Weiner, 1979). When the errors are grouped in this way, they resemble error patterns of young children who are developing their phonological systems. Phonologists attribute these patterns in normal children to operation of **processes** that simplify adult forms children are unable to produce (Ingram, 1976, 1981). Examples of such patterns are omission of final consonants in CVC words, called a final consonant deletion process, or substituting stops for fricative sounds, labelled as a stopping process. As noted, these patterns are called **phonological processes** by linguists. The resemblance between the error patterns of normal and articulatory-defective children has encouraged speech-language pathologists to view the articulatory disorders as phonologically based and the articulation errors as phonological errors. Consequently, speech and hearing professionals are rapidly adopting the label *phonological disorders* in place of *functional articulation disorders*. As with other factors that might have been causal in nature, however, the terms *phonological processes* and *phonological disorders* have not been shown to be etiologically useful; they are descriptive terms. As descriptive terms to indicate error patterns and show relationships between errors, the labels are useful.

*phon. proc.*
*1) final cons. del. proc.*
*2) Stopping proc.*

*phon dis ≈ fxn artic dis*

Although no causal relationships have been uncovered, individuals interested in articulation problems have proposed possible causes and subsequently developed models that could explain the nature of articulation disorders. As a result, several approaches to functional articulation disorders have emerged. Needless to say, most approaches are somewhat mixed in that no one cause is purported to be wholly responsible. Rather, proponents may suggest one strong causal factor accompanied by other less strong, but still influential, factors contributing to the disorder. Emphasis in most approaches is placed on the nature of the articulation problem (is it a motor problem? a perceptual problem?) more than on what caused the problem originally. A brief discussion of some major models follows. You should note, however, that these models are placed into broadly defined categories, and each category includes input from a number of specific conceptualizations, differing from each other on one or more dimensions.

### Discrimination Models

The most common model for a number of years, and perhaps today, was developed by Van Riper and Irwin (1958), and subsequently expanded (Van Riper, 1978). According to this model, the underlying problem in articulation disorders is poor **sound discrimination;** that is, the individual is not able to match the auditory feedback from her own productions with the auditory patterns others produce. She is unable to discriminate between her error production and the correct production of the same sound by others. This failure to discriminate may be caused by a number of factors (such as slow physical maturation, or listening to other family members who misarticulate), but the authors do not specifically identify the factors. In remediation, particular attention is paid to training the person with an articulatory defect to hear acoustic differences, evaluate the adequacy of her productions in comparison to standard productions, and modify error productions until they match the standard.

Another conceptualization that emphasizes discrimination and has some resemblance to Van Riper's (1978) model is described by Winitz (1975, 1984). In his most recent model, Winitz (1984) relates discrimination to the child's underlying phonological structure, and this relationship is revealed by testing the child's perception or ability to distinguish between speech sounds. If a child fails to discriminate between sounds, the inference is that his underlying phonological structure is not the same as the adult's structure; hence, perceptual practice is required. If the discrimination is accurate when tested, then one can assume that the child can make the appropriate perceptual judgment, but this does not necessarily mean these distinctions are used in the child's speech. A breakdown may occur on one or more of several levels: (a) the child cannot make the discrimination; (b) the child can make the discrimination, but has acquired a special phonological rule that changes the discrimination he is able to make in production; (c) articulatory constraints prohibit producing what the child hears; and (d) the child's implicit learning strategy leads him not to attend to what he perceives. Winitz does not specifically state that there is a causal relationship between discrimination and production, but suggests instead that there is a strong relationship between the two.

Support for a relationship between speech-sound discrimination and articulation disorders has been offered in some studies. Although equivocal findings have been reported, the inconclusive results have been attributed to an improper emphasis in some of the studies (Bernthal & Bankson, 1988; Monnin, 1984). Several problems with the discrimination tasks (tests) and their administration have been pointed out, but two main problems are emphasized. First, many of the studies tested a general speech-sound discrimination ability, not discrimination of the specific error sounds involved. Second, the children were asked to discriminate sounds produced by other individuals rather than by themselves. As pointed out by Monnin (1984), when articulatory-defective children are asked to discriminate between their specific error sounds and the target sounds, and additionally, when they are asked to judge the adequacy of their own productions, they perform more poorly than they do on externally presented and general discrimination tasks. Thus, Monnin suggests that there is a relationship between speech-sound discrimination and misarticulation if proper tests and procedures are used.

Other conceptualizations of articulation disorders may include discrimination as one component, but it does not constitute the major theme. Therefore, the extent to which discrimination training is provided differs from one professional to another. For example, in Hodson's (1986) phonological processes model for treating articulation disorders, the child is exposed to periods of auditory bombardment of the target sound.

There is another group of models in which discrimination is not considered to be an important variable contributing to the functional articulation problem. In these approaches, emphasis is placed on training correct production with no specific discrimination training administered. These conceptualizations are discussed next.

## Production Models

Undoubtedly, articulation involves, at least in part, the learning of a motor skill. An articulation disorder is not necessarily a case of motor disability; nevertheless, articulation consists of fine motor movements that need to be coordinated precisely if speech is to be accurate. Several experts consider the motor component to be the important variable in treatment of functional articulation disorders.

*Review chapter 3 for details on the many muscles and organs involved in articulation.*

Probably the best known model in this category is the one conceptualized by McDonald (1964). In this model, children with articulation errors are thought to be arrested at some stage in sensory-motor development. The model does not suggest that learning and other variables do not influence the articulation pattern they present; rather, it suggests that the primary problem is the sensory-motor arrest to which other factors may be contributing. McDonald contends that the syllable, not the isolated sound, is the smallest unit of speech. McDonald envisages articulation as a series of overlapping movements in which the tongue, lips, and other articulatory muscles and structures are moving almost simultaneously as a person

*The size of the speech unit has become an issue in speech science, linguistics, and speech pathology, and is yet to be resolved.*

produces a word. Essentially, sounds are not produced sequentially, one at a time in a word, but rather they overlap with each other. For example, the lips are beginning to protrude in preparation for producing the /u/ during production of the /t/ in the word *true*.

Presently, basic research appears to support, at least in part, McDonald's viewpoint regarding overlapping movements of the articulators in the form of coarticulation. Studies of coarticulation show that articulators begin to move to form a particular sound long before it is produced audibly (Daniloff & Hammarberg, 1973; Sharf & Ohde, 1981). This coarticulation occurs in other than syllable-size contexts, as proposed by McDonald; however, it occurs across word and sentence boundaries too. Speech-language pathologists are frequently encouraged to take advantage of the phenomenon of coarticulation in training (Kent, 1982; Winitz, 1975). It has been proposed that some sounds can be used to form facilitating contexts for acquisition of particular target sounds. For example, if /s/ is taught in the context of /t/, as in the word *stay*, the /t/ may make acquisition of /s/ easier than if the /s/ were followed by some other sound. Therefore, the /t/ is thought to be a facilitating context for learning to produce /s/.

If a child can produce a target sound correctly in some contexts, these contexts may be used in training by pairing a correctly produced context with an incorrectly produced context (Irwin & Weston, 1975). Contextual influence is a major component in McDonald's sensory-motor approach. An error sound will probably be produced correctly in some phonetic contexts because children's error productions are usually inconsistent. If production of the error sound is tested in a sufficient number of syllables, the sounds will probably be produced correctly in one or more of them. To find contexts in which a child might produce the target sound correctly, McDonald (1964) designed a test in which each sound is tested in a variety of word pairs (contexts) to help find the context(s) in which production is correct.

**Facilitative** coarticulatory influences in remediation have been investigated in experimental (Elbert & McReynolds, 1975, 1978; Hoffman, 1983) and descriptive research (Diedrich, 1984). Unfortunately, coarticulatory effects in training have not been demonstrated. Findings indicate that there are no universal facilitative contexts in which target sounds should be trained. Coarticulation has not been shown to be an important variable for choosing training item contexts.

Most motor skill learning models rely on sensory-motor feedback from all modalities. An example of such a program, with the addition of cognition, is one presented by Shelton in Shelton and McReynolds (1979). Much of Shelton's research has been based on principles involved in development of skilled motor performance. He has discussed a perceptual-motor learning model in which perceptual and cognitive factors are also emphasized. The model has been described by Ruscello (1984) in its expanded form. Although motor skill practice still receives its share of attention, perception and cognition play more important roles. Cognitively, production of sounds is planned prior to the articulation, and perceptually, the individual attends to feedback from all modalities to determine if the production was accurate. With sufficient variety in the contexts in which a sound is produced, the individual forms a **motor schema,** an internalized rule for sound production that dictates the range of variation allowed for producing the target sound in a variety of contexts.

Another conceptualization fitting into the production model is application of operant conditioning to articulation remediation (Garrett, 1973; Mowrer, 1973, 1978). In this approach, the accent is on careful programming in remediation to obtain maximal changes as efficiently as possible. The goals and procedures are operationally defined and specified, as are response and training criteria (Bernthal & Bankson, 1988). Reinforcement is used to define shaping procedures carefully. Many ready-made programs for articulation remediation are founded on the principles of operant conditioning (programmed instruction) and are available commercially (Costello, 1977; Gerber, 1977).

Needless to say, a number of motor skills learning principles have been incorporated into specific articulation remediation plans by individual speech-language pathologists. It is not unusual, for example, for speech-language pathologists to offer detailed phonetic instructions on tongue placement or lip postures during the course of training a new sound. Feedback on the child's response is also common practice in training.

## Linguistic Theory

Linguistic models were developed later than were the discrimination and production models; however, linguistic information was not ignored in the two earlier models. In fact, reference is made to linguistics in both. The impact of linguistic theory on language acquisition and treatment of language disorders is well recognized and familiar to most speech-language pathologists. This is less true for articulation. It was only when professionals realized that phonology, as one component of language, was being neglected in the onslaught of interest in morphology, syntax, semantics, and pragmatics that a revival of interest in phonology occurred (Ingram, 1976). Attention is being devoted to the relevance of linguistic theory to the understanding of functional articulation disorders. The first two linguistic concepts that aroused the interest of speech-language pathologists were **distinctive features** and **phonological processes.** Phonological theory in the form of generative phonology has carried linguistic concepts even further. These concepts will be discussed individually.

Distinctive feature theory has been explained in chapter 2. Therefore, only a brief review of the concept will be provided, sufficient to bring to attention the principle components of the theory. Distinctive feature analysis has been applied to the description of articulation errors (Grunwell, 1982; McReynolds & Engmann, 1975; Singh & Frank, 1972). Some (Bernthal & Bankson, 1988) have questioned the use of an abstract linguistic concept to describe a concrete articulatory event. The issue is a legitimate one, and the pros and cons for using distinctive features continue to be discussed. Sommers (1983), for example, presents evidence of the usefulness of distinctive feature analysis, as does Grunwell (1982) and Blache (1982). Perhaps the debate concerning which system, if any, is appropriate for analyzing articulation errors is less important than the concept of applying features for descriptive purposes. To give a rather simple example, the production of /b/ involves, among other things, bringing the lips together firmly, building up air pressure behind the lips, forcing the lips open with a burst of air, and vibrating the vocal folds (voicing). All of these articulatory gestures might be thought of as articulatory features that compose the /b/ sound. Each sound is composed of several features that, when grouped together, comprise a phoneme. The interesting thing about features is that any one feature is present in several sounds; this common feature defines the relationship among a number of sounds. For example, voicing is a feature of /b, d, g, z, v, ð/ and others. Because the sounds are all voiced, they form a class of voiced sounds. Other features function similarly in that they establish relationships between sounds.

Regardless of which theoretical system is used, application of feature theory to functional articulation problems enables us to describe a problem in terms of feature errors, which in turn helps to reveal relationships among error sounds. By comparing the features of the target sound with those of the error sound, one can determine which features are in error. If, for instance, a child produced /p/ for /b/, /t/ for /d/, /k/ for /g/, and /f/ for /v/, it would be possible to say that in all these errors, she is substituting a voiceless sound for a voiced sound. Obviously, her error is on voicing, a feature that is necessary to production of the /b/, /d/, /g/, and /v/. What the child needs to learn is to produce both the voiced and voiceless sounds in a cognate pair, that is, /p/ and /b/, /t/ and /d/, /k/ and /g/, /f/ and /v/, thereby acquiring the voiced and voiceless contrast. Possibly, because the problem is a feature error rather than unrelated errors on a number of individual sounds, the contrast can be trained in just one or two pairs and the voicing feature may transfer to the remaining pairs without specific training on each. It is this concept of relationships among error sounds that distinctive feature analysis has contributed to our view of articulation disorders.

The kind of generalization promised by looking at the features within error sounds instead of looking at each error sound individually has been obtained when feature contrasts are trained (Bunce & Ruder, 1981; Costello & Onstine, 1976; McReynolds & Bennett, 1972). When first introduced, however, the idea that error sounds are related and share some common attributes was a unique one for speech-language pathologists interested in articulation disorders.

Following the introduction of distinctive feature analysis to articulation errors, another kind of phonological analysis, phonological process analysis, gained attention. This conceptualization generated more interest than distinctive feature analysis in speech-language pathology. Like distinctive feature analysis, phonological process analysis draws attention to relationships among error sounds, but in a different form. The idea behind process analysis can be described briefly.

Articulation errors, particularly in children with multiple errors, frequently fall into **patterns**; a child may show a pattern of omitting most final consonants in words, or always substituting stops for fricatives, and so on. It is suggested that these patterns reflect phonological processes that may represent the way children simplify production of sounds they are unable to produce correctly (Edwards & Shriberg, 1983; Hodson, 1986; Ingram, 1976; Shriberg & Kwiatkowski, 1980; Weiner, 1979). To state it another way, children use phonological processes to simplify difficult productions. To illustrate, we might say that a child omits final consonants in words because they are difficult for him to produce; that is, the child is using the process of *final consonant deletion.* Application of phonological processes simplifies productions and results in articulation errors.

A phonological process is not applied to just one sound, but to several sounds. Returning to the process of final consonant deletion, several sounds may be affected. A child may omit the /t/ in words that end with /t/, such as *cat, put, let;* he may also omit the /p/ in words ending in /p/, such as *cup, mop, flip.* All final /f/ and /s/ sounds may be omitted in the same way. Consequently, final consonant deletion affects the /t/, /p/, /f/, and /s/ sounds; therefore, it is a general process (McReynolds & Elbert, 1981a, 1981b). Because it is general and the errors are systematic, relationships among the error sounds are revealed in a process analysis. Different sounds are affected in a similar manner by one process, which demonstrates how the sounds are related. Supposedly, the transfer principle demonstrated in distinctive feature training holds true for training directed at processes in that all affected sounds need not be trained individually. The speech-language pathologist should be able to focus training on elimination of a process, say, final consonant deletion, in only one or two of the affected sounds. When the process is eliminated on those sounds, it should also disappear from the remaining affected sounds without additional training. To date, a few training studies have been conducted to determine whether transfer occurs if training is directed at elimination of processes (McReynolds & Elbert, 1981b, 1984; Powell & Elbert, 1984; Weiner, 1981). Results have been equivocal in that McReynolds and Elbert were unable to show such generalization, but Weiner and Powell and Elbert did.

A number of issues have been raised regarding the reality of processes as defined by most individuals advocating process analysis. The issue is partly related to the theoretical foundation for explaining the nature and form of processes. For example, the theory of natural phonology (Edwards & Shriberg, 1983) makes one assumption about the nature of phonological processes, whereas the theory of generative phonology makes another (Elbert, Dinnsen, & Weismer, 1984). Still others who apply phonological process analysis to misarticulations make no assumptions about the nature of processes, applying the analysis simply to describe the kinds of error patterns in the child's speech (Hodson, 1986). The question has to do with whether the standard for the child is the adult form of the word, or whether her **underlying representation** may be different from the adult form (Elbert, Dinnsen, & Weismer, 1984). For example, if the child never produces a final consonant, or if she doesn't produce the sound in another form of the word, it is difficult to justify the presence of a process. Let us say that a child does not produce final consonants in words such as *dog, bat,* and *take.* She says, [do], [bæ], [te]. How do we know that the child even knows that these words end in /g/, /t/, and /k/, respectively? The implication in some process analyses is that the child knows the adult forms for the words and chooses to omit the /g/, /t/, and /k/. But without evidence, it is not possible to assume this. The child's underlying form for the words may be different from the adult form; therefore, she may not be applying final consonant deletion. We gain some confidence in thinking that a process is operating if in other forms of the words a child demonstrates an awareness that the words contain the /g/, /t/, and /k/. In this example, when tested, the child produces *doggy, batty,* and *taking.* Elbert et al. suggest that the current phonological process analyses assume that the child's underlying representation is the adult's form of the word, but do not test to see if this is true.

A number of phonological process analysis manuals are available commercially (Hodson, 1986; Ingram, 1981; Kahn & Lewis, 1986; Shriberg & Kwiatkowski, 1980; Weiner, 1979). Each manual presents a list of processes and specifies the procedures to follow in conducting a phonological process analysis. It has been pointed out that the number of processes differs from one manual to another, and the definitions do not always coincide (Edwards & Shriberg, 1983); however, the categories of processes are similar. The contribution of process analysis to treatment plans is unclear simply because more attention has been devoted to the procedure for analysis than to remediation. As in other approaches, speech-language pathologists develop their own treatments for eliminating processes (Hodson, 1984; Shriberg & Kwiatkowski, 1980; Weiner, 1981).

The literature on phonological analysis is growing rapidly. Study of phonological acquisition is an active area of research, and we can anticipate that findings from this research will continue to influence our views of articulation disorders. As mentioned earlier, many speech-language pathologists have exchanged the label *functional articulation disorders* for *phonological disorders*. Because training studies are few in number, it is not possible to evaluate the usefulness of phonological methodology and principles to remediation of articulation problems (McReynolds, 1988).

## Miscellaneous Models

Many other models or approaches to articulation disorders are available. For example, some earlier viewpoints stressed the importance of clients' psychological attitude (Backus & Beasley, 1951; Hahn, 1961). In these approaches, clients were not administered direct articulation training. Instead, they were counseled first until they were motivated to change their articulation, and only then received instructions for correct sound production.

It is tempting to say that there are probably as many different approaches as there are clinicians treating misarticulations (Perkins, 1983; Winitz, 1984); however, most treatments can be placed in one of the first three models described here: the discrimination model, the production model, or the linguistic model. These are not discrete models; they frequently overlap and/or include common components. For example, almost all of the treatments in each category employ some operant conditioning principles.

## Summary

Regardless of the speech-language pathologist's theoretical position concerning the cause or causes of functional articulation disorders or the nature of the disorder, most speech-language pathologists do not adhere strictly to any one theory or model of functional articulation disorders. Indeed, there are few "pure" models; the majority are eclectic, incorporating ideas and variables that appear sound or have been evaluated through controlled research. Etiological factors seldom play an important role in planning remediation programs, perhaps because they aren't readily identified. Customarily, too, speech-language pathologists use what they have learned from experience. We must work with the tools and materials available to us: the professional's behavior and the child's or adult's articulation.

As noted, the overlap among approaches is partly a function of research. Earlier we mentioned that many variables have been studied for causal relationships, but none were found to be etiologically important; however, a few of the variables can contribute useful information for understanding articulation problems. These variables are included in evaluations to help determine if an articulation problem is present and how severe it is. Some clinicians use the information in a prognostic sense, while many use the information to plan remediation programs. Later we will discuss articulation evaluation and how these variables influence our decisions. Before moving to evaluation, the variables and their role will be summarized briefly.

# Articulation and Other Variables

### Speech-Sound Discrimination

Some of the problems and discrepancies in the studies of speech-sound discrimination were discussed in the section on discrimination models. No doubt, speech-sound discrimination is one of the variables that has aroused the most attention. From seeking a relationship between general speech-sound discrimination and articulation, the research has moved to discrimination of individual children's specific error sounds and self-evaluation of error productions (Monnin, 1984). On the whole, this latter kind of discrimination research has been more consistent in showing a relationship between discrimination and production, and providing a better rationale for evaluating discrimination during assessment.

### Physical Variables

A number of variables besides structure are included in this category because they all relate to an organic, physiological, or neurologic factor in articulation problems. The interest in physical attributes arises logically from the relationships found between articulation and structure in children with cleft palate; children with other orofacial anomalies; or individuals with dysarthria, cerebral palsy, and oral apraxia. It was thought that children may not present obvious signs of organicity but may still have subtle physical problems. Some of the variables explored include oral structures such as lips, teeth, palate, and tongue. Motor skills related to those structures have also been investigated, as have oral sensory functions and hearing. In general, it has been found that physical characteristics need to be obviously and severely impaired before they are associated with articulation problems. Among sensory factors, hearing is of prime importance; skills such as oral-sensory form recognition, although at times poorer in individuals with poor articulation, are not related directly to impaired articulation.

### Subject-Environmental Variables

Subject characteristics originally received a great deal of attention as factors that might help explain articulation disorders. Among the characteristics investigated were age, sex, personality, and intelligence. To summarize the research, age is a factor only in that older children have fewer articulation problems than younger ones. According to developmental norms, by the age of 8 children have learned to produce all the sounds of their language, and if articulation errors persist past that age, they will probably be more difficult to eliminate. As for sex, intelligence, and personality, they are not important variables as long as they are within a broadly defined range of normality.

Similar findings have been obtained for external factors such as socioeconomic level. Language, however, is gaining importance with regard to articulation errors (Aram & Kamhi, 1982; Panagos, 1982; Shelton & McReynolds, 1979; Shriberg, 1982). Children with multiple articulation errors often evidence concomitant language problems. The presence of a language problem is sometimes defined by the speech-language pathologist's view of articulation disorders. For example, if articulation errors are viewed linguistically, articulation is synonomous with phonology, and phonology is one component of language. Thus, articulation disorders are phonological disorders. It follows that a phonological disorder must be a language disorder, and, as such, is a problem in learning the rules—the organization—of the community language.

## Other Related Variables

The variables discussed thus far constitute the most logical ones to associate with articulation and its disorder. Others have been considered—for instance, auditory memory, general and fine motor skills, and educational history and performance. At times, these may be important enough to be considered in assessment, even though they contribute peripherally, if at all, to the articulation problem. Now that we know more about some of the factors needing attention, we will go on to describe the evaluation procedures for diagnosing presence of an articulation disorder.

# EVALUATION

Evaluation of a child or adult with a possible articulation disorder is a critical process, with more than one important purpose. As we have seen, the first step is an evaluation to determine whether the individual does indeed have an articulation problem warranting attention. Second, if the initial evaluation indicates the presence of a problem, the speech-language pathologist conducts a more complete assessment that includes an in-depth exploration of the person's background and articulatory status. Results of a properly conducted comprehensive evaluation will help the professional understand and describe the problem, outline an effective remediation program, and make some educated guesses regarding the kind and degree of improvement to be expected.

## Initial Procedure

The first decision is whether the child or adult presents an articulation problem severe enough to warrant a more complete evaluation. In many cases, this question has already been answered by other referral sources. In the case of children, parents may be concerned about their child's speech and intelligibility, or teachers may refer children for evaluation. Other sources for referral are dentists or pediatricians who are concerned that a child is slow in developing speech. Adults frequently refer themselves for evaluation because they are concerned about their own speech.

In the public school, referrals may come after the speech-language pathologist has conducted a **screening** of children in the lower grades, or of all children in the school if the school has had no speech services. Screening may take one of several forms. Many professionals prefer to converse casually and briefly with each child on topics of interest to the children. They may ask the children their names, addresses, and when their birthdays are. Frequently each child is requested to count until stopped, or as far as he can. At other times, the children are requested to name the days of the week, and older children may read short passages, such as "My Grandfather" (Darley, Aronson, & Brown, 1975). These passages are chosen because they contain a representative sample of consonants and vowels in the English language, and the speech-language pathologist listens for the child's production of the sounds.

Published articulation screening tests are also available for this purpose. A number of complete articulation tests have a screening version. For example, the Templin-Darley Test of Articulation (Templin & Darley, 1969) has 141 items for testing consonants, vowels, diphthongs, and blends. From those 141 items, 50 have been set aside for screening purposes. One simple and briefly administered instrument that can be used for screening is the Predictive Screening Test of Articulation (Van Riper & Erickson, 1969). This test is designed to predict whether first-grade children will need treatment to correct their articulation errors or whether they will correct their articulation disorders without assistance. It can be administered within a matter of minutes, but the test applies only to first-grade children.

When a screening test indicates that a child's or adult's problem is severe enough to warrant further evaluation, we move on to diagnostic procedures.

## Background Information (Case History)

The extent of the case history information collected will depend on the severity of the problem. For example, if a child is identified in a school screening as having an articulation disorder on only one or two sounds, the speech-language pathologist may choose to obtain only a minimum amount of background information. On the other hand, if a child is referred by other sources, or is found in screening to be unintelligible, the professional will want to obtain as much information as possible. The amount of information sought on each person is based on an estimate of the need for detailed information.

In the initial interview with an adult, or with the parent if the client is a child, it is important to try to establish an understanding of the person's or the parent's view of the problem. The speech-language pathologist should establish effective communication with the adult or the child's parents and the child herself, for in remediation their cooperation is essential if changes are to take place. Thus, a case history is important not only to obtain information on the variables that contribute to the articulation problem, but to get an idea of the variables that are of concern to the people involved.

In some cases, it is essential that the speech-language pathologist obtain information from other professionals such as teachers, psychologists, nurses, social workers, and physicians to gain a better understanding of the problem. When several professionals are involved and after each individual's report has been read, the specialists most concerned about the person may gather to discuss their insights into the problems. They may attempt to formulate a plan together for intervention that will serve the person's needs the best. One of the specialists, the one most closely concerned, may assume primary responsibility for the overall treatment program.

*Remember that P.L. 94-142 currently mandates a team approach to assessing and remediating the deficits shown by school-age handicapped children.*

After a case history has been obtained, the speech-language pathologist will administer tests to obtain a comprehensive profile of the communication problem (or problems) and to gather information for planning remediation. The measures may include tests of skills thought to be indirectly related to articulation, as well as direct measurement of articulatory behavior. We will examine some of the indirect measures next.

## Performance on Related Skills

From all indications, if a clinician evaluates discrimination, an internal discrimination test brings in more useful information than a general speech-sound discrimination test. Recall that **internal discrimination testing** consists of asking the child to discriminate between his specific error sounds and the target sounds, and/or to judge the accuracy of his own productions. Monnin (1984) has explained some of the problems in administering discrimination tests that rely on live presentations. She mentions, for example, that it is essential that the child understand the task; hence, the instructions used are critical. In addition, the clinician's productions are susceptible to variation if the items are presented live. When administering discrimination tests, the speech-language pathologist is aware of these and other possible problems, and examines the results accordingly. Clinicians may administer either an identification test or a discrimination test, depending on the purpose of the test. Usually, the discrimination test requires a same/different judgment of two items presented orally, whereas in an **identification task,** the child is asked to select a phoneme category. In this task, a picture is named and the child points to the picture named in the presence of two or more that differ from each other minimally, for example, *bat, cat, hat.* Both kinds of tests are available. Examples of discrimination tests are the Auditory Discrimination Test (Wepman, 1973) and the Boston University Speech Sound Discrimina-

*Speech-sound discrimination has been discussed briefly in the description of discrimination approaches to functional articulation disorders.*

tion Test (Pronovost, 1953). Identification tests include the Goldman-Fristoe-Woodcock Test of Auditory Discrimination (Goldman, Fristoe, & Woodcock, 1970), and the Washington Speech Sound Discrimination Test (Prather, Minor, Addicott, & Sunderland, 1971).

### Physical Sensory Variables

Other related skills for evaluation consist of the structural, sensory factors and motor skills discussed in the previous section. Factors that seem related to articulation to some degree will be discussed in relation to evaluation.

It was pointed out that structural anomalies need to be rather apparent before they have a strong impact on articulation. Nevertheless, to rule out the possibility of these kinds of problems, the speech-language pathologist conducts an **oral-peripheral** examination. In this examination the speech-language pathologist examines alignment of the teeth, for example, overbite, underbite, openbite. The clinician also looks for missing teeth that might interfere with articulation. The child's hard and soft palate are checked to see if there are any signs of clefts or submucous clefts. The lips and tongue are examined for size and movement. For tongue movement, the child performs a diadochokinetic task in which nonsense syllables such as /pa-ta-ka/ are produced as rapidly as possible for a specific period of time.

Some speech-language pathologists also check for a condition called *tongue thrust*. They believe that some people exert undue pressure against the teeth, which results in malocclusion and possible articulation disorder. The posture is sometimes changed through training. Tongue thrust is a controversial issue (Mason & Proffit, 1974); however, training is thought by some to be beneficial. The Joint Committee on Dentistry and Speech Pathology-Audiology (1975) has published a statement recommending that tongue thrust treatment not be used routinely and that it should be considered an experimental procedure. Perhaps well-controlled research will contribute more information on this issue in the future (Hanson, 1983).

Although individuals with poor articulation do not always recognize forms placed in the mouth as well as normal speakers, oral form recognition is not checked by many clinicians. This is because research has not demonstrated a relationship between articulation and oral form recognition.

*This is called* oral *stereognosis.*

A sensory variable that is of extreme importance is hearing; it is routinely tested. The screening may be conducted by the speech-language pathologist. If a complete hearing test is mandatory, an audiologist may administer the test. Hearing impairment has been shown to affect a person's ability to articulate sounds, particularly the fricatives (Calvert, 1982).

### Subject-Environmental Variables

Subject and environmental variables include age, sex, socioeconomic level, intelligence, personality, educational achievement, and language. Of these, language has been found to be most closely related to articulation disorders, and speech-language pathologists often examine this behavior during evaluation. Language may be measured, but it is less important when children have only one, two, or three error sounds. Children who are unintelligible usually are unintelligible because of both language and articulation problems.

Clinicians who view articulation disorders as phonological impairments are apt to test language more often, even with moderate articulation cases. They obtain conversational samples and perform a syntactic as well as a phonological analysis to examine how a child organizes her linguistic system in language production and reception. Other speech-language pathologists administer commercially available tests to obtain a general picture of the child's linguistic performance, or to rule out the presence of a language disorder. If the test instrument reveals a possible language problem, the speech-language pathologist may choose to conduct a more in-depth linguistic analysis. Many language tests are available to measure both comprehension and production. Three widely used tests are the Peabody Picture Vocabulary Test (Dunn, 1965), Carrow Elicited Language Inventory (Carrow, 1974) and Test for Auditory Comprehension of Language (Carrow, 1973a, b).

## Articulation Assessment

The purpose of the articulation assessment is to obtain as many samples of a person's speech as are necessary to allow an accurate profile of the production of vowels and consonants. More attention is directed toward consonants because of their importance to intelligibility. If an evaluation of the problem in terms of phonological components is desired, production of the sounds in language contexts is obtained.

## Articulation Sample

Ideally, the speech-language pathologist should get samples of speech in spontaneous conversation, naming pictures, and imitation of words modeled by the examiner. This information helps show if the same sound (the test sound) is produced differently in the three kinds of samples. If an older child or an adult is the client, reading is added to the list.

Speech-language pathologists have always attempted to obtain conversational samples as well as responses to structured tests items, but conversational samples have become more important for two reasons. First, we are accumulating data that indicate differences in production of consonants and vowels in conversation and in single words, as in naming pictures (Faircloth & Blasdell, 1979). Second, a phonological analysis requires contextual information, and cannot be performed on isolated sounds independent of the phonetic environment (Ingram, 1983; McReynolds & Elbert, 1981a;

Shriberg, 1980). The production of sounds in single words provides one kind of information about the client's articulation ability, but does not represent habitual articulation in everyday speech. Conversational samples give a more accurate picture of an individual's usual articulation, and reveal if the production of the test sound is affected by the phonetic context in which it is produced. The movement from one sound to another is captured in conversational speech because coarticulation and phonological constraints occur not only within single words, but across word boundaries.

Several problems would be encountered, however, if the speech-language pathologist were to rely totally on conversational samples for information on production of all speech sounds. The primary problem is that some sounds are so infrequent in our language that we would need an enormous sample to evaluate all the sounds. In addition, scoring or transcribing productions from a conversational sample is time consuming. Finally, speech-language pathologists usually like to obtain several productions of any one sound, particularly if the sound appears in more than one position in a word. Since production may differ as a function of position in a word or syllable, it is preferable to obtain production of the same sound in releasing and arresting position in syllable and word contexts (for instance, /m/ in the words *mop, dummy,* and *zoom*). To fulfill that requirement, a large conversational sample would be necessary. The larger the sample, the more time consuming is the analysis of error productions. Therefore, professionals most often use articulation tests to assess articulation, at least initially, and in some cases solely. Such testing provides sufficient information for planning remediation. It is safe to say that the articulation test is the major vehicle used for assessing articulation disorders. Other measures are generally used to supplement the articulation test results. We will now take a brief look at a few commonly used tests.

*For example, the /ʒ/ in the word* azure *is found in only a few words.*

## Articulation Tests

Almost all commercially available tests sample articulation in picture-naming responses. The pictures are of items that can be named by a single word. Each consonant is tested in three positions: initial (*sun*), medial (*bicycle*), and final (*bus*). During testing, the child or adult is shown a picture and asked to name it. The speech-language pathologist records the response on score sheets provided in the testing kit.

In many tests, several forms for recording productions are available to the professional, who selects the one most suitable for his purpose. One simple way to record responses is to note whether the target sound was correctly or incorrectly produced, giving a "right" or "wrong" score. Another recording form is a notation indicating whether the response was a distortion, substitution, or omission (DSO). An example scoring sheet from a conventional articulation test, the Photo Articulation Test (Pendergast et al., 1984), is presented in Figure 7.2. The test consists of presenting single pictures in which the target sound is to be produced in the initial (sun), medial (pencil), and final (house) positions in words. A DSO scoring system is used and stimulability is recorded.

In some DSO scoring, the substitutions are specified; that is, the professional records the incorrect sound produced for the test sound. A final way of scoring responses is a transcription of the productions. Transcribing a production requires the speech-language pathologist to write exactly what the child or adult said on the score sheet. Usually the symbols of the International Phonetic Alphabet (IPA) are used for transcription. IPA transcription demands greater skill than other forms of response scoring, but the detailed information can often be put to use developing treatment plans. The trend is toward transcribing the responses as carefully as possible, so that the speech-language pathologist has a clear idea of how the person is using the articulators in producing errors. In addition, current linguistic approaches to articulation disorders require close phonetic transcription to specify errors explicitly. For a phonological analysis, the clinician must know what the child produces or how she responds to the target sound(s) to specify the rule in operation in her phonological system. For example, if a process such as stopping is to be revealed, the speech-language pathologist must be able to write (transcribe) exactly what the child produces when fricatives are tested—[piʃ] for [fiʃ], [pɪt] for [fɪt], [ted] for [sed].

*This book uses IPA transcription symbols.*

Commercially available articulation tests come in slightly different forms, but they are essentially designed to elicit similar responses. For example, in the Templin-Darley Articulation Test (Templin & Darley, 1969), a mixture of stimuli is used. At times a sentence completion form is presented. The speech-language pathologist shows a picture, begins describing it, and allows the child or adult to finish the sentence by supplying the word depicted by the picture (*Wash your hands with _____*). Questions are also asked (*What swims in water?*). The picture portion of the Templin-Darley is suitable for testing younger children, while for older persons a sentence form is available. The client reads a sentence containing words with the target sound. For instance, a sentence used to test the /s/ sound is *Sam helped a passenger get on the bus.* Many tests simply require the person to look at the picture and answer the question, What is it?

The Goldman-Fristoe Test of Articulation (Goldman & Fristoe, 1972) is often used for articulation testing, as is the Photo Articulation Test (Pendergast, Dickey, Selmar, & Sodor, 1984) and the Arizona Articulation Proficiency Scale (Fudala, 1974). The tests are similar in many ways, yet each one has a particular purpose in addition to the general purpose of assessing articulation accuracy. For example, the Arizona Articulation Proficiency Scale (AAPS) is based on the premise that the more frequently a misarticulation occurs in speech, the more severe is the articulation problem. Therefore, the AAPS gives a numerical scale of articulation proficiency by weighing misarticulations in terms of how frequently each sound occurs in American speech. As in

# PAT RECORDING SHEET

|  |  | Year | Month | Day |
|---|---|---|---|---|
| Name _____ | Date | ___ | ___ | ___ |
| School _____ Grade ___ Room ___ | Birth | ___ | ___ | ___ |
| Teacher _____ Examiner _____ | Age | ___ | ___ | ___ |

Key: *omission* ( − ); *substitution* (write phonetic symbol of sound substituted); *severity of distortion* (D1), (D2), (D3); *ability to say Supplementary Test Words* (circle previous error); *ability to imitate* (circle symbol in "Sound" column).

| Sound | Photograph | I | M | F | Vowels, Diph. | | Comments |
|---|---|---|---|---|---|---|---|
| | **I** | | | | **III** | | |
| s | saw[1], pencil[2], house[3] | | | | au | house[3] | |
| s bl | spoon[4], skates[5], stars[6] | | | | | | |
| z | zipper[7], scissors[8], keys[9] | | | | | | |
| ʃ | shoe[10], station[11], fish[12] | | | | u | shoe[10] | |
| tʃ | chair[13], matches[14], sandwich[15] | | | | | | |
| dʒ | jars[16], angels[17], orange[18] | | | | | | |
| t | table[19], potatoes[20], hat[21] | | | | æ | hat[21] | |
| d | dog[22], ladder[23], bed[24] | | | | ɔ | dog[22] | |
| n | nails[25], bananas[26], can[27] | | | | ə | bananas[26] | |
| l | lamp[28], balloons[29], bell[30] | | | | ɛ | bell[30] | |
| l bl | blocks[31], clock[32], flag[33] | | | | ɑ | blocks[31] | |
| θ | thumb[34], toothbrush[35], teeth[36] | | | | i | teeth[36] | |
| r | radio[37], carrots[38], car[39] | | | | | | |
| r bl | brush[40], crayons[41], train[42] | | | | e | train[42] | |
| k | cat[43], crackers[44], cake[45] | | | | ɝ-ə | crackers[44] | |
| g | gum[46], wagon[47], egg[48] | | | | ʌ | gum[46] | |
| | **II** | | | | | | |
| f | fork[49], elephant[50], knife[51] | | | | | | |
| v | vacuum[52], TV[53], glove[54] | | | | ju | vacuum[52] | |
| p | pie[55], apples[56], cup[57] | | | | aɪ | pie[55] | |
| b | book[58], baby[59], bathtub[60] | | | | ʊ | book[58] | |
| m | monkey[61], hammer[62], comb[63] | | | | o | comb[63] | |
| w-hw | witch[64], flowers[65], whistle[66] | | | Initial | ɪ | witch[64] | |
| | **I** | | | | | | |
| ð | this, that[67]; feathers[67]; bathe | | | | | | |
| h-ŋ | hanger[68], hanger[68], swing[69] | | | | | | |
| j | yes, thank you | | | | | | |
| ʒ | measure, beige | | | | | | |
| | (story)[70-72] | | | | ɔɪ | boy[70] | |
| | | | | | ɝ-ɜ | bird[70] | |

**SCORE**

*Sounds*

I Tongue _____
II Lip _____
III Vowels _____

Total _____

**Figure 7.2** PAT recording sheet. (*Note: From* Photo Articulation Test *by Kathleen Pendergast et al., 1984, Danville, Illinois: The Interstate Printers and Publishers, Inc. Used with permission of the publisher.*)

most articulation tests, the child is shown a picture and the examiner says, "Tell me what they are." The test has pictures that can be used to elicit spontaneous conversation and a sentence form that can be read by the client. Recording takes the form of a DSO scoring: substitutions are transcribed, sound omissions are indicated by a dash and distortions by an X. Each consonant and vowel has a value, assigned according to studies at Bell Laboratories that determined the number of times the sound probably would occur in 100 consecutive speech sounds. The error values of each sound are added and recorded in a total consonant score and total vowel score box. The two scores are added and the total is subtracted from 100 to obtain the AAPS total score. The proficiency of the speech is judged according to categories of scores. For example, a score from 70 to 84.5 is interpreted as "speech that is intelligible with careful listening," and a score from 60 to 69.5 means that understanding the speech is difficult. The test provides one way for a clinician to determine if a child needs to be placed in therapy. Most of the other tests use developmental norms as standards; that is, if the client being tested falls within the range of normal children's errors, then training might be delayed, but if, for example, the child's articulation is a standard deviation below the norm, she is probably a candidate for remediation.

A somewhat different kind of test was developed by McDonald (1964). *Refer to the description of his approach to articulation disorders earlier in this chapter.* A sound is tested in only two positions instead of three, as an arresting sound in a syllable and as a releasing sound in a syllable. Each consonant and vowel included in the test is sampled in approximately 48 contexts. Each sound is tested in two-syllable contexts in which the syllables are formed by two one-syllable words. The words are names for two pictures displayed side by side. For instance, in a sample on /s/ items, pairs of words such as *cup-sun, tub-sun, kite-sun,* and so forth, are presented to test the /s/ in a releasing position in a syllable. The /s/ forms an arresting position in word pairs such as *house-pipe, house-bell,* and *house-tie.* McDonald developed these numerous contexts to give the person an opportunity to produce the target sound correctly if it is present in the repertoire in some phonetic context.

The Fisher-Logemann Test (Fisher & Logemann, 1971) was developed with distinctive features in mind, but is more accurately characterized as a place, voice, and manner test and analysis procedure. As in most standard articulation tests, pictures are named, but the responses are analyzed according to place, voice, and manner errors. Narrow phonetic transcription of the responses is required to identify the features in error.

Other articulation tests (Developmental Articulation Test, Henja, 1968; Integrated Articulation Test, Irwin, 1972) are also available. In addition, some speech-language pathologists develop their own articulation tests using pictures from books or magazines.

## Stimulability Testing

In addition to eliciting spontaneous picture naming, speech-language pathologists test children and adults for their ability to imitate correct production of their error sound or sounds. This procedure is known as **stimulability** testing (Carter & Buck, 1958), and was introduced into evaluation procedures by Milisen (1954). The speech-language pathologist provides a model in words, syllables, phrases, and isolation. Frequently the model is accompanied by instructions or other help concerning placement of the articulators for production of the sounds. Stimulability can be used to discover if the individual has the phonetic ability to produce the sound, and is also used for prognosis. It is one of the variables found relevant to articulation disorders, principally as a predictive tool. Children who can imitate their error sounds correctly are thought to present a favorable prognosis. Speech-language pathologists may decide to delay treatment of stimulable children, with the expectation that correct production may develop without direct training. Even when stimulability information is not used predictively, a child's performance on this task assists in planning treatment, especially with regard to procedures for initial training steps. For example, training imitation is unnecessary because the child already imitates well. Involved instructions on production are not needed because the child knows how to produce the sound. Stimulable children are expected to move through treatment more rapidly than unstimulable children.

Not all speech-language pathologists have equal faith in the usefulness of stimulability as a predictive measure. Results from an analysis of data gathered in a field study of articulation assessment and treatment in public schools prompted Diedrich (1983) to question the usefulness of stimulability performance for planning treatment. Partly because of the lack of congruence in definitions of stimulability and in the procedures to measure it in the studies reported in the literature, Diedrich questioned the usefulness of stimulability in clinical management. The strongest objection was that the stimulability data were derived from group studies, and the individual variability found in children with articulation disorders makes prediction uncertain for any one child.

## Conversational Sample

In addition to the articulation and stimulability tests, a conversational sample may be recorded for purposes of phonological analysis. For hesitant children, pictures are presented to elicit spontaneous speech. Speech-language pathologists learn to provide cues and prompts that work effectively for obtaining speech from children.

# Use of Evaluation Information

A number of results from the evaluation can be used in decision making. Traditionally, the determination that an individual has an articulation disorder is based on a combination of factors. A few of the most important include (a) the person's age, (b) the number of sounds in error, (c) the consistency of error productions, (d) the form of error, (e) stimulability, and (f) dialectal distinctions. We will discuss the use of each of these factors.

With almost all children, speech-language pathologists use a developmental norm analysis to determine whether the sounds in error are produced correctly by most children of comparable age. If they are not, the professional may decide that the problem does not warrant treatment. In this case, the child is frequently placed on a list to be rechecked within a few months or a year to determine whether the correct production has developed. If the sounds in error are sounds that most children younger than the client are producing correctly, however, the speech-language pathologist will probably decide that treatment is warranted. Developmental norms are less useful for older children and adults in deciding if training is needed. When developmental norms are used in the analysis and if they are the primary determiners, the speech-language pathologist will sequence training on the basis of sound acquisition. Sounds that are acquired early will be trained before later-appearing sounds. As discussed earlier in the chapter, however, developmental norms should be used with caution.

Although age comparison is important, other factors are used in conjunction with the developmental timetable. Among these may be the number of error sounds in the person's repertoire. Customarily, a child or adult with many sounds in error would be considered to be more urgently in need of treatment than a person with only one or two sounds in error. But that decision also depends on the form of the error and whether the incorrect productions are consistent. If the child has an **inconsistent error,** producing both correct and incorrect forms of a target sound, the correct sound may be in a transition stage. It is possible that the correct production, which is now unstable, will stabilize without training. And if the error sound appears more in the form of a distortion than a substitution or an omission, the correct production may emerge in time without direct training. One other variable is considered in sifting through the information obtained during evaluation—stimulability. If the child produced the sound correctly in imitation, training may be delayed to give the correct production an opportunity to emerge without training.

All of these variables are weighted singly and in combination to determine if an articulation problem is severe enough to require treatment. Information on other factors will influence the decision as well. Among these are the cultural and/or dialectal variations that are acceptable in the speech community in which the child or adult lives. People living in the South produce the vowels differently from people living in northern states, and Northeasterners drop the /r/ after vowels. Black English Vernacular accounts for some articulatory differences from Standard English (see chapter 4). These differences in a number of minority groups may not constitute an

*Dialectical variations in speech are discussed in chapter 4.*

articulation disorder, particularly if they are not contrary to the speech practices of a given community. Speech-language pathologists must keep these variations in mind when diagnosing articulation disorders.

Consideration must also be given to the person's own concern about his articulation or, if the client is a child, concern expressed by parents or teachers. If these individuals feel that the articulation errors render the person unintelligible, the speech-language pathologist must consider these concerns in evaluating the articulation errors. In addition, reports from other sources that articulation errors interfere with intelligibility will influence decisions by the speech-language pathologist. A factor of some importance in many cases is the person's own motivation for changing his articulation pattern.

## Linguistically Derived Analyses

More in-depth analyses of evaluation results are used by those who believe that articulation problems arise from linguistic deficits more than other sources. Because these professionals suspect that a system is operating to account for the errors and that the errors are related to each other, their analyses are directed to revealing these relationships. As we saw earlier, two kinds of analyses may be performed: (a) a distinctive feature analysis (McReynolds & Engmann, 1975) and (b) a phonological process analysis (Hodson, 1986; Ingram, 1981; Shriberg & Kwiatkowski, 1980; Weiner, 1979). A third has been proposed (Elbert & Gierut, 1986). It is a phonological knowledge analysis, and it is designed to obtain evidence of the form for the child's underlying representation and an in-depth examination of the entire phonological system.

In a distinctive feature analysis, features composing the target sound are compared to the features composing the error sound replacing the target sound. The purpose is to identify the one feature, or the few features, that are in error and account for a number of error sounds. If any such features are found, the speech-language pathologist would use the analysis results to select the features to be trained contrastively. For example, if a child were found to substitute discontinuant sounds such as /tʃ/, /dʒ/, /t/, and /p/ for continuant sounds such as /ʃ/, /ð/, /s/, and /f/, then the child would be trained to establish the discontinuant and continuant feature contrast in a pair of sounds that differ only on that feature. In our example, the pair might be the /tʃ/ and /ʃ/ sounds. Except for the features of continuancy and noncontinuancy, these two sounds are composed of the same articulatory features. Because distinctive feature analysis is time consuming, many speech-language pathologists have not used it unless a child has several error sounds that are difficult to explain without seeking a common factor among them. With the introduction of computer programs that can complete the analysis (Blache, 1982; Driscoll & Driscoll, 1984) in a short time, however, the analysis is becoming more practical.

Another form of feature analysis is a place, manner, voicing analysis. These features are familiar to speech-language pathologists because these phonetic features are used to describe the consonants of our language phonetically. The Fisher-Logemann Articulation Test (Fisher & Logemann, 1971) uses a place, manner, voicing analysis to examine error patterns such as the production of voiceless sounds for voiced sounds or front sounds for back sounds, (/p, t/ for /k, g/).

The error profiles that emerge from feature analyses may differ somewhat depending on the feature system used. Features are often categorized by authors according to the derivation of the features, for example, acoustic, perceptual, articulatory, or linguistic abstractions. Nevertheless, all systems allow identification of error patterns and commonalities among the errors.

A phonological process analysis is usually applied to segments rather than features. In this analysis, all errors are categorized under the processes that appear to fit the description of the process (for example, all words in which the final consonant is omitted are placed in the final consonant deletion process; all words in which fricatives are replaced by stops are classified as being operated on by the process of stopping). The analysis is usually performed on a conversational speech sample because processes are context-sensitive, although sometimes pictures requiring single-word responses are used (Weiner, 1979), as in traditional articulation testing. For example, a final consonant deletion process can be demonstrated only in contexts requiring final consonants, as in words. After each word in the sample is carefully analyzed for processes (there are 8 to 40 or more processes possible, depending on the author), the speech-language pathologist selects the processes, one by one, that will be targets in remediation. The goal in treatment is to eliminate the processes because these simplification processes are responsible for the articulation errors.

An example of the form used to summarize a child's processes in Weiner's (1979) phonological process analysis is presented in Figure 7.3. Weiner separates the processes into three categories, syllable structure processes, harmony processes, and feature contrast processes. Listed under each category are the specific processes accounting for the simplifications indicated in the category titles. Thus, if errors reveal that the child does not produce final consonants, omits one of the consonants in clusters, or does not produce both syllables in two-syllable words, he is simplifying the structure of syllables in three ways. Weiner has designed a computer program to analyze phonological processes (Weiner, 1984b), as has Hodson (1986).

One extension of the phonological process analysis requires an even more in-depth examination of the speech sample. In this analysis the speech-language pathologist seeks to learn more details about the child's phonological knowledge in general (Elbert, Dinnsen, & Weismer, 1984). One purpose is to determine whether the child's underlying representation is the adult form or the child's own form, and how the contrasts in the child's

PROCESS PROFILE

Name _____ Age _____

Birthdate _____

Date _____

| | Proportion of test processes | Frequency of nontest processes | Process decision |
|---|---|---|---|
| **Phonetic Inventory** | | | |

| Present | Absent |
|---|---|
| h w j l r | |
| p b t d k g | |
| tʃ dʒ | |
| f v θ ð s z ʃ ʒ | |
| m n ŋ | |
| | |

Syllable Structure Processes

| Process | Proportion of test processes | Frequency of nontest processes | Process decision |
|---|---|---|---|
| Deletion of final consonants (1) | 8 | | |
| Cluster reduction (4) | 28 | | |
| Weak syllable deletion (3) | 6 | ■ | |
| Glottal replacement (2) | 8 | | |
| **Harmony Processes** | | | |
| Labial assimilation (4) | 8 | | |
| Alveolar assimilation (5) | 6 | | |
| Velar assimilation (3) | 8 | | |
| Prevocalic voicing (1) | 8 | | |
| Final consonant devoicing (2) | 8 | | |
| **Feature Contrast Processes** | | | |
| Stopping (1) | 8 | | |
| Gliding of fricatives (3) | 6 | | |
| Affrication (2) | 8 | | |
| Fronting (4) | 8 | | |
| Denasalization (5) | 8 | | |
| Gliding of liquids (6) | 8 | | |
| Vocalization (7) | 8 | | |

Descriptions of other processes, e.g., manner assimilation, nonfinal devoicing, neutralization, etc.

_____
_____
_____
_____
_____
_____

**Figure 7.3** Process profile. (*Note: From* Phonological Process Analysis, *by F. F. Weiner, 1979. Austin, TX: PRO-ED Inc. Copyright 1979 by PRO-ED Inc. Reprinted by permission.*)

system are applied. The analysis requires elicitation of forms derived from the errors and may include perceptual testing. Standardized tests for phonological process analysis are not available, but step-by-step procedures for conducting the analysis are available in a number of manuals (Hodson, 1986; Ingram, 1981; Kahn & Lewis, 1986; Shriberg & Kwiatkowski, 1980; Weiner, 1979), as well as computer programs that can complete the analysis for the clinician. Customarily, linguistic analyses are reserved for children with multiple articulation errors who are unintelligible or verge on unintelligibility in their speech. If done by hand, the analyses are time consuming. To conduct an adequate in-depth analysis, knowledge of phonemic and phonetic transcription is essential, and some background in linguistic concepts and terminology is helpful. (To obtain the background, see Parker, *Linguistics for Nonlinguists,* 1986.)

## Summary

We have described a number of analysis procedures and variables to be taken into account in planning remediation, including

> analysis based on developmental sequence of sounds
>
> analysis of distortions, substitutions, and omissions
>
> analysis based on distinctive features and place, manner, voicing
>
> phonological process analysis
>
> analysis of child's phonological knowledge

Variables that will influence the plans, in addition to the results on the analysis, include

> chronological age
>
> stimulability
>
> consistency
>
> number of errors
>
> the form of the error sound
>
> dialectal influences
>
> client concern and motivation

The speech-language pathologist attempts to place information derived from all of these measures into perspective. Decisions about which sounds to train, where training should begin, and how training should proceed are usually founded on information from a combination of the factors.

## Evaluation Report

When all the data from the initial interview and the audiological, peripheral, and other tests are in, and the articulation analysis has been completed, a summary speech evaluation report is written. The purposes of the report are to (a) indicate whether the person has an articulation disorder; (b) describe the articulation carefully; (c) make some statements, if applicable, about etiology and prognosis; and (d) make recommendations regarding the kind of training most suitable for the individual. If other professionals have been involved in the evaluation, copies of the report are distributed to them. When the evaluation report has been completed and treatment is indicated, a remediation program based on the recommendations is developed. Remediation is considered next.

# REMEDIATION

We have already seen that speech-language pathologists emphasize testing of the variables most relevant to their particular viewpoint concerning the nature of articulation problems. Remediation programs are subject to the same biases. In addition, other variables enter into decisions about the direction training should take. For example, speech-language pathologists may choose specific procedures from a variety of approaches to develop a treatment package. Some tailor treatment programs to meet the needs of individual clients. Others administer similar treatment to everyone, regardless of the history, the nature of the problem, or the pattern of each person's articulation errors. Professionals differ in their opinions about whether the articulation errors should be treated directly or indirectly. If indirectly, treatment may be aimed at causes or other problems thought to be responsible for, or to contribute heavily to, the articulation problem. Undoubtedly, approaches to remediation are numerous (Perkins, 1983; Winitz, 1984) and depend somewhat on the training received by the speech-language pathologist in her academic program. Little research has been devoted to careful evaluation of the approaches or models proposed and used; therefore, we cannot suggest that any one or several programs are more effective than others.

## General Principles

Although, on the surface, diversity in remediation programs seems the status quo, there is some agreement on broad principles underlying treatment programs. Ordinarily, intervention is viewed in terms of **learning** principles (Bernthal & Bankson, 1988; Weiss, Lillywhite, & Gordon, 1980). Remediation may be thought of as training in learning a motor skill, discrimination skill, articulatory response, or phonological rule, but regardless of what is thought to be trained—that is, the content of what is learned—it is generally recognized that learning takes place during treatment. Therefore, learning principles are used.

Treatment is usually divided into at least two phases, acquisition and generalization. Alternatively, some authors refer to three phases: acquisition, habituation, and automatization, or acquisition, generalization, and maintenance. The phases are not discrete stages in which one is readily separated from the others. In fact, evidence is beginning to accumulate that generalization, the goal of training, is best achieved if planned for from the beginning of treatment (McReynolds, 1987). Nevertheless, it is more functional to talk about remediation in terms of phases for descriptive purposes, as long as it is understood that there is overlap across phases, and the sequence is not uniformly followed in all cases. In the first phase, then, the person is made aware of how a sound is produced correctly and is provided with deliberate practice in producing the sound at a conscious level. In the second phase, the person gradually learns to produce the sound effortlessly in a variety of contexts and situations.

## Acquisition Training

Acquisition training consists of graduated training steps during which the child or adult is taught to produce the target sound consciously. Some clinicians train one target sound at a time, while others train several target sounds from an error pattern simultaneously (Bernthal & Bankson, 1988; Hodson, 1984; Schmidt, 1984). During training, the person is guided carefully through a series of graduated steps, from an incorrect production to approximation of the target response, and finally to the correct response (Bernthal & Bankson, 1988; Sommers, 1983; Van Riper, 1978; Weiss, Lillywhite, & Gordon, 1980). Not only is the specific response developed gradually, so are the contexts in which the response is produced. For example, the progression may be from learning to produce the target sound in isolation, to learning to produce it in more complex units in a sequence from syllables to words to phrases and sentences. A sequence may also be followed in the kind of stimuli presented and the kind of response required. For example, in initial phases, if needed, the person is given a model of the sound and asked to imitate the model. When the imitation is accurate, the speech-language pathologist may shift control to spontaneous production of the target sound. This may be done in a number of ways; most commonly, pictures with the target sound in the names are presented, and the child responds to them. Control can be shifted from picture naming to supplying a word with the target sound in a sentence completion form or to reading (if the child can read). Adults may go directly from imitating to reading.

Within this general framework, speech-language pathologists apply their own specific procedures. The approach used largely depends on the model of articulation disorders adhered to by the clinician. Each model has one or more specific components derived directly from the particular model. Nevertheless, many of the components used in the majority of treatment

*A general outline of training phases is found in Table 7.3.*

programs are similar or even identical. What the components accomplish is open to interpretation by individual clinicians. For instance, all treatment programs present the target sound in a variety of phonetic contexts, for example, the /s/ in initial, medial, and final positions in words; surrounded by different vowels as in *sad, soap, miss,* and so on; and in clusters such as *st, sp, sk,* and so on. It is customary to incorporate the /s/ words in phrases or sentences (*The boy sits quietly*) in later phases of training. If the clinician works within a perceptual-motor skill model, the practice is interpreted in light of establishing a motor schema; within a phonological disorders model, the practice is interpreted as establishing a phonological rule. Thus, there are a number of general procedures that cut across all models and can be applied to all clients, but there are also a few that reflect the model from which articulation is viewed. A few of the specific treatments from the models discussed earlier are briefly described in the next section.

## Perceptual-Motor Skill Treatment

The emphasis in this treatment approach is on drill-like activities in which the target sound is produced in a variety of phonetic contexts. Progression is from isolated sounds, to syllables, words, phrases, and finally to conversational speech. In terms of elicitation, the progression is from imitation to spontaneous speech. In the early phases of remediation, the child is requested to think about how the sound should be produced before producing it deliberately and slowly. As production becomes easier and more automatic, deliberate thought and movement can be relinquished. Target sound practice continues in the various phonetic contexts with an increase in speech production. In the automatization (final) stage, the child is producing the target sound effortlessly and unconsciously.

## Discrimination Models

In these models, regardless of the unit or skill thought to be in the process of acquisition, discrimination or perceptual training is the key ingredient. The child may start with discrimination of externally produced stimuli, for example, the clinician presents the target sound compared with the child's error production of the target. The child is trained to identify correct from incorrect productions as they are presented by the clinician or on tape. Gradually, the child learns to judge his own productions as correct or incorrect. At first, the child may listen to his productions of the target sound in words as they are recorded on tape. The child is then asked to self-monitor by evaluating his articulation live immediately after the word is produced. In other words, monitoring and feedback are gradually shifted from the clinician to the child. When discrimination is judged to be accurate, production training on the target sound is initiated. Although the discrimination phase usually does not extend over a long time period, Winitz (1984) suggests that it can last as long as a year or more.

## Phonological Disorders

In phonological disorders models in which processes compose the central target, a number of different treatments have been developed. The target in all treatments is elimination of processes. It is not particularly important that the target sound selected to help eliminate the process is produced correctly. In fact, adherents of the phonological process approach take pains to point out that it is not relevant, as long as there is evidence that the process is being eliminated. Adherents have individual treatments for eliminating processes. In one approach, for example, several sounds are targeted for work simultaneously and in cycles (Hodson, 1986). The phonological patterns (processes) that need to be treated are addressed in succession. Cycles last from 6 to 16 weeks, and the target sounds may still be in error from one cycle to another. Various procedures, most of them similar to procedures used in the other models, are incorporated into the treatment. For example, auditory stimulation, phonetic placement cues, self-monitoring, a variety of phonetic contexts for target sound production practice, and feedback are all procedures that have been used for many years in different models, and they are included in Hodson's phonological process treatment.

Another popular approach to elimination of phonological processes is the minimal contrast procedure. In one such treatment, the child is taught to produce two sounds that differ minimally in syllables or words. For example, if elimination of a final consonant deletion process is the target, the child may be taught to produce a vowel alone (/a/) and then with a consonant (/ab/) in an alternating fashion. The contrast is between /a/ and /ab/. Other consonants are exchanged for the /b/ as training progresses and the vowel also changes.

A frequently used contrast procedure is one in which the child is presented with two pictures. The picture names differ minimally, for example, *boat* and *bow*. The child is asked to name one of the pictures and request that the clinician pick it up. If the child deletes final consonants, both picture names will be produced as *bow*. If the child intended to say *boat* but produced *bow*, the clinician picks up the picture of the *bow*. When the error is noted, the clinician tells the child how the word should be produced and gives phonetic placement instruction, a bit of discrimination practice, and modeling and imitation. Again, many of the procedures are the same as those incorporated into treatments from other models.

As these brief descriptions indicate, many procedures are similar across conceptualizations of the nature of articulation disorders. Although we have learned a great deal from application of new theories to articulation disorders, it seems reasonable to suggest that all that is presented as new is not really new. For example, the traditional concept of estimating severity of the articulation problem by noting the number of sounds in error, the consistency of the error in a child's speech, and the stimulability of target sounds has now been incorporated into procedures for analyzing a child's phonological knowledge. In a similar fashion, traditional analyses took into consideration aspects such as inventory constraints (How many sounds does the child produce correctly?), as well as position and contextual constraints and morphophonemic alternations (Is the sound produced correctly in the initial, medial and final positions in the test words?). The terms are new, but many of the aspects taken into consideration are familiar. We have learned new ways to organize articulation information, and the new organization allows interpretations that may help in planning remediation programs. The changes appear to be more in the way we interpret data, however, than in the data we gather during articulation assessment and the procedures we develop for remediation.

Regardless of the approach, evaluation is designed for the purpose of allowing the clinician to select a target sound for training. The selection may be strongly influenced by the theoretical perspectives held by the clinician, but once treatment begins, the procedures are often identical.

An outline of a remediation plan is presented in Table 7.3. Depending on results from analyses of error consistency, stimulability, processes, and other measures, the clinician decides where the client should begin training. For example, if the client is stimulable on the target sound in words, training need not be provided on imitation of isolated sounds or syllables, but can begin on word imitation.

### Technology and Articulation

Technological advances in the form of computer software for speech disorders are evident in articulation and phonological disorders. In assessment, several programs are offered that would make the more tedious and time-consuming analyses more efficient. For example, Blache (1982) and Driscoll and Driscoll (1984) offer distinctive feature analyses. Weiner (1984b, 1985) has a phonological process analysis and a program for minimal contrast therapy on a computer disk. Other error analysis and articulation intervention programs are available (Fitch, 1985a, 1985b; Hood, 1984). Undoubtedly, the software for both assessment and remediation will continue to increase.

## Generalization

Articulation remediation, of course, has the goal of changing error sounds to correct sounds that are used in everyday speech in all situations. After the sound has been trained so that the person can produce it readily, attention shifts to generalization of the sound to a variety of contexts, situations, and

**Table 7.3**  General Outline of Remediation Phases and Materials Used

I. Acquisition
  A. Imitative production
    1. Responses
      a. Isolated sound
      b. Syllables—Sounds in initial, medial, final positions
      c. Words—Sounds in initial, medial, final positions
    2. Materials
      a. Clinician produces model
      b. Pictures
  B. Spontaneous production
    1. Responses
      a. Words
      b. Phrases
      c. Sentences
    2. Materials
      a. Pictures
      b. Completion sentences
      c. Short stories
II. Automatization or generalization phase
  A. Conversations with speech-language pathologist on topics of interest
  B. Conversation with speech-language pathologist in setting other than clinic or school
  C. Conversations with other individuals in clinic or school
  D. Conversations with other individuals in other settings
III. Maintenance
  A. Gradual withdrawal of stimuli present in clinic
  B. Gradual introduction of stimuli from the environment into the clinic

persons. We do not know much about how best to effect generalization (McReynolds, 1981, 1987, 1988a, 1988b; McReynolds & Spradlin, 1988; Rockman & Elbert, 1984). Therefore, speech-language pathologists attempt to conduct carryover work by shifting from highly structured to less structured lessons involving reading or conversational speech. Occasionally professionals will bring in other people to participate in the sessions to encourage carryover of the correct articulation with other individuals. They also ask classroom teachers to remind a child or, if the client is an adult, ask family members to be alert to the person's articulation. We must be careful to caution others not to overdo their help, however, so that the person does not become overly self-conscious about the problem. Self-consciousness could result in the person talking less, which defeats the purpose of the treatment program.

The newer linguistic approaches to articulation disorders offer an opportunity to structure training so that untrained sounds and contexts may generalize. Recall that both the distinctive feature and the phonological disorders approaches assume that a system with rules is operating. Thus, as in language, each item affected by a rule need not be trained individually to change the rule. Instead, training on a few examplars might lead to a change in the remaining items affected by the rule. The linguistic models are appealing in terms of the possibility of obtaining generalization with minimal training; however, data for this generalization are not abundant. Generalization has been shown to occur when features are trained (Costello & Onstine, 1976; McReynolds & Bennett, 1972), but conflicting results of generalization from phonological process training have been published (Elbert, 1988; McReynolds & Elbert, 1981b, 1984; Powell & Elbert, 1984; Weiner, 1981).

Procedures for maintenance of corrected sounds have not been specifically studied experimentally, although maintenance has been followed descriptively in a few studies. Variables important to maintenance have therefore not been identified. Procedures suggested for this phase include gradual and sequential withdrawal of stimuli associated with the training situation in the clinic room, or gradual introduction of stimuli from the environment into the clinic situation (McReynolds & Kearns, 1983).

In summary, remediation is an individual process for most speech-language pathologists. Mostly, it depends on each person's biases with regard to the nature of functional articulation disorders. Nevertheless, most speech-language pathologists, when they are exposed to procedures that have been shown to be effective, will incorporate them into the framework of their remediation principles. At this point, procedures used in acquisition training are more specific and exact than are procedures that will facilitate generalization and maintenance of the newly acquired target sound.

As we have seen already, of primary importance to any therapeutic endeavor is trust and understanding between the person with a problem and the helping professional. This is true in treatment of articulation disorders, too. The speech-language pathologist should put forth every effort to gain the child's or adult's cooperation. This is best done by recognizing that the client is a person to be respected, entitled to courteous treatment and understanding at all times; understanding each person's unique needs; and adjusting training so that it suits those needs. It is profitable to spend time encouraging the person to become an active participant in the remediation process, which will encourage motivation to change the articulation pattern that is in error.

# CONCLUSION

Articulation problems are successfully identified, assessed, and treated. Many methods are used for these purposes, all with some degree of effectiveness. The complexity of articulation and articulation problems has gained greater recognition. This awareness in turn has generated issues that need to be addressed in carefully controlled research studies. It has also resulted in new and exciting approaches to understanding and treating articulation and phonological disorders.

## STUDY QUESTIONS

1. What factors are considered in determining how severely intelligibility is affected in articulation problems?
2. The term *functional articulation disorders* has been replaced with the term *phonological disorder*. What is the problem implied in the term *phonological disorder?*
3. Name three analysis procedures that have been based on linguistic theory.
4. Name the components comprising the new model of articulation as a perceptual-motor skill.
5. How are phonological processes identified in articulation assessment?
6. Why should the clinician sample a child's articulation in spontaneous conversational speech as well as on structured single-word tests?
7. If a child produces an error sound in an inconsistent manner, what possibilities should the clinician consider?

## SELECTED READINGS

Edwards, M. L., & Shriberg, L. (1983). *Phonology: Applications in communicative disorders.* San Diego: College-Hill Press.

Elbert, M., Dinnsen, D. A., & Weismer, G. (1984). Phonological theory and the misarticulating child. *ASHA Monograph, 22.* Rockville, MD: American Speech-Language-Hearing Association.

McReynolds, L. V. (1987). Articulation disorders of unknown etiology and their remediation. In N. Lass, L. V. McReynolds, J. Northern, & D. Yoder (Eds.), *Handbook of speech-language pathology and audiology.* Toronto: B. C. Decker.

Winitz, H. (Ed.). (1984). *Treating articulation disorders: For clinicians by clinicians.* Baltimore: University Park Press.

# CHAPTER EIGHT

# Voice Disorders

## G. PAUL MOORE

### MYTHS AND REALITIES

- *Myth:* The vocal cords are similar to violin strings.
- *Reality:* The vocal cords are not cords or strings. They are composed of muscles and related tissue, and are somewhat similar to the lips of the mouth. They are frequently called *vocal lips* or *vocal folds.*
- *Myth:* The vocal folds are located vertically in the throat.
- *Reality:* The vocal folds are approximately horizontal when a person is sitting or standing erect. They are within the larynx and extend from just behind the Adam's apple backward to the arytenoid cartilages.
- *Myth:* Vocal sound is caused by vibration of the vocal folds, which results from nerve impulses from the brain to the vocal folds.
- *Reality:* Vocal sound is produced by vibration of the vocal folds, which are activated by the breath stream as it flows through the larynx.
- *Myth:* Each vowel sound requires a specific pattern of vocal fold vibration.
- *Reality:* The sound produced by the vocal folds is not any particular vowel; it is undifferentiated. Vowel sounds result from distinctive resonance patterns produced by the adjustments of the tongue and other structures

in the respiratory tract above the glottis. The resonance bands or emphases that are unique for each vowel are called *formants*.

■ *Myth:* The larynx is necessary for the production of speech.

■ *Reality:* Highly intelligible speech can be produced by persons who have had the larynx removed. Any complex sound put into the upper respiratory tract can be used for oral communication.

■ *Myth:* Girls do not have a voice change at adolescence.

■ *Reality:* Voice change in girls is not as obvious as that in boys, but a lowering of pitch does occur and is accompanied by a change in quality.

■ *Myth:* Boys and girls are equally liable to develop vocal nodules.

■ *Reality:* Clinical observation indicates that relatively more prepubertal boys, and postpubertal girls develop vocal nodules.

■ *Myth:* Paralyzed vocal folds cannot vibrate.

■ *Reality:* Vibration of the vocal folds is caused by the flow of air through the larynx. Paralyzed vocal folds usually are flexible. If a paralyzed fold rests where the breath stream can disturb it, it will vibrate almost as well as a nonparalyzed fold.

$V$OICE problems include deviations that may impair both speaking and singing. These problems go back thousands of years. They exist among persons of all ages and sometimes are seriously handicapping. Their prevalence and long history have led to many myths about voice production and disorders. A few have been listed here to introduce you to the area of voice and its problems. Voice deviations are all around you. Start listening to your acquaintances, to waitresses and store clerks, athletes when they are interviewed on radio or TV, coaches, and teachers. Many will have some variety of hoarseness or other voice deviation. The following case study introduces you to a likeable high school coach whose voice started to interfere with both his work and family life.

*Keith, a 27-year-old high school football coach and teacher in excellent physical condition, referred himself to the speech and hearing clinic with a moderately severe breathy, hoarse voice and intermittent moments of total voice loss. His pitch range was limited to the low notes in his potential range. He had lost the higher notes with progression of the voice disorder. The coach reported that he was verbal, which was confirmed by the fact that he talked almost continuously during the evaluation.*

*A medical report showed typical bilateral vocal nodules of moderate size. Both vocal folds were slightly inflamed. Keith reported a long history of hoarseness. He had always been active physically and vocally, and noted that the hoarseness had recently become worse. An older friend and coach also had a hoarse voice and a laryngeal tumor of some sort that required surgery. This experience frightened Keith into attending to his problem.*

*His typical daily routine began at 5:00 A.M. with 7 miles of jogging. At 6:30, he conducted football practice, which continued until the start of the regular school schedule. He taught five classes each day in which he lectured most of the time. After school there was more football practice and sometimes he held private classes in gymnastics. He arrived home around 8:00 P.M.; after dinner, he often read bedtime stories to his 3-year-old son. During those evenings when his team had a football game, he shouted and yelled almost continuously throughout the game. His voice was always extremely hoarse following a game.*

*A diagnosis of moderately severe breathy-hoarseness with intermittent loss of voice resulting from medium-size, bilateral vocal nodules was made. These lesions were caused by excessive vocal use and abuse in his occupation as coach and teacher.*

*Keith lived in a region where he could not obtain direct aid from a speech-language pathologist. Consequently, we planned a program with him that contained the following: (a) detailed description of the nature and causes of vocal nodules—this information was presented at the time of the voice evaluation with the aid of photographs of vocal nodules and the playing of his voice recording, and the need to eliminate vocal abuse and reduce speaking to a minimum was stressed; (b) review of the work situation to identify places where vocal abuse could be reduced—this discussion resulted in the following actions: elimination of all except essential speaking (he put himself on almost complete silence for 10 days), introduction of a whistle and bull horn for signalling and giving instructions on the football field, alteration of his classroom methods (use students in instruction, more written work, and the like), and restraint of vocal output during games.*

*After 1 month, Keith returned to the clinic for re-evaluation. His voice had improved substantially, and although the nodules were still present, the general inflammation had subsided and the nodules were somewhat smaller. A continuation of the same therapy regimen was recommended. Subsequent evaluations over the next several months revealed continued improvement except for temporary setbacks following games during which he had yelled.*

*One of the most important changes affecting the ultimate management of this voice problem was in Keith's perception of his role as a coach. He came to realize that his excessive yelling was an extension of his own participation in the sport. During the games and practice sessions, he partially reverted to his playing days through his shouting and excessive verbal output. When his thinking became more mature, Keith was able to exert appropriate control of his voice.*

Have you ever heard a voice with any intermittent **aphonia,** hoarseness, nasality, breathiness? What would you, as a speech-language pathologist, do with and for the man whose voice and case summary were presented? Discovering answers to questions about voice problems is the goal for this chapter.

*Aphonia is complete loss of voice.*

## VOICE PROBLEMS AMONG COMMUNICATION DISORDERS

Many people are difficult to understand or have speech that is unpleasant or unattractive to hear. Some omit or distort certain sounds of the language; others substitute one sound for another; this type of speech, of course, is an articulation disorder. Other individuals speak with many interruptions in the flow of speech, with pauses where they do not belong and with meaningless repetitions of sounds or words. You recognize this problem as *stuttering.* The pitch of the voice of still others is inappropriate. For a man it might be too high; for a woman, too low. Some have voices that are too weak; others, too loud. Still others have voice quality deviations such as hoarseness or too much nasal resonance. The last three kinds of deviations—pitch, loudness, and quality—are customarily classified as voice disorders. These problems sometimes exist by themselves, but frequently they are combined with other voice or speech problems to form a complex communication disorder. The speech-language pathologist must be prepared to manage each or all, regardless of their combinations.

*See chapter 7.*

*See chapter 9.*

*pitch*
*loudness*
*quality*

## Normal and Abnormal Voice

How can voice disorders be recognized? How are they determined? Perhaps the easiest way to get at the question is to try to define the "normal" voice. Experience tells us that there are many normal voices. We distinguish the voices of babies, children, adolescents, adult men and women, and aged men and women. Each of these groups has distinctive characteristics, and they are different from each other, yet they are "normal" as long as they meet our expectations for the group. On the other hand, when the pitch, loudness, or quality of a voice differs from that which is customary in the voices of others of the same age, sex, or cultural background, we classify it as deviant or defective. Obviously, the listener's personal criteria, which are derived from training and experience, are the bases for these judgments. Almost everyone will consider an extremely hoarse voice to be defective, but there are many degrees of hoarseness. Where on the continuum from severely defective to excellent will a particular voice be placed? The listener must make the judgment. Though everyone has a set of criteria for vocal excellence, your evaluation skills will improve with training. Consequently, it is essential that people dealing with speech-language pathology learn to listen definitively. There are instruments now available that assist listening by objectively measuring pitch, loudness, and some aspects of quality.

## Prevalence of Voice Disorders

How many voice problems are there in the population? Many surveys have been made of school populations, but there are no firm figures for the general adult population. The studies in the schools report wide variations that range from a few percent to 20% or more (Milisen, 1971, p. 628; Senturia & Wilson, 1968; Silverman & Zimmer, 1975). These differences probably result from variables such as the grade levels surveyed, the procedures used to gather and evaluate data, the criteria used, and possibly the cultural environment. Children in the lower grades usually have more deviations than older children (Baynes, 1966; Sauchelli, 1979). When we consider all the variables, we can see that selecting even an approximate estimate of the number of voice problems in the schools is arbitrary; however, we need some reasonable estimate to use as a basis for planning remedial programs. Consequently, a compromise, based on the largest survey thus far reported, justifies our accepting 6% as a reasonable estimate (Senturia & Wilson, 1968).

Voice disorders are heard frequently in the adult population, but since these problems rarely interfere with understanding what is said, lay people pay relatively little attention to most of them. One reason probably is that acute temporary conditions such as colds, laryngitis, and other upper respiratory disturbances that cause hoarseness, breathiness, hyponasality, and other vocal variations are so common they are not a source of concern. Unfortunately the chronic and sometimes serious diseases that affect the same areas and cause the same types of vocal deviations also tend to be ignored.

A voice—whether it is good, poor, or in between—tends to be identified with the person who uses it. Many people have a strong resistance to change, even when the voice is seriously defective. A contrasting attitude is found universally among persons who depend on their voices in their work. **Dysphonias,** whether resulting from disease or from no apparent organic cause, can be a source of great concern. When income or social acceptance is threatened, they are highly motivated to correct the problem. Many singers, teachers, lawyers, actors, politicians, and preachers seek help for voice problems. There are also many persons in various other professional groups

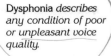

Dysphonia *describes any condition of poor or unpleasant voice quality.*

who are vitally concerned with voice and its production. These specialists include teachers of singers, teachers of speakers, speech-language pathologists, linguists, phoneticians, laryngologists, psychiatrists, and electrical and acoustical engineers. Voice is an enormously complex phenomenon. Those who are primarily concerned with the remediation and prevention of voice disorders are fortunate that there is so much help.

## PHONATION AND THE LARYNX

The squalling of a newborn baby is music to the parents and others in attendance, but the voice cannot properly be called *musical.* The infant fills his lungs with air and expels it vigorously. As the air rushes out, the vocal folds in the larynx come together and are forced to flutter. This vibration rapidly interrupts what would otherwise be a relatively continuous, rushing breath stream. The rapid interruptions of the air flow create pressure changes or sound waves in the air, which radiate in all directions from the infant's mouth and stimulate the ears of the listeners. As the infant matures, he learns to vary the vocal sound to express hunger, pain, discomfort, or pleasure—by cooing, squealing, and laughing. Additional refinement in voice production occurs with the acquisition of language, which is linked to the parallel maturation of the complex hearing, vision, neural, and muscle systems.

All persons involved with the training or remediation of voice should have a basic understanding of both the structure and function of the larynx. Read carefully chapter 3 and note particularly the sections on respiration and phonation.

Some of the vocal sounds produced by infants and adults are musical; others give the impression of roughness or noise that is often called *hoarseness.* Sometimes there is also a sound of the breath flow that is identified as *breathiness.* Occasionally, also, speech sounds that should come out through the nose do not do so, or the opposite may occur and sounds that should exit from the mouth seem to come from the nose. Almost everyone appreciates a musical voice, and most recognize nasality, hoarseness, or other deviant voices. Recognition and identification are important, but speech-language pathologists must also know what happens in the speech mechanism when normal and abnormal voices are produced. They must be able to answer questions such as What happens in the larynx when a musical tone is produced? How do the vocal folds create hoarseness? What is the basis for breathiness? Why is some speech denasal? Why do some sounds escape abnormally through the nose?

The musical, pleasant, or smooth vocal tone that is considered to be the normal voice occurs when the vocal folds vibrate regularly; that is, the glottis is opened and closed in regular intervals to alternately stop and start the air flow. This action creates a series of evenly spaced pressure waves that stimulate the ear mechanisms in comparable sequences. When this normal or musical voice is produced, the vocal folds move through a series of vibratory cycles in which they separate, then come back together again and remain in contact a brief instant. This normal vibratory cycle can be seen in Figure 3.15 on page 94.

If the normal voice slides up or down the musical scale, each succeeding vibratory period is progressively shorter for the upward glide and longer for the downward glide. This type of pitch change is called **glissando** by singers. The important features of these normal phonatory vibrations are regularity in successive cycles and continuous progressive change; that is, there is no random irregularity in the length or amplitude of the vibration from one cycle to the next. When randomness of vibratory period, and consequently of the sound wave, does occur in successive vibrations, the voice is heard as hoarse.

The vocal folds may also produce a breathy voice, a voice that sounds as though it combines a whisper with vocal tone. This type of sound occurs when the vocal folds vibrate without complete glottal closure. The vibratory cycles are composed of opening and closing phases in which the vocal folds move laterally and medially, but do not meet along their entire lengths. Normal speaking contains frequent moments of breathy sound, as when a vowel follows an /h/ or other unvoiced consonant. Some voices are predominantly or continuously breathy, however, and that categorizes them as abnormal.

## PARALLEL PERCEPTUAL AND PHYSICAL FACTORS

So far we have seen that the vocal folds can vibrate slowly or rapidly to create pitch changes, release a sequence of breath pulses under greater or lesser pressure to produce corresponding differences in loudness, or vibrate regularly or irregularly and with various other differences to create several phonatory qualities. These changes in vibration are not haphazard; they have causes. There are underlying physical principles that determine pitch, loudness, and quality.

## Pitch—Frequency

*Pitch* is a perceptual concept that refers to a musical scale. When a tone goes from a lower to a higher pitch, the vibrator, whether violin string, clarinet reed, or vocal folds, increases its frequency. **Frequency,** when referring to sound, is a physical concept that indicates the number of vibrations within a period of time. Raising the pitch, that is, increasing the frequency in a musical instrument such as a violin, occurs when elasticity (or tension) is increased, when the mass of the vibrator is made smaller, or when the length of a vibrator is shortened without changing its elasticity or mass. The pitch of the voice is raised when the vocal folds are elongated. This adjustment accom-

*Remember, the word that means vibration cycles per second is Hertz (Hz).*

plishes two changes. First, it increases the tension or elasticity (which is defined as the relative speed of return of an object to its position of rest after it has been displaced). Second, elongation reduces the mass of the vocal folds at all points along their length. Lengthening the vibrator to raise pitch may seem at first to contradict the idea that a shorter vibrator produces a higher frequency. When the vocal folds are elongated, however, the increased tension and reduced mass counter the length factor and cause a higher frequency. You can observe the same phenomenon by stretching and plucking a rubber band.

## Loudness—Amplitude

*Loudness* is a perceptual concept that has a physical parallel in the amplitude of motion of the air molecules against the tympanic membrane. When the sound wave, which is represented by the forward and backward movement of the air molecules, displaces the membrane a greater distance, the sound is said to be louder. Variation in amplitude is generated at the glottis by a combination of breath pressure and manner of vibration of the vocal folds. When the subglottal air pressure is relatively large and the resistance to glottal opening is substantial, the air is released in brief spurts that have both high velocity and high volume. When a high-energy pulse hits the air above the glottis, it moves the molecules a greater distance than when the pulse has a lower volume-velocity combination. This greater distance is in effect a greater amplitude, which is propagated in the sound wave and heard as a louder sound.

## Quality—Complexity

The quality of voice cannot be completely separated from pitch and loudness, but the word *quality* designates the audible features of a voice that distinguish it from another voice when both are at the same pitch and loudness. The perceptual concept of quality has a parallel physical representation in the complexity of the sound wave. Another way to express complexity is by referring to the number and relative intensities of the partial tones that constitute the sound.

Almost all the sounds we hear are complex sounds. An uncomplex, single, or pure tone is the kind that comes from a tuning fork or pure tone audiometer. When two or more tuning forks are sounded at the same time, the combined sound is complex. There are many other complex sounds, some of which contain **noise.** Some of these are the normal fricative sounds such as /f, v, θ, ð, s, z/. Noise is also a frequent component of hoarse and breathy voices. If several tuning forks are sounding and another is added, the quality of the sound will change. The quality of the sound will also change if one or more of the forks is made to produce a louder sound. As stated above,

*In technical use, noise is complex sound composed of irregular vibrations, to which a pure pitch cannot be assigned.*

the quality of a sound is determined by the number and relative intensities of the partials that compose it.

The complex sound that is *voice* is determined by the way the glottal pulse is released and the modifications of that pulse sound in the pharynx, mouth, and nose. Not all of the vibratory factors are known, but we have reason to believe that the speed of opening and closing of the glottis during vibration, the length of the closed phase in the vibration cycle, and the undulatory configurations of the vocal fold margins influence the number and intensities of the partial tones.

## RESONANCE

*A sonogram is a graph of a sound or sounds, produced by a special electromechanical device.*

*There are many other resonance distortions possible; they are discussed later in this chapter.*

The sound generated in the larynx is modified by a process called **resonance.** As the complex sound passes through the upper respiratory tract, some of the partials are enhanced and others are suppressed. Perhaps the most obvious resonance effect is in the formation of vowels. The partials that are emphasized become apparent as formants that can be displayed by **sonograms** and other means of analysis. Each vowel requires a unique positioning of the tongue and other structures; that is, the /i/ sound in *see* cannot be made when the mouth and tongue are adjusted for /a/ as in *father.* Sometimes the structures are impaired by paralysis or physical deformity, which alters the resonance patterns and creates speech or voice defects. For example, if the velopharyngeal closure cannot be made, sound comes out of both mouth and nose when only the oral route is normal. This open velopharyngeal port produces a hypernasal sound in the speech.

Resonance is a physical phenomenon that occurs in cavities and elastic structures. The air in the respiratory tract is elastic; when the pulses from the glottis enter the airway, they strike adjacent air molecules, which causes them in turn to bump the next molecules, and then the next, and so on. This process creates longitudinal waves that are propagated through the air. After the molecules are displaced, they tend to return to their positions of rest; that is, they tend to oscillate forward and backward. If another pulse comes along, however, the molecules are disturbed again, sometimes before they reach their rest or neutral positions. When a series of impulses occurs, the fluctuations create what we call a *sound wave.* The fronts or advancing parts of the wave cycles travel in all possible directions. They run into the walls and other structures in the upper respiratory cavities and bounce back in widening circles, much like water waves in a tub or pool. Sound waves are even reflected by openings such as the channels between the tongue and palate and the lips. The reflected waves encounter the oncoming waves with varying effects. When waves traveling in opposite directions are moving the molecules in the same back-and-forth directions, the movement is enhanced and the waves become bigger. When the oncoming and reflected waves impinge on the molecules in opposite directions, however, the motion is cancelled and no energy is transmitted. This simplified example explains what happens when a pure tone or a partial in a complex sound is resonated or suppressed. When *augmentation* occurs, the amplitude of the wave is increased and the sound is louder. In contrast, *cancellation* represses both the wave motion and the sound. In the case of the vowel sounds, augmentation and suppression create the formants that determine the phonemes.

By extending this image into the act of speaking, you can be overwhelmed by the potential variations in wave configurations that accompany the changing resonator adjustments. The complexity of the sound may be increased when an organic defect or paralysis is present. The resonance phenomenon persists as a physical occurrence, but the sounds produced are atypical. Consequently, they constitute either an articulation or voice disorder.

Another factor that relates to resonance and has an influence on vocal sounds is *absorption*. When a resonator has hard walls, as in a brass tube, its response characteristics are different from those found in a soft-walled cavity. The hard-walled space resonates only sounds that are at or close to its resonance frequency. In contrast, a soft-walled resonator responds to a broadened range of frequencies around the central frequency of the resonator. When you consider the changes in the linings of the nose, mouth, and pharynx related to moisture and dryness, excess mucus secretion, and abnormal contraction of the muscles, you can easily see the significance of this concept for the speech-language pathologist.

These comments about phonation and resonance imply that they are interrelated in voice production, even though they are distinct functions. This interrelation of the two processes is demonstrated in the production of vowel sounds. The distinction between phonation and resonance is illustrated by the fact that a person may have her larynx removed and still learn to speak. The requirement for speech without a larynx is a sound source that can substitute for the pharynx. Any complex sound in the voice range that can be put into the mouth or pharynx will form intelligible speech when you perform the customary articulatory movements and adjustments.

*The possibility of substituting another sound source for the larynx is discussed in some detail later in the chapter.*

## FACTORS THAT INFLUENCE VOCAL FOLD VIBRATION AND VOICE

We have seen that vocal sound is specifically and closely associated with the way the vocal folds and the resonators function. There is always a reason for a faulty voice and the associated abnormal function that causes it. Some of the causes influence vocal fold positioning and degree of glottal closure, others affect the vibrations of the folds themselves, and many simultaneously impair both positioning and vibration. The underlying factors that influence these laryngeal adjustments and vibration include psychogenic disorders and functional problems, and organic disorders such as paralysis and joint diseases, injury, and debilitating diseases and masses (tumors, cysts, edema, etc.).

## Problems Related to Nonorganic Factors

Voice problems frequently occur when there is no observable disease or structural defect. These disorders presume psychosocial problems or situations that cause atypical behavior of the voice-producing mechanism. Aphonia may occur when a person does not want to speak or sing; however, nonorganic aphonia and dysphonia are more apt to be unconsciously related to stress and anxiety. Emotional problems associated with overwhelming situations at home or at work or school may incapacitate the laryngeal function enough to prevent phonation. There are other instances when a true temporary laryngeal disease creates an aphonia that persists after full biological function has been restored. Possibly the aphonia provides a protection or relief somewhere in the individual's life and is, therefore, extended. However, prolonged aphonia following recovery from an organic laryngeal disorder sometimes results in an inability to adduct the vocal folds sufficiently for phonation. Some voices are aphonic all the time, but that degree of voicelessness is rare. Usually aphonia is intermittent; the voice often alternates irregularly between aphonia and dysphonia, which may be breathy-sounding or hoarse. The implication is that the laryngeal conditions contributing to one type of voice may also cause others when subtle changes in breath flow or muscle contractions occur.

Dysphonia of the breathy type, which signals vocal fold vibration without a closed phase, may also be associated with home or work environments where an extremely quiet voice is required. This type of speaking can easily become habitual. A similar condition and voice may be developed by young women in high school and college who try to emulate actresses and entertainers. In our culture, the breathy, low-pitched, female voice is often interpreted as "sexy."

*As in articulation and other disorders, a functional voice disorder has no known physical cause.*

Another type of functional dysphonia occurs when the vocal folds are squeezed together so tightly that they cannot vibrate normally. The adjustment resembles the laryngeal closure in the first stage of a cough. When overadduction occurs, the vocal sound may be quite hoarse and low-pitched, as heard in some of the stereotyped gang bosses shown in films. Occasionally the ventricular folds are adducted more or less completely and forced to vibrate. The voice usually is quite hoarse. The several forms of hoarseness associated with excessive closure of the glottis are called *hyperfunctional dysphonia* in the literature (Boone, 1983; Froeschels, 1952).

## Problems Related to Organic Factors

*An organic impairment is one which has a physical cause.*

Many voice disorders are caused by **organic** impairments. Treatment of the underlying problem is usually the responsibility of medical specialties such as otolaryngology, endocrinology, or neurology. If a person with a voice disorder comes to a speech-language pathologist for assistance without previous *hyperfunctional dysphonia* (handwritten annotation)

attention by a physician, the individual with the problem must be referred for proper medical diagnosis and appropriate treatment. Subsequently, if voice therapy is indicated, the speech-language pathologist should relate the plan for the remedial voice program to both the underlying problem and the medical treatment used. Consequently, the speech-language pathologist must have a basic knowledge of the common diseases, disabilities, and medical treatments related to the voice-producing mechanism.

## Paralysis

A common organic cause for the failure of the vocal folds to close the glottis completely is paralysis, which usually results from impairment of the nerve supply. Paralysis is a disorder in which a muscle loses the ability to contract; consequently, the structures to which paralyzed muscles are attached cannot be moved voluntarily. A paralyzed vocal fold can be vibrated almost as well as a healthy one, however, when it rests where the air stream can disturb it. In unilateral paralysis, the healthy fold usually can approach its paralyzed mate and thereby narrow the glottis enough to cause the air stream to set the folds vibrating. The closer the folds approximate each other, the louder and less breathy the sound. In bilateral paralysis, both folds often rest in paramedian positions, which provides the condition for an almost normal voice. Unfortunately, the airway is usually compromised, breathing becomes difficult, and surgical intervention is necessary to ensure an airway.

Ankylosis, or impairment of arytenoid movement resulting from stiffness or fixation at the cricoarytenoid joint, is another cause for incomplete glottal closure and a breathy voice. If cancer, arthritis, or some other inflammatory joint disease prevents adduction and abduction, the function of the impaired larynx is essentially the same as that which accompanies paralysis. The amount of glottal opening varies among individuals, and the severity of the vocal deviations corresponds to the degree of opening.

*ankylosis, fixation, cricoarytenoid joint – incomplete glottis closure, breathy voice* (handwritten annotation)

## Trauma and Surgical Modification

Occasionally movements of one or both arytenoid cartilages are limited or prevented by trauma. If the cartilages of the larynx are fractured in an automobile or motorcycle accident, they may heal in such a way that normal motion is not possible. The accompanying voice, of course, varies with the type and extent of the physical alteration.

The trauma problem is illustrated by the case of an 18-year-old student who was in a motorcycle accident. He was riding through a forest at dusk when he struck a chain that had been stretched across the trail at neck height. His larynx was crushed, but surgeons realigned the broken cartilages and placed a special splint called a **stent** into the larynx to support the parts while they healed. After the stent was removed, both vocal folds remained in

*stent – splint for larynx* (handwritten annotation)

lateral positions, causing a wide open glottis and total aphonia. Some months later, the right vocal fold regained the ability to adduct and abduct normally, but the left arytenoid cartilage and vocal fold remained somewhat lateralized. With the restoration of a partial glottal closure, some vibration could be achieved, producing a weak and breathy but serviceable voice.

A laryngectomy *is surgery to remove the larynx.*

A similar case occurred in which the larynx was crushed so severely it could not be preserved. Consequently, a total **laryngectomy** was performed. This young man developed excellent esophageal speech. Additional information about speech without a larynx can be found later in the chapter.

### Debilitating Diseases and Conditions

Incomplete or inadequate glottal closure can be caused by weak muscle contraction. A common cause of muscle weakness and relatively quick fatigue is anemia. This disorder results from an inadequate blood supply to muscles, organs, and other body parts. People who are chronically fatigued or who tire quickly with exertion often reflect this condition in the voice, which tends to be weak and breathy.

Anemia may also contribute to vocal weakness through its effect on the muscles of respiration. Since the loudness of voice is directly related to breath pressure, and since breath pressure is determined by expiratory force exerted by the thoracic and abdominal muscles, it follows that fatigue of these muscles will diminish the vocal energy.

Myasthenia *means a muscle without strength.*

Myasthenia can interfere with gross adduction and also the finer adjustments of the intrinsic laryngeal muscles. The term *myasthenia laryngis* was introduced by Jackson and Jackson (1937) to refer to muscles that are more or less chronically fatigued and tire readily.

### Protruding Masses

Closure of the glottis can be prevented by tumors or granulomas between the arytenoid cartilages or along the glottal borders. These abnormal structures interfere mechanically and result in an incompletely closed glottis or atypical vibration.

## LOCALIZED LESIONS AND OTHER DISORDERS

Frequently the conditions that impair glottal adjustment have a local influence on one or both vocal folds to cause voice abnormalities. Earlier in this chapter, we mentioned that hoarseness can be caused by random variations in the consecutive vibrations of the vocal folds. One cause for this vibration is abnormal increase or decrease in the size or mass of one or both vocal folds. Aronson (1980) summarized the effects of mass lesions:

Mass lesions of the vocal folds ... produce one or more of the following pathologic changes.

1. Increase the mass or bulk of the vocal folds or immediately surrounding tissues.
2. Alter their shape.
3. Restrict their mobility.
4. Change their tension.
5. Modify the size or shape, or both, of the glottic, supraglottic, or infraglottic airway.
6. Prevent the vocal folds from approximating completely along their anterior margins.
7. Result in excessive tightness of approximation. (p. 57)

What are these masses that can influence the vocal folds, their vibration, and the voice? A few of the common ones need to be well understood by the speech-language pathologist. You must always remember, however, that an abnormal voice and the aberrant vibrations associated with it can have a variety of causes. You cannot diagnose a specific disease by the sound of the voice. A mass on a vocal fold exerts its influence variably according to its location, size, and firmness.

## Tumors

Tumors usually come to mind first when you think about mass lesions of the vocal folds, but what is a tumor? The word *tumor,* like the word *automobile,* has a broad meaning encompassing many types. *Tumor* has been defined as a "neoplasm (new growth); an abnormal mass of tissue that grows more rapidly than normal and continues to grow after the stimuli which initiated the new growth cease" (*Stedman's,* 1976). They can be either benign or malignant. A *benign* ("kind") tumor is "one that does not form **metastases** and does not invade and destroy adjacent normal tissue" (*Stedman's,* 1976). *Malignant* means evil: "cancer; a tumor invading surrounding tissues and usually capable of producing metastases, likely to recur after attempted removal and to cause death of the host unless adequately treated" (*Stedman's,* 1976).

Metastasis *means the transfer or migration of a disease from one location to another and the establishment of the disease in the new location.*

## Polyp

A polyp is a benign tumor commonly found in the larynx. This term is also broad in its meaning. **Polyp** "is a general descriptive term used with reference to any mass of tissue that bulges or projects outward, or upward, from the normal surface level" (*Stedman's,* 1976). It may be broad-based (*sessile*) or be attached by a stalk (*pedunculated*).

If a polyp protrudes from the glottal border of a vocal fold, it tends to interfere with contact between the folds during vibration. The result may be a breathiness in the voice. If the polyp is large, it may rest partially on the opposite vocal fold, where it interferes with vibration. It may become an auxiliary vibrator contributing to the hoarseness.

## Vocal Nodules

**Vocal nodules,** often referred to as *singer's nodes* or *screamer's nodes,* are a type of polyp. Vocal nodules are usually small, sessile, slightly pink or grayish-white protrusions located bilaterally, opposite each other at the junction of the anterior and middle thirds of the entire length of the vocal folds. This position is the same as the midpoint of the membranous section of the vocal folds. The location of the nodules probably identifies the place of greatest trauma during vocal fold vibration.

These lesions tend to develop in people who yell themselves hoarse at football games or who abuse their voices with other types of excessive use. The vocal abuse causes swelling that reduces the flexibility of the vocal folds, tends to increase their contact at the swollen areas, and may also prevent total glottal closure. Swelling usually disappears in 24 to 36 hours with rest and moderate use. When vocal misuse continues, however, as with people who talk excessively, yell often, or sing abusively (as in some popular entertainment groups), the swelling persists, tissue changes occur, and the traumatized area becomes organized, circumscribed, and protuberant. The larynx pictured in Figure 8.1 shows vocal nodules in a 21-year-old woman.

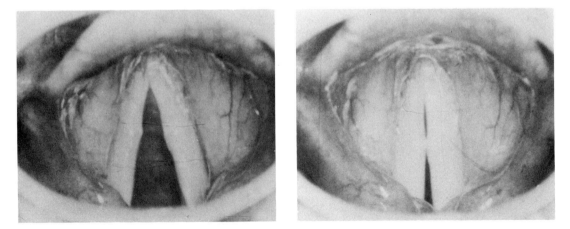

**Figure 8.1** Well-defined vocal nodules in a 21-year-old female. These lesions were caused by a combination of yelling, singing, and excessive talking. The voice was breathy-hoarse.

The abusive vocal behavior associated with vocal nodules can be caused by both psychological and social factors. The typical child with nodules is a younger sibling who fights verbally with his brothers and sisters. He is usually competitive, aggressive, interested in sports, vocally loud, and has some personality adjustment problems. Aronson (1980) observes that the factors related to vocal nodules in children are basically similar to those in adults.

## Papillomata

Papilla *means nipplelike.*

There are two general kinds of **papillomata;** one kind is hard, the other soft. An example of a hard papilloma is the common wart. The soft papillomata do not look like warts, but instead tend to be glistening, pinkish-white, and irregular. These lesions arise from the mucous membranes and may be found in the pharynx, trachea, and at other sites, including the larynx. "Papillomata are the most common laryngeal tumors of childhood; and although their presence is not unusual at birth, they are most often discovered between the ages of 2 and 4" (Aronson, 1980, p. 60). When these lesions are located on the vocal folds, they usually cause dysphonia; the type and severity of the voice deviation is related to the size and location of the lesion.

## Carcinoma

A **carcinoma** (a type of cancer) is a malignant tumor and is indeed an evil thing. It can grow on one or both vocal folds and affect their vibration much as do polyps or papillomata. It is not possible to distinguish among carcinoma, polyps, papillomata, and the like, by the sounds produced. They all simply alter the manner in which the vocal folds are positioned and vibrate. Each can disrupt the behavior in the same way. The etiology of carcinoma is not known, but there is a well-established positive statistical relationship between laryngeal cancer and smoking. The chance of developing laryngeal cancer is increased substantially when alcohol is combined with smoking (Snidecor, 1962, 1971; Webb & Irving, 1964).

Carcinoma, which is a cancer that develops from surface tissue, may grow subtlely in the larynx and not become apparent until it produces a change in the voice. This vocal change often appears early in the course of the disease and provides an opportunity for early, and frequently successful, treatment. Therapy is the responsibility of physicians, but their treatment may leave a condition that requires the services of a speech-language pathologist.

## Edema

-itis *means inflammation.*

An edema is a swelling caused by excessive fluid in the tissues. Its presence in the larynx signals a number of possible problems, which include vocal abuse, laryngitis, localized diseases, and systemic disorders such as endo-

**Edematous** *means filled with fluid or swollen.*

crine disturbances. The amount of swelling can vary from minimal to extensive, involving one or both entire vocal folds. When it is minimal, it may lower the pitch slightly as the result of increased mass and change in compliance. When swelling increases moderately, it can cause some changes in the vibration sequences, leading to hoarseness. When edema becomes so extensive that the vocal folds are greatly enlarged, the arytenoid cartilages may be prevented from adducting, which could leave an opening between them and cause a breathy hoarseness. With this degree of swelling, the vocal folds may also be pressed together so tightly that they cannot vibrate. Edema is not a disease, but a symptom that can be caused by various etiologic factors.

## Contact Ulcer

Another laryngeal disorder that is causally related to the way a person speaks and may produce vocal deviations is contact ulcer. Vigorous glottal closure sometimes traumatizes the mucosal covering of the vocal processes or other contacting areas of the arytenoids, causing an ulcer (a sore) to form on one or both cartilages. Frequently, as inflammatory processes continue, granulation tissue develops on the ulcer. The granulation may become large enough to prevent complete glottal closure. There is some evidence that gastric reflux is a predisposing factor (Cherry & Margulies, 1968; Chodosh, 1977; Delahunty & Cherry, 1968).

## Laryngeal Web

**Congenital** *means present at birth.*

**Laryngeal web** refers to a membrane, extending usually from one vocal fold to the other. It may occur also at the level of the ventricular folds or below the glottis and be either **congenital** or composed of scar tissue resulting from injury or surgical procedures. Webs can vary in size from a small bit of tissue to a membrane that completely occupies the glottis. When the web is extensive, it will impair respiration and require surgical intervention. When it is smaller, it may cause stridorous breathing or hoarseness, or even aphonia. The presence of the smallest congenital webs may not become apparent until a child attempts to talk. The voice may be hoarse and have a higher than normal pitch. This condition is another in which the laryngeal surgeon and speech-language pathologist must work together.

The effects of a laryngeal web and other problems are illustrated in the case of an 11-year-old boy in the fourth grade who had hypernasality and a high-pitched voice. The other children called him "squeaky" as a result of his unusual voice and ridiculed him. The hypernasality reduced his intelligibility somewhat and contributed to his communication problem. All these conditions led to withdrawal from his schoolmates and reclusiveness.

The child was examined by several physicians over a period of years. They reported a **bifid uvula** (divided in two parts) and a normal larynx. The probable cause for the nasality was recognized as the uvular defect, but the speech-language pathologist who worked with the boy became convinced that there was also some laryngeal abnormality causing the high pitch. She arranged for another laryngeal examination. On this attempt, a small web was exposed between the true vocal folds at the anterior commissure. Appropriate laryngological procedures eliminated the web and provided the basis for a normal voice, which the speech-language pathologist was able to help the boy develop and stabilize. The hypernasality was reduced through speech therapy, and the boy's personality improved markedly.

## Cysts

A *cyst* is "a closed bladder-like sac formed in animal tissues, containing fluid or semifluid morbid matter" (*American,* 1951). Sometimes they develop on a true vocal fold, as illustrated in Figure 8.2. When a cyst is on the glottal border, the voice is usually breathy and soft, similar to that heard with a polyp or other protrusion.

## VOICE DISORDERS RELATED TO RESONANCE DEVIATIONS

The discussions in the preceding section emphasize phonatory problems; that is, voice disorders originating at the sound source. In the case report of the 11-year-old boy with a congenital web and bifid uvula, however, we

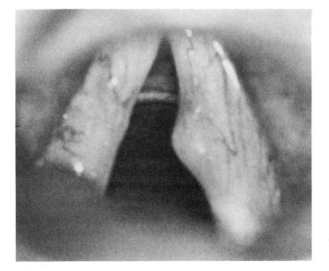

**Figure 8.2**   A cyst on the left vocal fold of an adult woman

referred to hypernasality, a resonance problem. Phonatory and resonance deviations may each cause voice disorders, but many vocal problems result from combinations of the two. Most resonance disorders can be characterized as either too much or too little nasal resonance. There are other types of resonance problems, but they are relatively unimportant in the present discussion.

## Hypernasality

*Chapter 11 discusses cleft palate in detail.*

When the sounds /m, n, ŋ/ come out through the nose, they are considered normal. When part or almost all of the other sounds of English escape through the nose, the result is atypical and is classified as abnormal. There are two types of **hypernasality** that are accompanied by nasal emission. A third uses the nasal spaces for resonance, but little or no sound is emitted from the nose.

One of these hypernasalities is caused by a continuous opening between the oral and nasal cavities. This speech often accompanies a cleft palate, a short palate, or paralyzed soft palate, and may be difficult to understand. People with these disorders may also have a noisy escape of air from the nose, particularly on the plosives and fricatives, sounds that normally require an increase in oral breath pressure.

A mild form of hypernasality is found in many speakers who habitually use an imprecise form of articulation. The problem is most obvious during rapid speaking; it is usually absent when vowels and other nonnasal sounds are produced in isolation. These persons sometimes present a mixture of hyper- and hyponasality. This tendency to mix the forms is increased when the adenoids are enlarged.

A second type of hypernasality is frequently referred to as *nasal twang*. The voice is related auditorially to the nasal area, but there is no audible air flow through the nose. Some regional dialects involve nasal twang, and there, of course, the voice is not considered to be abnormal. Country and bluegrass singing are often characterized by this sound. The twang hypernasality is caused by reduction of the size of the velopharyngeal opening in association with constriction of the pharyngeal and laryngeal muscles. It is almost without exception a learned vocal quality.

The third type of hypernasality sounds a little like the twang, but it is caused by an obstruction in the anterior part of the nasal spaces. It can be produced intentionally by pinching the nostrils closed and attempting to talk through your nose. When the nasal passages are occluded anteriorly and sound is allowed to enter the nasal cavities through an open velopharyngeal port, the posterior part of the nasal spaces and the nasopharynx resonate the sound jointly with the oral-pharyngeal space. The sound is emitted from the mouth.

## Hyponasality

Another type of resonance problem related to the nose is called **hyponasality** or *denasality*. As the name implies, there is less than the expected amount of nasal resonance, which results from an occlusion of the nasal spaces either in the nasopharynx or at the posterior part of the nose. Almost everyone has had this type of voice with a severe head cold. When denasality is chronic, however, it is usually caused by enlargement of the adenoids.

## ASSESSMENT AND DIAGNOSIS

Speech-language pathology is a direct, active clinical profession. The speech-language pathologist's major objective is to provide effective therapy that will enable an individual with a speech or voice problem to speak more normally or adequately. To develop rational therapy, the speech-language pathologist must understand the structure and function of the vocal mechanism and the disorders that may impair that mechanism. We have now sketched those factors. To know *about* it is not enough, however; you must also have a knowledge of *how to*. How to develop therapy begins with an assessment of the voice and a diagnosis, or determination of its cause, whenever possible. Starting therapy without a diagnosis is a lot like starting on an automobile trip in a strange place without a map.

The procedures of assessment and diagnosis of voice disorders are not codified into one best system, but a plan that works reasonably well can be described as having five steps: (1) listening; (2) looking; (3) asking questions, that is, obtaining a history; (4) seeking the help of specialists in other fields as necessary; and (5) assembling the data and establishing a diagnosis.

## Listening

Earlier in this chapter, you were urged to listen to the voices of your associates and strangers and to your own voice. Now that we have described many of the causes of voice problems, you should be able to listen with greater precision and to have some insight into related causes.

The voice pathologist's ear is her most useful instrument; it recognizes when the pitch goes upward or downward on the musical scale, the sound is loud or soft, and the voice quality deviates from normal. It does not, however, measure how much change or deviation is present, nor does it remember vocal sounds over a period of time. There are a number of manufactured instruments on the market that will precisely display pitch (frequency), loudness (intensity), breath flow, duration, and some of the components of quality to aid the clinician and the client in both diagnosis and therapy (Baken, 1987; Hirano, 1981; Stemple, 1984). Most of these instruments allow measurement, which means that changes over time can be monitored and compared. The amount of vocal improvement or regression reveals the effectiveness of therapy or, possibly, the progression of disease. New instruments are being developed and many of them are related to computers. There is not enough space here to describe them, but this fact is not detrimental at this stage in your training. More efficient and more user-friendly instruments will be available when you take advanced training. The most widely used aid now in both diagnosis and therapy is the sound recorder. It is essential and since it has been available for so long, almost every school system and clinic will have such equipment.

How should you go about listening to a voice that may be defective or atypical? You should listen to a variety of samples to assess its conversational characteristics, customary pitch and pitch range, usual loudness, and phonatory and resonance qualities. A simple method of listening to a voice is to record it. This procedure not only gives you an opportunity to hear the voice in its customary state, it also establishes a permanent record for reference.

By the time the speech-language pathologist has heard the voice samples from preliminary conversations and during the recording, he should be able to describe the major features of the problem and its probable source, that is, the larynx, resonance areas, or both. Any other deviations in speaking, such as articulatory abnormalities, should be noted also.

## Looking

Usually what you hear is not an adequate basis for assessment; observation of the organs and structures that produce the voice is also necessary. The speech that comes from a person's mouth is only as good as the motions and adjustments of the structures that produce the speech.

Looking means observing the size, shape, color, and mobility (where applicable) of the face, lips, teeth (and mandible), tongue, hard and soft palate, pharynx, and larynx. Casual observation of the face while the child or adult talks and smiles will usually identify asymmetries or sluggish movements. The purpose here is to identify weakness or paralysis that may have a relationship to the speech or voice disorder. Looking at the regularity and occlusal relationships of the teeth can also be valuable. This type of observation, as well as noting other internal structures, can be aided by a flashlight.

Observe your own face and mouth in a mirror. Note the features of your lips, tongue, the way your teeth occlude; watch your soft palate when you yawn and produce various sounds. Try to see your palatine tonsils. The vocal folds cannot be seen when looking directly into the mouth; however, a trained person can view them with the aid of a small mirror, similar to that used by a dentist, when it is placed in the pharynx. Look carefully at the vocal fold images in this chapter and chapter 3. They were all made with the aid of a mirror. Self-observation of the structures used in speaking is a first step toward diagnostic observation of persons with voice and speech problems.

## History

The history of a voice disorder often contributes greatly to the planning and conduct of the remedial program. In those instances where the cause of the problem is obvious, such as an accident, surgery, or a specific disease, the collection of background data will concentrate primarily on current attitudes about the problem, expressed need for remedial help, motivation, and capacity to undertake a remedial program. When the cause of the vocal difficulty is not evident, however, careful questioning is essential. The speech-language pathologist attempts to obtain the following five types of information: (1) the individual's opinion of the nature and seriousness of the problem; (2) the start and course of development of the problem, including previous speech treatment; (3) medical and health history; (4) family structure and interrelationships; and (5) history of voice and speech deviations in the family. Answers to these questions will tell how precisely the child or adult perceives the problem as compared with what the examiner has heard and seen. It will also reveal the length of time the disorder has been present, plus the suddenness or gradualness of onset. Learning about previous remedial experience will give insight into the concern for the problem felt by the person and the family. The medical and health history, particularly prior to and around the time the voice problem seemed to begin, may reveal not just the diseases that could have influenced voice production, but also the feelings of the family toward the person and the problem. The family structure, including the number of siblings, the position of a child in the sequence of children, and the stability of the family, will reveal the presence or absence of verbal competition and compatibility. These factors are often associated with vocal abuse and voice disorders. When voice disorders are apparently present from birth, as evident in the cry sound or stridorous breathing, the etiology may be developmental lag, structural abnormality, or disease. The developmental and structural deviations may be inherited, and questioning sometimes reveals voice problems elsewhere in the family.

*In cases where you are assessing a child, you may have to obtain the history from the parents.*

Obtaining a thorough case history requires broad knowledge about speech and voice disorders and skill in formulating questions. It is a process designed to aid the person with the problem, but she may not always perceive it as such. Questioning is an art that improves with self-evaluated experience.

*It can be facilitated by careful reading of the pertinent books listed at the end of the chapter.*

## Referral

As we have seen, voice disorders have different and often quite complicated etiologies. This chapter has suggested that the causes may be found in heredity, disease, injury, learning ability, family structure, environmental models, or a combination. While speech-language pathologists are required to know the potential significance of etiologic factors, they are not qualified to explore all of them. Fortunately, there are skillful professional colleagues in special areas of medicine, psychology, and education who are ready to help. Frequently, a complete diagnosis of a voice disorder cannot be made until one or more of the specialists has contributed his or her evaluation.

## Summary and Diagnosis

The cause of voice disorders can usually be determined when the description of the vocal sound is evaluated along with observations made by the speech-language pathologist and physician, and with information from the history. Of course, during the voice evaluation, the examiner constantly relates what is heard with what is seen and reported, so that establishing a diagnosis may not require a separate, formal assembly process. When referral data are not available at the time of vocal assessment and several persons are involved in the evaluation, however, a systematic amalgamation of information is desirable. The first focus is on a description of the voice and an indication of its relative severity; second, a statement should be made of pertinent medical, social, and psychological information; finally, an opinion should be stated that indicates the probable causal chain. The case study and recording presented at the beginning of this chapter illustrate a typical summary and diagnosis.

## THERAPY FOR VOICE DISORDERS

The real reason for learning about voice disorders and their causes is to help prevent or remedy these disorders. We have seen that voice problems almost always occur when the vocal folds vibrate abnormally or when the resonators are shaped or linked atypically. The altered vibration and resonance can be caused either by organic changes affecting the size, shape, texture, tonicity, and position of the critical structures, or by learned changes, which can also determine position as well as dimensions and contractile tensions in the antagonistic muscle groups. The organic changes originate in disease, heredity, injury, and aging; the learned changes are based on speech models, personal beliefs, and methods of adjustment to environmental requirements and stresses. Obviously, the organic and nonorganic causes are frequently intertwined. Whenever possible, therapy is directed toward the underlying causal factors. Sometimes the direct causes are no longer active or are not amenable to change. Consequently, therapy must often be directed partly or entirely to symptoms. Unfortunately, the term *voice therapy* is synonymous with *voice exercises* for many people. Voice exercises *are* important, but they constitute only a small part of voice therapy. One of the major objectives of

*For an example, see the case study at the beginning of the chapter.*

this chapter is to stress that vocal rehabilitation is an overall process affecting the individual's health and lifestyle as well as the voice itself.

Therapy for voice disorders combines three distinct but interdependent procedures. One is medical, which includes surgery, radiation, medication, and psychiatry; the second is environmental, which encompasses both modification of the environment for the benefit of the child or adult and the related program of helping the individual adjust to the environment; the third is direct vocal rehabilitation, which includes the training activities for reducing the disorder and improving the voice.

## Medical Approach

Surgical treatment may completely eliminate a voice problem, or it may unavoidably leave an impaired structure and a voice defect. In this situation, voice rehabilitation may help the person achieve maximum effectiveness with the structures that remain.

Medications and other nonsurgical techniques may help cure a disease or bring a condition such as anemia or allergic response under control, thereby restoring physical vigor or reducing swelling. This kind of aid provides a more normal vocal mechanism and the possibility of a normal voice.

## Environmental Approach

Earlier in this chapter we suggested that school or employment and living environments sometimes cause people to use their voices excessively or traumatically and thereby create behavioral or organic changes in the larynx that produce voice disorders. Environments may also contain physical irritants or allergens that are detrimental to the larynx or resonators and consequently cause problems.

Voice therapy must consider, and when possible alter, these detrimental factors. One procedure that can be used where appropriate is consultations with the family, teachers, or employer to explain the effects of vocal abuse and to gain cooperation in reducing the amount and loudness of the individual's speaking, yelling, and singing. Air pollution from particulates, dust, pollen, and the like, can often be reduced by the use of air conditioners or masks.

## Direct Approach

Many and varied activities can be employed by the speech-language pathologist working directly with a person who has a voice disorder. These procedures constitute the therapy of the clinical sessions and transition into independent practice and daily use. For convenience, the activities are

*Whole books have been written on each of these seven items; the discussion here is limited to concepts involved.*

grouped under the following seven headings, listed alphabetically: listening skills, mental hygiene, physical hygiene, posture and movement, regulation of breathing for voice, relaxation, and voice training.

## Listening Skills

Most of us do not hear our own voices as others hear them when we speak or sing. We are almost always surprised (and frequently shocked) when we hear a recording of our voices for the first time. Fortunately, clinical experience shows that a person usually is not doomed forever with a faulty voice; it can be improved (Van Riper, 1972).

Teaching a person to listen is an important and early step in voice therapy. The process should be systematic, and usually begins with pitch recognition and discrimination. Identifying pitch differences can be followed by attempts by the child or adult to match them. A great number of recorded instrumental and animal sounds can be introduced when recognition deficits are severe.

## Mental Hygiene

This old-fashioned term, which has been replaced in current literature by *mental health,* is used here on purpose to parallel the concept of physical hygiene. It implies healthy thinking and the means of both achieving and maintaining it. Everyone must confront problems and decisions, and some form of resolution is always made, whether appropriate or inappropriate. When people have a way to resolve difficulties, they do it easily and appropriately. When they do not have a "normal" or acceptable solution, they may acquire some substitute such as withdrawal, aggressive behavior, worrying, or a voice disorder.

Many people with voice disorders do not understand what is happening in the larynx or resonators when they produce deviant sounds. They also do not readily associate their vocal disorders with their anxieties and frustrations. Careful explanations using diagrams, photographs, and models or other illustrations where appropriate often help people understand their problem. Detailed descriptions also provide insight that can lead to modified behavior or relief of anxiety about possible disease. The person who is worried or anxious about his or her voice or state of health will tend to be hypertense and will have poor control over the voice.

Another procedure in mental hygiene is careful, sympathetic, unhurried listening by the speech-language pathologist. When the person learns that what he says is held in strict confidence, he may reveal worries, frustrations, and anxieties that adversely affect his life and his voice. Many of these problems are not deep-seated or of long duration, but they can interfere with the restoration of a normal voice. With proper management by the speech-language pathologist, the basic problems can often be talked through with relief and voice restoration.

You may wonder about the appropriateness of using interviewing, counseling, and guidance techniques in therapy for voice disorders. This concern is appropriate because it should encourage you to seek instruction in these techniques of clinical psychology. They are essential. Aronson (1980) expressed the need in the following statement:

> Any in-depth study of voice disorders forces us to conclude that so long as clinicians obtain privileged information from patients; so long as people have voice problems because of <u>life stress and interpersonal conflict</u>; so long as voice disorders produce anxiety, depression, embarrassment, and self-consciousness; so long as patients need a sympathetic person with whom they can discuss their distress, will speech pathologists need to consider their training incomplete until they have learned the basics of psychological interviewing and counseling. (p. 239)

*In this aspect, treatment of voice disorders is no different from treatment of any other speech or language problems. See the other chapters in parts III and IV of this book.*

## Physical Hygiene

Good physical hygiene encompasses those activities and practices that promote good health. The presumptions underlying our emphasis on physical well-being are that a healthy person learns more easily, her muscles respond more readily, she has greater stamina, and her respiratory system is more efficient. Conversely, muscles that lose tonus and strength as the result of sedentary living, poor diet, or illness are less capable of performing properly than when they are strong and in good condition. Voices of weakened or ill persons reflect their disabilities. The speech-language pathologist can contribute to the health of the child or adult by encouraging a proper diet, adequate rest, and sufficient exercise. Many persons with voice disorders, particularly functional disorders, are not aware of the potential relationship of the voice to physical health.

## Posture and Movement

Good posture could be considered an aspect of physical hygiene, but it is so vital in voice therapy that it deserves special emphasis. The term *good posture* as used here means maximum efficiency in body movement and positioning. It does not mean a rigid military position.

People who have sedentary occupations without compensatory physical activity typically lose strength in the muscles of the abdomen, back, and legs. This weakening allows the anterior abdominal wall to protrude and the shoulders to droop forward. When these persons stand or walk, the abdominal protrusion and shoulder droop are often accompanied by a rounded upper back, forward head carriage, and a forward curving of the lumbar spine. This postural change tends to interfere with respiratory efficiency.

The speech-language pathologist can help a person improve posture by encouraging him to institute a physical education program at a local physical fitness center, or at least do routine daily calisthenics at home. Poor posture and reduced tonus of the skeletal muscles cannot be identified as a direct cause of voice disorders, but general physical fitness certainly will augment the remedial process.

## Regulation of Breathing for Voice

The process of breathing and its role in phonation has been described in chapter 3. Sometimes voice problems are caused by or related to breath pressure, air flow and the manner of breathing. The movements of the body mechanisms that control breathing can be modified; breathing for speaking and singing can be made more efficient through training. The literature in the area of voice and diction is rich with guidance and exercises.

## Relaxation

Many voice problems are associated with too much tension in the muscles used in speaking, a condition that is often found in other muscles throughout the body. Earlier in the chapter, we referred to stressful situations causing excess muscle tension. The resolution of conditions causing anxiety, worry, and the like, is certainly important in reducing such tension, but the satisfactory management of psychogenic factors often is not possible. The reduction of psychological and social pressures may leave a void; many people would not know how to relax, even when they had nothing specific to cause heightened tension. Consequently, direct and specific training in relaxation is usually helpful and often necessary in the management of a variety of voice problems.

There are many procedures in use today through which people try to achieve a state of relaxation. For general purposes, *relaxation* is defined as the absence of muscle contraction. This state can be induced throughout the entire body, where it is used as therapy for both muscular and circulatory hypertension, digestive disorders, "nervousness," and a host of other illnesses. The techniques commonly used to achieve relaxation can be grouped into four categories: (1) meditation and/or deep breathing, (2) biofeedback, (3) suggestion, and (4) muscle sense with voluntary reduction of contraction.

Meditation techniques emphasize quiet surroundings and a mental state of peacefulness and calm. Deep breathing and various postures are often employed to help achieve the desired state. Biofeedback makes use of the phenomenon of electrical activity in muscles, which is directly proportional to the degree of muscle contraction. When sensors (small electrodes) are placed on the skin (usually the forehead) and the sensed excitation is amplified and connected to a meter or other responder, an individual can be informed visually or audibly of the extent of muscle contraction. This feedback monitoring allows the person to learn how to reduce undesirable muscle contraction. Relaxation by suggestion is an old procedure that depends on imagination. The person pictures himself in a quiet, peaceful place, or imagines his arms, legs, hands, feet, and so forth, as being either heavy or light. Often an instructor who is guiding the relaxation procedure heightens the effect of suggestion by directing attention to, for example, heaviness in the arms and legs, while speaking in a quiet, monotonous voice. The fourth listed technique, which teaches the person to become aware of muscle contraction and to release the tension, is called *progressive relaxation* and is associated most closely with Jacobson (1976). Jacobson developed a a systematic procedure in which each of the major muscle groups is contracted, one at a time in a progressive sequence, usually beginning with the arms, so that the sensation of the particular contraction can be identified and voluntarily released. As a person practices relaxation, the amount of tension progressively diminishes; practice facilitates relaxation. A refinement of total body relaxation is called *differential relaxation*. In this process, the individual learns to recognize and release muscle contractions in a limited area such as the face or an arm. The objective step-by-step, sensory approach of the Jacobson procedure associated with the differential relaxation feature has caused progressive relaxation to be widely used in speech-language pathology.

*We urge you to read one of the Jacobson books or chapter 7 in Moncur and Brackett (1974).*

## Voice Training

The six procedures of the direct approach we have discussed so far have not included much discussion of the voice proper and what can be done to rehabilitate or improve it. The first six procedures focus on the reduction or elimination of both mental and physical impediments to efficient voice production. In contrast, vocal training is designed to improve the voice to the maximum extent possible. Some of the rehabilitative procedures that are used most commonly include eliminating vocal abuse, finding the best sounds, reducing excessively tense phonation, increasing phonatory efficiency, modifying vocal pitch, increasing vocal loudness, and altering vocal resonance.

*Eliminating vocal abuse.* As long as vocal abuse or excessive vocal use is present, exercises for vocal improvement that do not address the abuse problem directly will have little beneficial effect. Eliminating vocal abuse begins with a careful analysis of the amount of loudness in the individual's habitual speech and singing. Subsequently, a prescription for the reduction of both the quantity of vocal use and the loudness level is developed. The plan is often implemented through the application of behavior modification techniques that have been particularly successful in the treatment of vocal nodules, which are a common result of vocal abuse. After eliminating the abuse, the previous faulty habits must be replaced by nonabusive voice production (Johnson, 1983, 1985).

*Finding the best sounds.*    Everyone (except someone who is mute) has a repertory of vocal sounds. Some sounds will be produced more easily and with better quality than others. The best sounds can be located by asking the child or adult to produce a variety of vowel sounds at low, medium, and high pitches, and with different loudness levels. The most pleasant or least effortful phonation is selected as a guide or target voice (Boone, 1983). The person is taught to feel and hear optimum production, and an effort is made to produce other sounds equally well. Finding the best voice is closely related to the listening training we have described.

   Finding the best voice is also related to a concept called *optimum pitch*. This term refers to a note or small cluster of notes on the musical scale at which vocal tone can be produced with relatively little effort and considerable loudness. Everyone has a pitch range that extends from a lowest to a highest note, extremes at which little or no change in loudness can be produced. As the pitch is moved upward from the lowest tone, the dynamic range (loudness) can be increased progressively with each scale step to a maximum. After the maximum, the dynamic range decreases with rising pitch. Vocal training increases the ranges of both pitch and loudness, but the average voice reaches its maximum dynamic range at four to five full tones above the lowest pitch (Coleman, Mabis, & Hinson, 1977; Damsté & Lerman, 1975; Schutte, 1980). This region is where the voice seems to be produced with maximum efficiency; it is the optimum pitch for speaking.

*Reducing excessively tense phonation.*    This type of phonation signals overly tight glottal closure during phonation, or excessive effort to close the glottis when an organic problem interferes. This pattern can usually be relieved by the combination of general relaxation and phonation drills that stress excessively breathy sounds, as in a vocalized sigh and aspirate initiation of vowel sounds (represented in sentences such as *Hold hope high, How high is his house?* and *He hid Harry's hat*).

*Increasing phonatory efficiency.*    Phonatory efficiency implies maximum balance between air supply and adjustment of the laryngeal mechanism. Stated negatively, if there is air waste or the vocal folds are adjusted with too much or too little glottal opening, phonatory efficiency is reduced. When excessive air escapes during phonation or, in contrast, when the inefficiency of phonation reflects a glottal closure that is too tight, efficiency may be increased by tone prolongation. In this type of drill, the individual practices vocalizing as long as possible on each breath, at various pitch and loudness levels, and while as relaxed as possible. The tonal drills can be extended into phrases and sentences, where the number of words on one breath can be gradually increased. As steady-tone phonation is extended and phrase length increases, there is usually an accompanying reduction in both laryngeal hyper- and hypofunctional phonation.

*Modifying vocal pitch.* Vocal pitch is abnormal when it is either higher or lower than the voice expected in most persons of the same age and sex as the speaker, or when it is monotonous. The high pitch, effeminate voice in men and low pitch, masculine voice in women can be serious social and economic handicaps. If medical examination reveals a normal larynx in the male, vocal retraining that includes intentional lowering of pitch, changing head position (such as tilting the head backward), prolongation of throat clearing sounds, and sometimes manual manipulation of the larynx usually produces improvement if the person really wants to change (Fawcus, 1986).

When the pitch of a woman's voice becomes low enough to cause her to be falsely identified as a male in telephone conversations, the basic problem is almost always a change in the vocal folds secondary to hormonal imbalance. Medical treatment may arrest the change, but does not reverse it. Voice therapy emphasizes forward articulatory adjustments of the tongue and female prosodic patterns, such as upward pitch changes in word stress.

When an individual speaks with little pitch variation, the voice may reflect an identity problem such as that of men who wish to sound "more masculine" by speaking monotonously at the bottom end of the pitch range. Another type of relatively inflexible, monotonous pitch pattern signals a listless, weak, or depressed person. If these individuals want to change their voices, they usually can do so through ear training, self-monitoring, and pitch flexibility drills of the type mentioned previously. Obviously, combinations of mental hygiene and pitch drills are needed.

*Increasing vocal loudness.* People who do not speak loudly enough for their needs do so for one or a combination of four reasons: (1) there is an organic problem that impairs normal function, (2) the person is shy and reticent about speaking, (3) there is a hearing loss, or (4) the person does not know how to use a big voice without damaging the mechanism. When an individual has an organic problem such as paralysis, a postsurgical condition, or some other disability that prevents glottal closure during vocal fold vibration, the voice may never be loud enough; however, we do have a few procedures that often prove helpful. One is greater air flow, which improves the approximation of the vocal folds by increasing the amplitude of their vibration. The **Bernoulli effect** probably contributes some additional medial deflection when the vocal folds approach each other.

Another suggestion made frequently for the improvement of vocal fold approximation is to tense the muscles of the arms or legs, which heightens the muscle tonus elsewhere in the body—including the larynx, where it can improve glottal closure. The person is instructed to squeeze the arm of the chair, pull upward on the seat of the chair, or try some similar isotonic exercise (Froeschels, Kastein, & Weiss, 1955).

*You might wish to review the suggestions for improving articulation in chapter 7.*

Further assistance for the person with a continuously weak voice is improvement in articulatory precision. When words are spoken with precise movements of the tongue, lips, and soft palate (this does not mean overly precise, pedantic speaking), the speech is easier to understand, and there is less demand on the phonatory mechanism. The person who is capable of producing adequately loud sound, but who is reluctant to speak with sufficient voice, usually needs help with personality adjustment and the development of more self-confidence. In addition to mental hygiene methods, there are some procedures that reduce the voice problem and contribute to self-confidence. One is supplying masking noise through headphones while the person reads aloud. This technique causes the speaker to use a louder voice unknowingly, which can be recorded and played back to the client to demonstrate that an adequate voice can be produced. Another approach is role playing with a play script or hand puppets to facilitate imitation of other characters and their voices.

The person who must be able to use a loud voice, such as a minister, lawyer, athletic coach, or actor, but who is unable to do so for more than a few minutes without feeling discomfort or becoming hoarse needs help in building a voice. Those who have this problem usually come to the speech-language pathologist with hypertense muscle adjustments in the larynx and also in the tongue, soft palate, and jaw. These adjustments are often accompanied by generalized, excessive muscular tension, poor posture, and respiratory habits that are inadequate for sustained loud speaking. These people also often have vocal nodules or chronic laryngitis.

Remediation is a long-term process. This fact often surprises or even irritates people with a problem; they want something done to them or for them immediately. They frequently find it difficult to accept the concept that whatever is done is done *with* them, not *to* them; remediation is a collaboration among client, speech-language pathologist, and other professionals. These hypertense people accept the fact that change and improvement in their tennis will take time and practice. But they fail to realize that the coordination needed for effective voice production is probably more subtle and less easily modified than movements of arms, legs, and torso. Voice therapy, particularly when designed to build a big voice, goes on 24 hours a day, 7 days a week.

The specific procedures to be instituted, in addition to explanation, relaxation, respiration, and posture, include drills for easy phonation, unvoiced-voiced fricative production at minimum and maximum intensities, and the drills for prolongation to increase the efficiency of breath usage. In addition to these exercises, practice should be gradually carried over into a large room such as an auditorium. When the person begins to practice the exercises in the large hall, she should phonate gently as though attempting to reach only the first few rows of seats. Gradually, over a period of weeks, as each loudness level becomes established, the loudness should be increased to reach successive rows. Efficient, relatively relaxed, loud voice for long periods of time is the ultimate objective.

*Altering vocal resonance.* The resonance characteristics of the vocal tract have a marked influence on the quality of the voice. Where organic variations do not interfere, resonance is modified primarily by movements of the tongue, positioning of the lips, opening or closing of the velopharyngeal valve, and changing the size of the pharynx. When the tongue is carried forward in the mouth, the voice has a "thin quality." Frequently, this faulty voice quality also features articulation of the back, lip-rounded vowels with broad smile or slit-shaped lip positions. The "thin voice" gives the impression of immaturity (Fisher, 1966). This voice is also characteristic of the effeminate male voice. In contrast, when the tongue is retracted, the voice tends to sound throaty. These resonance problems can be relieved with exercises in which the person is taught to sense the tongue positions and hear the deviant sounds by exaggerating the malpositions and distorted sounds. Of course, the woman who uses a thin voice to wheedle her father or boyfriend, or who is reluctant to accept a more mature role, will need to change her perceptions of herself. The effeminate male will also need counseling to help him recognize the abnormal impression he conveys. The voice and diction literature contains many useful drills (Fisher, 1966; Moncur & Brackett, 1974).

The throaty quality is heard most frequently in men, particularly those who attempt to speak near the bottom of their pitch ranges. Direct drills that stress front vowels are beneficial, particularly when used with the bilabial and lingua-alveolar consonants.

The most obvious resonance disorders are hyper- and hyponasality. *See chapter 11.* When hypernasality is present without an apparent organic cause, the speech usually responds to voice treatment. The basic objective, of course, is to achieve closure of the velopharyngeal port at the proper time. You are urged to study chapter 11 and to recall the discussion about resonance deviations presented in this chapter. Please remember also that the separation of communication disorders into chapters is simply an academic way to treat the material systematically. Real individuals with communication problems usually do not fit into neat categories. Their complex problems often require management through the combination of material in many chapters.

So far, we have emphasized reducing excessive nasal resonance. Occasionally a person needs to increase nasal resonance. Usually denasality is associated with an obstruction in the nasal passages or nasopharynx. In some cases, however, medical treatment cannot remedy the situation, or the person maintains a denasality that was learned by imitation. Increase in appropriate nasal resonance requires ear training and drills for emphasizing the /m, n, ŋ/ sounds. Humming each of these sounds, combining them with vowels, and intentional, vigorous exhalation through the nose usually produce results. Additional practice should be conducted with phrases and sentences that are rich in the nasal sounds.

## SPEECH WITHOUT A LARYNX

Earlier in this chapter, in the review of the relationship between phonation and resonance, we described the larynx as the generator of linguistically undifferentiated sound that is modified into meaningful speech by the movements and positions of the organs of resonance and articulation. We also said that any complex sound could substitute for the laryngeal sound if it were put into the upper airway. Loss of the larynx occurs usually as the result of surgical treatment for cancer or, occasionally, from injury that requires laryngectomy as a life-preserving measure.

Removal of the larynx alters the structures in the anterior part of the neck. The changes are suggested in Figures 8.3 and 8.4. The dashed line surrounding the laryngeal area indicates the parts that would be removed if a laryngectomy were performed on the person represented. A **stoma,** or

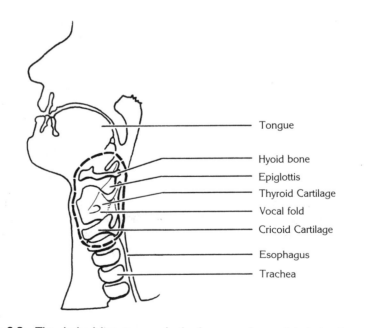

**Figure 8.3** The dashed line surrounds the larynx and associated structures that probably would be removed in a total laryngectomy.

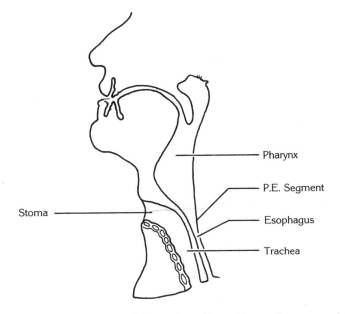

**Figure 8.4** Estimated changes of the neck profile and internal structures following the laryngectomy presumed in Figure 8.3. The opening to the trachea and lungs for respiration is the stoma. The passageway between the mouth and stomach for food and fluids can be followed through the pharynx and the P-E segment and into the esophagus. The airway and food-fluid channels are completely separate.

opening, is created in the lower front of the neck. The trachea is attached to this stoma and the person breathes through it. The changes are shown schematically in Figure 8.4. The complete separation between the airway to the lungs and the alimentary tract, specifically the mouth, pharynx, and esophagus, can be seen readily.

   After the larynx has been removed, the laryngectomized person has three possible substitute sound sources that can be used for speaking: first, the natural vibrator at the junction between the pharynx and esophagus with which the belch, burp, or eructation sounds are made; second, an artificial larynx instrument; and third, surgical modification that either constructs a vibrator from remaining tissue or, in combination with an artificial device, creates a source of sound.

*The unique speech problems of the laryngectomized justifies extra study; see the books by Case, 1984; Diedrich and Yongstrom, 1966; and Salmon and Goldstein, 1978.*

## Esophageal Speech

A natural sound source is present in the neck area of almost everyone. This voice generator is usually located at the junction between the pharynx and esophagus, an area sometimes called the **P-E (pharyngeo-esophageal) segment.** The sound is produced when air in the esophagus is forced through the constriction at the P-E segment, causing it to vibrate. The air is released in a sequence of puffs that create sound pressure waves similar to those produced at the vocal folds. The esophageal sound can be used in speaking if it is prolonged and available when needed. The requirement, then, is to learn to take air into the esophagus and return it with sound when desired.

## Artificial Larynges

Artificial larynges can be classified according to their source of power: pneumatic and electronic. The pneumatic instruments use pulmonary air; are handheld; and have an air supply tube, sound source, and sound-conducting tube. An example of such an instrument can be seen in Figure 8.5. When a **laryngectomee** speaks with one of these instruments, he holds the air supply tube against the stoma to conduct the exhaled air to the sound source, which is located in the capsule displayed in the figure. The capsule contains a vibrator, either a reed or a broad rubber band, that is activated by the air flow. The sound that is generated is conducted into the mouth through a small tube that passes between the lips and opens above the tongue in the vault of the mouth. Intelligible speech is produced by articulating in the usual manner.

The electronic artificial larynges are more common than the pneumatic instruments primarily because they are easier to use and maintain. These

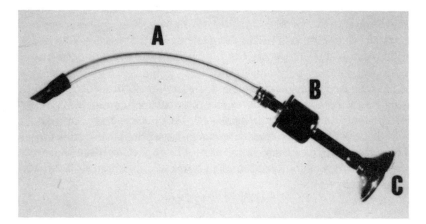

**Figure 8.5** Tokyo artificial larynx, one type of pneumatic instrument. The user places the stoma cover C firmly over the stoma thereby directing the exhaled breath to B, the vibrator chamber, where the "voice" is generated. The sound then passes through the tube A into the mouth, where it is articulated into speech.

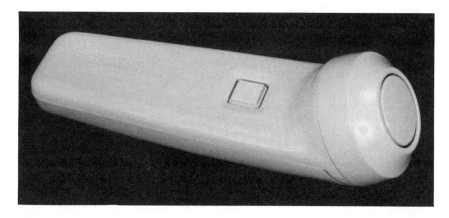

**Figure 8.6**   The Western Electric Electronic Artificial Larynx contains a battery, and an electronic circuit that activates the disc shown at the right end of the unit. The square button in the handle is the on-off switch. The disc is held firmly against the neck, allowing the sound to be transmitted into the pharynx for speech.

units take several forms according to the manufacturers' designs, but their function in speaking is similar. One commonly used instrument is pictured in Figure 8.6. A battery and associated circuit, which are located in the handle, vibrate a small disc at one end. This generates a buzzing sound that can be turned on and off with a thumb switch, and in some models the pitch can be varied. When a laryngectomized person speaks with this type of instrument, she places the sound-producing end firmly against the upper part of the neck at a location that has been experimentally determined to produce the loudest speech. The sound passes through the skin and other tissues of the neck into the pharynx and mouth, where it is available for speech.

Another device that conducts the sound from an earphone-type sounder through a tube into the mouth is shown in Figure 8.7. The speaker unit is held in the user's hand and can be turned on and off with a push-button switch. The power for the unit comes from a battery carried in a pocket or other convenient container. A variant of this concept has a speaker unit mounted in the bowl of a tobacco pipe or cigarette holder and uses the stem to transmit the sound into the mouth. These units have not been widely used; they are mentioned here to suggest the range of aids developed to help the laryngectomee.

## Surgical Procedures

Many surgical procedures to aid voice production have been developed with varying degrees of success. Some reconstruct a vibrator, a pseudoglottis, at the laryngeal site from the remaining tissue and this is activated by the

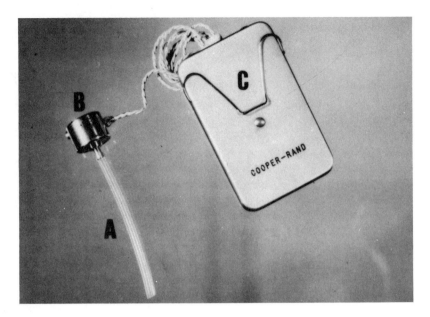

**Figure 8.7** The Cooper-Rand electronic speech aid generates sound with a battery-powered buzzer that feeds its sound into a flexible tube opening into the mouth. The illustration shows the battery case E, which is carried in a pocket; the sounder B with a control switch; and the mouth tube A.

pulmonary air. Others incorporate an external device with a reed-type vibrator through which the pulmonary air flows to create a sound that is carried back into the pharynx through a small tube passing through a surgically created opening in the neck. A third surgical procedure, and the most widely used, employs a **shunt (fistula),** a tunnel that connects the trachea with the esophagus. This channel allows the pulmonary air to pass from the trachea into the esophagus and up through the P-E constriction, where vibration occurs to create sound. (See Figures 8.8 and 8.9.)

Shunts tend to close, consequently they are kept open by the insertion of a plastic tube that permits relatively easy flow of the breath when the tracheal stoma is closed. Figure 8.8 illustrates the location and shapes of two of the several types of prostheses, either of which would be used alone. Figure 8.9 indicates the route of the air when the stoma is intentionally closed by the thumb or a special valve. The drawings reveal slits at the inner ends of the prostheses. These are one-way valves that allow the exhaled air to pass into the esophagus and prevent food and liquids from going the other way into the trachea. Since air from the lungs activates the vibrator, the length of sentences and fluency can be similar to speaking with a normal larynx. A "tracheostoma" valve may be placed at the stoma, instead of a thumb, to direct the air through the fistula for speaking. The valve allows inhalation and exhalation for ordinary respiration, but a sudden slight increase in airflow to initiate speech closes the valve, thereby causing the breath to flow through the fistula. The valve will also open completely to accommodate a cough. The shunt procedure helps many laryngectomized persons to speak well, and it frees both hands for ordinary activities, but it is not for everyone.

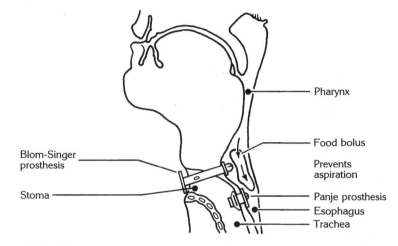

**Figure 8.8**   Schematic illustration of the placement of the Blom-Singer (Singer & Blom, 1980) and Panje speech aid prostheses. The two would never be placed concurrently. They extend from the posterior tracheal wall into the esophagus. The illustration shows a bulging of the pharyngeal-esophageal area to accommodate a bolus of food and to make the point that the prostheses prevent the passage of food into the trachea.

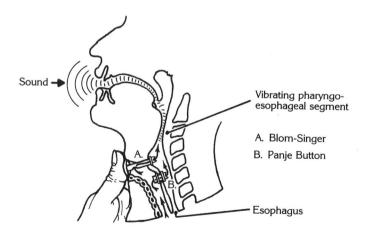

**Figure 8.9**   This sketch illustrates the flow of air from the trachea through the prostheses into the esophagus when the stoma is covered by a thumb. An attempt is made also to suggest vibration of the P-E segment and sound waves passing through the pharynx and mouth to the outside.

Postsurgical structural conditions may prevent its use. Removing, cleaning, and reinserting the prostheses requires dexterity and personal management that may be beyond the capacity of some patients.

No alaryngeal form of speaking is as desirable as normal speech, but any of the forms, when used well, can be extremely serviceable. In addition to the short phrases of esophageal speech and the atypical vocal quality and pitch accompanying all substitute voice production, a further limitation with surgical reconstructions and artificial larynges is the need to use one hand to assist the voice production when there is no tracheostoma valve. One offsetting advantage of the reconstructions and artificial larynges is the capacity to use normal phrasing. Almost all alaryngeal speech lacks pitch variation; the exceptions are among the few esophageal and fistula speakers, who achieve some pitch change.

The most frustrating problem for all alaryngeal speakers is low vocal intensity. Trying to compete with ordinary social and environmental noises is difficult and fatiguing. It is also difficult for alaryngeal speakers to communicate with hearing-impaired spouses and others. Another difficult and sometimes embarrassing problem is trying to speak while eating. Swallowing food temporarily prevents the use of the esophagus and P-E segment for speech. Working with the laryngectomized person requires patience, understanding, and sensitivity to these social components of a physical problem.

## CONCLUSION

Voice disorders, which encompass abnormalities of pitch, loudness, and quality, are found among people of all ages. The atypical voice can arise either at the sound source, usually the larynx, or in the resonators, the spaces of the upper respiratory tract. For various reasons, the sound generator or the resonators may not function normally. These malfunctions are not capricious—they have causes, but the causes are not always apparent. There is much evidence that the factors underlying faulty operation of the vocal mechanism are extremely varied. They range from psychosocial disorders that show themselves in atypical adjustments and movements of the organs of communication, to structural modification of these organs by disease or trauma.

Remedial programs for voice disorders must recognize the etiologies in each individual case and attempt to modify those causes where possible. Therapy programs must also incorporate the means for increasing function to maximum efficiency. The full restoration or development of normal voice is not always possible, but usually we have remedial techniques available that can at least facilitate more intelligible speech; more normal vocal sound; and more efficient, trauma-free voice production. In a society such as ours, which depends heavily on spoken communication, every step toward better communication is a valuable contribution.

*[handwritten top margin: (vocal nodules) vocal abuse causes swelling flexibility decreases tends to increase of folds + tends to contact at the swollen their areas + may prevent total glottal closure]*

## STUDY QUESTIONS

1. Many untrained, young singers of popular music destroy their voices within a period of 2 or 3 years. Can you trace the probable sequence of events and changes that might occur in a hypothetical singer who develops hoarseness? *[handwritten: muscle tension not excessive]*

2. What is a relaxed state? Name several methods that may be used to help an individual become relaxed. *[handwritten: 1) meditation &/or deep breathing 2) biofeedback 3) suggestion 4) muscle sense w/ vol. of control]*

3. When a person sings up the scale, what adjustments take place at the vocal folds? What changes in frequency occur? *(272)*

4. What are the structural and functional conditions that usually cause hypernasality? *[handwritten: 1. continuous opening between oral & nasal cavities — cleft palate, paralyzed palate 2. nasal twang — learned]*

5. What kinds of vocal use can be classified as vocal abuse? *[handwritten: — excessive use — excessive loudness]*

6. Explain how it is possible for a person to speak after the larynx has been removed. *[handwritten: artificial larynges, using P.E. junction esophageal speech, surgical ... between larynx & esophagus]*

7. Why do voice deviations tend to be of less concern within the general population than other communication problems, such as stuttering and articulation disorders? *[handwritten: Probably because the person is intelligible]*

*[handwritten right margin: If the swelling persists, tissue changes occur & the traumatized area becomes organized, circumscribed & protuberant]*

## SELECTED READINGS

Andrews, M. L. (1986). *Voice therapy for children.* New York and London: Longman Inc.

Boone, D. R. (1983). *The voice and voice therapy* (3rd ed.). Englewood Cliffs, N.J.: Prentice-Hall.

Moore, G. P. (1971). *Organic voice disorders.* Englewood Cliffs, N.J.: Prentice-Hall.

Perkins, W. H. (Ed.) (1983). *Current therapy of communication disorders: Voice disorders.* New York: Thieme-Stratton, Inc.

Wilson, D. K. (1987). *Voice problems of children* (3rd ed.). Baltimore: Williams and Wilkins.

*[handwritten calculations right margin: 305 −266 = 39 ; 3 ) 39 = 13]*

# CHAPTER NINE

# Disorders of Fluency

## GEORGE H. SHAMES

## MYTHS AND REALITIES

- *Myth:* Stutterers are not as intelligent as nonstutterers.
- *Reality:* There are no significant differences in intelligence between stutterers and nonstutterers.
- *Myth:* Stutterers cannot hear as well as nonstutterers, and that is why many people speak more loudly to them.
- *Reality:* Stutterers hear as well as anyone else, but some people believe that if they talk louder, it will be helpful to the stutterer.
- *Myth:* Stutterers are destined to stutter all their lives.
- *Reality:* Experience reveals that most stutterers recover spontaneously from their stuttering before starting school, and that a large number of older stutterers no longer stutter as a result of therapy.
- *Myth:* Stuttering is inherited.
- *Reality:* Stuttering runs in families, but there are no "hard data" to support conclusively a theory of inheritance.
- *Myth:* Stuttering is generally learned by imitating playmates who stutter during childhood.
- *Reality:* There are no data to support this common idea.
- *Myth:* Stuttering in a child is a result of sins committed by their parents.

- *Reality:* This is a common superstition held by some parents that they are being punished by God for their transgressions.
- *Myth:* Stutterers are basically inferior to nonstutterers.
- *Reality:* Research on birth history, personality, EEG, physiology, blood chemistry, and general development shows that stutterers are not significantly different from nonstutterers.
- *Myth:* Stutterers are all pretty much alike in terms of their feelings, beliefs, and the way they talk.
- *Reality:* Stutterers are as different from one another in terms of their feelings, beliefs, and ways of talking as nonstutterers.
- *Myth:* Stutterers like to have listeners finish saying what they started during their instances of stuttering.
- *Reality:* Most stutterers consistently report that they resent these actions by a listener, but instead want to be listened to in a patient way.

STUTTERING is a complicated multidimensional communication problem. There is an overt, easy to see, easy to hear side of the problem. But there is also a covert, private side of the problem involving the feelings of the stutterer, the feelings of his listeners and family, and often their attempts to deny its existence. There is a mutual self-consciousness that develops and is expressed, sometimes subtly and sometimes blatantly. Both stutterers and their listeners engage in a type of conspiracy of silence about stuttering, with each often helping the other to avoid a confrontation, acknowledgement, and acceptance of this problem. Society's penalties for stuttering, though unintentional, are often quite harsh and intolerant, as well as intolerable. One of the most difficult things about this problem is not knowing with any confidence what causes it, and hence, being left with unanswered questions of "where did it come from" and "why me." The myths listed above reflect this state of affairs. These are commonly encountered misunderstandings that focus on views about the original cause of stuttering, how the stutterer and his listeners feel, and how to be helpful. In spite of these misunderstandings and not knowing the cause of stuttering, children, adults, and their families have been helped a great deal with this problem by professional speech-language pathologists. This chapter on stuttering provides the understanding and realities that constitute the groundwork to help you refine your skills as a participant in that process.

*When she first came to the clinic, Laura was 30 years old. She was a college graduate, trained as an occupational therapist. She had then been married for 10 years and had three children—8, 5, and 2. Her husband was a young, successful attorney with offices in a large Eastern city some 30 miles from the small urban community in which the family resided. Laura had worked, but never as an occupational therapist. Before her marriage, she had worked for a short time on an assembly line in a factory and as a waitress while in college. She had applied for a job as an occupational therapist only once and was turned down, she felt, because of her speech. She never again applied for such a position. Laura was graceful, poised, mature, and articulate; she would be considered an attractive and sensitive person. She had an open and ready smile for her children and her husband, and an easy and comfortable manner with them. During her first interview, however, we could see the traces of sadness in her face and eyes. She projected a sense of helplessness that elicited a great deal of nurturing from those around her. Two years before, soon after the birth of her third child, she had become extremely depressed and attempted to commit suicide, but it was considered more of a gesture than a bona fide attempt. Her psychiatric therapy was brief and apparently successful. Laura attributed her depression in part to having a severe stuttering problem.*

*As she related the history of her stuttering, she openly cried when recalling how, in her childhood, her parents had forbidden her to talk when guests were in the home. Her embarrassment, sadness, and anger over these thoughts overwhelmed her. Wherever she went, she carried little index cards on which she had written brief messages as substitutes for oral communication, in case she needed information, was lost, or was in an emergency situation that required communication. She reported that on one occasion, in an airport, she had wandered around for 30 minutes trying to locate a gate and flight without talking or asking for help. She had finally found her destination in silence. She tearfully stated that, because she stuttered, she could never say thank you to people, who as a result thought she was rude, aloof, or ungrateful. She never used the phone, depended on her husband for talking, shopping, and so on, and constantly stayed at her husband's side during social outings. She felt she was a failure as the wife of a professional and as a mother. She recognized her overdependence on others and how she had benefited from her own posture of helplessness.*

*She reported several previous encounters with therapy for her problem. These ranged from parent counseling, psychiatric therapy, and hypnosis, to more traditional speech therapy in schools, hospitals, and universities. She had been in and out of therapy for about 25 years. Although her hopes for help had been dashed many times, and she carried the scars of many years of disappointment and futility, she was still more hopeful than skeptical. She came in for her initial interview literally pleading for freedom from her agonies, both public and private, about her stuttering.*

*One could not help but be impressed with her motivation, need for support, and fragility as she was about to initiate still another duel with her problem. It was with this awareness of her and a sense of my own responsibility that I joined her in this clinical relationship.*

The brief case report that you just read may seem unusually dramatic. After all, a disorder of fluency, in this case, stuttering, is not typically a matter of life and death. But it is most certainly a matter of the quality of life. Volumes could be filled with horror stories associated with the problem of stuttering. This problem can eat away at one's sense of well-being, personal adequacy, and confidence. The longer it persists, the more it feeds on itself, as stutterers attempt to hide their problem to avoid social stigma and embarrassment. The joys of life, communicating with other human beings, sharing oneself intimately with loved ones, accepting and valuing oneself—the things that nonstutterers take for granted in their daily life—can be major crises for a person who stutters. For the stutterer, his circumstances at times appear to have no exit, and he often gives up all hope for ever reversing this problem. We see people who are literally choking on their own helplessness.

How does this problem arise? How does a seemingly normally developing youngster, in an apparently normally evolving family, eventually find himself in such a complicated set of circumstances?

In our examinations of articulation and voice, we have seen that a broad range of characteristics can be considered "normal," and that the line between "normal" and "disordered" is often blurred, depending, as it does, on the opinion of the evaluator, the reactions of the person being evaluated, and those of the other important people in his life. This is also the case with disorders of **fluency.** Fluent speech contains all the appropriate nuances of meaning associated with variations of rhythm, phrasing, stress, inflection, and speed, without inappropriate pauses, interjections, or fragmenting of the communication act. We use the term for people who speak a foreign language—"Oh, yes, Jonathan speaks four languages fluently." We readily accept many forms of disfluency, such as pauses to edit and compose utterances. We accept interjections like "um" and "uh" while a speaker gathers his thoughts. We accept the fragmenting associated with being interrupted, and the repetitions of sounds and words of an excited speaker. Clearly, not all **disfluencies** are part of a disorder or a problem. But we also recognize some limit to acceptable disfluency, and once a speaker goes outside of these broad, imprecise boundaries, we say she has a fluency disorder. Fluency disorders, like other communication disorders, come in an array of types, forms, and circumstances, and they cause a broad array of reactions in both listeners and speakers.

Finding the line between normal disfluency and fluency disorders can be quite difficult. Most normal disfluencies are either repetitions of whole words, or pauses and interjections. But if a speaker repeats words quite frequently

*Disfluencies include pauses, hesitations, interjections, prolongations, and repetitions that interrupt the smooth flow of speech. Some professionals use* disfluency *and* dysfluency *interchangeably.*

or repeats the same word again and again in the same utterance, his speech may be considered abnormal. If his pauses are too frequent or too long, they may also be considered abnormal. As listeners, we are accustomed to hearing speech in a certain way, which lets us respond to the content of the message. But sometimes we find ourselves paying attention to how the speaker is talking instead. If we are paying attention to the disfluencies in the speaker's speech, then the speaker may have crossed the line over to "disorder." Listener reactions are a significant dimension of a fluency disorder. These reactions may vary greatly from culture to culture. What may be considered a stuttering disorder in the United States may not necessarily be considered a disorder in Camaroon, Japan, or Italy.

Fluency disorders are seen in both children and adults. They can be associated with neurological and physical problems such as cerebrovascular accidents (strokes), cerebral palsy, epilepsy, and other forms of brain damage, as well as mental retardation. One type of problem that should be differentiated from stuttering is the fluency disorder of **cluttering.** Cluttering is a fluency problem that is characterized by rapid, staccato speech, sometimes monotonous, sometimes so telescoped in nature as to be unintelligible. This particular fluency problem often occurs with few clues about its cause or origin. Clutterers are known to have emotional reactions to their type of speech and often avoid talking as a result. In this sense, cluttering is seen as being similar to stuttering. One theory (Weiss, 1964) is that stuttering and cluttering often occur in the same individual, and that stuttering has its origins in cluttering. The anxiety of the speaker about rapid speech—cluttering—results in tension, avoidance of additional forms of disfluency, and attempts to overcome the cluttering. These reactions to cluttering are the events we call stuttering. In a more recent review and research of the problem of cluttering, St. Louis et al. (1985) pointed out the difficulties that exist in defining cluttering and identifying it as an entity unto itself, as well as pinpointing its cause. Although both clutterers and stutterers emit whole-word and phrase repetitions in their speech, clutterers appear to emit far less sound and syllable repetitions. Also, the clutterers showed significantly more language problems, especially incomplete utterances and lower linguistic complexity. The similarities in the symptoms of stuttering and cluttering have often resulted in confusion and misdiagnosis. In essence, Weiss says that cluttering causes stuttering. As we shall see, however, there are many ideas about the origins of stuttering, and, for the most part, they do not relate stuttering and cluttering in any direct way.

Stuttering is the major subcategory of fluency disorders. It is a problem for approximately 1% of the population, over 2,000,000 children and adults in the United States. The latest statistics reveal that in some locales in the United States, prevalence is as high as 2.1%. Prevalence data outside of the United States ranges up to 4.7% in the British West Indies (Bloodstein, 1987). About 85% of all cases of stuttering start during the preschool years. Boys

*Cluttering is characterized by rapid speech, often so rapid as to be unintelligible. The speaker may clip off speech sounds, omit sounds and words, and fire rapid bursts of speech—almost with the speed of a machine gun. The exact causes of cluttering have not been identified, but it may have physical as well as emotional components.*

*See chapters 12–14.*

outnumber girls who stutter by a ratio of 4:1. But a study of American blacks by Goldman (1967) showed a ratio of 2:1, males over females, suggesting the operation of cultural effects on this problem. About 80% of those who have stuttered at one time or another spontaneously recover from it (Sheehan & Martyn, 1966).

*For this reason, we will often use "he" in reference to a single stutterer.*

The longer stuttering persists, the more likely it is that associated emotional problems will develop. As listeners react to a developing stutterer's speech, the young stutterer also reacts to his speech and to the reactions of others. He may feel embarrassed, guilty, frustrated, angry. Many stutterers come to feel helpless, which often damages their sense of personal value. Stuttering frequently leads to confusion and to social and emotional conflicts for the child or adult speaker, for his family, friends, teachers, and anyone else who interacts with him. Thus, the normal disfluency that is a relatively simple and effortless developmental milestone can be transformed into a serious social, emotional, and communicative handicap. It can profoundly affect an individual's self-concept, sense of worth, goals, aspirations, expectations, and basic style of coping with life.

Many stutterers respond to their problem by being overaggressive, denying its existence, projecting reactions in listeners, or feeling anxious and timid. They often avoid talking or any social circumstances where talking is expected, to the point of socially isolating themselves. A child's potential for an education, occupation, and fulfilling social and emotional life can be seriously reduced by long-term, persistent stuttering. Stuttering can easily become the focal point around which a person and his family organize their lives. The speech-language pathologist, therefore, must address this problem within all of the individual's developmental, familial, and social contexts.

# DEFINITION

For a definition to be functional, it should account for all instances of a particular phenomenon and, at the same time, provide boundaries or limits that differentiate or distinguish that phenomenon from all other phenomena of a similar nature. A definition is important in measurement for research purposes, in clinical diagnosis, and in assessment of effectiveness of therapy and clinical management. For each of these purposes, we must be able to know when a person is or is not stuttering, when he does or does not have a problem, whether clinical intervention is appropriate, what the nature of that clinical intervention should be in terms of prevention or therapy, whether and how much therapeutic gain has been achieved, and whether relapse has occurred.

As we shall see, there are probably as many definitions of stuttering as there are theorists, researchers, clinicians, and stutterers. Some definitions focus on describing what happens during an instance of stuttering, both overtly and covertly; others focus on the dynamics, functions, and alleged purposes of stuttering. Still others focus on the effects of stuttering on the speaker and his listeners. Some definitions reflect the cause or origins of stuttering. We might refer to some of these definitions as _unidimensional_ in that they tend to focus on a single or limited aspect of the problem. For example, we see definitions such as:

- Stuttering is a psychoneurosis caused by fixation at an early psychosexual stage of development.
- Stuttering is a psychological difficulty characterized by morbidity of social consciousness.
- Stuttering is a symptom of an underlying emotional problem and is a conversion neurosis.
- Stuttering is a lack of cerebral dominance.

Each of these broadly based definitions of stuttering shifts the problem into a more generic category of theory, with implications for its origins and treatment. Other definitions focus on overt behavioral characteristics. Such definitions have stated:

- Stuttering is a deviation of ongoing fluency in speech.
- Stuttering is a rhythm disorder.

Such broad sweeps about the speaking behavior of a person would ultimately include all speakers, since nonstutterers also exhibit such fluency and rhythm characteristics.

Some definitions try to combine some of the separate issues of overt and covert, behavioral and emotional, and interpersonal and social dimensions of stuttering into a more cohesive summation. Four of the definitions most frequently invoked by researchers and clinicians have been offered by Johnson, Van Riper, Wingate and Sheehan. Johnson (cited in Bloodstein, 1987) defined stuttering as an anticipatory, hypertonic avoidance reaction, due to misevaluations of normal disfluency. He felt that stuttering was what a speaker did in his attempts to avoid nonfluency. Wingate (1964) stated that stuttering is (a) frequent disruptions in the fluency of verbal expression, (b) sometimes accompanied by accessory struggle and tension in speech-related and nonspeech-related structures, and (c) in the presence of emotional states and excitement (both negative and positive) that may or may not relate to the act of talking. Van Riper (1971) stated that a stuttering behavior consists of a word improperly patterned in time and the speaker's reaction thereto. Sheehan (1958a) defined stuttering as an approach-avoidance conflict. He stated that stutterers had the desire both to talk and to remain silent. Anxiety builds up about each of these, and the stutterer vacillates in between. When these opposing forces are equivalent, the conflict is manifested as an instance of stuttering.

These four definitions are examples of attempts to include information about the speaker and his stuttering behaviors, reactions, feelings, and their origins. The more expansive and cohesive the definition of stuttering becomes in an attempt to account for all instances of its occurrence, the less precise it becomes in its application to the variations of individual stutterers. It also becomes less delimiting, and therefore less functional in distinguishing stuttering from other types of speech and speech problems.

A precise, quantitative definition of stuttering is therefore difficult to present. Stuttering is a multidimensional problem. Some aspects lend themselves to reliable and quantitative measurement, while other aspects are more elusive. Perhaps stuttering is best characterized as a cluster of particular speech behaviors, feelings, beliefs, self-concepts, and social interactions. The components of the problem vary from person to person. In each person, they influence one another to generate a complicated problem involving disruptions of speech and the associated reactions. The speech-language pathologist must deal with the emotional and social problems, as well as the disordered speech itself.

Stuttering affects the fluent, smooth, and effortless flow of words emitted by a speaker, and has long been recognized as a problem. This complex and unusual disorder has perplexed the victims and their families, as well as professionals, from the days of Moses and Demosthenes to the present. We still do not know what causes stuttering, and effective therapy for it has been quite elusive.

Stutterers present a wide variety of symptoms, both visible and hidden. Overtly, they may repeat sounds or words; prevent their vocal cords from vibrating, resulting in a block or absence of sound; or prolong sounds abnormally. In addition, they may show secondary behaviors, such as eye blinking, head jerking, or facial grimaces. Many stutterers show a great deal of muscular tension and forcing when they try to speak. Covertly, they may substitute words, talk indirectly around a topic, or reply with incorrect information to avoid certain words. We must be careful not to categorize a stuttering problem as mild, moderate, or severe based on overt behavior alone. A stutterer with only covert behaviors may have as many difficulties as one who has an overtly severe problem. Although other people may not recognize the person as a stutterer, he may be avoiding speaking situations or may be giving incorrect information to avoid stutterering. For example, stutterers have reported giving an incorrect name when asked, ordering hamburger when they wanted steak, and answering "I don't know" to questions as simple as "What is your address?" The problem of stuttering can have an extreme effect on a person's life, whether or not the problem appears severe on the surface. Bloodstein (1987, pp. 9–10) ultimately summarizes our current dilemma about the definition of stuttering by calling it "whatever is perceived as stuttering by a reliable observer who has relatively good agreement with others."

*See chapter 4 for a discussion of some cultural differences in stuttering symptoms.*

## BASIC ISSUES AND QUESTIONS

As an area of study, stuttering has had a varied history. If we were to attempt to write that history, we would need to consider several simultaneous developments that at times interacted, and at other times were quite independent of one another. The simultaneous developments in the theory, research, and clinical management of stuttering parallel many developments in the behavioral, biomedical, and clinical sciences. We are still trying to answer one basic question—does one learn to stutter or does one inherit the condition (or tendency)? This question relates to a number of other significant questions. If stuttering is a neurosis, what are its basic personality characteristics? What are the psychodynamics? If it is learned, how is it learned? Are there basic physiologic and organic factors operating together to contribute to its development? What are the roles of anxiety, family, and culture in the development and maintenance of stuttering?

These theoretical questions have led researchers to ask whether stutterers as a group differ from fluent speakers by any identifiable characteristics. Are there certain characteristics, which distinctly and uniquely differentiate stutterers from nonstutterers, that could give us clues to the cause of stuttering? These questions leave us unsure about clinical management. Do we attempt to identify and treat the cause of stuttering, or do we treat its symptoms, independent of its cause? Do we treat the emotional aspects or the motor aspects of the problem? If both, then in what sequence? Can we apply the principles learned in experimental laboratories to the clinical management of the problem?

In addition to these substantive questions about stuttering are a number of methodological questions about the general area of research and clinical observation and measurement. Issues such as what you observe and measure, as well as when and where you observe, are basic to our research and clinical strategies. Some clinicians and researchers observe and quantify forms, frequencies, and durations of disfluency; others attempt to measure listeners' holistic reactions to the naturalness of speech, including fluent as well as disfluent utterances (Ingham et al., 1985a, 1985b; Ingham & Onslow, 1985; Martin et al., 1984). Another issue is the representativeness of observations, with a focus on whether or not stutterers should be aware that they are being observed. It appears that covert and overt observations each have advantages and disadvantages (Ingham, 1975b).

Still another issue deals with developing a quantitative as well as qualitative definition of relapse (Shames, 1981; Shames & Rubin, 1986), in terms of speech, vigilance, feelings and attitudes, phases of therapy, and sources of information, which quite naturally leads to the need for strategies to deal with relapse. These are some of the many issues and questions that continue to face the theorist, researcher, clinician, and stutterer.

# THEORIES OF CAUSATION

As with other communication disorders, we can generally classify the numerous theories of stuttering as being based on inheritance, child development, neurosis, and learning and conditioning. These categories of theories overlap somewhat, and a specific theory may fit into more than one category.

## Cerebral Dominance

The Orton-Travis theory of cerebral dominance (Orton & Travis, 1929) is one of the better known dysphemic theories of the cause of stuttering. It states that a child is predisposed to stutter because neither side of the brain is dominant in controlling the motor activities involved in talking. Although the theory was popular and generated great interest, evidence does not support it. The research evidence is equivocal, and the clinical results of therapy associated with this theory (encouraging unilateral motor activity) have been found wanting.

*Dysphemic theories view stuttering as a symptom of some inner, underlying, complicating neurophysiologic or biological disorder.*

## Biochemical and Physiological Theories

West (1958) also viewed stuttering as involving an inherited predisposition. He felt that it was primarily a convulsive disorder, related to epilepsy, with instances of stuttering being seizures that could be triggered by emotional stress. West related his theory to a blood-sugar imbalance observed in stutterers while they were stuttering. This theory in particular is associated with a great deal of research on basal metabolism, blood chemistry, brain waves, twinning, and neurophysiologic correlates to stuttering.

Related theories have been developed by Adams (1978); Perkins, Ruder, Johnson, and Michael (1976); Schwartz (1974); and Wingate (1969). These researchers discuss the physiological and aerodynamic events occurring in the vocal tract during speech, and view stuttering as problems with phonation, respiration, and articulation. Adams, Wingate, Perkins, and colleagues separately discuss the problem in terms of phonetic transitions that make it difficult for the stutterer to start, time, and sustain air flow and voicing in coordination with articulation. Freeman and Ushijima (1978) suggest both discoordination and excessive tension in the laryngeal area as factors in stuttering, while Conture, McCall, and Brewer (1977) suggest that stutterers mismanage their laryngeal activity and that "laryngeal stuttering" covaries with "oral stuttering."

Schwartz discusses the possibility of an uninhibited airway dilatation reflex, which is the stuttering **block.** Whereas Schwartz feels that there may be a genetic predisposition to this problem, Adams leans toward an explanation of **classical conditioning.**

*In reference to stuttering, a block is a complete or partial interruption of the smooth flow of speech.*

All of these studies have been reviewed by Bloodstein (1987). His general conclusions are that "the results of this type of research do not appear to demonstrate conclusively that the average stutterer exhibits any clinical pathology within the range of the factors that have been investigated." The few differences that have been reported in cardiovascular functioning and metabolic rate, as well as autonomic reflexes and brain potentials, have not been confirmed.

Much earlier, Hill (1944a, 1944b) concluded that suspected physiological and biochemical differences between stutterers and nonstutterers could just as easily be caused by excitement, emotion, muscle effort, or fatigue. The theories of Wingate and Adams, however, dealing with abnormal laryngeal activity, are still new and tentative. They may lead to a broader understanding of the dynamics and cause of stuttering. Starkweather (1982) has provided a critical review of this area and has raised serious questions about the validity of a vocalic theory of stuttering.

## Genetic Theory

It is difficult to attribute the development of any trait or behavior solely to effects of genetics or the environment because all traits develop in some context. The question is how to determine the relative contributions of each—in this instance, to the problem of stuttering (Kidd, 1977). We have not yet been able to identify any biochemical defects as a cause for stuttering, and it seems unlikely that we will do so in the foreseeable future. Even if such a defect were to be discovered, determining its contribution to the development of stuttering would be difficult because of confounding by environmental factors. We do have, however, research models that have been applied to the data on the concentration of stuttering in families. Those data sometimes enable us to predict stuttering and suggest that there may be an important genetic basis for this problem. A study by Farber (1981) of identical twins raised apart provides significant data that do *not* support a genetic theory of stuttering. Of the 95 sets of identical twins that she studied, Farber identified 5 with stuttering. In each of these cases, only one member of the pair stuttered. We still need research to sort out these genetic factors and apply them clinically.

## Diagnosogenic-Semantogenic Theory

Perhaps the most widely embraced theory of the cause of stuttering is Wendell Johnson's diagnosogenic-semantogenic theory (Johnson, 1938, 1942, 1944, 1961). This theory has been called a developmental theory (Ainsworth, 1945) and an "anticipatory struggle" theory (Bloodstein, 1975). Following his research and interviews with parents of young stuttering and nonstuttering children, Johnson stated:

> Practically every case of stuttering was originally diagnosed ... by usually one or both of the child's parents. What these laymen had diagnosed as stuttering was by and large indistinguishable from the hesitations and repetitions known to be characteristic of the normal speech of young children. ... Stuttering as a definite disorder was found to occur, not before being diagnosed, but after being diagnosed. (1944, pp. 330ff.)

In Johnson's view, this diagnosis by the parents creates an environment of "difference" and "handicap." The child soon begins to speak abnormally in response to the parents' anxieties, pressures, help, criticisms, and corrections. Both child and parents respond to the idea of handicap more than to the child's speaking behavior. As Johnson stated so aptly, stuttering begins not in the child's mouth but in the parent's ear.

This theory inspired a great deal of research. We have a large amount of evidence showing that most normal young children exhibit disfluent speech (Davis, 1939, 1940; Winitz, 1961). We also know that parents of stutterers are sometimes anxious and perfectionistic and have high standards; however, there is some question about the dynamics of the "original diagnosis" (Bloodstein, 1975). And there are serious questions about whether calling attention to disfluency necessarily results in an increase in its frequency (Wingate, 1959).

Outgrowths of Johnson's diagnosogenic-semantogenic theory include ideas dealing with stutterers' feelings that they are helpless and victimized (Williams, 1957), as well as the concept of stuttering as anticipatory struggle (Bloodstein, 1958). The theory also directly influenced cognitive therapy, which focuses on faulty beliefs about self-control and the reinforcing payoffs of stuttering (Rubin & Culatta, 1971).

## Neurotic Theories

The neurotic theories of the causes of stuttering focus on a number of different personality and psychological attributes of stutterers. Through observation, interviews, projective tests, and paper-and-pencil tests, attempts have been made to understand the stutterer's personality; psychodynamics; social adjustment; and inner, unconscious needs. Stuttering has been viewed as a need for oral gratification, a need for anal gratification, a covert expression of hostility, an inhibition of threatening feelings and messages, a fear of castration, repressed aggression and hostility, a device for gaining attention and sympathy, and an excuse for failure. According to these theories, stuttering can become a well-integrated, purposeful defense against some threatening idea. From a psychoanalytic point of view, stuttering acts as a mechanism to repress unwanted or threatening feelings (Abbott, 1947; Barbara, 1954; Glauber, 1958; Travis, 1957).

Research on these ideas has had a spotty history. Formal tests given to stutterers to identify their unique personality characteristics suffer from problems of validity and reliability, while observations of behavior suffer from the theoretical biases and subjectivity of the observers. Goodstein (1958) reviewed the research literature dealing with the personalities of stutterers. He concluded that the research suffered from design and procedural problems and that the results were not conclusive. Neurotic theories, then, might best be evaluated in terms of their utility in clinical management, rather than in research activity. Psychoanalysis and traditional psychotherapy for the problem of stuttering, especially in adults, have not been effective on a large scale.

## Conditioning Theories

*Systematic desensitization refers to a process whereby the stutterer learns to do something (for example, relax) that competes with his anxiety about talking.*

As applied to stuttering, classical conditioning theories suggest that an originally unconditioned breakdown in speech fluency becomes associated with a speaker's anxiety about talking. If this happens often enough, the person will stutter in any anxiety-provoking circumstances; the stuttering becomes classically conditioned. Wolpe's (1958) view of stuttering as a symptom of classically conditioned speech fears led him to use systematic desensitization in therapy. Techniques of systematic desensitization include **counterconditioning** and **reciprocal inhibition.** The stutterer, who has learned to stutter, learns not to. This, in turn, influenced Brutten and Shoemaker (1967), who formulated a two-factor theory of stuttering. They state that speech disruptions, triggered by autonomic fear reactions, are classically conditioned responses to speech, talking situations, listeners, and so on. They see the nonspeech behaviors of stutterers (the muscle tension, blinking eyes, grimaces, etc.) as being operantly conditioned. These behaviors are designed to avoid stuttering or to cope with fluency failures.

We have seen that stuttering is often (if not always) associated with anxiety. Some theorists feel that anxiety reduction is an important component of the conditioning process that results in stuttering. One such theory sees Johnson's view of stutterers as doing those things that would avoid stuttering or would avoid negative listener reactions as the core of the problem (Wischner, 1950, 1952a, 1952b); that is, stutterers build up fears before they begin to speak. Once they have spoken (stuttered), those fears are reduced simply because the problem is no longer in front of them. This reduction in anxiety reinforces the stuttering.

Sheehan (1953, 1958a, 1958b) applied approach-avoidance conflict theory to the problem of stuttering. In this theory, the stutterer is seen as vacillating between the desire to speak and the desire not to speak. The stutterer also vacillates between wanting to be silent and wanting not to be silent. When the drive to avoid talking is stronger, he is silent. When the drive to approach talking is stronger, he is fluent. When the drives are equal, he is in conflict and he stutters. According to Sheehan, whether they choose to be silent or choose to talk, stutterers are reinforced for their choices by an immediate reduction in their anxieties.

Still another group of theories are derived from operant conditioning. Flanagan, Goldiamond, and Azrin (1958) demonstrated that stuttering could be increased and decreased in the laboratory as a function of its consequences. At least some overt stuttering behaviors could be controlled through operant conditioning. Based partly on these experiments, Shames and Sherrick (1963) analyzed and discussed various hypotheses relating Johnson's diagnosogenic theory to **operant conditioning.** They found continuity between the conditioning processes operating in normal disfluency and those operating in stuttering.

Another spinoff from the Flanagan et al. research was a group of several therapies known as *rate control therapies.* These techniques use delayed auditory feedback as a vehicle for initially changing a stutterer's speech (Curlee & Perkins, 1969; Goldiamond, 1965; Ingham & Andrews, 1973; Perkins, 1973a, 1973b; Ryan & Van Kirk, 1974; Shames & Florance, 1980).

The Shames and Sherrick theoretical analysis also led to several therapies that apply operant conditioning techniques within clinical interviews. Shames, Egolf, and Rhodes (1969) demonstrated that the specific content of stutterers' speech in therapy could be increased by reinforcing the content with verbal approval, or reduced with mild, verbal disapproval. Other research has dealt with parent-child verbal interactions (how parents and children talk to each other) (Kasprisin-Burrelli, Egolf, & Shames, 1972; Shames & Egolf, 1971, 1976). This research showed that it is possible to change the way parents and children verbally interact and to reduce stuttering with these tactics. These results can be interpreted to mean that stuttering is reinforced on an individualized basis in parent-child verbal interactions.

A persistent question in the study of stuttering has been the role of **punishment** in its development. For years, under the influence of Johnson's diagnosogenic theory, it was generally felt that parents' punishment of, or attention to, the normal disfluencies of their children aggravated the problem and led to the development of stuttering. Some operant conditioning research (Siegel, 1970) has shown, however, that stuttering and disfluency can be reduced by punishment. Thus, there has been a professional as well as humanitarian conflict about the role and function of punishment in stuttering and its management.

*In the terminology of operant conditioning, punishment is the opposite of reinforcement; that is, it denotes a consequence that weakens the preceding behavior.*

The cause or causes of stuttering have not been established, although there have been many studies of its symptoms and correlates, and tactics for modifying it. The methods of therapy have grown, and we have improved our success rates in spite of our basic lack of understanding of the cause(s) of stuttering. We cannot help but wonder how much further along we might be in its prevention and management if such knowledge were available.

## NORMAL DISFLUENCY

A speaker produces 14 phonemes per second, using about 100 muscles that require 100 motor units apiece ($100 \times 100 \times 14$). Complex motor behavior results (Darley, Aronson, & Brown, 1975). The act of speech is enormously complicated. Lenneberg (1967) has conservatively estimated that there are 140,000 neural events required for each second of motor speech production.

Because of the difficulty and complexity of learning to talk and learning language, young children often make errors. Normal disfluency may begin in the infant's early babbling. As he begins to imitate the rates, rhythms, sequences, and melody of his language, usually during his second year, a child may use jargon as he plays; that is, he may utter a stream of nonsense syllables, but use the inflections and stress of developed language. This may well be a "fluency rehearsal" state for the child, as we hear smooth transitions from nonsense syllable to nonsense syllable, many of which resemble adult patterns of fluency. But as they move from babbling to early jargon to early speech, some children develop a pattern of disfluency that makes their speech difficult to understand or calls attention to itself. Thus, rather than the normal disfluency of occasional pauses and repeated words, these children may use more distracting repetitions of syllables. It is not atypical that, as a child begins to develop longer and more linguistically complicated utterances, an increase in disfluency is observed. This usually occurs between the ages of 2 ½ and 3 ½ years, and is characterized by an increase in effortless repetitions of words (and syllables). More words and syllables are repeated, and more repetitions per word unit may occur. This has come to be known as **developmental disfluency.** How long developmental disfluency continues varies from child to child—sometimes weeks, sometimes months, and then it typically disappears.

When parents decide whether disfluency in a child is to be considered normal or not, a complicated judgment is involved; it includes the use of an imaginary **norm** that represents the way most children talk. It is obvious that, depending on the particular experience of the adult, this norm or baseline can vary greatly, with the result that the speech behavior of the same child is evaluated differently by different listeners, one deciding that the child's speech is normal and the other that it is not. It may be that, in some instances, the only difference between normal and abnormal disfluency is the attitude or decision of the listener, rather than any formal or discriminate properties in the child's speech.

Davis (1939, 1940) and Winitz (1961) have suggested that speech disfluencies in diverse forms such as repetitions, prolongations, interjections, and pauses occur relatively often in young children. Repetitions have been the most frequently observed form, as the repetition of codified speech is a part of the child's repertoire by the age of 2 years. These repetitions may be whole words, parts of words, or several words or phrases. The repetitions of whole words and of several words or a phrase are more often thought to be characteristic of the normal development process, while syllable repetitions or part-word repetitions more often result in the diagnosis of stuttering.

It seems that the breaking up of the rhythm of a single word constitutes a greater departure from the basic rhythms of language than the rhythm breaks associated with whole-word and phrase repetitions. The symbolic meaning of an utterance and its intelligibility may be only minimally distorted in whole-word and phrase repetition, while these qualities are seriously impaired in syllable repetition. These factors may be quite potent in deciding that syllable repetition constitutes a disfluency problem, while whole-word and phrase repetition are normal disfluencies. As a result, speech clinicians watch for part-word repetition as a danger signal, while whole-word and phrase repetitions may often be evaluated as normal in the absence of unusual environmental circumstances.

The conditions associated with the original emission and early development of disfluencies in the speech of infants are still obscure and in need of detailed observation. It is possible that the repetitions observed in what is called disfluency in later life may be related to the vocal behavior of infants during their early speech development, such as in babbling and syllable chaining. Winitz's observations of repetitions in the vocal behavior of infants offer data to support such a hypothesis.

It is also possible that the physiologic characteristics of the human organism are such that speech disfluencies are a "wired-in" characteristic. Structured speech, after all, is an adjunctive function of organs having other basic biologic functions, and hence, speech appears within the limitations imposed by these other functions. We must pause and hesitate, if only to inhale. Thinking of speech disfluency as a function of a physiologic predisposition of humans may suggest that disfluency should be expected and, therefore, has a general aura of normality about it.

This is not a necessary conclusion. Although the physiologic restrictions imposed may, in fact, result in the fundamental rhythms and rates of speech that are a part of language, logically these physiologic constraints would appear in the form of normal pauses and hesitations in speech. It is difficult to connect them with any of the forms of speech repetitions. These repetitions, on the contrary, appear to be acquired or learned responses, some of which may constitute problems and some of which may not.

Let us now look at a few illustrations of what may be considered normal disfluency. It has been observed that the verbal behavior of a speaker varies in response to actions by a listener such as looking, nodding, smiling, speaking, or doing something for the speaker. We infer that these consequent activities reinforce the speaker because we observe that the speaker continues to speak as long as these activities continue. We also observe that the speaker's behavior diminishes in strength when these activities are no longer forthcoming.

It is possible to view the repetition response as a special class of verbal response, whose initial appearance may have a basis entirely foreign to its development as disfluency. For example, a speaker may repeat a statement to make sure that it has been heard correctly. After several occasions of such repetitions, the speaker is "reinforced for repetitions," and on future occasions the repetitions may increase in number.

Speakers often compose, edit, and prompt themselves while speaking. Discrete, staccato speech units of varying sizes and dimensions are punctuated by pauses, during which it is thought that the processes of composition and editing go on. The emission of speech and its composition and editing appear to be almost simultaneous activities. As a speaker hears and feels himself speak, he monitors what he hears and feels. Sometimes he changes and corrects certain aspects of his utterances such as articulation, pitch, rhythm, or combination of phonemes. These changes and corrections are often heard as short repetitions of sounds, syllables, or words. It is believed that these composing and editing processes result primarily from the continuous feedback and monitoring of speech behavior. These processes may be among the prime factors in the disfluencies of young children who are still linguistically immature and actively involved in developing language skills.

Related to the processes of editing and composing is yet another possible function of speech disfluencies: obtaining and holding the attention of a listener. The composing process may also be partly under the control of the attending listener. As long as attending is forthcoming, composition and speech emission continue. When attending is withdrawn, speech and presumably composition diminish. It is possible that the repetition response may serve to hold the attention of the listener during composition. Therefore, while a child is composing, he may emit repetitions to fill the silence produced by pauses for composition, and to prevent the listener from interpreting those pauses as cues for speaking. Such repeated interjections as *uh, ah,* and *um* are frequently encountered in the speech of adults as well as children. In fact, often when a speaker fails to use such repetitions to fill pauses during composition, the pauses are mistakenly identified as signals to the listener that the speaker has terminated that particular utterance. If the listener then chooses to speak, he may be embarrassed to find himself in the role of an interrupter.

## DISFLUENCY ASSOCIATED WITH ENVIRONMENTAL PRESSURE

As mentioned earlier, a decision about the normality of disfluency involves the judgment that professional intervention is necessary to modify the speech behavior of the child. This judgment is based in part on the attitudes of the child's listeners and in part on the speech emitted by the child. Such a decision for the professional also involves an evaluation of environmental factors that may influence the child's speech. The abnormality is not viewed only with reference to the speech behavior of the child, but, just as importantly, with reference to the child's environment. The abnormality may be in events going on around the child, to which the child may be reacting normally. If this is the case, the child's disfluency may be considered a normal reaction to an abnormal environment. Professional intervention to modify the child's speech under these circumstances is not necessarily directed toward the child, but rather toward modifying the factors in his environment that influence his emission of speech disfluencies. Like **normal** disfluency, that which is related to environmental pressure appears to be primarily learned, orderly, and under the control of variables that can be specified in the environment.

The research referred to earlier by Davis, which suggested that certain forms of disfluency were normal and to be expected, contained some additional and important information about the circumstances for the emission of disfluencies. Davis observed that repetitions, which were the most common form of disfluency, seemed to be related to getting attention, directing someone else's activities, trying to gain an object, coercing, seeking status, giving and seeking information, criticizing, seeking a privilege, or trying to obtain social acceptance. Nearly all of these occasions involve a type of verbal behavior that is controlled by a listener's consequent reactions. Such utterances may be used when the child is in a specific state of deprivation or is aversively stimulated (exposed to a situation that he avoids, withdraws from, tries to terminate, dislikes, or that appears to make him uncomfortable).

Typically, the listener does something for the speaker or gives something to the speaker. The listener's behavior can have the effect of increasing the likelihood of a particular form of verbal behavior by the speaker on future occasions of similar aversive stimulation or deprivation. An example is the young child who falls and either is hurt or becomes frightened. He shouts, "Mommy, mommy, hurt, hurt, up, up!" This is followed by the child's mother coming, lifting him, and soothing him. The child has indicated to his mother the behavior that will reinforce his utterance. In the future, if the child wants his mother to lift him up, he may emit the same form of verbal behavior. Davis's observations suggest that a relation between repetition responses and occasions of aversive stimulation or states of deprivation should be studied.

Clinically, one must judge whether a particular state of deprivation or aversive stimulation resulting in speech disfluency should be reduced or modified, or whether such a situation is a normal part of everyday living. If it is the latter, then some speech clinicians directly involve the child in desensitization activities that gradually make him more tolerant of these pressures.

There may, however, be times when, even under normal environmental circumstances, a decision is made to reduce normal pressures temporarily, to the point where they are nonfunctional. In such instances, few if any demands are made on the child as a temporary measure during a particularly critical stage of speech disfluency. Such clinical strategies are often difficult to implement in the complex system of a family or social community. They also have to be closely monitored and gradually terminated. It should be recognized that such strategies, if not used properly, run the risk of begetting a spoiled child who develops unrealistic views and maladaptive behavior relative to his role in society and the demands and constraints he should expect in this regard.

It should also be pointed out that the demanding behavior of a child on the occasion of physical or social deprivation or aversive stimulation is usually strengthened in a somewhat haphazard, variable manner by parents. Often the demands of a child are satisfied at the convenience of the adult. Such a variable pattern of **reinforcement** may accomplish two things. One of these is to establish the child's behavior so strongly that it may be resistant to extinction. Data from experimental behavior laboratories suggest that such is the case for variable interval schedules of reinforcement. Second, this pattern of reinforcement may result in sustaining the social deprivations operating for the child at a consistently high level, thereby increasing the probability of a particular response that has reduced a deprivation in the past. These factors can become active variables in speech disfluency if speech repetitions become connected with the variable reinforcement of these demands. If these connections occur frequently, the speech repetitions may appear in greater strength because they are being reinforced on the same schedule as the child's verbal behavior of demanding, commanding, and asking questions. An example might be the parent who delays responding to a child's first utterance because of the inconvenience of doing so. The child may then repeat the utterance several times, until the repetition becomes undesirable to the parent. The parent finally comes to the child's rescue and does whatever he has demanded, perhaps unaware that he is not only doing something for his child, but also teaching him to repeat.

Another function of speech repetition may be found in relation to aversive stimuli. A child may show avoidance of certain unpleasant conditions by his verbal behavior. The speech repetition response may be used to postpone or avoid aversive, painful conditions known to be associated with a forthcoming portion of the verbal response. For example, if aversive consequences follow a lie or the admission of responsibility for a socially unacceptable act, the child may be observed trying to postpone or avoid that crucial aversive part of his utterance by repeating an interjection or repeating a word or a phrase prior to such a response.

A final illustration of a commonly encountered environmental pressure associated with disfluency, which is usually amenable to professional intervention, is the problem of competition for talking time in the home. Children typically learn quite early that two people in conversation do not talk at exactly the same time. The silence of the conversational partner serves as the occasion for one's speech, while the sound of the partner's voice calls for silence and listening on one's part. Sometimes, however, the conversational partner's silence is only a short pause while she is composing her response and is not meant to be a cue for the child to speak. If the child speaks on this occasion, it is likely that the first speaker will interrupt him. This in turn will result in the child's silence, since the partner's voice has become an occasion for his silence. If this happens frequently enough, repetitions and long pauses may become a recurring pattern in the child's speech. The child must determine when a silence in his conversational partner is merely a pause and when it is a signal for him to speak (without interruption). If the speech patterns of the partner are persistently of the sort described, the child may emit the first sound and wait briefly for the interruption. If the interruption is not forthcoming, he repeats the first sound as part of the originally intended message unit and continues with the remainder of his utterances. The repetition response may be maintained in great strength under such circumstances.

Family case histories and clinical observations reveal many other specific occasions for disfluency involving aversive stimulation and states of deprivation in the child's environment. These include maintaining too high a level of excitement and activity, requiring too fast a pace of activity—both verbal and nonverbal—in the family, pressuring the child for answers to questions, unconsciously arranging situations that are consistently frustrating for the child, using inconsistent and confusing child-rearing practices, permitting highly charged emotional interactions between parents to occur in front of the child, consciously or unconsciously allowing the teasing or frightening of the child, failing to give the child adequate attention (sometimes due to parents' persistent absenteeism from the home), and causing the child to experience rapidly changing environments (as in families who move a great deal).

Fluency and disfluency may be two separate classes of speech responses. Each may have its own history of original emission (fluency in early jargon and disfluency in early repetitious babbling) and of later reinforcement and **stimulus control.** The two classes of response coexist, but compete in time and physiology for their behavioral occurrence. You cannot be fluent and disfluent at the same exact instant. Both responses are a part of normal speech development and are elements in the speaking repertoires of normal nonstuttering as well as stuttering children and adults (Shames, 1968).

# THE DEVELOPMENT OF STUTTERING

Bloodstein (1960a, 1960b) describes four general phases of development of stuttering. These phases may overlap, and there is a great deal of individual variation. In its earliest phase, phase 1, the stuttering is episodic, occurring most often when the child is upset, has a great deal to say, or is under pressure to communicate. The stuttering is characterized mostly by repetitions of words or syllables at the beginning of an utterance, on function as well as content words. In this phase, the child usually shows little concern about or reaction to the speech disfluencies.

In phase 2, the stuttering has become more chronic, and the child thinks of himself as a stutterer. The stuttering occurs on the major parts of speech, increasing under conditions of excitement or rapid speech. The child still shows little concern about his difficulties in talking. This phase is usually characteristic of elementary school children.

In phase 3, the stuttering may vary with specific situations. The stutterer may regard certain sounds and words as more difficult than others. He may avoid saying certain words and substitute easier words in their place. There is little avoidance of talking situations, and no outward evidence of embarrassment. The child may show the beginnings of anticipatory stuttering, however, and react with irritation to his difficulty.

In phase 4, the stutterer fearfully anticipates stuttering; fears words, sounds, and situations; has frequent word substitutions; avoids speech situations; and feels afraid, embarrassed, and helpless. This phase is usually seen in late adolescence and adulthood.

Van Riper (1954) has suggested a three-stage development process: primary, transitional, and secondary stuttering. Primary stuttering is the effortless repetition and prolongations of speech, which Johnson called normal disfluency. The transitional stage is characterized by repetitions and prolongations that are faster, longer, and less regular in occurrence. Some children also begin to struggle and feel frustrated. This stage is sometimes followed by the third stage, secondary stuttering, which is characterized by struggle reactions, fear, and avoidance. Van Riper (1971) has modified this original view of development by discussing how stuttering changes over time. He has identified four tracks of development, change, and probable ultimate outcome. A given child will show only one of these patterns, progressing through the track sequentially. The four tracks are generally differentiated by age and nature of onset; form, frequency and duration of disfluencies; loci of disfluencies; awareness and reactions of the speaker; presence of muscular tension; consistency and situational variations of the disfluency; and presence of word and situational fears.

## THE ASSESSMENT PROCESS

There is no one right way to assess a stuttering problem. The choice of tactics will vary with the problems presented by the stutterer. These may vary from person to person, with the theoretical and professional training of the speech-language pathologist, and with the interpersonal styles of both participants.

For the speech-language pathologist, the diagnosis of stuttering requires a sensitivity to many factors. Diagnosis is not just a determination that a child repeats words or parts of words, hesitates, or prolongs or struggles with a sound. It is also important to determine the consistency of the speech response, its history, and the consistency of the circumstances for its emission, such as specific antecedent events and consequent reactions by listeners. This information will help to differentiate among normal disfluency, disfluency that is a reaction to unusual environmental pressures, and stuttering.

The differentiation among these three clinical entities is the major task for the diagnostician. There seems to be fairly universal acceptance of normal disfluency in young children; that is, during normal speech development, it is expected that young children will exhibit breaks in the rhythm of their speech, resulting in various forms of disfluency. This is viewed as a normal aspect of speech behavior and not as a problem requiring professional intervention.

Differentiating normal disfluency from disfluency associated with environmental pressure may be difficult. Often the forms and frequencies of speech disfluency are similar, and they do not differentiate the two types of disfluency. Adams (1980) states that the child who can be considered normally disfluent has 9 or fewer disfluencies per 100 words uttered, primarily emits whole-word and phrase repetitions as well as revisions, shows no effort or tension in initiating an utterance, and does not substitute the **schwa** for the appropriate vowel in part-word repetitions. The differentiating factors may be in the child's home environment, and therefore require the clinician's assessment of that environment. A child should not be expected to outgrow a highly pressurized environment. Professional intervention that focuses on reducing these pressures may be warranted.

Curlee (1980), in a review that cited Van Riper (1971) suggested the following criteria:

1. Part-word repetitions of two or more units per repetition on 2% or more words uttered. An increased tempo of repetitions and use of the schwa for vowels in the word as well as vocal tension.
2. Prolongations longer than one second on 2% or more of the words uttered. Abrupt termination of prolongations, increases in pitch and loudness.
3. Involuntary blockings or hesitations longer than two seconds in the flow of speech.
4. Body movements, eye blinks, lip and jaw tremors, and signs of struggle that are associated with disfluencies.
5. Emotional reactions and avoidance behaviors associated with speaking.
6. Using speech as a reason for poor performance.
7. Variations in frequency and severity of speech disruptions with changes in speaking situations.

These seven criteria have generally been employed, and one or more of these behaviors are commonly observed and differentiate stuttering from normal disfluency, or from disfluency related to environmental pressure.

*The* schwa *is the ultimate reduced vowel /ə/, which is unstressed, lax or short, and midcentral. It can achieve the minimal duration for a vowel sound.*

It is common to hear clinicians ask questions such as:

- What was the occasion for your child's disfluency?
- What was going on just prior to the stuttering?
- How often do these circumstances occur?
- What did you observe?
- Does it always look like that or does it vary?
- What do you do when this happens?
- What, in general, seems to happen as a result of your child's speech behavior?

These are typical questions asked during an initial evaluation of stuttering. They are designed to tap an important source of information: the observations that parents make during their daily contacts with their children. Reflected in these clinical questions is a focus on antecedent events, forms of speech responses, and consequent events. The questions suggest that the antecedent event evokes disfluency or stuttering, and also that the consequent event, in the form of a listener's reaction, strengthens or fixes the child's speech responses.

The most valid and reliable assessment procedures are based on direct observation. With direct observation, we need not worry about the memory lapses of parents, about distortions of the extent of the problem, or about intervening theoretical interpretations by previous speech-language pathologists. If we limit our assessment to observing current behaviors, however, we may lose the overall historical development of the problem or any long-term pattern of behaving, feeling, and interacting. At best, any assessment procedure is a short-term compromise. Recognizing that we cannot directly observe everything that is currently happening, go back and watch the problem develop, or see the person fantasize or get angry or frustrated, we try to sample the client's and family's behaviors, feelings, interactions, and personality. We do this with direct observation, interviews, and tests, trying to tap representative and pertinent dimensions of the problem. Most of the time, this process of substituting small samples for long-term observation during an evaluation is recognized as a compromise. Most speech-language pathologists talk about assessment as being a long-term, ongoing process, continuing even through therapy. They temper their formal test interpretations with information gained during the therapy process.

The speech-language pathologist's personal view of the causes of stuttering will affect the assessment process (and the therapy process as well). This view of etiology should provide guidance about evaluation and a description of the problem. If the original causes of the problem and reasons for its maintenance are significant elements in the theory, and if they are to be dealt with in therapy, they ought to be part of the basic description of the problem. On the other hand, if these factors are not significant targets during therapy, then the search for causes may have little purpose. From the general description, we should be able to develop a general strategy of therapy, including short-term and long-term goals, as well as special tactical procedures. No matter what the speech-language pathologist thinks about the causes of stuttering, certain types of questions need to be asked during the assessment.

## Description of the Problem and Baseline Measurement

The evaluation of the stutterer includes a description of the disordered behavior. Many speech-language pathologists tally the frequency and type of stuttered words during spontaneous speech or oral reading. The severity of the problem may also be assessed using a rating scale or descriptive categories such as mild, moderate, or severe. Other behavioral baselines used include measurement of talking time, speech content selection, and secondary symptoms. Ingham (1984) reported on the value of rating the stutterer's "naturalness" of talking as a more holistic description of the problem.

An interview with the person or family often provides information regarding the current impact of the problem on the person's social and school or vocational life, as well as his self-concept. Further exploration of certain personality variables may be important for planning therapy. During therapy, adults, especially, may be encouraged to take risks in revealing their feelings about themselves and about people they know and love. They may be confronted with their own rigid feelings about their problems. For these reasons, the speech-language pathologist needs a feeling for the client's tolerance of ambiguity, his rigidity or flexibility, and how comfortable he is taking risks. These variables can be assessed, and may help indicate how the client will handle the stress associated with personal change during therapy. How does the person see himself? If he sees himself as a helpless victim of fate, controlled by his environment, and is a person who needs a lot of support and nurturance, he may require different treatment than a person who feels in control of himself and his life. It may be important to understand these types of personality differences before therapy begins, so that appropriate treatment can be offered and the potential for success improved. The coping and defense mechanisms the person has developed to help him adjust to stuttering may influence the rate of change. The person who has used his stuttering as the primary excuse for his failures or fears may need more time in therapy, progressing more slowly than someone with a more realistic self-concept.

Assessment of the environment may play an important part in understanding the current problem. Especially when evaluating the young child, the speech-language pathologist may wish to examine the specific events that occur before and just after incidents of stuttering. Analyzing video- or audiotape samples of parent-child interaction in the home and therapy setting may be time well spent. The environment of the adult stutterer may also contribute to **prognosis.** Factors such as resistance to progress from the spouse and time or job constraints may affect therapy. Unfortunately, these factors may be difficult to assess at first.

The client's reinforcement history may have a strong impact on the current problem as well as on the prognosis. Generally, the longer the person has had the problem, the worse the prognosis. Many adolescents experience more difficulty in therapy than many adults, however, perhaps because it is harder for them to admit that they are different from their peers. From previous therapy experiences, the older client may have developed negative attitudes toward the problem, as well as toward his own ability to succeed and change. These attitudes may influence the prognosis and treatment. As with evaluating personality, assessment of a case history is dynamic. It does not end after the first session, but actively continues on the parts of both therapist and client throughout therapy.

The speech-language pathologist's approach to causation may lead him to certain questions during the assessment. At the same time, a preoccupation with causation can create clinical near-sightedness. For example, if you believe that the stuttering is the result of irrational beliefs, then you may evaluate how the person talks about and characterizes the problem. If you believe that the environment may affect the development and maintenance of the problem, you may choose to do a home analysis. If you see stuttering as a learned behavior, you may elect to obtain baseline behavioral tallies. In general, any speech problem is complex, affecting all aspects of the person's life. The wise speech-language pathologist keeps an open mind during the assessment, and remains vigilant and attentive about any behavior, attitude, or belief that may contribute to the current difficulties.

## Treatment Plan and Prognosis

During the assessment, the speech-language pathologist determines a general treatment plan. For the young, he may plan to spend a great deal of time with the parents in the home and clinic. The goal may be to manipulate the child's environment rather than to directly treat the child. For older clients, the professional may decide to describe the proposed treatment as completely as possible in advance, giving the client the opportunity to make a knowledgeable and informed choice to enroll in therapy.

Questions regarding prognosis may also be raised during the assessment. The prospective client (or the child's parent) is often concerned with issues such as the chances of success, and length, frequency, and cost of therapy. Although these questions can be of vital importance to the person, they are usually difficult to answer directly or precisely. Generally, each person

progresses through the therapeutic process differently. Nevertheless, predicting outcome and duration of treatment is important. The baseline measures
made before therapy may be helpful here. Variables such as how the person
views his ability to control his destiny, his tendency to reinforce himself, ability
to cope with stress, and speech characteristics may predict how rapidly he
will make progress.

# THERAPY FOR STUTTERING

There are probably as many perspectives toward therapy for stuttering as
toward its causation. Some of our ideas have changed, while others have
remained fairly constant over time. As you might expect, the ideas that have
remained constant are generally those that have proven to be effective. In
general, the approach to treatment will depend first and foremost on the age
of the stutterer; different techniques are used for young children, who are just
developing the problem, than for adolescents and adults, who have had
fluency problems (and often unsuccessful therapy) for years.

## Therapy for the Young Developing Stutterer

Therapeutic strategies for the preschool, developing stutterer have been fairly
constant and have had high success rates. There are several approaches to
therapeutic intervention for early stuttering—environmental manipulation,
direct work with the child, psychological therapy, desensitization therapy,
parent-child interaction therapy, fluency-shaping behavioral therapy, and
parent and family counseling. The choice of approaches in individual cases
depends on the results of an assessment of the problem. Some of the
strategies can be used in combination with each other, and some may also
be useful for more advanced stages of the problem in older stutterers. A
critical variable in dealing with young children is always the family—the
family can either reinforce or counteract the efforts of the speech-language
pathologist.

### Environmental Manipulation

Environmental manipulation is a therapeutic procedure that focuses on
those variables operating in the child's environment thought to be contributing to the maintenance of the stuttering. Through both direct observation
and parent and family conferences, the speech-language pathologist tries to
identify these factors and to change the child's environment so that their
function in maintaining stuttering is reduced or eliminated. Variables that can
affect stuttering include:

1. General excitement level in the home
2. Fast-paced activity

3. Communicative stress

4. Competition for talking time

5. Social and emotional deprivation

6. Sibling rivalry

7. Excessive speech interruptions, and talking attempts aborted by family members

8. Standards and expectations that are unrealistically high or low

9. Inconsistent discipline

10. Too much or too little structure for acceptable child behavior

11. Lack of availability of parents

12. Excessive pressure to talk and to perform

13. Arguing and hostility among members of the family

14. Negative verbal interactions between the child and the family

15. Use of the child as a scapegoat, or displacement of family problems onto the child

Clearly, the list could be much longer. Each of these variables could be potent in maintaining stuttering. And each, if reversed, could help eliminate stuttering. By helping a family become aware of these elements and their effects on the child's fluency, helping each family member to determine his or her own individual influence, and establishing a high priority for changing the child's environment, the speech-language pathologist may be able to reduce or eliminate the stuttering. But to accomplish this, the family has to agree on the goal—to eliminate the child's stuttering. The needs of each family member and their direct influences on the child's fluency have to be reconciled with the process of changing the family environment. Often this process opens up new and unexpected problems that relate to the child's speech. It may also lead to interpersonal or psychological problems of the family. The speech-language pathologist should be prepared to deal with these problems or refer the family for appropriate intervention, such as family therapy, marital counseling, or psychological therapy.

Gregory (1986) combines family counseling and environmental manipulation in ways that recognize individual differences in family dynamics and in responses to treatment. He analyzes the parents' concerns and feelings, and the interactions between them and the disfluent child. Based on the evaluation, he has formulated three treatment strategies. One involves preventive parent counseling, during which only the parents are seen four times to analyze and modify the environment. A second strategy involves prescriptive parent counseling, when the parents and child are seen for four to eight weekly sessions. This is recommended if the child is showing borderline disfluencies. The third treatment involves seeing the child two to four times a week, with two counseling sessions per week with the parents. The third treatment is recommended if the child's borderline disfluencies have existed for a year or longer.

Johnson (1980) mobilizes the parents in a home program where their attention is restricted to their child's speech only when it is fluent (thereby eliminating any accidental reinforcement of disfluency), and they provide a model of slowed down, effortless speech for their child.

## Direct Therapy

Direct therapy involves actively and regularly seeing the young, developing stutterer for therapy. Sometimes this means working directly on the speech symptoms of the child, but more often it means seeing the child while working indirectly on disfluency behavior. The theoretical assumption is that the child's stuttering is symptomatic of a more basic underlying problem, usually of a psychological and interpersonal nature.

*Psychological therapy.* Children who are thought to have psychological or emotional problems that affect stuttering may be referred to play therapy or psychiatric therapy. These therapies assume that the disfluent speech is a symptom of a deeper, underlying, psychodynamic problem. Little attention is given to the speech symptom per se. Rather, the focus is on the child's psychological coping and defense mechanisms, personality development, anxieties, other feelings, and interpersonal relationships. Advocates of this approach believe that, through the theoretical perspectives and clinical tactics of these therapies, psychological problems will be eliminated, thereby eliminating the symptoms of stuttering. These therapies, of course, are carried out by trained specialists.

Some children have been helped by these psychologically oriented therapies, but, for the most part, they have not been effective in reducing or eliminating stuttering behavior. There might be some value to psychotherapy, however, as an adjunct to other forms of speech therapy (Bloodstein, 1975).

*Desensitization therapy.* Another form of direct work with the child, but not on the child's speech disfluency, is desensitization therapy (developed by Egland, cited in Van Riper, 1954). The theory behind this therapy is similar to the theory that underlies environmental manipulation. The child's stuttering is a response to environmental stresses. A distinction is made, however, between unusual or unreasonable stress (the criterion for electing environmental manipulation) and the expected or reasonable stress found in the typical family situation. Stuttering that is judged to be a response to normal stress may be reduced by increasing the child's tolerance for stress. Desensitization therapy attempts to increase gradually the child's tolerance for stress. This is usually done in individual activities—often play—that reduce disfluency to its lowest level, known as the *basal level of disfluency.* Often stuttering can be completely eliminated during these activities. The speech-language pathologist keeps as many stress factors as possible out of the activity. The desensitization sessions might involve eliminating talking altogether and interacting nonverbally, not asking direct questions, silent parallel play, avoiding stressful content themes while talking, maintaining a low excitement level, maintaining a slow pace of interaction, and so on. Gradually, the speech-language pathologist reintroduces these stress factors (usually identified by watching the child interacting with family members and by conferring with parents) into the therapy session. The professional closely monitors the child's behavior for signs of emotional reactions and tries to stop just short of precipitating speech disfluency. This (introduction of stress followed by reduction) may happen three or four times in a session. The speech-language pathologist introduces more stress into each session without precipitating stuttering, with the goal of extending the child's tolerance for the process. In this way, the child is desensitized to these normal stresses. Eventually, family members may be brought into the session to help the child generalize the fluency to the home environment, where these stresses probably occur naturally. The child is gradually nurtured into the normal stress of the family. The family can learn this nurturing process and become amenable to it, and even to reducing some of the stress, when the goal is helping to change the child rather than changing something about themselves.

***Parent-child verbal interaction therapy.*** Related to the tactics of desensitization therapy is a therapy based on parent-child verbal interactions (Shames & Egolf, 1976). The assumption underlying this therapy is that childhood disfluencies develop in the social context of verbal interactions with parents, with the parents inadvertently reinforcing and maintaining the child's disfluency. After observing specific and individual parent-child verbal interactions, the speech-language pathologist can mirror-image the process and do just the opposite of what the parent was observed to do following instances of disfluency. When the child's stuttering is reduced to 1% or less (determined by the number of words stuttered divided by the number of words uttered) with the speech-language pathologist, the parents are intro- duced into the therapy to learn the more productive forms of verbal interaction with their child and to use them in the home.

***Fluency-shaping behavioral therapy.*** For many years, under the influence of the diagnosogenic-semantogenic theory of stuttering, direct work on the speech of young stutterers was avoided. Experts thought that direct work on a young child's early stuttering could result in awareness of disfluency by the child, anxieties and guilt, and a feeling of being different. There is logic to this line of thought, especially if the focus of direct therapy is on stuttering and its acceptance and control. Some therapies have been developed, however, that focus on fluency, that is, on helping children learn to do those things while talking that nonstuttering children do.

Williams (1979) has developed a therapy that emphasizes easy, normal talking and encourages children to attend to the smooth and easy behavior they are capable of performing. The therapy developed by Ryan and Van Kirk (1974) gradually increases the length and complexity (GILCU—gradual increase in length and complexity of utterance) of the child's utterances. Webster (1980) developed a therapy that focused on the gentle onset of an utterance. Curlee and Perkins (1969) developed a rate control program, and Perkins went on to develop a program for replacing stuttering with normal-sounding monitored speech. Shames and Florance (1980) have developed a slowed-down speech pattern keyed to continuous phonation between words and shaped to normal processes of speaking behavior. The Ryan-Van Kirk and the Shames-Florance therapies also organize a system of reinforcement to facilitate generalization to the child's everyday environment (Ryan & Van Kirk, 1974; Shames & Florance, 1980).

*Parent and family counseling.*　　We have just seen that many aspects of the child's environment cut to the core of the family and its individual members. Identifying and ultimately changing some family behavior patterns might well require a close and caring counseling relationship for the group as a whole, as well as for its individual members. To meet the final goal, the needs of the family as well as the child must be considered. Parent and family counseling is designed to help family members understand how their behaviors and feelings interact with those of the stutterer, and to recognize, accept, and act on these feelings.

In some instances, the speech-language pathologist may feel that the speech of the child is within the boundaries of normal disfluency, but the anxieties and concerns of the parents persist. Parent concern is then a legitimate target for therapeutic intervention. This intervention is not simply a matter of providing parents with information about normal developmental disfluency. The speech-language pathologist also acknowledges and deals with the parents' feelings. The parents, not the child, are the clients. The focus may start on the child, but the counseling situation often redefines the problems and issues in terms of the parents and their histories, interactions, feelings, and behaviors, with a much broader perspective than speech and/or parenting. Therapy starts to focus on the parents as individuals.

Interviewing and counseling skills, as well as knowledge of stuttering, child management, and family dynamics, are prerequisites for this type of therapeutic intervention. Without these skills, the speech-language pathologist might serve the family better by a referral to a professional who has the proper training and skills. The combination of parent and family counseling with environmental manipulation probably represents the highest rate of therapeutic success for the problem of stuttering. This success may be due to the short history of the child's stuttering problem, and its early form and development.

Cooper (1984), over a period of 20 years, developed a therapy entitled Personalized Fluency Control Therapy (PFCT). The goal is "the feeling of fluency control." It focuses on attitudes, feelings, and interpersonal relationships, as well as fluency inducing gestures and the confrontation of those behaviors and feelings that either impede or facilitate the client's modification of behavior.

Riley and Riley (1984) developed a multidisciplinary approach to the neurological, attitudinal, and environmental components of stuttering in children. A fluency monitoring program is employed by parents for non-chronic stutterers, sometimes for as long as two years, to determine changes in the frequency and form of disfluency. Analysis of the child's home, family counseling, and environmental manipulation are important components of this approach to the child's problem. If abnormal disfluencies are still present, direct modification procedures are employed, sometimes with voluntary fluent stuttering included in the process.

Shine (1984) developed a direct fluency training program for children ages 3 to 12. The goal is to change the child's basic pattern of speaking so that he uses his speech mechanisms in ways that are incompatible with stuttering. The therapy addresses developing appropriate processes of respiration, phonation, resonance, and articulation. Environmental stresses are also modified as the child learns an easy speaking voice.

## Therapy for Advanced Stuttering

Advanced stuttering can be much more complicated than early stuttering in its dynamics, overt symptoms, hidden aspects, and interpersonal and psychological correlates. The problem has existed longer, and thus the stutterer, his family, and his listeners have had more opportunity to develop reactions to the stuttering. Most advanced stutterers develop many coping strategies in their attempts to handle the problem. The stutterer's speech is typically characterized by muscular tension and forcing, fragmenting of utterances, and superfluous motor activity. He is painfully aware of his speech and of reactions to it. He may be embarrassed, or feel inferior, guilty, hostile, anxious, aggressive, or timid as he vacillates between approaching and avoiding talking. Given the motor and emotional complexities of a problem that feeds on itself, it is not surprising that the therapies for this problem have also vacillated between the mysterious, the complex, and the simplistic.

Therapy for advanced stuttering has ranged from tactics such as putting stones in the mouth, oral surgery, waving the hand rhythmically in the air, "chewing" one's breath stream, superstitious incantations, deliberate stuttering, and electric shock, to psychotherapy, biofeedback, controlled fluent stuttering, and sophisticated conditioning techniques. Within each of these broad therapeutic techniques, there have been numerous variations and combinations involving counseling, desensitization, stuttering controls, and fluency inducing procedures. Space in a single chapter does not permit detailed discussion of these various therapies. Many are no longer in use. We will discuss a few because they may illustrate some specific issues and principles about therapy.

Variations in therapeutic practice are partly a function of how the problem has been defined and perceived theoretically. If stuttering is seen as a symptom of anxiety, then therapy will deal with anxiety. If stuttering is seen as an anticipatory struggle, then therapy will deal with the stutterer's expectancies. If stuttering is seen as being conditioned, then therapy will deal with components of the conditioning model.

When we talk about therapeutic practice, we include several components that are critical to overall clinical management:

1. General goals of therapy
2. Tactics of therapy:
   a. Target behaviors
   b. Style of therapy
   c. Self-management
   d. Transfer and maintenance
3. Follow-up studies

## General Goals of Therapy

The goals of a therapy program are a function of how the problem is perceived, and the goals should be reflected in the therapeutic tactics used. Generally, the goals of therapy focus on:

- changing the way the stutterer talks
- changing the way the stutterer feels
- changing the way the stutterer interacts with the environment

Within these broad categories, we find much polarization of thinking. In the past, for example, some therapies assumed stuttering was a chronic and permanent condition that would be aggravated by any therapeutic attempt to reduce or eliminate it. Stutterers were counseled to accept their problem. These therapies employed tactics of negative practice (Dunlap, 1932), voluntary stuttering (Bryngelson, 1955), and controlled and fluent stuttering (Van Riper, 1954). Therapy on stutterers' anxieties was also part of these programs. Advocates felt that, by learning to control stuttering and to stutter voluntarily, stutterers would develop a sense of control over their behavior that would result in their not feeling helpless and anxious. These therapies generally had the reduction or elimination of avoidance behaviors as their major goal. They focus on, for example, word fears and word substitutions, circumlocution, the use of starters and postponements, repeated interjected phrases ("you know", "you see", "well") that avoid or hide stuttering, situational avoidances, fear of using the telephone, remaining silent, or social isolation. Such therapies have become known as anti-avoidance therapies because the therapy confronts any and all avoidance activities by the stutterer with a view toward their elimination.

Other therapies have as their primary goal the reduction of anxiety about speech. These would include systematic desensitization (Brutten & Shoemaker, 1967; Lanyon, 1969), psychotherapy (Barbara, 1954; Glauber, 1958; Travis, 1957), semantic-based therapy (Bloodstein, 1975; Johnson, 1933; Shames et al., 1969; Williams, 1957), and role enactment (Sheehan, 1975).

Some therapies were more prominently concerned with developing stutter-free speech. These are known as fluency shaping or fluency inducing therapies (Curlee & Perkins, 1969; Goldiamond, 1965; Ingham & Andrews, 1973; Ingham & Onslow, 1985; Ryan & Van Kirk, 1974; Shames, 1987; Shames & Florance, 1980; Webster, 1980).

Some have used delayed auditory feedback, computerized feedback about gentle onset of phonation, continuous phonation, increasing the length and complexity of utterances, prolonged speech, and vibro-tactile feedback of phonation. Ingham and Onslow (1985) developed a therapy that provides frequent and systematically scheduled feedback to the stutterer about how natural his speech sounds. The stutterer is instructed only to make his speech sound more natural. This feedback is a numerical rating of naturalness provided in response to speech that is already free of stuttering but may not sound natural, perhaps because of the procedures used to institute stutter-free speech.

Some of these therapies have used devices and instrumentation to enhance speech that is stutter-free. These devices have employed auditory masking, delayed auditory feedback of the speaker's speech, information about the speaker's breathing patterns, pattern of initiating phonation, and vibro-tactile sensory feedback of phonation. There is also a device for use in outside social transfer activities. Figures 9.1 to 9.5 show how some of these devices are used.

All of the therapies for advanced stuttering seem to have in common a concern for helping the stutterer change the quality of his interpersonal relationships, although a great variety of tactics are used to accomplish this. With the accumulation of stutter-free talking time, the person's expectations should eventually change from anticipating stuttering to anticipating fluency, which results in a reduction of speech anxieties and hence, greater comfort in social interactions. At the least, the stutterer's post-therapy speech status will cease to be a factor in his interpersonal relationships. On paper, this sounds reasonable. With new talking skills, the stutterer should be in a better

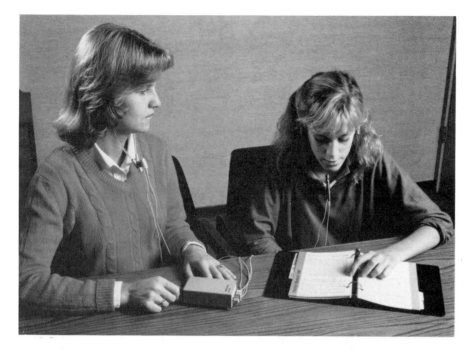

**Figure 9.1** Client using DAF (delayed auditory feedback) during reading in a therapy session. (*Note: Courtesy of Phonic Ear, Inc., Mill Valley, CA.*)

position to relate, socialize, and interpret the nature and quality of his relationships without stuttering being a factor. Our society tends to put high value on being gregarious, outgoing, and talkative, with much less value on being relatively quiet and deliberative. Naturally, the person should be comfortable in both circumstances, and should make choices according to his comfort rather than superimposed expectations.

*Transfer and maintenance.* Most of the early therapies for advanced stuttering that focused on learning to accept and control stuttering paid a great deal of attention to transferring these skills, behaviors, and attitudes to the stutterer's nonclinical environments. Often the bravery and resolve that operated in the clinic room had to be carefully moved into the stutterer's outside world, or the new skills would not be functional in any real-life situation. The transfer of these new skills might meet with resistance from the stutterer, especially when the stuttering had been emotionally useful. Therefore, in these programs, stutterers were given talking assignments, homework, and situational desensitization experiences to facilitate their carryover.

Unlike the older therapies, some of the newer therapies that emphasize fluency-inducing behaviors focus primarily on tactics for initially changing

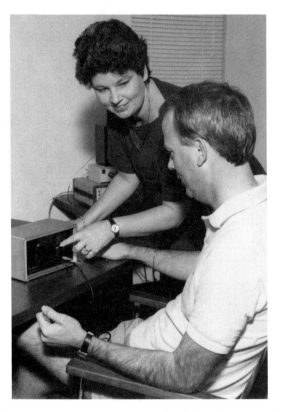

**Figure 9.2**  Client using voice monitor to evaluate his voice onsets in the precision fluency shaping program. (*Note: Courtesy of Hollins Communication Research Institute, Hollins College, Roanoke, VA.*)

the stutterer's speech in the clinic, with much less attention to transfer and maintenance. Therapeutic regimes that do not consider the issues of transfer and maintenance can be criticized as being nothing more than laboratory exercises in fluency, with little or no impact on the real problem. Any effective therapy program must involve transfer, and several of the fluency-inducing therapies have developed strategies to address this important aspect of therapy.

One technique mobilizes the stutterer's family, friends, and teachers as agents of reinforcement in the therapy for children (Ryan and Van Kirk, 1974). The child is scheduled for a series of nonclinical experiences under reinforcement contingencies that are carried out by people in the home, at school, and so on.

In another technique, the stutterer systematically rates himself on how well he monitored his new speaking skills during the day (Perkins, 1973b).

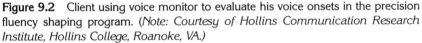

The stutterer would rate his breath-stream management, prosody, rate of speech, and self-confidence. If the ratings were low on any of these components, the stutterer would give extra attention to that component in practice and conversational settings.

Another approach invokes the principles and use of behavioral contracting (Shames & Florance, 1980). The stutterer commits himself in advance to monitoring his stutter-free speaking behaviors in a progressively expanding array of comfortable social and emotional circumstances, using explicit self-reinforcement procedures. The contract is generated daily by the client. It spells out in detail where, when, to whom, and for how long he will monitor his speech. The stutterer also rates the difficulty level of the contract and evaluates his performance. Gradually, the detailed contract is expanded in time, duration, frequency, and difficulty. Eventually, most of the stutterer's talking time is deliberately monitored under his own self-regulated contingencies.

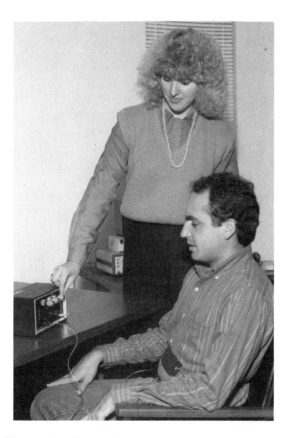

**Figure 9.3** Client using the respiration monitor to control respiration. (*Note: Courtesy of Hollins Communication Institute, Hollins College, Roanoke, VA.*)

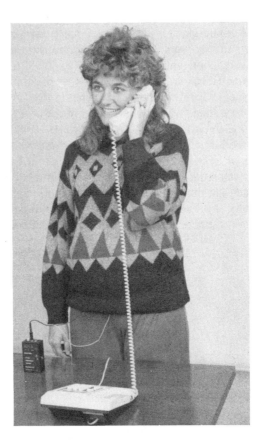

**Figure 9.4**   Client in transfer-carryover activities—on the telephone with the PVFD (personal vibro-tactile feedback device). (*Note: Courtesy of Vocaltech, Inc., Pittsburgh, PA.*)

Depending on the stutterer and his disposition toward self-management, a balance among these types of transfer activities and processes may be the most effective way to approach this critical phase of therapy.

*Counseling.*   Another tactic found in most therapies is counseling. Counseling does not mean "lecturing" a stutterer about himself. Rather, it refers to providing an opportunity for the person to explore, verbalize, think, and express his feelings about himself and his problems, about his therapy, about the process of changing, about his expectations and fears about the future, and about anything else that is of significance for him. The process is usually a client-centered one that respects the individual's potential for finding solutions. It encourages the person to take the responsibility for setting the topical agenda and for setting the pace for talking about himself and his problem. As we have seen, therapeutic change can bring with it stress and, therefore, the need for a caring companion through the change process. Therapeutic change may also be directly related to how susceptible the client is to the influences of the therapist (Strupp, 1962, 1972). As the client learns to trust the therapist and learns that the therapist will not abuse him, some powerful bonds of affection may develop between them. It is out of this climate of trust and love that the client makes changes in himself. Although the client may bring his own "will to recover" to the therapeutic experience, it is this powerful and close interpersonal relationship that nurtures and sustains that will through the sometimes painful aspects of therapy.

In the total clinical management of advanced stuttering, there is little doubt that counseling is a necessary component. Changes in speech are accomplished through direct teaching processes, the clinical relationship,

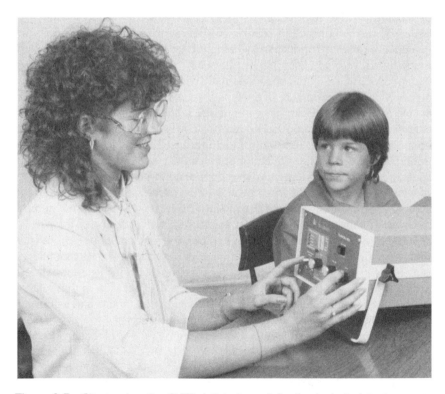

**Figure 9.5** Client using the CVFD (clinical vocal feedback device) in therapy to monitor phonation. (*Note: Courtesy of Vocaltech, Inc., Pittsburgh, PA.*)

and the support of a caring speech-language pathologist. The self-understanding that emerges from the counseling process can be a powerful and effective facilitating force in providing for the total needs of the stutterer in therapy.

## Maintenance and Relapse

When a stutterer first enters therapy, he is capable of many different kinds of behaviors, of having many different kinds of feelings, and of generating many different kinds of interactions and reactions in his environment. Some of these are desirable and productive, and contribute to the stutterer's happiness and well-being. Others may be undesirable and nonproductive, and contribute to feelings of despair and desolation.

As a result of therapy, the desirable and productive behaviors and feelings should become more prominent, while the undesirable and nonproductive behaviors and feelings should become less functional. At any point, however, each of us is capable of bringing out any part of ourselves, depending on the circumstances of the moment. This directly relates to issues of maintenance and relapse in therapy for stuttering. There is no quantitative criterion for deciding whether or not a relapse has occurred. How many times, with what frequency, duration, form, and time intervals after therapy does it take to constitute a relapse? In spite of the problem of precisely defining the nature of a relapse, we can say that relapses occur with an alarming and discouraging frequency following therapy for advanced stuttering. Those behaviors called *relapse* come under the same behavioral controls that any other behavior does (Shames, 1979). At any time, before, during, and after therapy, the stutterer can stutter, use monitored stutter-free speech, and speak without stuttering or monitoring speech. The probability of each of these behaviors may be a function of the events occurring at the time. Our evaluation of their desirability (related to the goals of therapy) dictates whether or not each instance is called *maintenance* or *relapse*.

There are a number of different possible explanations for relapse (Boberg, Howie, & Woods, 1979). One rather pessimistic view is that relapse is a part of the human condition and occurs almost invariably after treatment for most (if not all) human behavior problems. Another view is that relapse might be prevented if clinic support were maintained longer and withdrawn more slowly. Still another view is that change in personality must take place before a lasting change in fluency will result. Another view is that, in intensive therapy programs, the stutterer cannot cope with the speed of changes in his speech and he therefore relapses. Boberg and colleagues further suggest three significant theoretical possibilities for relapse. One is that stutterers use small disfluencies that are barely recognizable in therapy, but grow in magnitude and form the seeds for later relapse after therapy ends. A second possibility is that posttherapy speech monitoring is a nonrewarding experi-

**Maintenance** *refers to the continued emission of the target behaviors acquired during formal therapy. It may also refer to the continuing experience of certain desirable feelings and social patterns that were acquired during therapy.* **Relapse** *refers to a return to the pretherapy state. It may also refer to substitution of new undesirable behaviors for the old ones.*

ence and is eventually not continued by the stutterer. Third is the inevitability of relapse if there is a heavy genetic and therefore physiological basis for stuttering in a given person.

Many experts have proposed techniques to promote maintenance. Ryan and Van Kirk (1974) encourage daily monitoring of stuttering, fading out home practice but continuing clinical contact for evaluation and reinstruction. Ingham and Andrews (1973) and Ingham (1975a) encourage the stutterer to continue practicing prolonged speech and to maintain clinical contact. Perkins (1971) suggests a continuation of periodic clinical contacts for speech practice and counseling. Webster (1980) encourages the initial overlearning of the behaviors necessary for fluent speech, with the goal of making these behaviors automatic. Shames and Florance (1980) tend to agree with Webster that the best way to combat relapse is to make behaviors that compete with stuttering automatic. They approach that goal not through initial overlearning, but through processes of generalization and systematic scheduling of unmonitored speech as a formal part of therapy.

Different therapies have reported different maintenance and relapse rates, ranging from 50% to over 90% maintenance, depending on the ages of the clients, the tactics used initially in changing the stutterers' speech, and whether transfer and maintenance procedures were employed. All therapies seem to have a significant drop-out rate. In spite of these data and the drop-out rates, we are making significant increases in successful therapeutic outcomes. The prognosis for the problem of stuttering has been undergoing a gradual change from pessimism to tempered optimism.

# PREVENTION

For many reasons, there has been no work directly attacking the issue of prevention of stuttering. Without any conclusive evidence about the etiology of stuttering, it is difficult to eliminate the causes. Unlike the medical sciences, we cannot immunize children against developing stuttering. From a humanitarian and ethical standpoint, we cannot attempt to cause a child to stutter (even if we knew how) because we are not certain that we could reverse the process. Direct research on the prevention of a problem that may have an environmental base is extremely difficult to conduct. Except for the genetic theory of stuttering, however, most theories imply a message of prevention.

Johnson's semantogenic theory (1944) tells us that if we can arrange the appropriate semantic environment relating to a child's normal, developmental disfluencies, stuttering could be prevented from developing. Shames and Egolf's work on parent-child verbal interactions (1976) suggests that, as a general preventive measure, positive verbal interactions between parents and children could prevent a stuttering problem. Both common sense and research tell us that part of the answer to prevention is in good child-rearing and parenting practices, along with providing parents with information about child development in general, and about speech and language development in particular. Perhaps the most successful preventive measures are those that pay attention to parents' concerns (well-founded or not) in conferences and counseling, so that any untoward factors operating in the home can be promptly and compassionately handled before they start to affect how fluently a child communicates.

## CONCLUSION

The problem of stuttering continues to present a number of challenges to theorists, researchers, speech-language pathologists, and stutterers themselves. The cause of the problem is still not clear. As a result, prevention has received almost no attention. The problem has had a history of controversy and inconsistency. Experts have argued and disagreed over its theory, causation, definition, dynamics, measurement, and clinical management. Emerging from all this controversy, however, has been a history of growth and improvement. Some parts of the problem are obvious and available for all to see; other parts are hidden and private. There are many facets to its study, understanding, and management. We can look at its behavioral, physiological, emotional, and interactional components. As these various components of the problem are conceptualized, integrated, and related to broader perspectives in the cognitive, developmental, behavioral, and biomedical sciences, the potential for the ultimate resolution of the problem is accordingly enhanced. There is much to do, and we have the resources to do it.

## STUDY QUESTIONS

1. Discuss the ways that a theory of the origins and dynamics of stuttering contributes to the management of stuttering.

2. How does therapy for early, preschool stages of stuttering differ from advanced stuttering in adults?

3. Discuss the similarities and differences (in theory, form, and circumstances of expression) of normal disfluency, disfluency in response to environmental pressure, and stuttering. What would you do about each?

4. Speech clinicians move in and out of various roles in providing therapy for stuttering. Give an example of how the clinician functions as a:
   a. teacher/instructor
   b. model or example
   c. reinforcer
   d. counselor

5. How would you determine the effectiveness of your therapy for stuttering? How and what would you evaluate with a specific client? with a large group of clients?

## SELECTED READINGS

Bloodstein, O. (1987). *A handbook on stuttering.* Chicago: National Easter Seal Society for Crippled Children and Adults.

Emerick, L., & Hamre, C. (1972). *An analysis of stuttering: Selected readings.* Danville, Ill.: Interstate Printers and Publishers.

Florance, C.L., & Shames, G.H. (1981). Stuttering treatment: Issues in transfer and maintenance. In J. North (Ed.) and W. Perkins (Guest Ed.), *Seminars, speech language hearing, strategies in stuttering therapy.* New York: Grune & Stratton.

McFall, R.M. (1977). Parameters of self monitoring. In R. Stewart (Ed.), *Behavioral self management, strategies, techniques and outcomes.* New York: Brunner/Mazel.

Sheehan, J.G. (1970). *Stuttering: Research and Therapy.* New York: Harper and Row.

Stewart, R. (1977). Self help group approach to self management. In R. Stewart (Ed.), *Behavioral self management, strategies, techniques and outcomes.* New York: Brunner/Mazel.

Strupp, H. (1962). Patient-doctor relationship; Psychotherapist in the therapeutic process. In H.J. Bachrach (Ed.), *Experimental foundations of clinical psychology.* New York: Basic Books.

Strupp, H. (1976). On the technology of psychotherapy. *Archives of general psychiatry, 26,* 270–278.

Van Riper, C. (1973). *The treatment of stuttering.* Englewood Cliffs, N.J.: Prentice-Hall.

# PART FIVE

# Disorders of Special Populations

# Hearing and Hearing Disorders

## F R E D   N .   M A R T I N

### MYTHS AND REALITIES

- *Myth:* Children's hearing cannot be tested until they are old enough to take voluntary tests.

- *Reality:* Infant screening certainly appears justified—it has been estimated that 1 neonate in 750 will have some degree of hearing impairment (Northern & Downs, 1984). Downs & Sterritt (1967) used a device that produces a high intensity tone at 3000 Hz to elicit startle responses from newborn infants. These responses generally come in the form of eye blinks, body movement, and other general startle reactions.

- *Myth:* Children with profound hearing losses cannot be taught to speak.

- *Reality:* The multisensory approach involves the predominant use of speech. Often called the aural/oral method, receptive communication is accomplished through amplification and speech reading. The emphasis is on listening.

- *Myth:* Hearing loss is merely a loss of the loudness of sounds. If sounds, such as speech, are made loud enough, they will become clear.

- *Reality:* Persons with sensorineural hearing losses usually evidence some distortion of the sounds that are presented to them, even if those sounds are above threshold. As a general rule, the greater the amount of sensorineural hearing loss, the greater is the distortion (although the extent of hearing loss, as shown on an audiogram, is not always an accurate predictor of speech discrimination ability). Because of the distortion of sound, word recognition scores are usually affected, and many clients have great difficulty in discriminating among the sounds of speech, even when those sounds are amply loud.

- *Myth:* People with sensorineural hearing losses should not wear hearing aids because they will only amplify distortion, and will not make speech easier to understand.
- *Reality:* It is unarguable that rehabilitation with amplification is more difficult for persons with sensorineural loss than for those with conductive loss, but it is precisely the challenge of rehabilitative audiology to restore maximum auditory function to those in greatest need.

E ACH of the popular myths has so far received only a short answer. The remainder of the chapter will provide much more detailed and professional answers. First, however, we shall look at a case history of a child with a subtle hearing loss, and follow her through the growth years. This type of case history is not atypical, but fortunately is encountered less frequently now.

*Violet had been a bright child, born to a family with no known history of hearing loss. When she was small, she was friendly and affectionate, but her parents wondered why her language skills were developing more slowly than would have been anticipated, based on her other development. Her speech and voice also lacked the precision of other children her age.*

*When she was 3 years old, Violet's parents asked her pediatrician whether there might be something wrong with the child. Their concerns were brushed aside, and they were made to feel that she was just a little slower than normal in her speech development and that she would be fine. Her hearing was judged to be normal when she turned around on hearing the pediatrician clap hands behind her back.*

*Violet's first-grade teacher wondered about the possibility of hearing loss, based on her behavior in class. Her parents were notified, and she had her hearing tested. Testing suggested the possibility of a hearing loss, and a conference was held between the clinician and Violet's father. The clinician explained that Violet had been inconsistent in her responses, and that the test results could not be considered valid. Violet was reprimanded by her father for what was perceived as her inattention, and she was returned to the sound suite for retesting.*

*Violet felt that she had disappointed her father by not responding each time a tone was presented to her. To succeed the second time, she watched* the face and movements of the tester carefully to search for any clue that a tone might be presented, even though she heard none of them. Violet had had her entire life to practice taking advantage of visual clues. At the end of a short time, the second test was concluded and Violet's father was told that she had done much better, her hearing was normal, and there was nothing to worry about.

It was not until 6 years later, at the age of 12, that Violet's hearing was finally retested. She was found to have normal hearing for low-pitched sounds, but a severe loss of hearing for high-pitched sounds, a condition she probably had her entire life. The energy of most environmental sounds is in the low-pitch range, so Violet naturally gave normal startle responses to sounds such as hand claps, door slams, and even the vowel sounds of speech. She could not hear high-pitched sounds well, causing her to miss many of the consonants that make speech intelligible.

Since Violet had been told when she was young that her hearing was normal, she simply assumed this to be the case. She wondered why students paid attention in class to teachers who just seemed to move their lips and make no sounds, but she assumed that this was somehow normal. When she did not understand, she assumed it was her own fault. She blamed all her scholastic and communication difficulties on herself.

At age 12, when Violet was finally fitted with a hearing aid, her life changed, and she realized for the first time what she had been missing. Today, she wears two in-the-ear hearing aids, and she is a successful graduate student preparing to be a teacher of deaf children. Because of her intelligence and despite the odds against it, she has excellent communicative skills, but her speech and voice betray her hearing loss to anyone accustomed to hearing what is sometimes called "deaf speech."

It is impossible to estimate the suffering that might have been avoided if Violet's hearing loss had been properly diagnosed when she was small. Violet has taken two of my audiology courses and realizes that her story is, fortunately, the exception rather than the rule. She bears no ill will against the people who failed to make the appropriate diagnosis earlier in her life. She does, however, vow to see that these kinds of oversights do not happen in any circumstances over which she has control.

# INTRODUCTION

If one were to ask the person in the street how human beings communicate, "speech" would be the most likely response. Surely, when pointed out, it would be acknowledged that concepts of language and hearing must also be involved, but communicative disorders are probably first thought of as speech disorders. It is because hearing is so integral a part of the communicative process that the editors of this book decided to include a chapter on hearing and its disorders.

It was Denes and Pinson (1963) who coined the term *speech chain.* They acknowledged that the communicative process begins first with a thought or concept in the mind of the communicator on the output side of the communication process. For the thought to become a message, linguistic coding (utilizing words, grammar, syntax, and the like) is required. This involves the use of specialized brain centers that allow for abstraction and symbolization.

The next step in the communicative chain of events involves articulation and phonation of the selected words. Since nature has not devised specialized organs for these functions, humans utilize those organs that have evolved for the purposes of chewing, swallowing, and breathing. Vibrations from these organs set up perturbations in the air around us, resulting in waves that travel in all directions from the source.

When the waves strike a human ear, the input process begins. Reception of these waves involves the peripheral hearing apparatus, but it has been correctly observed that we do not hear with our ears but with our brains. The auditory mechanism is a system that utilizes the waves around us to carry a message to our brains for **decoding,** the process of deducing a thought or message from oral (or written) language. The decoder must come up with the same message that the encoder intended. It is little wonder why "failure to communicate" is such a common explanation for why humans do not get along with one another.

When a breakdown occurs in the generation of a thought to be transmitted, production of linguistic coding, or articulation or phonation of the intended phonemes (speech sounds), communication on the output side is affected. Speech-language pathologists are the specialists who deal with such disorders. Any interference with the propagation of the waves from the speaker's lips to the listener's ears results in a reduction of the loudness or distortion of the signal. Abnormalities of the peripheral auditory system also result in alterations of the loudness or fidelity of an acoustic message, and it is the clinical audiologist, with otologists (physicians who specialize in diseases of the ear), who remediate such disorders. When disease or damage occurs in the specialized areas of the brain designed for decoding acoustic messages, speech-language pathologists and audiologists combine their skills to help the patient.

*For details of the concepts of language and language disorders, see chapters 2, 5, and 6.*

*See chapters 5, 6, and 12 to learn about therapeutic measures.*

Audiologists and speech-language pathologists share common roots. Their basic educations are parallel, and it is not until graduate training that they separate into specialized coursework. Specific interests and goals put them on different but parallel tracks, which come together when the needs of hearing-impaired individuals present themselves. The fundamental knowledge of each specialty is shared, along with trained expertise in the remediation of hearing-impaired persons.

# THE NATURE OF SOUND

We live in a gaseous environment, air. In air, the molecules are spread far apart, and, as long as there is heat, they move about randomly, colliding, and retaining a certain amount of elasticity. Of course, similar molecular activity exists in liquids and solids, but in those environments, the molecules are packed much more closely together than in air.

When any vibration, from a violin string, a tuning fork, human vocal cords, occurs in air, the result of that vibration is an impingement upon the surrounding air molecules. These air molecules are then pushed more closely together than would normally be the case; they are condensed (compressed), leaving behind them areas where the molecules are fewer in number. The result is a partial vacuum, called a *rarefaction*. The alternate condensations and rarefactions are called *pressure waves*. An example of a simple pressure wave, which is the result of back and forth vibration, may be seen in part A of Figure 10.1.

It is convenient to think of sound waves as a form of projected circular motion (part B of Figure 10.1), and these projected circles can be broken down, like any circles, into 360°. Zero degrees is the point on the wave of minimum molecular movement; 90° is the point of maximum compression;

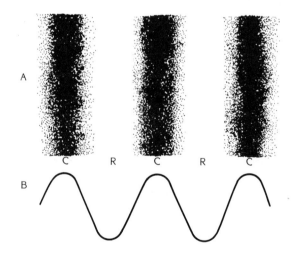

**Figure 10.1** Simple wave motion in air. In part A, "C" represents areas of compression, where air molecules are packed closely together; "R" represents areas of rarefaction, where the molecules are further apart. In part B, the pressure waves are displayed as they change over time (projected circular motion). (*Note. From Frederick N. Martin,* Introduction to Audiology, *3/e,* © *1986, p. 16. Reprinted by permission of Prentice-Hall, Inc., Englewood Cliffs, New Jersey.*)

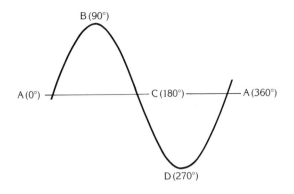

**Figure 10.2**   Denotation of a sine wave in 360°. (*Note. From Frederick N. Martin, Introduction to Audiology, 3/e,* © *1986, p. 18. Reprinted by permission of Prentice-Hall, Inc., Englewood Cliffs, New Jersey.)*

180° is at the same height as 0° as the pressure wave moves in time and space to 270°, which is maximum rarefaction (Figure 10.2). Trigonometry allows mathematical computations with circles, including measurements of angles, which can be examined in terms of their sines, cosines and tangents. Since the sines of these angles are used often when examining sound waves, they are often referred to as sine or sinusoidal waves. The height of a wave, that is the point to which it moves maximally, is called its *amplitude.* The amount of force or energy per unit volume of air is called **intensity.** The number of compressions and rarefactions in a time period is referred to as **frequency.**

## Intensity

We have seen that the *intensity* of a sine wave is related to its amplitude. Because of the extreme range of intensities to which the human ear is capable of responding (from barely audible to extremely loud), a linear system of intensity measurement is impractical. For this reason, the decibel (¹⁄₁₀ of a bel, named for Alexander Graham Bell) is used. The **decibel** (dB) expresses a ratio between two sound pressures or two sound powers. The decibel scale, therefore, is logarithmic rather than linear.

Since the expression of sound intensity is made in decibels, the reference must be specified. To talk of 50 dB or 100 dB is meaningless. Common references for the decibel include *sound pressure level* (SPL), which implies a pressure reference of 20 μPa (micropascals), supposedly the intensity at which normal young adult ears can barely detect a sound. A sound intensity great enough to cause physical pain or discomfort to the human ear is about 140 dB SPL (a ratio of 100,000,000,000,000:1). Another common decibel reference in audiology is *hearing level* (HL), where the zero reference is the intensity at which normal ears can barely detect the presence of a variety of frequencies through a single earphone. The sound pressure level required for 0 dB HL is slightly different for different frequencies. *Sensation level* (SL) means the number of decibels above the point where an individual can barely hear a tone. Therefore, a 50 dB HL tone, presented to a person who can barely hear that tone at 15 dB HL, is heard at 35 dB SL. The term *sensation level* is somewhat misleading because the *sensation* implies something to do with how the ear perceives a sound, rather than the number of decibels above threshold.

*Special scales for rating loudness have been developed.*

As the intensity of a sound is increased, the pressure of the wave is also increased, and the sound appears to increase in loudness. It is important not to think of the two phenomena as one—loudness (a subjective or psychological experience) is influenced by intensity (an objective or physical phenomenon). A scale of the intensities of some everyday sounds is shown in Table 10.1.

# Frequency

The *frequency* of a sound is the number of back and forth vibrations made in a single time period. It is convenient to use one second for this purpose. The number of complete compressions and rarefactions of a wave through 360° is called one cycle, and the frequency of a wave is described in terms

**Table 10.1**   Scale of Intensities for Ordinary Environmental Sounds

|  |  |
|---|---|
| 0 dB | Just audible sound |
| 10 dB | Soft rustle of leaves |
| 20 dB | A whisper at 4 feet |
| 30 dB | A quiet street in the evening with no traffic |
| 40 dB | Night noices in a city |
| 50 dB | A quiet automobile 10 feet away |
| 60 dB | Department store |
| 70 dB | Busy traffic |
| 60 to 70 dB | Normal conversation at 3 feet |
| 80 dB | Heavy traffic |
| 80 to 90 dB | Niagara Falls |
| 90 dB | A pneumatic drill 10 feet away |
| 100 dB | A riveter 35 feet away |
| 110 dB | Hi-fi phonograph with a 10 watt amplifier, 10 feet away |
| 115 dB | Hammering on a steel plate 2 feet away |

*Note.* The decibel reference is 20 μPa.

*Source.* Data from Van Bergeijk, Pierce, and David, 1960.

of *cycles per second* (cps). Because of the major contributions of Heinrich Hertz, the 19th century German physicist, his name is often used to mean cycles per second. Therefore, if 100 complete cycles occur in one second, the frequency is said to be 100 cps, or 100 **hertz** (Hz).

Frequency has a relationship to pitch in the same way that intensity is related to loudness. As the frequency of a sound increases, so does its pitch, but once again, frequency is a physical measurement and pitch is its psychological counterpart. To say that a sound has a pitch of 1000 Hz is as inaccurate as referring to loudness in decibels.

*Like loudness, pitch scales have been developed that show the subjective "highness" and "lowness" of sounds.*

The human ear has a frequency range that is extremely wide, from about 20 to 20,000 Hz. While it is unlikely that other animals can hear sounds below our lower frequency limit (infrasonic) there are those, such as bats, dolphins, and whales, that can hear well above our upper frequency limit (ultrasonic). This high-frequency hearing capability allows some animals to generate and bounce high-frequency sound waves off surfaces so they can be "echolo-cated." In the evolution of the human auditory system, our high-frequency hearing ability seems to have been lost, but there is evidence that the ability to respond to ultrasonic vibrations still exists in our brains, a vestige from a survival need we no longer have.

When a sound has only one frequency, it is said to be a pure tone. Equal multiples of the frequency of a pure tone are said to be *overtones* or *harmonics,* and the lowest frequency in a complex wave is called the *fundamental frequency.* Given a composite wave including 100, 200, and 300 Hz, 100 Hz is the fundamental, 200 Hz is the second harmonic, 300 Hz is the third harmonic, and so forth.

Pure tones do not exist in nature. They can be generated by whistles and tuning forks, but the closest human beings can come to generating a pure tone is to purse their lips and whistle. What we hear all around us is a series of complex tones. The complex sound that is of greatest acoustical interest to us is speech.

## Acoustics of Speech

From an acoustical viewpoint, speech is a complex wave that is constantly changing. The sounds of speech are divided into different classifications. Vowels, for example, are complex waves that tend to repeat their waveforms over time. An analysis of vowel sounds, using a device called a sound spectrograph, shows that the fundamental frequency of the wave is deter-mined by the fundamental frequency of the larynx (voice box), and all other sounds produced are equal multiples of that frequency. The length and cross-sectional areas of the vocal tract (determined largely by the height and position of the tongue) act as filters. The energy peaks at different harmonics, known as *formants,* that determine the characteristics of specific vowel sounds. The first and second formants usually provide enough information to make each vowel recognizable. Spoken English vowels are not limited to the five vowels as written. Rather, they take on a number of different pronunciations, a fact that makes learning English as a second language quite formidable. Semivowels in English are shorter in duration and fewer in number than are vowels. They include the sounds /w/, /r/, /l/, and /y/. Recognizing the acoustic difference between /r/ and /l/ requires the presence of a third formant.

The bulk of English sounds are made up of consonants. Each of the consonants varies to some degree in its production (and perception), based on the influence of other phonemes (speech sounds) with which it is juxtaposed. For example, the phoneme /t/ is different in words like *too, hat, butter,* and *must.* Each of these variations is called an *allophone.* Vowel sounds produce the bulk of the energy (intensity) of speech, while consonants provide most of the intelligibility. As mentioned in the story of Violet, persons with hearing difficulty in the higher frequencies, with normal low-frequency sensitivity, often can hear the vowel components of speech, but miss many of the consonants. All audiologists have heard many times the complaint, "I can hear, but I can't understand the words."

Some of the consonant sounds can be differentiated from each other based on whether their *resonances* (natural frequencies) are produced orally or nasally. All vowel sounds in English are oral, as are all consonants except the nasals /m/, /n/, and /ŋ/. Vowel sounds are said to be voiced because they are normally produced while the vocal cords are vibrating. Many of the consonant sounds have voiced and voiceless (whispered) partners (*cognates*). These cognate pairs are articulated the same way, but vary from each other based on voicing. Examples are /p/ and /b/, /t/ and /d/, and /s/ and /z/.

The production and ultimate perception of speech are influenced by elements of **prosody**. These include pitch, intonation, loudness, stress, duration, rhythm, tempo, and quality. Disorders of hearing may interfere with perception of the prosodic elements of speech, as well as its articulation. This contributes to what has been called the *deaf speech* of persons with severe to profound hearing losses.

## DISORDERS OF HEARING

For the most part, disorders of hearing will be examined in this chapter as a function of the time in life when they have their onset: prenatally (before birth), perinatally (at the time of birth), and postnatally (following birth). We will also cover the most common disorders by progressing in the same way that an acoustical signal progresses, beginning at the outer ear and culminating in the brain. To begin, a cross-sectional drawing of the human ear is shown in Figure 10.3.

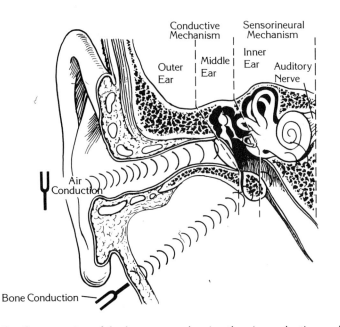

**Figure 10.3**   Cross section of the human ear showing the air conduction and bone conduction pathways. (*Note. From Frederick N. Martin,* Introduction to Audiology, *3/e, © 1986, p. 2. Reprinted by permission of Prentice-Hall, Inc., Englewood Cliffs, New Jersey.*)

## The Outer Ear

A simplified drawing of the outer ear is shown in Figure 10.4. It can be seen that the outer ear is comprised of an external appendage called the auricle (pinna), whose function is to funnel sounds down the external auditory canal to the tympanic membrane. The tympanic membrane is commonly called the eardrum, which is technically incorrect because the "drum" is actually the entire middle ear and the tympanic membrane is the drum head. The external ear canal is lined with skin, and its outer portion contains several glands that produce earwax (cerumen).

Many of the disorders that affect the outer ear do not appear to affect hearing. There may be some people who believe that damage to, or absence of, the pinna is more of a cosmetic than an auditory problem and, indeed, measurement of hearing through earphones ignores the contribution of the pinna to human hearing. In fact, the pinna is an excellent gatherer of high-frequency sounds from the environment so that they can be funneled into the external ear canal, and loss of the pinna can create significant difficulties in auditory localization. Hearing loss in the outer ear is called

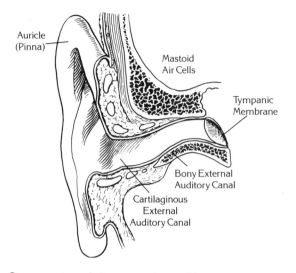

**Figure 10.4**  Cross section of the external ear. (*Note. From Frederick N. Martin, Principles of Audiology: A Study Guide,* © *1984. Reprinted by permission of University Park Press, Baltimore, Maryland.*)

**conductive,** and is caused either by blockage of the canal or damage to the tympanic membrane.

### Prenatal Causes of Hearing Loss in the Outer Ear

Pinnas may be missing or malformed because of the influence of the genetic makeup of one or both parents. The same is true of the external auditory canal, which may be totally or partially blocked (atresia). Illnesses or the ingestion of drugs, sometimes before fertilization (on the part of fathers as well as mothers) and sometimes after fertilization, can produce defects.

### Perinatal Causes of Hearing Loss in the Outer Ear

When the outer ear is affected at the time of birth, it is probably because of the trauma from violent uterine contractions. At times, during difficult deliveries, forceps may be used that inadvertently traumatize the external ear. Trauma can cause atresias and/or malformed pinnas.

### Postnatal Causes of Hearing Loss in the Outer Ear

Because they protrude from the sides of the head, pinnas are susceptible to damage from a number of sources, including burns, frostbite, and skin cancer, all of which can result in total or partial removal of a pinna. Trauma from a variety of sources can damage and malform a pinna. The cauliflower ear is sometimes the badge of merit for the prizefighter.

For reasons that have been debated but not entirely agreed upon, children are fond of putting small objects into their ears. Although less common, this is seen in adults as well. When the occluding object blocks off the passage of sound in the external auditory canal, a hearing loss may occur. Removal of such objects is imperative, and is usually best performed by an ear specialist who has the lighting, instrumentation, and expertise required for such maneuvers. I have seen the simple removal of a bean from a small child's ear result in extreme damage and great pain when not done properly.

Earwax (cerumen) is a normal substance found in the outer portions of external ear canals. Its presence is probably to keep insects and foreign substances from approaching the tympanic membrane. Normally the wax migrates naturally toward the opening of the canal. When occlusion takes place because of excessive wax, it is often because the individual has packed it down in attempting to remove it with an object like a cotton swab. Such removal is highly inadvisable and is best left to nature, or, if wax occlusion occurs, to the otologist.

Infections of the external ear are common, especially in warm, damp climates. These are dermatological disturbances and can be treated medically. If left untreated, they will result in the piling up of debris within the canal, and a great deal of pain along with hearing loss can ensue. Audiologists frequently find that they cannot determine the extent of a hearing loss produced by an external ear infection because the swelling and pain do not permit placing earphones on the infected ear(s).

The tympanic membrane vibrates sympathetically with sounds in the external auditory canal. If it is thickened or scarred by repeated disease of the ear, or if it is perforated by trauma or disease, its natural functions can be altered or lost. **Trauma** can include an instrument, sudden changes in air or water pressure, a blow to the head, or intense sound. There are several excellent plastic surgery procedures available to close tympanic membrane perforations, and they should be considered whenever possible. Under certain circumstances, these operations cannot be performed, but the indications for surgery must always be decided by the appropriate physician.

Tumors, both benign and malignant, can form in the external auditory canal. When they are observed by hearing or speech clinicians, the patient should be referred for immediate medical consultation. It is not until the size of a growth in the canal impedes the passage of sound waves that a hearing loss takes place, but hearing loss is not the primary concern when medical referral is made in the case of tumors.

## The Middle Ear

The middle ear is a tiny air-filled space, the lining of which is mucous membrane, similar to that found in the nose, throat, and sinuses. In normal ears, it is closed off from the external auditory canal by the tympanic membrane. Since the air in the middle ear is constantly being absorbed by the mucous membrane that lines it, and since any membrane vibrates best when the air pressure is the same on both sides, there must be a means to replenish the air in the middle ear space. The eustachian tube, which connects the middle ear to the nasopharynx (where the nose and throat join) is normally closed, but opens during such actions as yawning and swallowing by the pull of four sets of muscles. When the tube is open, atmospheric pressure is restored to the middle ear space.

Since the outer ear is filled with air and the inner ear is filled with fluid, the impedances (opposition to energy flow) of the two systems are different. Without the middle ear to match the impedances, many sounds that strike the tympanic membrane would bounce off or be distorted and weakened before they reached the inner ear. The matching of impedances is accomplished in two ways. First, the area of the tympanic membrane is about 22 times larger than the area of the oval window, the membranous entry to the inner ear. This step-down ratio increases the pressure from tympanic membrane to oval window in much the same way that water pressure is increased in a garden hose when a thumb is placed over the end. Second, impedance matching is provided by the lever action of the middle ear bones. A diagram of the middle ear is shown in Figure 10.5. The middle ear contains the three smallest bones in the human body, the ossicles. The ossicles in

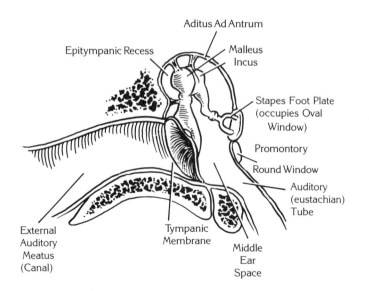

**Figure 10.5** Cross section of the middle ear. (*Note. From Frederick N. Martin, Principles of Audiology: A Study Guide, © 1984. Reprinted by permission of University Park Press, Baltimore, Maryland.*)

each middle ear are called the malleus, incus, and stapes. The fact that the malleus, the largest of the ossicles, moves like a lever on a fulcrum also increases the energy that passes through the middle ear. The outer ear is primarily a place of acoustical energy; the middle ear deals primarily with mechanical energy.

## Prenatal Causes of Hearing Loss in the Middle Ear

A variety of genetic disorders have been associated with abnormalities of the middle ear. Sometimes a congenital malformation of the middle ear is seen with no other symptoms. At other times middle ear anomalies are part of a syndrome, including craniofacial pathologies.

*Chapter 11 discusses cleft palate, an example of a congenital craniofacial abnormality.*

## Perinatal Causes of Hearing Loss in the Middle Ear

Damage to the middle ear at the time of birth is relatively unusual. Severe trauma from violent uterine contractions or forceps, while they could conceivably damage the middle ear, would undoubtedly result in other severe damage to the fetus.

## Postnatal Causes of Hearing Loss in the Middle Ear

The largest single cause of hearing loss, not only in the middle ear but in general, is **otitis media,** infection of the middle ear space. These infections are quite common in children as a result of upper respiratory infections, but they are seen often in adults as well. The infectious organisms may gain access to the middle ear space through the eustachian tube, by way of the bloodstream, or through a perforation of the tympanic membrane. Before the advent of antibiotics, it was quite common for persistent otitis media to result in an infection of the mastoid bone (mastoiditis), with serious threat to the health and life of the patient because of the danger of infectious spread to the brain. In those earlier days, surgery was the course of treatment for chronic otitis media, which often resulted in disfigurement of the middle ear and permanent hearing loss. Mastoiditis is still common in Third World countries and among the poverty stricken in the United States.

Otitis media must be thought of first from the medical perspective, and second from the point of view of hearing loss with its concurrent communicative implications. Medical treatment is primarily directed at alleviation of the dangers of infection, and second at improvement in hearing. Surgery can be performed to close a perforation of the tympanic membrane, which can improve hearing sensitivity, and, more importantly, protect the middle ear from agents in the air that could irritate or infect the middle ear. Surgery should never be performed to close off a middle ear that is actively infected.

Although fluid in the middle ear is the hallmark of otitis media, there are times when the fluid itself is noninfectious. When eustachian tube function is altered, the system that maintains equal air pressure between the outer and middle ears is affected. This results in a drop in middle ear pressure and the suctioning of fluid from the moist mucous membrane that lines its walls. This condition is called *secretory otitis media,* and it is often the result of closure of the eustachian tube because of overgrown adenoids, allergy, or pathology of the muscles and nerves that pull the eustachian tube open. Poor eustachian tube function is common in infancy and early childhood.

A common surgical procedure performed on patients with fluid in the middle ear is lancing the tympanic membrane with a slender, sharp knife to relieve the pressure and pain. This procedure is called **myringotomy.** Myringotomies are customarily performed on children under light anesthesia in a hospital, or as part of an adenoidectomy-tonsillectomy procedure. Myringotomies are often done on adults in the physician's office and, while somewhat painful, the procedure is quite brief, and relief from the discomfort is almost immediate.

After the tympanic membrane has been lanced and the fluid suctioned out of the middle ear space, it is common practice to place a small ventilating tube through the incision. This tube usually remains in place for several months. Though the patient must be careful to keep water out of the external ear because of the possibility of introducing infection into the middle ear, the tube usually does an excellent job of performing as a kind of artificial eustachian tube. The use of pressure-equalizing (PE) tubes has been popular for three decades, especially with small children.

Since otitis media is so common in children, it is often discovered during routine hearing testing by speech-language pathologists when they perform therapy for communicative disorders that have nothing to do with hearing loss. In such situations, the clinician can become an advocate for the child by performing or requesting tests that point to the presence of a middle ear abnormality.

Otitis media in small children may have consequences beyond temporary hearing loss, pain, and discomfort. Northern and Downs (1984, pp. 10–18) discuss the possible effects of even mild conductive hearing losses on the language development of small children. This condition is called minimal auditory deprivation (MAD) syndrome, and it is of concern to many clinicians. It is possible that there is damage to the brain cells developing in babies during the occasions of mild hearing loss because of lack of sensory stimulation.

Otosclerosis, a condition seen primarily in adults, is caused by a growth of new bone that interferes with the vibrations of the stapes (the tiniest bone in the human body). This condition is interesting for two reasons: it is more common in women than in men, and it is largely restricted to Caucasians.

The development of the surgical microscope has led to a number of operative procedures for alleviation of hearing loss from otosclerosis.

Any condition that causes damage to the middle ear system can produce a hearing loss. This includes burns, trauma, tumors, and a host of other pathologies. Whenever there is a suggestion of a middle ear disorder, medical consultation is mandated.

## The Inner Ear

The inner ear (Figure 10.6) is often called a labyrinth because of its resemblance to a winding and twisting cave. It is comprised of two portions. The vestibular portion is responsible for balance and equilibrium. The cochlear portion functions as a transducer, which converts the mechanical energy of the middle ear into an electrochemical signal that can be sent to the brain for processing. While the fluids (there are at least two) of the two branches of the inner ear are connected, the functions of each part are quite different. The cochlea is a pressure-sensitive system, while the vestibule is a motion-sensitive system. Even with all its moving parts and complex functions, the inner ear is the size of a small pea.

### Prenatal Causes of Inner Ear Hearing Loss

Prenatal factors producing hearing loss are more common in the inner ear than in the outer or middle ears. Prenatal factors include genetic disorders in isolation or in conjunction with other abnormalities. Not all hereditary hearing

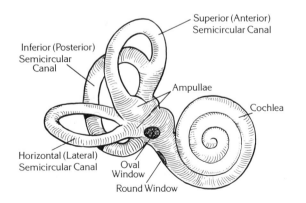

**Figure 10.6**  Diagram of the inner ear. (*Note. From Frederick N. Martin,* Principles of Audiology: A Study Guide, © *1984. Reprinted by permission of University Park Press, Baltimore, Maryland.*)

losses are evident at the time of birth. Some, called hereditodegenerative, are progressive and begin some time after birth.

Many of the factors that produce cochlear hearing loss, such as deprivation of oxygen to the fetus (anoxia), also produce damage to the central nervous system. For this reason, it is not uncommon to find hearing loss in association with conditions such as mental retardation and cerebral palsy. Other prenatal causes include maternal viral infections, such as cytomegalovirus (one of the herpes viruses) and rubella (German measles), which can produce a variety of other abnormalities to organs such as the brain, heart, and eye. Other causes of prenatal cochlear hearing losses are blood incompatibilities between the mother and fetus. Best known among these disorders is Rh incompatibility.

## Perinatal Causes of Inner Ear Hearing Loss

The birth process itself may be harmful to the inner ear. Children considered to be in medical distress may be placed on what has come to be called the *high-risk register*. While not all hospitals agree on which conditions put a newborn at risk for hearing loss, the following criteria have become common (Gerkin, 1984): (1) family history of hearing loss; (2) maternal viral infections during pregnancy (including rubella, cytomegalovirus, herpes, syphilis, toxoplasmosis); (3) craniofacial abnormalities (including cleft lip and palate; oddities of the pinna, throat, etc.); (4) low birthweight (less than 1500 grams, or approximately $3\frac{1}{2}$ pounds); (5) hyperbilirubinemia (high levels of liver bile in the blood); (6) meningitis; and (7) asphyxia, coma, or seizures. Chief among the perinatal complications is anoxia. When the delicate cells of the inner ear are starved of oxygen, they may be killed or damaged.

## Postnatal Causes of Inner Ear Hearing Loss

Otitis media, usually associated with hearing loss in the middle ear, is also a common cause of cochlear hearing loss after birth. Many viral infections, such as mumps and measles (rubeola—the 10-day variety, not to be confused with rubella), are associated with adventitious hearing loss, along with bacterial meningitis.

Damage to the cochlea by noise is commonly seen in older children or adults. While many industrial plants with high noise levels have established hearing conservation programs (thanks in large measure to federal laws designed to protect workers on the job), humans have discovered other ways to traumatize their sensitive cochleas with noise. Stereo headphones, including the portable ones worn by runners, cyclists, motorists, and others, are often implicated in noise-induced hearing loss.

Some acquired cochlear hearing losses have a sudden onset in one ear only. Many of these conditions are associated with vertigo. Two common causes are spasm of the internal auditory artery (the only artery carrying blood to the inner ear) and Meniere's disease. These conditions are frequently debilitating to the patient, and require prompt medical attention when symptoms are first noticed.

As the world's population is given to increased longevity, it can be expected that more persons will show hearing losses associated with age. The name given to age-induced hearing loss is *presbycusis,* and can usually be found in males by their early sixties and females by their late sixties. With increased medical and sociological interest in the phenomena associated with aging, more is being learned about communicative disorders related to aging. Age-related changes that occur in the central nervous system complicate the receptive communication problems of the elderly.

## The Auditory Nerve and the Brain

Nerve impulses from the cochlea reach the centers in the brain responsible for receptive auditory communication by way of the auditory nerve and a series of way stations in the brain. Damage to the auditory nerve usually produces pronounced difficulties in hearing and in discriminating speech. Damage to the auditory centers in the brain affects processing of auditory information, but does not always manifest a loss of hearing sensitivity. Beyond the auditory nerve, many of the brain centers that receive, process, and transmit impulses are duplicated on both sides of the brain. This redundancy is partially responsible for our specialized abilities to hear and understand speech in difficult listening situations where there are competing messages or noisy backgrounds. Often people complain of listening difficulties that go unheeded because hearing sensitivity remains normal, while speech recognition is subtlely impaired.

### Prenatal Causes of Hearing Loss
### in the Auditory Nerve and the Brain

Many of the etiologies of prenatal causes of cochlear disorders are the same for the central nervous system. Common causes include some of the maternal viral infections and genetic disorders. Evidence about the effects on the development of the central nervous system of substances ingested or inhaled by parents before and during pregnancy is growing.

### Perinatal Causes of Hearing Loss
### in the Auditory Nerve and the Brain

Trauma to the head during birth by violent uterine contractions or the use of forceps may produce damage to the brain. Other conditions that produce interruption of blood with its oxygen supply (such as umbilical strangulation) can cause brain damage. Many of the perinatal etiologies of cochlear hearing disorders also manifest in abnormalities of the central nervous system.

### Postnatal Causes of Hearing Loss in the Auditory Nerve and the Brain

Common causes of damage to the brain after birth include trauma (automobile accidents and gunshot wounds are frequent in this category) and the formation of tumors. Many of the tumors, especially of the auditory nerve, are benign and can be removed by a trained surgeon. When tumors are removed from the auditory nerve, it is common for the hearing to be completely lost from that side, even if only a mild loss was seen preoperatively. Hearing can only occasionally be preserved.

The advent of new imaging techniques, such as computerized tomography (CAT-scanning) and magnetic resonance imaging (MRI), have made the diagnosis of brain lesions more objective. Since these important and expensive diagnostic tests must be ordered by a physician, it is the responsibility of the audiologist to call to medical attention any hearing test results that suggest a lesion beyond the cochlea.

Presbycusis (hearing loss due to aging) was mentioned earlier as a cause of cochlear dysfunction. Many of the delicate inner ear structures are lost and not replaced during the aging process. Brain cells are replaced more slowly than most other cells in the body, and there is a point during aging when more brain cells are lost than are replaced. This process is unique to the individual, and may begin for some people during their twenties.

## THE MEASUREMENT OF HEARING

Early hearing tests took a variety of forms, such as the clicking of coins or use of soft speech. The introduction of tuning fork tests in the middle of the last century added an element of qualitativeness. It was not until the development of the pure tone audiometer that quantitative measurements of hearing could be made. Using audiometers allows the comparison of the auditory thresholds of clients, measured in decibels, to the thresholds of normal hearing persons. *Threshold* may be defined as the level of a sound so soft that it can just barely be perceived, perhaps 50% of the times it is presented. The manufacturers of audiometers use data established in 1969 by the American National Standards Institute (ANSI) to determine zero decibels hearing level. When an audiometer is set to 0 dB HL, the level of the sound from the earphone is just intense enough to be at the threshold of an average, normal hearing, young adult.

Although some financial compensation regulations require conversion of hearing loss data to a percentage, it is not a concept that is useful to people in understanding their hearing problems. There are still clinicians who attempt to explain hearing loss as a percentage of normal hearing, but this concept is not considered scientifically valid. Despite the fact that many people wish to know what percent of their hearing they have lost, the concept is almost meaningless, and this should be explained to the parties involved.

## Pure Tone Audiometry

When testing with pure tone audiometry, the client is instructed to signal (raising one hand is common) every time a tone is presented, even if the tone is barely audible. When working with special populations, such as children, the infirm, mentally retarded, or the multihandicapped, voluntary responses are often difficult to obtain, and special techniques must be developed to elicit responses that suggest auditory threshold. Figure 10.7 shows a small child signaling that he has heard a tone by raising his hand, presumably when the tone is barely audible.

The results of pure tone tests are customarily shown on a special graph called an **audiogram**. This graph is unusual because numbers are smaller near the top and grow larger near the bottom. The auditory threshold for each frequency (shown across the top of the graph) is indicated by the number of decibels required to reach the threshold for that frequency (shown

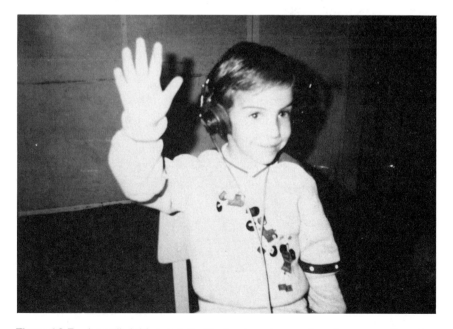

**Figure 10.7**   A small child signals that he has heard a pure tone from an audiometer.

along the side of the graph). The intensity range on most audiograms is from − 10 to 110 dB HL. The frequency range, in octave and midoctave points, is from 125 to 8000 Hz.

## Air Conduction

Tests by **air conduction** are accomplished by placing earphones over the pinnas of the outer ears. Sound waves are carried through the outer ear and middle ear, converted to electrochemical energy in the inner ear, and transmitted to the brain by the auditory nerve. The drawing of a cutaway of the ear in Figure 10.3 illustrates the air conduction pathway. Test results are shown by placing a red circle for the right ear and a blue X for the left ear beneath the frequency being tested and next to the number of decibels required to find threshold. Normal hearing shows a range from − 10 to 15 dB HL. Remember that 0 dB HL does not mean the absence of a sound, but rather the intensity at which normal hearers can barely hear that sound. Minus 10 dB HL represents hearing sensitivity slightly more acute than what is normally expected, but there are normal dispersions around the mean any time numbers are averaged. There is, therefore, a range of intensities at which thresholds may be found for normal hearers.

## Bone Conduction

Tests by **bone conduction** were designed to bypass the outer and middle ears, and measure only the integrity of the inner ear (Figure 10.3). In practice, bone conduction is less simple than just stated, but it can be understood this way for now. Bone conduction thresholds are obtained by placing a special vibrator on the head, usually on the mastoid process behind the pinna. The bone conduction vibrator stimulates the inner ear by literally distorting the skull. Thresholds are obtained in the same manner for bone conduction as for air conduction, and are usually graphed using a red symbol for the right ear and a blue symbol for the left. Persons interpreting test results should always consult the audiogram's legend to be certain they are interpreting the symbols correctly. The symbols recommended by ASHA are shown in Figure 10.8. Normal hearing persons will show hearing thresholds at 15 dB HL or less for all frequencies, for both air and bone conduction. An example of an audiogram for a normal hearing person is shown in Figure 10.9. The shaded area in the approximate center (also shown on the other illustrative audiograms in this chapter) is the range of intensities and frequencies within which most speech sounds are produced. Because of its shape, this area is often called the *speech banana.*

## Speech Audiometry

Because pure tones do not exist in nature, and because the most common complaint clients make about their hearing is that they have difficulty hearing

| Modality | Ear* | | |
|---|---|---|---|
| | Right | Both | Left |
| Air Conduction — Earphones<br>Unmasked<br>Masked | | | |
| Bone Conduction — Mastoid<br>Unmasked<br>Masked | | | |
| Bone Conduction — Forehead<br>Unmasked<br>Masked | | | |
| Air Conduction — Sound Field | | S | |

*The fine vertical lines represent the vertical axis of an audiogram.

| Modality | Ear* | | |
|---|---|---|---|
| | Right | Both | Left |
| Air Conduction — Earphones<br>Unmasked<br>Masked | | | |
| Bone Conduction — Mastoid<br>Unmasked<br>Masked | | | |
| Bone Conduction — Forehead<br>Unmasked<br>Masked | | | |
| Air Conduction — Sound Field | | S | |

**Figure 10.8** Symbols for use in pure tone audiometry, as recommended by the American Speech-Language-Hearing Association (1974).

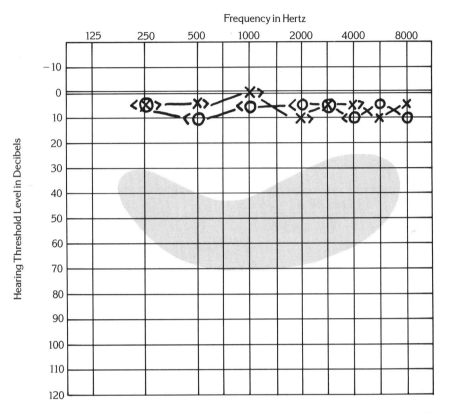

**Figure 10.9** Audiogram illustrating normal hearing in both ears. Note that all thresholds are 10 dB HL or lower (better) for all frequencies in both ears, by both air and bone conduction.

speech, the development of speech audiometers was inevitable. There are many measurements of audition that have been made possible through speech audiometry. The most common is the speech reception threshold (SRT)—the point at which speech can barely be heard and understood about 50% of the time. The SRT is not only a measurement of hearing loss for speech (a normal SRT is in the − 10 to 15 dB HL range), but compares favorably with the pure tone average (PTA) of the thresholds obtained at 500, 1000, and 2000 Hz. Therefore, the SRT is often a reliable check of the pure tone audiogram.

Another speech threshold commonly measured is the speech detection threshold (SDT), often called the speech awareness threshold (SAT). The SDT is the lowest level, in decibels, at which an individual can barely detect the presence of speech and recognize it as speech. SDTs usually require about 10 dB less intensity than do SRTs.

Since so many hearing-impaired clients complain that they can hear speech, but have difficulty in understanding it, a routine audiological examination today includes tests of speech discrimination (recognition). There are many discrimination tests available, but detailed descriptions of the stimuli and procedures are beyond the intended scope of this chapter. Suffice it to say that each test leaves something to be desired in the determination of an individual's speech discrimination abilities, although each can be useful in its own way. Speech discrimination is most commonly measured using special lists of monosyllabic words, and results are scored in terms of the percentage of the words that are correctly identified.

# Nonbehavioral Audiometry

Since many clients seen for hearing evaluations either cannot or will not cooperate by giving reliable responses to sounds, there has always been a desire for a procedure that did not require voluntary responses. Throughout the short history of modern audiometry, a number of electrophysiological approaches have been used.

## Auditory-Evoked Potentials

For several decades, emphasis has been placed on **auditory-evoked potentials:** introducing tones or clicks via earphones, and measuring the electrical responses to these stimuli with electrode pickups on the scalp. These procedures are based on electroencephalography. The rapid development of modern computers has allowed for signal averaging of the tiny microvoltages that are received from the head, so that the random, ongoing electrical signals from the brain do not obscure the responses to the acoustic signals. Most popular today is the auditory brainstem response (ABR) technique, which allows for measurement of responses that occur in the first 10 milliseconds following the rapid presentation of a series of clicks. While ABR has been a useful tool for estimating hearing sensitivity for the mid- to high-frequency range, even in tiny babies, and for diagnosing lesion sites in the auditory system, it has some limitations. Experts in this area agree that ABR should not be viewed as a test of hearing, but rather as a measurement of synchronous neural activity in the central auditory nervous system in response to a series of clicks. Like all diagnostic procedures, the effectiveness of ABR must be kept in proper perspective, but there is little doubt that some variation of this procedure will remain as an essential part of diagnostic audiology for some time.

## Acoustic Immittance

Modern technology has made it possible to take measurements that the founders of audiology would have considered amazing only a few short decades ago. Chief among these is the measurement of the impedance of sound waves in the plane of the tympanic membrane. Theoretically, when the tympanic membrane or the chain of ossicles in the middle ear become stiff, or when fluid is present in the middle ear, a conductive hearing loss exists because less sound is admitted to the middle ear, and more sound is reflected from the surface of the tympanic membrane. It is now possible to determine the relationship between the *admittance* of a sound to the middle ear and the *impedance* placed in the pathway of the sound. The term used to describe these phenomena is **acoustic immittance** (*immittance* is a combination of the two words). Tests of acoustic immittance take three general forms: static immittance, tympanometry, and measurements of the acoustic reflex.

Static immittance is measured in either cubic centimeters (cc)—when describing the opposition to energy flow into the middle ear—or millimhos (mmhos)—when describing the admittance of sound into the middle ear. The two measurements are reciprocal—as one increases, the other decreases. Due to the wide range of variability, the overlap in immittance values between normal and abnormal ears has resulted in static immittance measures being less helpful in diagnosis than had earlier been anticipated.

**Tympanometry** is the plotting of a function that measures the compliance of the tympanic membrane as the pressure placed against it is varied. The resulting graph is called a *tympanogram* (see Figure 10.10). A probe assembly is placed into the external ear canal (in the same manner when taking static immittance measurements). This assembly introduces a continuous "probe" tone to the tympanic membrane, and a microphone senses the amount of energy reflected from the membrane. An air pressure pump then introduces against the membrane a positive air pressure, which forces it gently in toward the middle ear and has the effect of partially clamping or immobilizing the middle ear system. The result of this positive pressure is a decrease in the compliance of the tympanic membrane and greater acoustic energy reflected from it. The pressure is gradually decreased until it reaches normal atmospheric pressure, and then is decreased further until it becomes slightly negative (a partial vacuum) in the external auditory canal.

Any vibrating membrane will be most compliant (mobile) when the air pressure is the same on both of its sides. This is also true of the tympanic membrane. Figure 10.10 illustrates the tympanogram (pressure/compliance function) of a person with a normal middle ear. Millimeters of water (mm $H_2O$) or decapascals (tenths of a pascal, or daPa) are customarily used as units of pressure. Notice that when the pressure in the outer ear is at zero mm $H_2O$, the tympanic membrane is maximally compliant. As both positive and negative air pressure are increased in the canal, the membrane becomes less compliant. Jerger (1970) has called this the *Type A tympanogram.*

A common type of tympanogram is seen in persons whose middle ear spaces are not properly ventilated by the eustachian tube. When this occurs, the pressure in the middle ear drops, and the tympanic membrane becomes

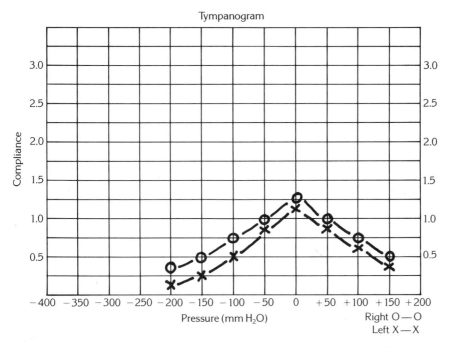

**Figure 10.10** Tympanogram showing normal pressure/compliance functions (Type A) for both ears. Note that the peaks of the curves (points of maximum compliance) are at 0 daPa (atmospheric pressure) for both ears.

most compliant when the artificially induced pressure in the outer ear is negative. This is Jerger's *Type C tympanogram,* and is shown in Figure 10.11.

When there is fluid in the normally air-filled middle ear, the pressure of this fluid becomes greater than what can be safely produced by the immittance device in the outer ear. In such cases, small or no changes in compliance of the tympanic membrane can be seen as pressure is varied from positive to negative. Jerger's *Type B tympanogram* (Figure 10.12) is extremely accurate in predicting fluid in the middle ear.

The acoustic reflex is the contraction of two small muscles in each middle ear, the tensor tympani muscle and the stapedius muscle. While several kinds of stimuli are thought to cause these muscles to contract, the stapedius in humans is known to contract in response to loud sounds. For most normal hearing individuals, a sound about 85 dB above threshold in one ear will produce a stapedial reflex in both ears. It is possible to monitor the stapedial reflex using the same probe that is used in static immittance and tympanometry. When the stapedial muscle contracts in response to sound, the acoustic immittance meter shows a decrease in the compliance of the tympanic membrane. Measurements of the acoustic reflex threshold

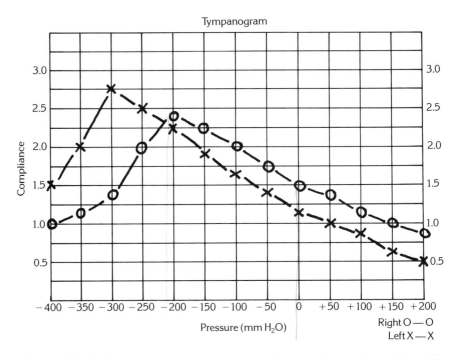

**Figure 10.11** Tympanogram showing retracted tympanic membrane (Type C). Note that the peaks of the curves are at −200 daPa (negative pressure) for both ears.

(ART), the number of decibels above the threshold of a client, can assist in the diagnosis of the type of hearing loss present, and, in many cases, the likely site of the pathology causing the loss.

The acoustic immittance battery, which includes static immittance, tympanometry, and acoustic reflex threshold measurements, has become an indispensable part of the diagnostic audiologic battery.

## TYPES OF HEARING LOSS

Hearing loss is usually divided into three general types: conductive, sensorineural, and mixed. A fourth category of central auditory disorders includes individuals whose lesions in the central auditory nervous system produce real but subtle symptoms. Central disorders often do not show up on routine hearing tests, but are identified by alert clinicians when taking a client history.

Experts do not completely agree about the handicapping effects of different degrees of hearing loss. Table 10.2 reflects my view. Although many people consider 25 dB HL to be the lower limit of normal hearing, many years of seeing clients with this amount of hearing loss have led me to conclude that this much hearing loss is handicapping. Indeed, there are people whose hearing levels are close to the 15 dB level, shown in Table 10.2 as representing the lower limit of normal hearing, who complain of a hearing

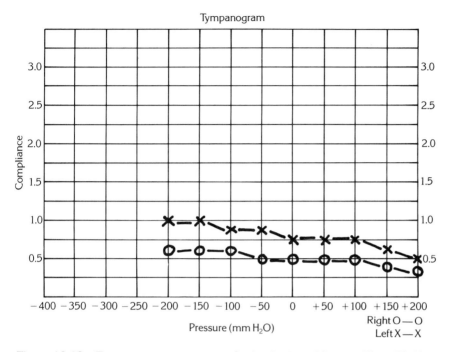

**Figure 10.12** Tympanogram suggesting fluid in both middle ears (Type B). Note that there are no peaks in these curves for either ear.

handicap. The wise clinician is guided more by the comments of the client than by arbitrary rules of thumb.

## Conductive Hearing Loss

Conductive hearing losses result from the interference of sound vibrations as they would normally pass through the outer and middle ear. These can be in

**Table 10.2** Degree of Hearing Impairment Based on the Average Thresholds Obtained at 500, 1000, and 2000 Hz.

| Pure Tone Average (dB) | Degree of Handicap |
|---|---|
| −10−15 | None |
| 16−25 | Slight |
| 26−40 | Mild |
| 41−65 | Moderate |
| 66−95 | Severe |
| >95 | Profound |

*Note.* Hearing levels are with reference to the ANSI 1969 standard.

the form of sound blocks, stiffness, or perforation of the tympanic membrane, or stiffness or interruption of the ossicular chain. Conductive losses usually result in an audiogram similar to the one in Figure 10.13, in which the air conduction thresholds are elevated (made poorer) in direct proportion to the amount of hearing loss found. Theoretically, since the inner ear and pathways beyond are unaffected in conductive hearing loss, the bone conduction thresholds should remain normal.

General rules in interpreting audiograms is that air conduction thresholds show the total amount of hearing loss present (the difference, in decibels, between 0 dB and the client's air conduction thresholds at each frequency); bone conduction thresholds show the amount of the hearing loss that is sensorineural (the difference, in decibels, between 0 dB and the

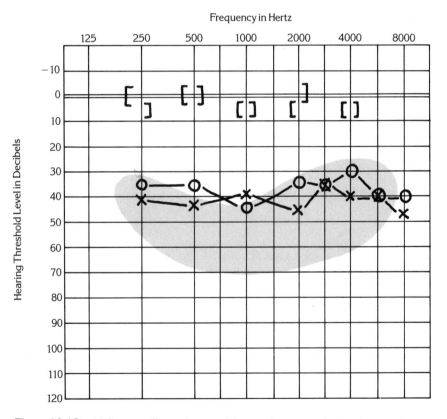

**Figure 10.13** Audiogram illustrating a mild to moderate conductive hearing loss in both ears. Note that, while the thresholds are above normal (poorer hearing—lower on the graph) for air conduction, they are normal for bone conduction.

client's bone conduction thresholds at each frequency); the air-bone gap (the difference between the client's thresholds by air conduction and bone conduction) shows the portion of the hearing loss that is conductive at each frequency. In conductive hearing losses, speech recognition (discrimination) SD P scores are usually quite high. The primary problem is in the loss of the energy of sound and not in the clarity.

## Sensorineural Hearing Loss

Hearing losses due to damage to the inner ear or the auditory nerve are called **sensorineural**. The term is rather general because one cannot tell from looking at an audiogram whether the problem is in the sensory or the neural portions of the ear. (An example of a sensorineural hearing loss is seen in Figure 10.14.) With sensorineural hearing losses, the amount of hearing loss by air conduction is approximately the same as the amount of loss by bone conduction. Persons with sensorineural hearing losses usually evidence some distortion of the sounds that are presented to them, even if those sounds are above threshold. As a general rule, the greater the amount of sensorineural hearing loss, the greater is the distortion, although the extent of hearing loss as shown on an audiogram is not always an accurate predictor of speech discrimination ability. Because of the distortion of sound, word recognition scores are usually affected, and many clients have great difficulty in discriminating among the sounds of speech, even when those sounds are amply loud.

## Mixed Hearing Loss

Conductive and sensorineural hearing losses are not mutually exclusive. Clients often exhibit symptoms of both types of losses, and this is referred to as **mixed hearing loss**. The causes of the sensorineural and conductive components of a mixed hearing loss may be the same, or each component may be of an entirely different cause. For example, a person may have a conductive hearing loss from wax accumulation in the external auditory canal, and damage to the inner ear from a loud noise. A mixed hearing loss is illustrated in the audiogram in Figure 10.15.

The amount of word recognition difficulty in a mixed hearing loss cannot be predicted based on the total amount of hearing loss present. Rather, it is the sensorineural component of a mixed hearing loss that determines the amount of distortion of speech sounds that will be present. Therefore, the bone conduction audiogram is the best indicator of how much difficulty a person may have in discriminating speech, even when it is amplified to the point where it is loud enough.

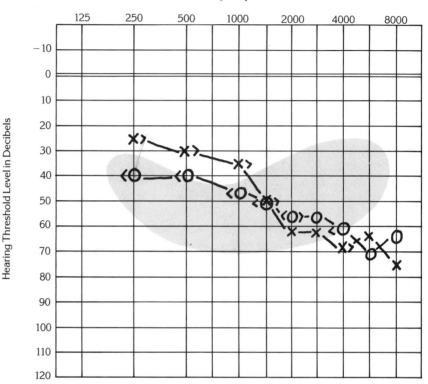

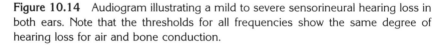

**Figure 10.14** Audiogram illustrating a mild to severe sensorineural hearing loss in both ears. Note that the thresholds for all frequencies show the same degree of hearing loss for air and bone conduction.

## IMPLICATIONS OF HEARING LOSS

The implications of a hearing loss are determined by several factors. Chief among these are the type and degree of loss, the contour of the audiogram, and the age at onset of the loss. Combinations of these factors make for varying degrees of optimism when prognostic statements are made about any hearing-impaired individual.

### Type of Hearing Loss

There is little argument that if one *had* to have a hearing loss, it would be better for that loss to be conductive than sensorineural. First of all, many conductive hearing losses are reversible by medical or surgical means. If the loss is permanent, word recognition is usually quite good. The client will benefit from the amplification provided by a hearing aid.

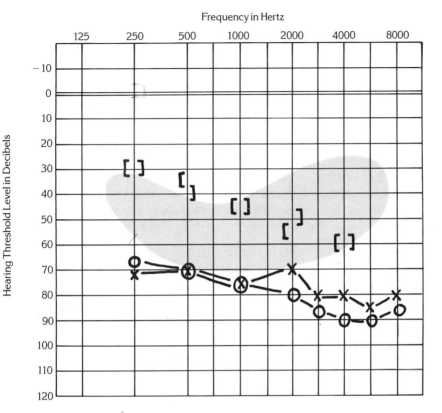

**Figure 10.15** Audiogram illustrating severe mixed hearing loss in both ears. Note that there is a greater loss of hearing for air conduction than there is for bone conduction, although both are abnormal.

Persons with sensorineural hearing losses, except in unusual circumstances, have problems that are irreversible. Their impaired speech recognition causes them difficulty in communicating, especially in noisy background situations or when there are several people talking at once. Sometimes these people are resistant to amplification because they find that simply making speech louder does not make it clearer. It is not known why clients with sensorineural hearing losses often do poorly with amplification. One reason would certainly be their word discrimination problems. It is also likely that disappointment results when expectations for help from a hearing aid have been too high. Clients with sensorineural hearing loss have a better chance adjusting to a hearing aid if they receive appropriate professional guidance and therapy.

There was a notion among physicians years ago, which is fortunately less popular today, that persons with sensorineural hearing loss should not wear hearing aids because what would be amplified is the distortion they already hear. It is unarguable that rehabilitation with amplification is more difficult for persons with sensorineural loss than for those with conductive loss, but it is precisely the challenge of rehabilitative audiology to do as much as possible to restore maximum auditory function to those in greatest need.

## Age of Onset of Hearing Loss

Naturally, the age at which a hearing loss begins can make a big difference in terms of the effects on the individual. One who develops hearing loss after speech and language have developed is said to have **postlingual hearing loss**. For such individuals, remediation must come in the form of *rehabilitation*. *Habilitation* is performed on children whose onset of hearing loss is **prelingual,** beginning before speech and language concepts have been formed. Speech, it must be remembered, is an imitative process best learned through the hearing sense.

It is generally agreed that the earlier in life a hearing loss can be detected, the better are the chances that a child can be taught communication through speech and hearing. Even if a different avenue of communication is chosen for the child, early detection almost always increases the potential for a child's learning. Having said this, it must then be asked, which kinds of screening methods should be used, and at what point in a child's life should they be attempted? There is no earlier time than when a child is in the hospital after birth, nor is there a more captive audience.

Infant screening certainly appears justified. It has been estimated that 1 neonate in 750 will have some degree of hearing impairment (Northern & Downs, 1984). Downs and Sterritt (1967) used a device that produces a high-intensity tone at 3000 Hz to elicit startle responses from newborn infants. These responses generally come in the form of eye blinks, body movement, and general startle reactions. Some of the difficulties inherent in such procedures include the large number of false positive responses (the appearance of a response when the sound has not been heard) and false negative responses (failure to respond when a sound has been heard). Additionally, there is the nagging problem of the expense of widespread screening procedures, and the question of who will perform the tests. When audiologists or trained nurses do neonatal hearing screening, the chances of accurate interpretations of responses are better than when the tests are done by volunteer laypersons or relatively uninformed professionals.

A number of ingenious devices have been developed for testing infants before they leave the hospital after birth. These include the Crib-O-Gram (Simmons, 1976; Simmons & Russ, 1974) and the neonatal auditory response cradle (Bennett, 1979). The basic concept involved with these devices is that a motion-sensing transducer picks up changes in body movement as they relate in time to the presentation of sounds. Computers can be used to separate body movements that are startle reactions to sound from random body movements. Research on these methods has both encouraged and discouraged their use.

The use of the auditory brainstem response (ABR) test has become increasingly popular in the hearing screening of infants. The procedure is complicated by the fact that the relative maturity of the central auditory nervous system can result in difficulty in interpreting responses. When doing ABR testing on young children, norms based on the age of the child must be calculated for responses because the relative maturity of the central auditory nervous system can affect them. The audiologist must consider not only the chronological ages of children to be tested (age 0 months at birth), but also their gestational ages (age 0 months at conception) because many babies at risk for hearing loss are premature.

Since the widespread use of neonatal hearing screening is impeded by both technical and financial obstacles, the conventional wisdom is to screen only those infants who are considered at risk for hearing loss. The Joint Committee on Infant Hearing Screening (1982) recommends the use of the high-risk register discussed earlier in this chapter. The earlier after onset a hearing loss is diagnosed, even when the loss is adventitious, the better is the prognosis for improved communication.

## REMEDIATION

Whenever a hearing loss is medically or surgically reversible, this is the treatment of choice. Audiologists and speech-language pathologists have a legal as well as a moral obligation to refer all clients with conductive and mixed hearing losses to appropriate medical specialists. Once medical treatment is either eliminated as a choice or is unsuccessfully attempted, the skills of the communication specialist are needed for auditory (re)habilitation.

### Counseling

The first words said to a client, or to the caretakers of a client, can critically influence all the treatment that follows. Evidence is mounting that families of hearing-impaired children may be severely shocked by the news that their child has an irreversible handicap. Once the word *deaf* has been used, the family often becomes incapable of processing information that follows. The audiologist may feel that the family needs a great deal of information about the child, but it does little good if the family cannot use this information. All of this contradicts parents' claims to want more information at the time of diagnosis than they presently get (Martin, George, O'Neal, & Daly, 1986).

We are also learning now that adults may be psychologically upset by the news that they have a hearing loss, even though one would assume that such news was anticipated. Though adults claim they want more information than they customarily receive about the options open to them, there is evidence that they too often have difficulty understanding that information when it is presented before they are psychologically prepared for it (Stevenson, Daly, & Martin, 1986).

Counseling of clients and their families should be considered an ongoing process, rather than a one-time sharing of information. Perhaps the best way to begin after hearing testing is completed is simply to ask what information the parties involved wish to receive. A surprising number of people do not wish details at that moment, but rather an overall impression of their hearing status and general implications.

In the case of children, many experts agree that having the caretakers observe or even take part in the testing allows them to be prepared when a severe hearing loss is discovered in the child. The audiologist might simply ask, "What was your impression of your child when those loud sounds were presented to him?" Parental response is often, "He didn't seem to hear them, did he?" Allowing the parent to assist in verbalizing the diagnosis can be helpful and may aid in reducing the trauma.

When the client involved is an older child or an adult, it is important that the diagnostic information be delivered to the client and not to persons accompanying the client to the evaluation. All too often, clinicians speak to parents of teenagers, children of the elderly, or spouses of the severely impaired. This can be insulting and demoralizing to the client.

As stated earlier, counseling is an ongoing process. The client and the family must feel confident about the clinician, but they must be allowed to make their own decisions in their own time, based on the information provided to them. Luterman (1987) points out that audiologists are willing far too often to step in as saviors of the family, making decisions, giving directions, and generally taking charge. It is Luterman's belief that such actions interfere with the maturation of the family because they, after all, should be the decision-making parties.

## Prosthetic Devices

A prosthesis is an artificial substitute for a missing or damaged body part or function. Prostheses may be cosmetic, such as the caps on teeth, or they may be functional, such as artificial limbs. Prosthetic devices for the hearing impaired used to be limited to hearing aids. Today there is a variety of listening devices, and their use has increased dramatically.

### Hearing Aids

The first consideration after diagnosis of a hearing loss is made should be whether or not to use a hearing aid. While not every hearing-impaired person can be helped with a hearing aid, dramatic improvements in electronic technology have vastly improved the options for amplification. Far more people can be helped with modern hearing aids than ever before.

Hearing aids are of five general designs (Figure 10.16). The traditional body instrument consists of a microphone, amplifier, transmitter, power supply, and other circuitry in one housing. A cord delivers the electrical impulse to a receiver (miniature loudspeaker), which is coupled to the ear by a custom plastic earmold. This type of instrument has become less popular in recent years because of technological advances in ear-level instruments. Ear-level or behind-the-ear (BTE) aids have many advantages over body aids, not the least of which is that they place the microphone (the input for the signal) on the head, where sounds are normally received, instead of the chest. Wearing two ear-level hearing aids often allows people to localize the source of a sound, and improves their ability to discriminate speech in the presence of background noise, competing messages, or other adverse listening conditions. The decision of monaural (one-ear) versus binaural (two-ear) fittings is an individual one, and, while there are no rules, most audiologists today believe that fitting binaurally should be the preferred approach unless there is some specific contraindication.

Once popular was the eyeglass hearing aid. For people who needed to wear both eyeglasses and hearing aids, the two could be combined into one instrument. One of the problems with such devices, of course, is that whenever the hearing aids are being repaired, the eyeglasses cannot be

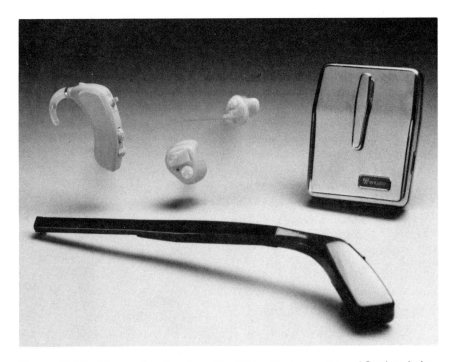

**Figure 10.16** Five modern hearing aids. (*Note. Photo courtesy of Starkey Laboratories, Austin, Texas.*)

worn, and vice versa. Eyeglass hearing aids are still manufactured, but are worn quite infrequently today.

Microcircuitry has allowed the development of hearing aids that can be worn entirely in the ear. Probably the original impetus for such instruments was their cosmetic value—they are often hardly noticeable. It has been learned that in-the-ear (ITE) aids take advantage of the natural sound gathering properties of the pinna, and their acoustic properties have been vastly improved. Some instruments, designed for fairly mild hearing losses, can be worn entirely in the canal (ITC). In-the-ear instruments now account for about 70% of hearing aids sold in the United States.

All the hearing aids described here are designed to present the amplified sound to the ear via a custom earmold. The earmold itself can be modified in many ways, which alters the response characteristics of the hearing aid and allows for emphasis of sound in certain frequency ranges, reduction of unwanted sensations of pressure in the ear, and so forth. There are some people who cannot wear air conduction instruments because of structural abnormalities of the external ear, drainage from the ears, or other causes. In such cases, it is possible to use a bone conduction receiver, which can be helpful to those suffering from conductive hearing loss. Most audiologists agree that air conduction is preferable when practicable.

## Cochlear Implants

Research has been underway for many years on the development of an implantable hearing device for clients who cannot derive benefit from conventional hearing aids because of the profound nature of their hearing losses. This goal has been met with the cochlear implant. Although these devices were originally restricted to profoundly impaired adults, the Federal Food and Drug Administration has recently approved implantation for profoundly hearing-impaired children.

Cochlear implants consist of one electrode or an array of electrodes that are placed surgically into the cochlea of the inner ear. The electrodes are attached to an internal receiver that is implanted in the bone behind the external ear. The acoustic signal is received by an externally worn microphone, which feeds a speech processor, which, in turn, amplifies and filters the sound and sends the electrical impulses to a transmitter than converts the signal to magnetic impulses. The connection between the external and internal components of the cochlear implant is made either by an induction system or by a direct, plug-in arrangement through the skin. When the cochlea is severely damaged, the cochlear implant can provide electrical stimulation to the auditory nerve for transmission to the brain.

Hopes are high for the potential use of cochlear implants, and more and more of this surgery is being performed. Of greatest importance is the careful selection of candidates for the procedure, along with extensive pre-

and postoperative counseling, training, and (re)habilitation. It is important for potential implant candidates and their caretakers to realize that normal hearing cannot be expected with these devices. Although they are becoming more popular, cochlear implants must still be regarded as experimental, and the completion of surgery marks the beginning, not the end, of the auditory rehabilitation process.

Although quite different from cochlear implants, a new implantable device called a temporal bone stimulator has been designed for persons with irreversible conductive hearing losses. A bone conduction vibrator is implanted in the temporal bone behind the pinna, and it is stimulated by an induction coil. Induction is provided by an externally worn hearing aid. The future for such devices is quite bright.

## Vibrotactile Aids

Many years ago, I saw a profoundly hearing-impaired client who had decided, on his own, that he could not hear and understand using a hearing aid, but the vibrations he felt from the receiver helped him to follow the rhythm and rate of speech so that his lipreading ability was improved. He changed from an air conduction receiver to a bone conduction receiver, and finally moved the bone conduction receiver to his wrist, where he could feel the vibrations better. He was surely ahead of his time, for only in recent years has interest been renewed in vibrotactile devices.

The outputs of vibrotactile aids can be placed on the backs or stomachs of small children, or worn on the hands or finger tips. Filters divide the input speech signal into separate bands so that vibrations are felt on different parts of the skin for different speech sounds. Once thought to be limited only to persons who had such severe hearing losses that they could not derive any benefit from a hearing aid, vibrotactile devices are worn by some children now in combination with conventional hearing aids. The eventual design of vibrotactile aids and their potential for helping the profoundly impaired, especially small children who have not grasped the concepts of speech, will be developed through the research efforts underway today.

## Assistive Listening Devices

Two problems for hearing-impaired persons are their distance from the sound source and the noise in the environment. Normally, the closer a person gets to a speaker, the louder the signal becomes. The greater the amount of background noise present, the more difficult the discrimination of speech becomes. Most people do best when the relationship in intensity between the primary signal and the unwanted background noise (called the *signal-to-noise ratio*) is favorable (that is, the signal is louder than the noise).

Many hearing aids contain circuitry that allows switching from the microphone to telephone position so that sound is picked up by an electromagnetic coil in the aid and bypasses the microphone, which therefore eliminates the noise in the room. This can be helpful to many hearing-aid wearers. There are several devices available that amplify the sounds coming from the telephone itself. Some of these simply fit over the receiver of the phone, and can be purchased at retail electronics outlets or the telephone company. Internal amplifiers can be obtained from most telephone companies. For people who need to use the telephone but do not derive benefit from the usual devices, it is possible to connect the phone to a teletype (TTY) arrangement so that communication with persons at the other end of the line who have the same device can be carried out by means of a keyboard.

An exciting stage in the development of technology to provide assistance to hearing-impaired persons is the advent of a new generation of assistive listening devices (ALDs). Some of these use lightwave technology for wearable, wireless earphones. These devices provide better sound fidelity than a hearing aid, and can be used for listening to the television and in theaters, meeting halls, churches, or other large rooms in which listening through a hearing aid can be difficult.

While many of the devices just described use infrared beams to carry the signals to a receiver, other kinds of technology are also available. Magnetic loops can be placed inside rooms and the signals can be received from the telephone pickups in wearable hearing aids. Speech can also be carried along frequency modulated (FM) signals directly to a wearable FM receiver, or to a receiver that is coupled to a hearing aid.

### Alerting Devices

For those people who cannot rely on their hearing for the alerting signals that normal hearing people take for granted, there are many instruments available. Some of these devices flash a light when a telephone or doorbell rings, a baby cries, a smoke or fire alarm goes off, or an alarm clock sounds. Some units convert these signals not into light, but into vibrations that are sent to a receiver placed beneath a bed pillow.

## Training Adults

Giolas (1982) points out that it is important to make a distinction between hearing impairment and hearing handicap. *Hearing impairment* refers to an organic hearing problem, while *hearing handicap* refers to the manner and degree to which the impairment affects a person's day-to-day communication. For this reason, Giolas believes that it is important to concentrate on the handicap, as the client perceives it, for aural rehabilitation to be effective.

In the past, aural rehabilitation consisted of a great deal of drilling. Emphasis was placed on lipreading (a better term is *speechreading* because the lips play only a part in the visual perception of speech) and on auditory retraining (listening to a variety of environmental, music, and speech sounds to practice their recognition and discrimination). Some aural rehabilitation today is practiced in the same way it was decades ago—the differences are in the use of more modern instrumentation for presenting stimuli.

Aural rehabilitation, it seems to me, should begin with the proper assessment of the hearing impairment (primarily by the clinician with the cooperation of the client), followed by assessment of the hearing handicap (primarily by the client with the assistance of the clinician). Rehabilitation can then proceed according to individual needs: providing amplification where appropriate, using group or private therapy, developing hearing handicap scales, learning communication strategies, maximizing visual and auditory cues, solving communication problems, and finding support groups such as Self-Help for Hard of Hearing People, Inc. (SHHH). The hearing-handicapped adult should receive the maximum amount of education in terms of what constitutes normal and impaired hearing, how the ear operates, what hearing test results mean, and the potential for rehabilitation.

## Training Children

Few challenges are greater than the education and training of prelingual, hearing-impaired children. When concepts of language have been learned before the onset of a hearing loss, the remediation must begin as quickly as possible to prevent the loss of language skills. Inappropriate delays are far too common. When a child is born with defective hearing, or acquires a hearing loss shortly after birth, language must be learned in a way different from normal. It was stressed earlier in this chapter that help should be delivered to such children as quickly as possible.

For many years, a philosophical battle has raged between two camps. The manualists believe that children with severe hearing losses should be taught, as early as possible, to use sign language so that they can learn to communicate quickly. The oralists believe that children should be taught to communicate through speech and hearing so that they can better integrate into the normal world of the hearing. The manualists claim that the deaf child does not belong (communicatively speaking) in the hearing world, and that manual communication is a more natural way for deaf children to learn. Prinz (1985) points out that the first sign of a deaf child comes earlier in life than the first word of a hearing child.

No resolution of the differences between the manual and oral approaches is forthcoming. A brief description of some of the methods used today for teaching children follows. It must be reiterated here that it is the caretakers of a small child who should decide on the system to be undertaken. The clinician must serve as a facilitator and educator, and must honor the decisions of the caretakers, even when a different decision might appear to be better for the child.

1. The multisensory approach involves the predominant use of speech. Often called the aural/oral method, receptive communication is accomplished through amplification and speechreading. The emphasis is on listening.

2. The unisensory (acoupedic) method makes predominant use of speech through listening. The child is denied visual input through speechreading to force improvement in auditory skills.

3. Fingerspelling (dactylology) is the use of a full set of letters and numbers created by different positions of the fingers. Words are spelled out as if written in air. Many sign language systems include fingerspelling for proper nouns and unknown signs. The Rochester Method utilizes fingerspelling and speech simultaneously, and each letter of every word is spelled out.

4. American Sign Language (Ameslan or ASL) has been called a natural language because it has its own grammatical structure (Fischer, 1982). ASL has certain advantages in terms of speed; it can be learned more quickly than other systems, and the communicative process itself is faster than other systems. Critics of ASL are quick to point out that this speed is often at the expense of important grammatic, syntactic, and cognitive elements of language.

5. Seeing Essential English (SEE 1) combines ASL with English; provides signs for the articles *a* and *the*; and includes the verb *to be,* which is omitted in ASL.

6. Signing Exact English (SEE 2), like SEE 1, follows English word order, but is less rigid in its rules than SEE 1. Users of ASL can communicate by SEE 2, but SEE 1 is more difficult.

7. Linguistics of Visual English (LOVE) is a system whose signs are identical to those in SEE 1 and SEE 2, but it is less comprehensive, and its written system is different from the other two methods. It is not used as often as SEE 1 and SEE 2.

8. Cued Speech involves a set of hand cues (near the mouth of a speaker), which augment recognition of phonetic elements (such as voicing) that are difficult for children to separate based on lipreading alone. Unlike sign language, the cues convey no communicative message by themselves. The response from the child can be in speech, sign, or a combination of the two.

9. Total Communication (TC) has become extremely popular in recent years. It is based on the concept that caretaker-child relationships are

improved when communication is achieved rapidly, and, therefore, rejects neither the manual nor the aural/oral approach, but combines the two. There are many unanswered questions about the efficacy of simultaneously speaking, signing, and fingerspelling to a child, but total communication is in widespread use today.

# CONCLUSION

No person involved professionally with people who have speech and language problems can escape dealing with the hearing impaired. The purpose of this chapter has been to introduce concepts associated with hearing and its impairment to those interested in the processes of communication and its breakdown. Since libraries contain many books related to hearing loss, it was ambitious to attempt to summarize, in one chapter, even the highlights of the science of audiology and its related fields. Nevertheless, it is hoped that this brief introduction will help spark interest in the science of audiology and in the needs of the hearing impaired.

# STUDY QUESTIONS

1. Why is it inaccurate to say, "Sound is 50 decibels loud," or, "Sound has a pitch of 1000 Hz"?
2. What is minimal auditory sensory deprivation syndrome? How does it relate conductive hearing loss in small children to language learning disorders?
3. What are the main causes of middle ear infections?
4. What significant factors place a child on the high-risk register for hearing loss?
5. List as many causes of hearing loss as you can. Divide them into categories of prenatal, perinatal, and postnatal, and conductive and sensorineural.
6. Sketch an audiogram illustrating a mild conductive hearing loss. Try to predict the probable speech reception threshold and speech discrimination scores.
7. What are the advantages and disadvantages of neonatal hearing screening?
8. What are some differences among traditional hearing aids, vibrotactile aids, and cochlear implants? For whom would the different types of devices be prescribed?
9. What are some differences between auditory rehabilitation and auditory habilitation?

10. List and describe some methods used in teaching profoundly hearing-impaired children.

## SELECTED READINGS

Luterman, D. M. (1979). *Counseling parents of hearing-impaired children.* Boston: Little Brown.

Martin, F. N. (Ed.) (1987). *Hearing disorders in children.* Austin: Pro-Ed.

Martin, F. N. (1986). *Introduction to audiology* (3rd ed.). Englewood Cliffs, N.J.: Prentice-Hall.

# CHAPTER ELEVEN

# Cleft Palate

## BETTY JANE McWILLIAMS

**MYTHS AND REALITIES**

- *Myth:* Facial disfigurement and palatal clefts are God's punishment for parental sins.
- *Reality:* Most clefts result from the interaction of genetics and environment.
- *Myth:* Cleft palates occur because of "marking," an example of which would be a pregnant woman seeing blood running down the upper lip of a suicide victim.
- *Reality:* Prenatal experiences such as "markings" have nothing to do with the baby's development.
- *Myth:* The deformity was caused by poor obstetrics.
- *Reality:* A cleft results from an alteration in embryogenesis between the 6th and 12th week of pregnancy. It has nothing to do with faulty obstetrical practices.
- *Myth:* Children with clefts are mentally retarded.
- *Reality:* Only if clefts are accompanied by other abnormalities or if there is a cleft of the palate only is there an increased risk for developmental problems, including mental retardation.

- *Myth:* The severity of facial deformity is an index of mental abilities.
- *Reality:* Individuals with severe facial deformities are sometimes brighter than others with little or no disfigurement.
- *Myth:* Children with clefts of the palate only are brighter than children with clefts of the lip and palate, and brighter even than children without clefts.
- *Reality:* There is no support at all for this view. While some are gifted, overall, they have an increased risk for developmental deficits.
- *Myth:* Most speech problems associated with cleft palates can be corrected by speech therapy.
- *Reality:* Many such problems are not treatable by behavioral means alone.
- *Myth:* There is a typical "cleft personality."
- *Reality:* While people with clefts must make obvious adjustments, they have a range of personalities just as people in general have.

THE many destructive myths surrounding congenital malformations of the face and oral cavity, including clefts, are difficult to eradicate, even though reality directly contradicts these old wives' tales that plague the lives of our patients and their parents and families. A well-informed speech-language pathologist is often in a unique position to provide information that may modify some of these harmful beliefs. In this chapter, the realities of cleft palate will be discussed first in relationship to a case history. The classification of clefts will then be presented with prevalence figures. This will be followed by information about etiology. Finally, diagnostic procedures and treatment approaches will be discussed. The case history that follows illustrates some of the realities.

*Martha, born with a cleft of the soft palate, was referred to the Cleft Palate Center at the age of 10 by her speech-language pathologist, who wanted suggestions for therapy to correct Martha's hypernasality. The original defect had been repaired by a plastic surgeon when Martha was 18 months old, and she had had no additional surgery. She had a history of middle-ear fluid, for which she had had several myringotomies with tubes, the first at 3 months of age. While she showed an air-bone gap, she responded to pure-tone testing at an average of 12 decibels (dB) in the left ear and 10 dB in the right. She had had no episodes of ear disease since age 5, and her hearing was stable. While she required periodic otological and audiological examinations, her hearing was not currently a problem for speech. Martha had a mild crossbite on the right, even though the* maxilla had not been affected by the cleft, and her tongue lateralized to the right when she produced sibilants. She was awaiting orthodontic attention.

Martha's receptive language had always been within normal limits, but she had used no expressive language until 4 months after the palate was repaired. Receptive language, as measured by the Test for Auditory Comprehension of Language (Carrow, 1973), was at the 65th percentile at age 4, and at the 70th by age 6. Expressive language, however, as measured by the Elicited Language Inventory (Carrow, 1974), yielded percentiles of only 9.8 at age 4 and 22.0 at age 6. During the preschool years, Martha showed slight reductions on all subtests of the Illinois Test of Psycholinguistic Abilities. By age 8, she was within normal limits. Her mental development had progressed much as her linguistic abilities had. At age 4, her verbal IQ on the Wechsler was 99, and her performance IQ 100. By age 8, her Wechsler verbal IQ had increased to 120, and her performance IQ to 117.

At age 10, Martha's speech was marked by consistent, moderate, visible, bilateral nasal emission on /p/ and /b/ (which were the only pressure consonants she could produce); severe hypernasality; slight hoarseness; and gross articulation errors, including omissions, pharyngeal fricatives, and glottal stops. She also had /r/ and /l/ immaturities. Her speech was only about 25% intelligible. On the Pittsburgh Screening Test, Weighted Values for Speech Symptoms, Martha's score of 18 was indicative of probable velopharyngeal incompetency, or the inability to separate the oral and nasal cavities during speech. Since speech therapy could not be expected to solve Martha's communication problems, the next step was to evaluate her velopharyngeal valving mechanism to learn how the soft palate and the posterior and lateral walls of the pharynx or throat worked together to separate the oral and nasal cavities during speech.

On Warren pressure-and-air-flow studies, performed while she spoke, Martha demonstrated an orifice area of 20 mm$^2$ on the word hamper. Multiview videofluroscopy showed a short soft palate with excellent patterns of movement; however, the soft palate never made contact with the posterior pharyngeal wall. The lateral pharyngeal walls moved about 50% of the distance toward midline. The basal view of the sphincter supported the lateral and frontal projections, and showed that closure was never achieved. Thus, the instrumental assessment of the velopharyngeal valve was consistent with speech data, and a pharyngeal flap designed to correct the incompetence was recommended and carried out.

After surgery, instrumental analysis demonstrated a velopharyngeal valving mechanism capable of achieving closure. Martha showed no air flow through the nostrils for /p/ and /b/, but it was impossible to predict what would occur on other consonants, which she still could not produce. Speech therapy was recommended for the elimination of gross *articulation errors and the correction of her immaturities. She was able to eliminate these errors with 6 months of therapy; however, she retained sibilant errors related to her dental malocclusion. Speech therapy was discontinued, and she was monitored at regular intervals until the completion of her orthodontic work. No additional therapy was required because the sibilant errors were easily modified after her orthodontic appliances were removed.*

*This case is like many that are presented for speech therapy. Without careful diagnosis, this child might have had therapy that could not have succeeded. Martha was fortunate that her structural and physiological limitations, clearly revealed in her speech pattern, were recognized and treated.*

# DEFINITIONS

A **cleft** is an elongated opening, especially one resulting from the failure of parts to fuse or merge early in prenatal development. Openings in the lip, the hard palate or roof of the mouth, and the soft palate represent a failure of structures to fuse or come together as they normally do between the 6th and 12th week of the mother's pregnancy. This failure to fuse may occur on one or both sides; it may involve only the lip, only the palate, or a combination of the two. Clefts may include the entire structure or only a part of it. Thus, babies with clefts are affected in different ways. Some clefts are associated with other congenital malformations, some of which occur predictably together and are classified as **syndromes** or phenotypic manifestations. When the traits that make up the phenotype affect the head, face, and oral structures, we refer to the syndromes, of which there are hundreds, as *craniofacial abnormalities.*

*A syndrome is a set of symptoms that occur together in predictable combinations of traits that we call phenotypes.*

# EXAMPLES

## Classification of Clefts

Clefts are of different types, and range from minimal to severe defects. A unilateral cleft lip may be a simple notch or a complete cleft extending through the dental arch on only one side, usually the left (Figures 11.1 and 11.2). When both sides and the nostril as well are affected, it is described as a bilateral complete cleft (Figure 11.3). A cleft palate without cleft lip is an isolated palatal cleft. If the dental arch is involved, the problem is described as a left, right, or bilateral complete cleft palate. The most common type of cleft is the unilateral complete cleft of the lip and palate. More severe clefts extend through portions of the face, as shown in Figure 11.4. Figure 11.5 presents a classification of the various types of clefts.

Of special interest to the speech-language pathologist is the **submucous cleft palate.** This is a true muscular cleft, but it is covered with a thin mucous

*A submucous cleft is a cleft in underlyingmuscle, and often in bone, with a thin mucous covering that may obscure the condition.*

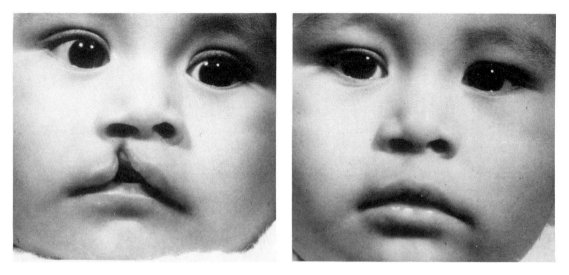

**Figure 11.1**   (a) Infant with a left incomplete cleft lip. (b) The same infant after lip repair.

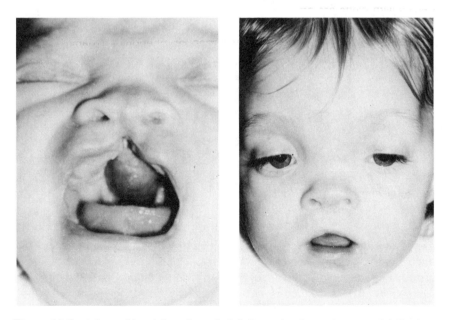

**Figure 11.2**   Infant with a left unilateral cleft lip and palate prior to and following surgery. Note the widely spaced eyes and the flattened nasal bridge, indicative of a craniofacial abnormality in addition to the cleft.

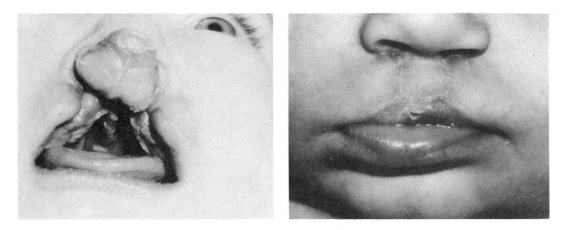

**Figure 11.3**   (a) Infant with bilateral complete cleft lip and palate. (b) The same infant after repair.

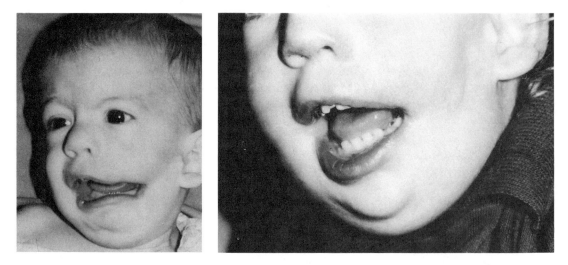

**Figure 11.4**   Infant with left lateral facial cleft before and after repair.

membrane that partially conceals the defect so that it is often overlooked, often until a speech problem persists into childhood. Not all submucous clefts cause speech problems, but those that do require the care provided for overt clefts. The submucous cleft can usually be identified by a careful examiner. The uvula may be bifid, so that it looks as if it is double. In reality, it has a small cleft. There may be a bluish line through the middle of the soft palate, where the muscles underlying the mucosa are separated, and there may be a notch in the posterior border of the hard palate that can be

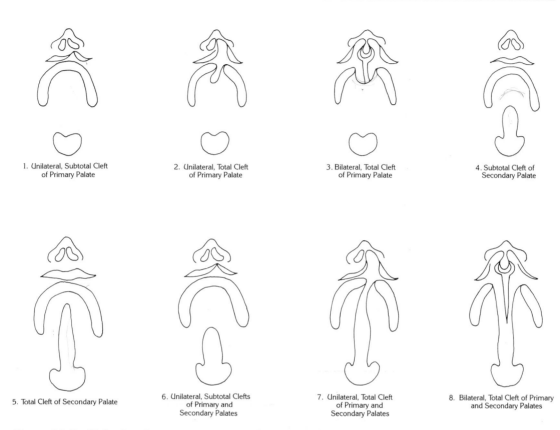

1. Unilateral, Subtotal Cleft of Primary Palate

2. Unilateral, Total Cleft of Primary Palate

3. Bilateral, Total Cleft of Primary Palate

4. Subtotal Cleft of Secondary Palate

5. Total Cleft of Secondary Palate

6. Unilateral, Subtotal Clefts of Primary and Secondary Palates

7. Unilateral, Total Cleft of Primary and Secondary Palates

8. Bilateral, Total Cleft of Primary and Secondary Palates

**Figure 11.5** Cleft classification proposed by Kernahan and Stark (1958), and adopted by the International Confederation for Plastic Surgery in 1967. (*Note: From "A New Classification for Cleft Lip and Cleft Palate" by D. A. Kernahan and R. B. Stark, 1958,* Plastic and Reconstructive Surgery, 22, *p. 435. Reprinted by permission.*)

palpated or felt. Speech-language pathologists often discover these anatomical variations and realize that the person needs the help of others before speech is likely to improve.

## Other Structural or Functional Deviations

The overt submucous cleft palate is not difficult to diagnose; however, there are other abnormalities that pose more serious problems. Kaplan, Jobe, and Chase (1969) described and illustrated some of these conditions. The space between the soft palate and the posterior pharyngeal wall may be deeper or wider than normal, so that the soft palate, often still capable of normal movement, cannot compensate. This condition is often diagnosed after an adnoidectomy. In some cases, the hard palate may be somewhat short, so that the soft palate is carried too far forward in the oral cavity to be effective, or the soft palate itself may be short. This latter condition may be associated with soft-palate musculature that is inserted into the hard palate instead of properly into the anterior part of the soft palate.

Other deviations include motor deficits, such as limited or poorly timed movement. These problems often require neurological consultation.

## Craniofacial Abnormalities

Craniofacial abnormalities are defects of the head and face, and they often include palatal abnormalities as well. These deformities take a variety of forms, and were once thought to be untreatable because of their extent and complexity. Corrective surgery is now relatively common (Christiansen & Evans, 1975; Marsh, 1986; and Tessier, 1971), and speech-language pathologists are encountering these problems more and more frequently. There are hundreds of such abnormalities, and the information about them is much too extensive to review here. Beginning speech-language pathologists will want to explore this topic in much greater depth to learn more about the associated communication problems (Cohen, 1978; McWilliams, 1984; Peterson-Falzone, 1973, 1988; Shprintzen, 1982; Siegel-Sadewitz & Shprintzen, 1982; Sparks, 1984). Figure 11.6 shows a child with Apert syndrome, an example of a craniofacial abnormality.

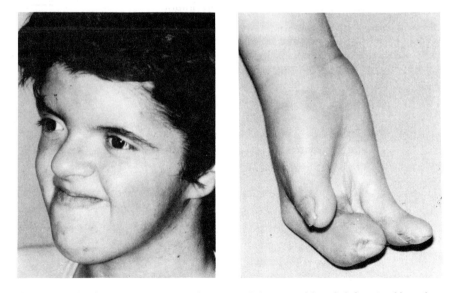

**Figure 11.6**   Child with Apert syndrome, and the typical hand deformity. Note the widely spaced eyes and the midface retrusion.

## PREVALENCE

Clefts, which affect more boys than girls, vary in frequency from one racial group to another, indeed from one report to another. There is agreement, however, that Orientals have the highest rate, about 1 in 500 births. Caucasians are in the midrange, with estimates from 1 in 750 to 1 in 1,000 births. Blacks are least likely to have clefts, with estimates for them ranging between 1 in 1,900 and 1 in 3,000 births. Clefts involve both the lip and palate about twice as often as the palate alone, although these statistics may be shifting somewhat to include more isolated palatal clefts. Syndromes occur much less frequently, and the prevalence varies from syndrome to syndrome.

## UNDERLYING MECHANISMS

It is easier to describe what happens, or fails to happen, to cause a cleft than it is to explain why. Parents are understandably concerned about the reasons why, and speech-language pathologists and other professional people must be sensitive to their questions and anxieties. Sometimes the myths discussed at the beginning of the chapter influence parental behavior, to the detriment of the child.

The developmental failures that cause clefts cannot be attributed to moral shortcomings of parents. Most clefts appear to be related to genetic factors interacting with an adverse environment. This means that the genetic programming of the developing infant predisposes it to some alteration in the growth pattern, and that the environment also contributes to the disruption. In some cases, especially syndromes, the cause appears to be purely genetic (Cohen, 1978). Genetic counseling is essential to any complete system of care, and speech-language pathologists should be well informed in this area so that they can discuss the issues with families and make wise referrals.

## DIAGNOSIS

### Developmental Background

A cleft in the palate has implications for early development that ultimately affect language and speech. While we are still struggling to understand these relationships completely, it is clear that they form the foundation for all diagnostic work.

### Feeding Problems

Feeding is usually the first hurdle for parents and infant, with protracted feeding times, limited intake of food, choking, and nasal regurgitation.

Speech-language pathologists often serve as the feeding specialists on the cleft palate team, and are eager to simplify the process so that the infant may use the oral structures successfully, and have a rewarding rather than a frustrating feeding experience. Successful feeding encourages quiet talking and cooing, which are the natural accompaniments of a pleasant experience shared by parent and child. Tension related to feeding may well disrupt early parent-child bonding, and negatively affect linguistic development.

Fortunately, it is usually possible to feed such babies successfully, and to lay a portion of the foundation for future verbal behavior. A simple, compressible bottle permits the parent to apply light pressure through a cross-cut nipple, which helps ease the formula or breast milk gently, while the infant is held in a sitting position. Satisfactory feeding should be reflected in adequate weight gain. Feeding intervention represents the earliest speech and language programming for cleft infants (Paradise & McWilliams, 1974).

## Middle-Ear Disease

*The* tensor veli palatini muscles *are responsible for opening the Eustachian tubes.*

This is present at birth in most infants with palatal clefts (Paradise, Bluestone, & Felder, 1969; Stool & Randall, 1967), but there is no increased risk when only cleft lip is present. The ear disease is variable, and may range from mild to severe. It seems to be related to the malfunctioning of the Eustachian tube, caused, at least in part, by an alteration in the action of the tensor veli palatini muscles.

*A myringotomy is a small incision in the tympanic membrane to permit drainage. Tympanostomy tubes, sometimes called pressure-equalization (p.e.) tubes, are inserted to permit aeration, pressure equalization, and drainage.*

The fluid in the middle ear causes mild conductive hearing losses of a fluctuating nature. If left untreated, the ear disease and associated hearing loss may worsen and lead to permanent hearing impairment. Theoretically, early, mild hearing loss can slow both language and articulatory development. While we know that ear disease improves in most cleft children as they get older, as it does in children generally, it is clear that we must strive for the best possible hearing as early as possible. Even with treatment, a few children retain persistent and recurring middle-ear disease into their teens and adulthood. Both **myringotomies** and antibiotics are employed to treat middle-ear disease, but myringotomies and aeration tubes are usually required prior to the first birthday—and often much earlier. The speech-language pathologist must be alert to the possibility of hearing loss, and to the need for frequent air- and bone-condition pure-tone testing, along with tympanometry. This topic is discussed in greater detail by McWilliams, Morris, and Shelton (1984).

## Psychosocial Problems

Psychosocial problems can also influence the way language and speech develop. This is true for all children, but the baby with structural problems of the oral cavity is undoubtedly at increased risk (McWilliams, Morris & Shelton, 1984). When the baby is born, parents are understandably disappointed, shocked, and grief-stricken. Yet, most data show that they usually recover quickly and accept their baby, the cleft, and themselves. Parents vary in their ability to cope with this particular problem, just as they vary in relationship to all problems (McWilliams, 1982; McWilliams, Morris & Shelton, 1984). Some will do well from the beginning, and a few will never accommodate. The speech-language pathologist must be sensitive to parents and the ways they interact with their children. A perceptive parent can encourage communicative skills better than a clinician can, while another may be destructive to all efforts to make communication functional. Communicative interaction does, after all, begin between parents and their children.

As for the children, there is no strong evidence that they are any more or less likely to be emotionally disturbed than are other children. This is not to imply that cleft children are never disturbed. Some are, and the implications for language and speech can be profound. The mother who punished her child when he began to say single words before his palate was repaired reinforced his not talking, and then could not understand why he did not immediately communicate verbally after surgery. She exemplifies the need for early counseling, with emphasis on language and speech development. The speech-language pathologist conducts guidance programs of this type, but is also alert to indicators of more serious problems requiring the cooperation of a psychiatrist, psychologist, or social worker.

While there is no evidence of a "cleft-palate personality," those with clefts and other structural abnormalities affecting the head and face are subject to unique problems imposed by a society that penalizes differences. These extra stresses may be especially marked during the school years, and may lead to withdrawal, impulse inhibition, altered interpersonal relationships, and lowered self-esteem (Richman & Eliason, 1986). The speech-language pathologist has an important role in helping to overcome these barriers to a full life and the acquisition of communicative skills (McWilliams, Morris & Shelton, 1984).

## Mental Development

This has also been a source of concern. Much of the literature reports that the ranges in IQ for children with clefts are lower than for unaffected children (McWilliams, Morris & Shelton, 1984; Richman & Eliason, 1986). Recent studies are more specific, however, and clarify issues that were previously obscured. On the average, children with clefts appear to have mental abilities that are not seriously different from those of other children. When other congenital abnormalities in addition to the clefts are present, or if the palatal cleft is isolated, the risk for deficits in intelligence is increased. Additionally, evidence shows that older children do significantly better on intelligence tests than do the same children in the preschool years (Musgrave, McWilliams, & Matthews, 1975), but that neither younger nor older cleft children, as a group, show the higher performance IQ than verbal IQ reported in the older studies (McWilliams & Matthews, 1979). Richman and Eliason (1986) summarize the literature in this area and make a strong case for the probability that about one-third of children with clefts, especially those with cleft palate only, have language-based learning disabilities resulting in underachievement in school and a higher than usual occurrence of reading problems.

## Language Development

*Chapter 2 reviews normal development.*

Influenced by all of these variables, language development is generally slower in children with cleft palates than in others (Lynch, 1986; McWilliams, Morris, & Shelton, 1984). The differences can be recognized in infancy, and account for many of the variations found in early mental development. If first words do not appear until between 20 and 24 months, the early developmental profile may be negatively affected.

These early language differences are less marked at later ages (Musgrave, McWilliams, & Matthews, 1975; Shames & Rubin, 1971). Mean sentence length remains shorter in comparison to peers, however, even though the longest sentences are likely to be appropriate for chronological age. Children with clefts, for still unexplained reasons, talk less than other children. Since this reduction in verbal output cuts across the entire cleft population, regardless of speech ability, the probable explanation lies in some aspect of self-esteem, or in the way much of society responds to their defects, which often encompass appearance, speech proficiency, or both.

Group data or measures of central tendency do not permit us to make predictions about individuals, who may not conform to group trends. Careful assessment of each individual is, therefore, essential.

## Articulation Development

When there is a cleft or velopharyngeal incompetence from other causes, articulation development is usually slow. This observation has been made repeatedly (Bzoch, 1959; Philips & Harrison, 1969; Van Demark, 1966; Van Demark, Morris, & Vandehaar, 1979). The delays are complicated, and the explanation is not always apparent. Part of the reason may be that coupling between the oral and nasal cavities does not permit the impounding of sufficient intraoral pressure for consonant production. Even early babbling is less rich than it is normally.

After surgery, if the velopharyngeal valve separates the oral and nasal cavities during speech, articulation, while slow in the early years, is often normal for chronological age by 5 or 6 years. Many speakers, however, have persistent articulation disorders into adulthood.

## Diagnostic Procedures

A diagnostic philosophy is imperative in understanding the many aspects of communication disorders associated with structural impairments. Almost anyone can recognize defective speech when they hear it, but a speech pathologist must be able to determine what is wrong and why. As Locke (1983) wisely noted, we have a tendency to label instead of explain, and to take our labels as explanations; yet successful treatment depends on accurate diagnosis.

When assessing verbal behavior in people with clefts, we must be aware that many do not have speech problems that are related directly to the cleft, and many have perfectly normal speech patterns. Over the past 25 years, success rates following initial surgery have ranged from a low of 12% to a high of 94%, with about 25% eventually having secondary surgical procedures to correct velopharyngeal incompetence. How many more might have profited is unknown. For those who do not develop speech at a high level of proficiency, a well-established diagnostic protocol is essential.

The initial evaluation always includes a complete case history, stressing the areas of known developmental difficulty for individuals with clefts or other abnormalities. This initial workup also explores language development as thoroughly as necessary to be certain that the basis for speech is intact and that any speech deficits found are not, in fact, linguistic in nature. A word of warning here. Sometimes children speak poorly for structural reasons, and they may elect to talk as little as possible to protect themselves against the social stigma attached to their speech. It would be a mistake to conclude that such children are language- rather than speech-impaired. On the other hand, it would be equally disastrous to fail to recognize a language-impaired child.

*Chapters 5 and 6 provide information about language assessment.*

The speech examination depends on the speech-language pathologist gaining control over an important instrument—his own ear. "The ultimate measure of the adequacy of the speech is always its effect on listeners, and it is here that the speech pathologist must begin" (McWilliams, 1980). It is the ear that will suggest what avenues should be explored and what instruments should be used. It is the ear that will determine the extent to which remedial procedures are indicated, and when they have succeeded or failed. For these reasons, speech-language pathologists must learn to be competent listeners. McWilliams and Philips (1979) have published a series of audio tapes designed to teach listening skills as they relate to velopharyngeal incompetency and associated disorders.

### Nasal Escape

This commonly occurs when velopharyngeal incompetence is present. Visible nasal escape on consonants other than /m, n, ŋ/ is the most minimal evidence of a poorly functioning valve. Nasal escape becomes a more serious problem when it is audible or when there is turbulence. Turbulence is an extra noise created when air passes through the velopharyngeal orifice

*Clinically significant nasal escape is air lost through the nasal passages on phonemes other than nasals.*

and encounters nasal obstruction. The fricatives, especially the voiceless sibilants, are more likely to be accompanied by some form of nasal escape than are the plosives, which can be produced with a somewhat larger velopharyngeal opening than can fricatives. Nasal escape that is visible on a mirror, but is not heard, and is accompanied by no other speech symptoms requires no intervention. Audible nasal escape and turbulence are distracting and are usually treated. In some cases, it will be necessary to improve both the valve and the nasal airway.

One should test specifically for nasal escape in the diagnostic evaluation. Hold a mirror under the nostrils to see if the individual is able to exhale freely from both nostrils. If that is not possible or if only a limited amount of air is visible, air escape during speech will not be any more obvious. It is then desirable to examine for nasal escape on nasals, where it is appropriate, and then on sibilants, other fricatives, and plosives because air loss may be more profound on some phonemes than others. It may also be apparent on blends, but not on single phonemes adjacent to vowels, rather than other consonants, particularly those requiring high intraoral pressure. Remember that the absence of nasal escape is not, by itself, proof of an intact velopharyngeal valve.

*A facial grimace is a ticlike movement of the nostrils or adjacent facial muscles, used in an attempt to reduce nasal air flow.*

Facial grimace sometimes occurs when there is significant nasal escape. A speaker may try to valve with the nostrils to cut off the air flow. This strategy is usually not effective, and the behavior is visually distracting. Examination for facial or nasal grimace is quite simple. It involves watching the speaker's face to see if collateral muscle activity occurs.

## Resonance

Resonance is an acoustical phenomenon that can be defined as "the vibratory response of a body or air-filled cavity to a frequency imposed upon it" (Wood, 1971). Resonance disorders are first recognized perceptually rather than instrumentally. There are several types, from limited nasal resonance to little or no oral resonance.

*Hypernasality is characterized by sound coming through the nose.*

Hypernasality is too much nasal resonance; it ranges from very mild to very severe. It is the characteristic most commonly associated with velopharyngeal incompetence. While hypernasality occurs on vowels, the vowels usually can be identified, and intelligibility is not seriously impaired unless the consonants are affected by the inability to create appropriate intraoral pressure. Since this frequently occurs in association with hypernasality, some writers avoid discussing hypernasality only and use other terms such as *nasalance* (Fletcher, 1978) or *nasalization* (Philips & Kent, 1984) to encompass a broader range of symptoms.

The speech-language pathologist listens to a speech sample and makes a judgment as to whether there is too much nasal resonance. A gross but simple test is to pinch the nostrils closed and listen for a shift in resonance from hypernasality to **cul-de-sac resonance.** Of course, this test is not effective when there is nasal blockage already influencing resonance. Such problems are discussed briefly below.

Whenever possible, determine the extent to which hypernasality is present. To do this, both clinicians and researchers use rating scales, even though such scales are difficult to apply reliably (Peterson-Falzone, 1986). These scales may include any number of points, but are more reliable if there are not too many choices. Thus, a 5- or a 7-point scale is often used, with 1 representing normal resonance and 5 or 7 identifying the most severe hypernasality.

Hypernasality and nasal escape are usually associated with velopharyngeal incompetence. Occasionally, however, an oral-nasal fistula will complicate the diagnosis. If there is a question about the possible role of a fistula, it can be closed with dental wax, chewing gum, or a temporary prosthesis as described by Bless, Ewanowski, and Dibbell (1980). It is then possible to assess speech perceptually and instrumentally with the fistula open and closed. Air loss may occur from one or both sources. There are few data-based reports on this issue.

Hyponasality is likely to be heard when the nasal passages are seriously obstructed, as with enlarged adenoids, a shallow pharynx (seen in some syndromes such as Apert), or blockage within the airways. The nasals /m, n, ŋ/ are the phonemes most influenced by nasal obstruction. They will approach, but not match, /b, d, and g/ because they will be produced with some residual characteristics of continuants and with the timing associated with the nasals. Testing involves listening to these particular phonemes and applying the cul-de-sac test as well. The obstruction is often great enough that there will be no shift from either or both nostrils. Sometimes a change will be heard with the constriction of one nostril but not with the other, and this finding helps to identify in which nostril the obstruction is to be found.

Speech-language pathologists may assume that, if hyponasality is present, velopharyngeal valving must be intact. This is not necessarily the case. The nasal obstruction may impede air flow that has not been cut off at that crucial valve, and hyponasality results. Opening the nasal passages under these circumstances is likely to reveal the inadequacy of the velopharyngeal valve.

Cul-de-sac resonance is a muffled quality that is created when there is velopharyngeal incompetence, through which energy and air enter the nasal passages that are obstructed anteriorly. If you repeat the sentence *Mike may make money* as you pinch your nostrils together, you will hear cul-de-sac resonance. Air pressure and flow studies will demonstrate the reduction in nasal air flow on nasals, and the evidences of cul-de-sac resonance can be heard in the speech pattern.

Hypo-hypernasality sometimes occur when air and energy that should be directed through the oral cavity are deflected through a deficient

*Cul-de-sac resonance is created by energy passing through a portal into a chamber that is closed on the opposite end.*

*An oral-nasal fistula is an opening from the palate into the nose.*

*A prosthesis is an appliance used to replace a missing part or to close an undesirable opening.*

velopharyngeal valve into a partially obstructed nasal airway. The quality of vowels becomes nasal, and there may even be visible nasal escape on high-pressure phonemes, especially /s/. The nasals lose some of their nasal characteristics, however, because the obstruction, although only partial, is too great to permit sufficient nasal transmission for the nasal phonemes. Thus, both characteristics can be heard in the speech pattern. The nasality will shift during the cul-de-sac test, but the nasal phonemes will show little if any alteration.

It is necessary to point out that children are often so resistant to and so embarrassed by the cul-de-sac test that they change vocal effort and invalidate the test. This will happen sometimes to children with perfectly normal velopharyngeal valves.

### Articulation Errors

Articulation errors associated with clefts and various other structural anomalies are more destructive to intelligibility than any other of the many speech characteristics. Articulation deficits spring from a wide variety of causes, all of which must be understood to diagnose and treat them accurately.

Maturational lags are one possible explanation for some articulation errors. You will recall that the child described in the case history had some articulatory errors that were attributable to slow maturation, and that such maturational lags are common in children with clefts. It would be a disservice to the child, however, to decide that problems traceable to anatomy or physiology were merely the result of slow development. Thus, it is necessary to discriminate accurately between what is clearly developmental and what is structural or physiological. Martha demonstrated both types of disordered articulation.

Hearing loss (usually mild conductive loss as previously mentioned), if untreated, seems to be partly responsible for at least some of the articulation deficits in cleft children. Hubbard, Paradise, McWilliams et al. (1985) reported better articulation in children who had had early and consistent ear care than in a carefully matched group whose ear care had been delayed. Thus, otological and audiological attention from birth is essential until ear disease has been eliminated and hearing stabilized.

*The **maxillary arch** is the upper dental arch. Midface deficiency results from a maxillary arch that is small and posterior to the mandibular or lower arch. This retarded development is sometimes thought to be related to the effects of surgery, but may be part of a syndrome.*

Maxillary arch collapse, midface deficiency, and missing teeth all may have adverse effects on articulation, especially sibilants, which may be distorted when the speaker attempts to close these anterior openings with the tongue or when the tongue cannot find alternative points of contact. Such errors are common in children and adults with clefts and craniofacial anomalies, and it is necessary that the causes be recognized and the basic one treated. Since speech therapy by itself has not been effective, we usually prefer to correct the anatomical defects as the first step. See Figure 11.6 on page 400 and Figure 11.7.

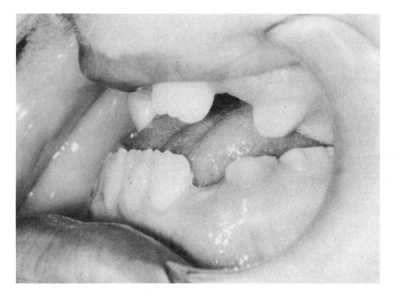

**Figure 11.7**   Tongue posture associated with midfacial deficiency, with disruption of relationships between the maxilla and the mandible.

Velopharyngeal incompetence is responsible for the articulation errors that we worry about most. These errors seem to increase in number and severity as the velopharyngeal opening present during speech gets larger. While this is far from a perfect relationship, small openings are usually less damaging than larger ones. Velopharyngeal competence is undoubtedly necessary for normal speech production (McWilliams, Morris, & Shelton, 1984; Morris, 1968; Shelton, Morris, & McWilliams, 1973). Many studies have shown that the consonant most sensitive to even small degrees of velopharyngeal incompetence is the voiceless continuant /s/. The other sibilants, the affricates, other fricatives, and finally the plosives are affected as valving deficits increase in size. If only /s/ is affected, the velopharyngeal incompetence is probably not severe. If plosives are involved, however, the probability is that the incompetence is moderate or severe. Plosive errors herald a larger opening than do sibilant errors (Subtelny & Subtelny, 1959).

If a speaker articulates accurately, retaining place and manner features in spite of reduced intraoral pressure, intelligibility can be excellent. Many speakers, however, find it either unacceptable or too difficult to keep up a conversational stream with so little intraoral pressure, and they compensate for the pressure losses by producing phonemes in other ways. We refer to this as *compensatory articulation.* It decreases intelligibility, and is difficult to eliminate because of the complexity of the substituted articulatory gestures. Warren (1986) suggests that these substitutions are attributable to the need to regulate pressures in the vocal tract.

*The* rugae *are the ridges on the dental arch behind the upper teeth.*

One of the simplest compensations is producing sibilants linguapalatally. Instead of placing the tongue tip against the **rugae** for /s/, the tongue is targeted to a position behind the dental arch, and the blade rather than the tip articulates with the most anterior portion of the hard palate. This creates a less distinct /s/, and the difference can be readily heard. Other speakers, often those with greater degrees of velopharyngeal incompetence, produce sibilants even more posteriorly, and may use the back of the tongue to interact with the posterior margin of the hard palate or with the soft palate. Backing errors may be even more pronounced when the posterior part of the tongue is elevated and the pharynx constricted for /s/, thus creating a pharyngeal fricative. These gross substitutions, which take many forms, have a sibilant quality, but are produced where there is access to as much pressure as possible.

When velopharyngeal incompetence is great enough to affect plosives, speakers may resort to still other compensatory strategies. They may do reasonably well with /p/ and /b/ by trapping buccal air behind the lips to make a plosivelike sound that is recognizable. The /t/ and /d/ are harder, and may be produced further back in a linguapalatal position. The /k/ and /g/ may be replaced by pharyngeal or glottal stops. Even fricatives may be produced glottally.

*The* glottal stop *is a coughlike sound. A plosive is produced by expelling air quickly through the approximated vocal cords.*

In any discussion of compensatory articulation, it is inevitable that some possibility will be overlooked, or that some adaptation never heard before will be missed. For this reason, we explore what a speaker is doing when she produces the various phonemes of our language. One example is the child who sniffed instead of attempting an oral /s/. The sniff had a sibilantlike character and avoided the necessity of high intraoral pressure, which was not available. Another is the woman who pooled saliva in the labial sulcus and forced it through her lower teeth into the oral cavity to approximate /s/.

*The* labial sulcus *is the trench that is seen when the lower lip is pulled away from the lower teeth.*

The speech-language pathologist should be aware that gross articulation errors may not be accompanied by nasal escape. The critical velopharyngeal valve is bypassed, and velopharyngeal closure is not required. Thus, the worst speakers may demonstrate little or no nasal escape, and you may be fooled into thinking that the mechanism is competent and that speech therapy could change the articulation patterns.

Gross errors constitute a subsystem of the English language. This subsystem incorporates nonstandard English sounds that can be produced by people who have velopharyngeal competence. In fact, in some sections of the country, glottal stops are used in certain combinations as part of standard English. An example is the New England glottal substitution in the word *bottle,* instead of the standard American form. The New Englander who does that however, has the competency to produce /t/ and /d/ when they occur in other contexts. This is not usually true of the person who uses glottal stops throughout his speech pattern to compensate for velopharyngeal incompetence. The problem with these gross errors is that, even after the velopharyngeal valve has been corrected, the system of gross errors will remain.

These patterns have been incorporated into phonology, and therapy will be required to teach new rules so that the individual can use the improved velopharyngeal valve effectively. If gross articulation errors are not present and there is only reduced intraoral pressure, improving the valve may be all that is required to improve speech. Once again, it is clear that differential diagnosis is required if we are to understand articulation errors, their potential for change with therapy alone, and the outcome that may be expected following modification of structure.

Formal articulation tests are as relevant to the diagnostic procedures used with these cases as they are for those with articulatory disorders in the absence of clefts. Articulation testing must go beyond the judgment that a phoneme is not in error. Differential diagnostic articulation testing implies that each error will be described in detail so that place and manner of production, along with idiosyncratic characteristics, are carefully noted. This information will assist in deciding what is responsible for particular articulation deficits.

*Chapter 7 discusses formal articulation tests.*

Articulation testing should be carried out using a small dental mirror to determine whether or not there is visible nasal escape on the various sounds or, of course, if the nature of the errors is such that nasal escape will probably not occur. The speech-language pathologist will also test for the patency of the nasal airway, listen for audible nasal escape and nasal turbulence, and record those characteristics in association with the phonemes on which they occur.

It is important when evaluating articulation to do stimulability testing. We want to know how much better an individual can do than she habitually does in conversation. Thus, we compare discrepancies between articulation heard in conversation and on formal articulation and stimulability tests. We cannot assume that, because an individual can produce a given consonant in one context, the potential for learning to produce it in conversational speech is automatically present. Keep in mind that a person with borderline velopharyngeal valving abilities can sometimes achieve a fleeting closure in the production of an isolated sound or of a single word, but cannot maintain closure during the rapid-fire muscular demands of free-flowing speech. Stimulability testing gives us some idea of the depth of the problem. If most of the phonemes can be produced, it may well be that speech therapy would be effective—after we have determined that the velopharyngeal valve is adequate to the task. On the other hand, it may be that a borderline valving mechanism can meet the speech demands in one situation, but cannot do so under more complex speaking conditions.

## Disorders of Phonation

Phonation disorders also occur in association with velopharyngeal incompetence. Vocal hyperfunction results when an attempt is made to reduce pressure loss and hypernasality by controlling the air stream at or below the larynx. Some speakers even retain as much air as possible, releasing just enough to produce a tense, strangulated voice of low volume. You may experience such a voice if you bear down on the diaphragm while you vocalize. You will also feel the larynx rise in the neck. This vocally abusive behavior may lead to hoarseness, often accompanied by periodic aphonia, and to bilateral vocal cord nodules (McWilliams, Bluestone, & Musgrave, 1969; McWilliams, Lavorato, & Bluestone, 1973). Other evidence of vocal stress include a hard attack on vowels, breathiness, and a significant reduction in loudness. This soft-voice syndrome is related in many cases to the loss of pressure through a defective valve, necessitating the compensatory regulation of subglottic pressure. Speaking at lower volumes requires less subglottic pressure than speaking at higher volumes, and results in proportionately less pressure loss through the velopharyngeal portal. Some speakers are unable to increase loudness (Bernthal & Buekelman, 1977), while others show an increase in hypernasality when they do so. These vocal responses to what is likely to be only borderline velopharyngeal incompetence provide additional evidence that the vocal mechanism is an interactive system, and that it is impossible to modify it at one level without influencing what occurs elsewhere. Thus, changes in the phonatory patterns are not surprising when you realize that the larynx is the first valve in a series of valves in the vocal tract.

Assessment of voice should be a routine part of the clinical evaluation of all those with structural defects. A first step is to decide whether or not vocal abuse is present, what the characteristics of the abuse are, and how susceptible the voice is to behavioral modification. See chapter 8 for a discussion of voice evaluation—the same methods apply here.

## Intelligibility

*Intelligibility refers to how well speech is understood.*

Intelligibility should be evaluated when speech is assessed to determine the severity of a communication impairment and what should be done about it. Speech may be intelligible, even with marked alterations in the way it is produced. On the other hand, aberrant production strategies may seriously reduce intelligibility.

An objective method of assessing intelligibility is to have a panel of listeners write down what they understand of a given speech sample and then to average the responses. This method, while useful in research, is too cumbersome and time consuming for routine clinical application. Intelligibility may also be assessed by using rating scales that place completely intelligible speech at number 1, and completely unintelligible speech at number 5, or perhaps number 7. Again, speech-language pathologists must develop rater reliability in the use of these scales because they are clinically useful in determining how handicapping a problem is only if the ratings are accurate. If speech is slightly defective but is generally intelligible, treatment might be less aggressive than if it is unintelligible.

It should be clear by this time that the speech problems associated with structural deficits are complex, and that careful diagnostic studies are necessary before intervening to help the individual speak more efficiently.

## Diagnostic Tools and Methods

### The Pittsburgh Screening Test, Weighted Values for Speech Symptoms

This test is a useful method of integrating information from the speech evaluation, and of using clinical data to make decisions about the adequacy of velopharyngeal valving. This instrument also provides a simple method for assessing changes in speech over time, and for documenting the effects of various methods of treatment. The system, together with the way in which the weighted scores have been found to relate to velopharyngeal integrity (McWilliams, Glaser, Philips et al., 1981), appears in Figure 11.8.

An oral examination is also required, even though it will not often be helpful in making decisions about velopharyngeal valving. The valve cannot be visualized by looking into the mouth because closure occurs well above what the eye can see; however, the examination of the oral cavity can provide information about other unusual structures or functions. In Apert, for example, the examiner is likely to see a high, narrow palate with excessive maxillary tissue, and what looks like a cleft but may not be. Earlier in the chapter, we described the submucous cleft palate, which can often be seen. The presence or absence of a gag reflex can also be determined. If a gag is not present, we would want to know more about motor integrity because it might affect speech production. We can also explore for oronasal fistulae and for dental abnormalities that may be related to the speech pattern. It is important to understand that the oral examination provides clues but does not permit decision making in the absence of other diagnostic data.

The assessment of velopharyngeal valving is an integral part of the clinical evaluation when a deficient mechanism is suspected. The score on the Pittsburgh Screening Test (McWilliams & Philips, 1979) will reliably predict valving problems, but it will be necessary to go beyond that to plan and execute treatment. Historically, many approaches, including blowing up a paper bag, puffing the cheeks, puffing the cheeks while the tongue is held by the examiner (Fox & Johns, 1970), measuring nasal escape, measuring the pressure created by blowing with nostrils open and closed, were used. All sought information about the ability to impound intraoral pressure, and all yielded less than accurate data about velopharyngeal valving.

Measurements of air pressure and flow as described by Warren and DuBois (1964) made a remarkable contribution to the assessment of velopharyngeal valving. This system measures intraoral pressure and nasal air flow during speech, and uses a hydrokinetic equation to translate the data into an estimate of the size of the velopharyngeal orifice. This technique has

| Nasal Emission | | Right | Left | (Add only side |
|---|---|---|---|---|
| Not present | | _____ 0 | _____ 0 | with |
| Inconsistent, visible | | _____ 1 | _____ 1 | highest value) |
| Consistent, visible | | _____ 2 | _____ 2 | |
| Nasal escape on nasals appropriate | | _____ 0 | _____ 0 | |
| Reduced | | _____ 0 | _____ 0 | |
| Absent | | _____ 0 | _____ 0 | |
| Audible or Turbulent | | | _____ 3 | Subtotals _____ |

Facial Grimace        _____ 2          _____

| Nasality | | Phonation | |
|---|---|---|---|
| Normal | _____ 0 | Normal | _____ 0 |
| Mild hypernasality | _____ 1 | Hoarseness or breathiness | |
| Moderate hypernasality | _____ 2–3 | Mild | _____ 1 |
| Severe hypernasality | _____ 4 | Moderate | _____ 2 |
| Hypo- and hypernasality | _____ 2 | Severe | _____ 3 |
| Cul de sac | _____ 2 | Reduced loudness | _____ 2 |
| Hyponasality | _____ 0 | Tension in system | _____ 3 |
| | | Other _____ | |
| Subtotal | _____ | + | _____ = _____ |

Articulation
| | |
|---|---|
| Normal | _____ 0 |
| Developmental errors | _____ 0 |
| Errors from other causes not related to VPI | _____ 0 |
| Errors related to anterior dentition | _____ 0 |
| Reduced intraoral pressure for sibilants | _____ 1 |
| Reduced intraoral pressure for other fricatives | _____ 2 |
| Reduced intraoral pressure for plosives | _____ 3 |
| Omission of fricatives or plosives | _____ 2 |
| Omission of fricatives or plosives plus hard glottal attack for vowels | _____ 3 |
| Linguapalatal or other backing errors on sibilants | _____ 2 |
| Pharyngeal fricatives, snorts, inhalation or exhalation substitutions | _____ 3 |
| Oral backing on plosives | _____ 3 |
| Glottal stops or glottal fricatives | _____ 4 |
| Nasal substitutions for pressure sounds | _____ 4 |

                                    _____

                        Total _____

Speech suggests a velopharyngeal valving mechanism that is:
| | | |
|---|---|---|
| _____ | 0 | Competent |
| _____ | 1–2 | Competent to borderline |
| _____ | 3–6 | Borderline to incompetent |
| _____ | 7 and up | Incompetent |

**Figure 11.8** Pittsburgh Screening Test—Weighted values for speech symptoms associated with velopharyngeal incompetence. *(Note: A modification of the form suggested by McWilliams and Philips, 1979.)*

414

been simplified recently by the introduction of the Perci (Warren, 1979) and the newer computer-assisted Perci II. Warren has suggested that orifice areas larger than 20 mm$^2$ are always associated with defective speech. This does not mean that speech is not defective at smaller openings. In fact, McWilliams et al. (1981) found that any orifice area greater than 5 mm$^2$ almost invariably had some speech characteristics suggestive of velopharyngeal valving deficits. The technique developed by Warren and DuBois does not provide information about the location of the deficit or the shape of the orifice. The technique is simple to use, however, and many speech-language pathologists find it helpful, especially in combination with other methods.

## Radiological Techniques

These techniques permit the visualization of the velopharyngeal valving mechanism, at least in part. The earliest method was still X rays or cephalometrics taken in lateral projection and showing the mechanism only in profile. This method does not show the sphincter itself, and there are other shortcomings as well. Speech is a dynamic event, and these studies are done during the production of a single phoneme, often the undemanding /a/. It is usually not clear where in the sound production the picture was taken. Therefore, it is uncertain whether an observed opening occurred during speech production or as the palate was moving away from or toward closure. If closure is seen, there is no evidence about what would happen under the more complex demands of connected discourse. Yet, some speech-language pathologists still use these films without reservation.

*Figure 11.9 shows a cephalometric X ray and two tracings—one of closure achieved on a normal /s/, and the other of the opening seen on an abnormal /s/.*

Cinefluoroscopy, or X ray recorded on motion picture film, was an improvement over cephalometrics. Cinefluoroscopy uses the lateral projection, but the part of the mechanism being studied is seen in action. Even with this added feature, what sometimes appears to be competence is not because closure is not achieved in the unseen lateral parts of the valve. In addition, exposure to radiation is a factor to consider, as it is with any X ray.

McWilliams and Girdany (1964) first used videofluoroscopy, X ray data recorded on videotape, for speech studies. This method had the advantages of reduced radiation, which permitted the study of longer speech samples, and of immediate playback. These dynamic examinations were first done in lateral projection so that parts of the valve were seen, but the entire valve was not visualized. They improved the technique by performing the lateral views with the neck in extension and by adding frontal views showing the lateral pharyngeal walls. When the neck is extended, the slight deepening of the pharyngeal space does, in borderline cases, unmask velopharyngeal incompetence that is not seen in the true lateral position (McWilliams, Musgrave, & Crozier, 1968). An advantage of both cine- and videofluoroscopy is that both provide information about the consistency of palatal and pharyngeal move-

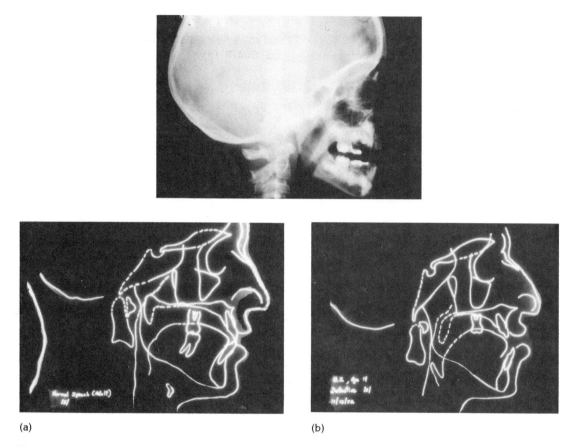

(a)                                                    (b)

**Figure 11.9**   Cephalometric X ray with two tracings, one showing a normal /s/ (a) and the other an /s/ produced with a velopharyngeal opening (b).

ments, timing in relationship to speech production, and the patterning of the movements. These factors are relevant because some speakers sound as if they have velopharyngeal incompetence when they do not have that precise problem. Instead, they have motor deficits that affect the way the palate and pharyngeal structures relate to each other during speech. A disadvantage of lateral projection is that it does not show the size, shape, or location of the orifice. The technique provides clinically useful information in many but not all cases.

Skolnick (1970) further developed videofluoroscopy by introducing multiview videofluoroscopy, an approach using lateral and frontal projections, but making increased use of the frontal view and adding the base view. Taken while the patient is in a sphinxlike position, the base view shows the orifice with the soft palate and the posterior and lateral pharyngeal walls. However, clinicians, including the speech-language pathologist who is active in interpretation of these studies, must synthesize data from all three views to make clinical judgments. Figure 11.10 is a schematic representation of the three views of the velopharyngeal valve derived from multiview fluoroscopy. The advantages of multiview videofluoroscopy are that it (a) shows the presence or absence of an opening between the nasal and oral cavities during speech, (b) provides reliable information about the size of the opening, (c) delineates the shape of the orifice, (d) shows velar and pharyngeal movements, and (e) allows the examiner to estimate the vertical position of the portal (by interpretation of the combined views). Videofluoroscopy offers one of the most satisfactory methods of studying velopharyngeal closure.

## Nasoendoscopy

This is another widely used technique, sometimes used by a speech-language pathologist with a physician in attendance. It incorporates a fiberoptic bundle encased in a fine tube that is passed through the nasal airway and positioned to reflect the velopharyngeal orifice, which the examiner can view through an external eyepiece. The intense light passing through the fiberoptic bundle permits the image to be photographed and recorded on videotape for a permanent record. This method has special attraction because it involves no radiation. Even with topical anesthesia, however, a few patients, particularly young children, find the procedure unacceptable. In spite of that, endoscopy is rightfully gaining in popularity.

The choice of assessment techniques depends on the preference of the individual clinic as well as on what is most readily available. While some

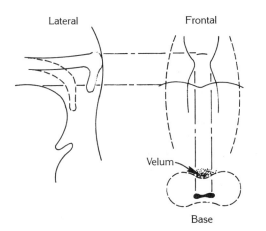

**Figure 11.10** Schematic representation of the three views used in multiview videofluoroscopy. (*Note: From "The Sphincteric Mechanism of Velopharyngeal Closure" by M. L. Skolnick, G. N. McCall, and M. Barnes, 1973,* Cleft Palate Journal, *10, p. 287. Reprinted by permission.*)

clinics continue to avoid instrumentation to assess velopharyngeal valving, the best evidence is that diagnosis cannot be completed without it. We do not yet have a single device that will provide all the information required. Thus, it is often desirable to use more than one and make interpretations based on combined data. Remember that Martha, whose case history was presented at the beginning of the chapter, had videofluoroscopy and aerodynamic studies, a combination that we find useful, often in conjunction with endoscopy. We use instrumentation because we want to know as much as possible about the nature of the problem, its causes, what can be done, and what the prognosis is. To ignore those necessities is to be guilty of administering treatment that may be inappropriate or even harmful and thus unethical.

# TREATMENT APPROACHES

The purpose of diagnosis is to have the information required for planning the best treatment. The communication specialist seeks care that will make effective communication possible. Several different types of intervention are available for those with clefts and related problems.

## Improving Velopharyngeal Valving

It is almost never possible, except in rare and unusual cases, to improve velopharyngeal valving through behavioral approaches alone. For this reason, speech-language pathologists must work with plastic surgeons and prosthodontists to improve the potential for the velopharyngeal valve to work effectively. One procedure frequently used is the **pharyngeal flap** operation. This surgery elevates a flap of tissue from the posterior pharyngeal wall, brings it forward, and attaches it to the soft palate. The goal is to make it possible for the lateral pharyngeal walls to close around the palato-flap structure and, probably, to lengthen the soft palate somewhat. Results from pharyngeal flaps have been promising and have often made normal speech possible. Like any other surgery, the success rate is not 100%, and it varies from one series of reported cases to another. We have never seen a patient made worse by this procedure, however, and most improve noticeably, many eventually acquiring normal speech.

Pharyngeal flaps usually result in a certain amount of mouth breathing and in frequent snoring at night. Sometimes speech may be hyponasal following the surgery, but in some cases this is only temporary until the edema or swelling subsides and healing is complete. While a pharyngeal flap can reduce hypernasality, it cannot change the gross articulation errors we talked about earlier, and speech therapy is often necessary to eliminate them.

A second approach to the correction of velopharyngeal incompetency is to build out the posterior pharyngeal wall or to increase palatal bulk. Various types of implants have been used, including teflon (Bluestone, Musgrave,

McWilliams, & Crozier, 1968; Bluestone, Musgrave, & McWilliams, 1968). Teflon injections have had their highest rates of success with people who show a small midcentral gap on basal view videofluoroscopy and small amounts of nasal air flow on pressure flow studies. When the only characteristic of the speech is a reduction in intraoral pressure, the injection, like the pharyngeal flap, is likely to make immediate and amazing changes in speech production. When there are gross articulatory errors, intervention through speech therapy will be necessary. Since teflon is not currently approved by the Food and Drug Administration (FDA) for our purposes, experimental work using other materials, including collagen, is now underway.

In rare instances, it is desirable to correct velopharyngeal incompetency with a prosthetic speech aid or a palatal lift. The prosthesis is a dental appliance made by a prosthodontist. It incorporates a bulb to close the space between the oral and nasal cavities. The palatal lift, on the other hand, is designed to elevate a soft palate that moves poorly, so that it can make contact with the posterior and lateral pharyngeal walls. Prosthetic speech aids are not used today as frequently as they once were, but they are still valuable and should be considered if surgery is contraindicated, or if there is any possibility that the bulb may stimulate pharyngeal wall movement. Figure 11.11 shows prosthetic speech aids with the bulb attachment. These aids are usually fitted in the presence of an experienced speech-language pathologist who can determine the proper placement and size of the bulb. Air pressure

*A prosthesis is an artificial replacement for a missing or underdeveloped part of the body.*

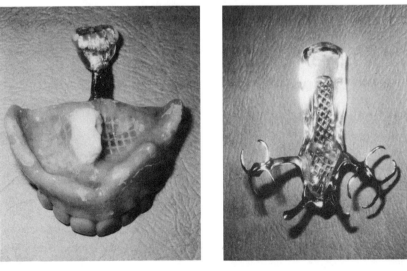

**Figure 11.11** Prosthetic speech aids—one with dentures, the other without. Note the posterior bulb that fills space and provides a contact for lateral and posterior pharyngeal wall movement.

and endoscopic studies are of help in this work, as is auditory evidence of a reduction in nasal air flow and of an increase in intraoral pressure.

## Correcting Dental Problems

Sometimes speech problems are related to maxillary or dental anomalies that can be corrected or improved. These defects include misaligned or missing teeth, maxillary collapse in the line of the cleft, midfacial deficiency, narrow maxilla, and small oral cavity. Some of the associated speech disorders respond poorly to speech therapy alone. Therefore, our preference is to correct the dental and structural problems as early as possible and to delay speech therapy for the affected phonemes. The speech-language pathologist will work closely with the prosthodontist, the orthodontist, and sometimes other dental specialists so that dental treatment and speech intervention can be coordinated.

When midfacial deficiency is present, the midface may be advanced surgically to bring it into a better relationship with the mandible. Properly aligned jaws provide the oral architecture required to house the tongue so that it can function efficiently for speech. Before surgery, the tongue rests between the extruded mandible and the retracted maxilla, so that it is difficult if not impossible to produce the tongue tip sounds accurately, even after a great deal of speech therapy. On the other hand, correcting these kinds of structural malrelationships often leads to spontaneous improvement in speech (Vallino, 1987).

The intent of this section is to explain some forms of intervention that should be considered before undertaking speech therapy. The speech-language pathologist must be able to recognize when a mechanism is functioning at its maximum and when therapy will probably not be beneficial. It takes a sophisticated and confident speech-language pathologist to understand that speech therapy is not for everyone who has a communication problem.

## Speech and Language Therapy

You have probably gathered that I am not a strong advocate of speech therapy for many problems associated with structural deformities. Therapy is appropriate under certain circumstances, however, and some of the choices are described here.

### Language Therapy

This form of therapy is often appropriate since palatal clefts and other structural defects are associated with mild delays in early language development. Parents need to learn positive methods of stimulation that they can use at home. Talking to babies, reading to them, describing activities that are going on in the household, and talking about the child's activities or play while they are going on are all techniques that parents use almost automatically, but in which they can be encouraged and reinforced to advantage.

As the child develops, small informal play groups may be helpful, particularly if there is too much isolation from other children. This kind of experience can often be accomplished informally in neighborhoods, or more formally in a cleft palate center or a regular nursery school.

Creative dramatics has also been used to increase the verbal output of children with clefts. Children sometimes begin this experience on a nonverbal level, but quickly initiate spoken language and eventually express many of their innermost feelings. This experience is fun and does not suggest that the children have something "wrong" with them—it is an interesting activity in which they can participate and from which an increase in verbal output has been demonstrated (Irwin & McWilliams, 1974).

Suggestions for dealing with early language development have been formalized and incorporated into clinical routine. These range from working primarily with parents to optimize their verbal interactions with their children, to more direct intervention with babies and preschoolers (Brookshire, Lynch, & Fox, 1980; Hahn, 1979; Lynch, 1986).

## Articulation Therapy

Although frequently necessary, there is some disagreement as to when and under what conditions articulation therapy should be introduced. Hoch, Golding-Kushner, Siegel-Sadewitz, and Shprintzen (1986) often recommend it to change gross variations such as backing errors, pharyngeal fricatives, and glottal stops, to more anterior oral productions, thus encouraging maximum velopharyngeal valving and movement in the lateral pharyngeal walls prior to a pharyngeal flap. Their rationale is that the need for a flap may sometimes be eliminated, or the flap may not have to be so wide, thus reducing the risk of hyponasality; and speech will be better immediately postoperatively if articulation has been improved beforehand. The contrasting view is that the gross errors are responses to an inadequate valving mechanism, and that the need to regulate pressure within the system makes such therapy difficult, at best, with a high probability of failure unless it can be established that the mechanism has greater potential than is demonstrated in habitual speech. Our preference is to correct a valve that is unequivocally incompetent before starting articulation therapy and to do trial therapy if there is reasonable doubt. This view is supported by Van Demark and Hardin (1986), who reported that speech therapy was effective in changing articulation patterns in 13 children treated intensively in a 6-week summer program, but that progress was much slower than had been anticipated. The children did not continue to improve, even though most continued in speech therapy. It is possible to spend an inordinate amount of time in therapy for only limited gains. The same philosophy applies to articulation patterns that are strongly influenced by max-

*See chapter 7.*

illary and dental architecture. Developmental errors can safely be treated just as they would be in any other child.

The principles underlying articulation therapy for patients with clefts are similar to those for anyone else. Response to stimulability testing will determine which phonemes are likely to respond best to therapy. Gross errors may not be readily stimulable, however, and will usually require attention to place of articulation (McWilliams, Morris, & Shelton, 1984). It is often useful to work from a whisper, aspirate, or voiceless phoneme to avoid hard glottal attacks (Hoch, Golding-Kushner, Siegel-Sadewitz, & Shprintzen, 1986; Morley, 1967). Articulation therapy is undoubtedly necessary more often than any other form of speech therapy for patients with clefts.

### Therapy to Establish Velopharyngeal Valving

This has long been attempted with only minimal results (McWilliams, Morris, & Shelton, 1984). More recently, however, biofeedback using endoscopy to visualize the sphincter during speech has been useful, especially for those who can achieve closure but do not habitually do so (Hoch, Golding-Kushner, Siegel-Sadewitz, & Shprintzen, 1986).

Articulation training has also been thought to influence velopharyngeal closure. Although Shelton, Chisum, et al. (1969) found no support for this contention, Hoch, Golding-Kushner, Siegel-Sadewitz, and Shprintzen (1986) have presented papers at meetings in which they put forth the thesis that articulation therapy does, in some cases, favorably influence velopharyngeal valving. This theory is most likely accurate for subjects who can but do not usually achieve closure.

Many other approaches continue to be applied, but supportive data as to their efficacy are either lacking or sparse. Students may wish to read about bulb-reduction therapy (Blakely & Porter, 1971; Weiss, 1971); lowering of a high-riding posterior tongue to increase the relative size of the oral cavity (McDonald & Koepp-Baker, 1951); and instrumental approaches, such as Tonar (Fletcher, 1978) and its successors, which provide feedback about "nasalance" and the shifts that may occur during therapy. These are all methods that still require systematic study and the delineation of the precise conditions under which they may be expected to be effective. To date, the most successful means of improving a significant velopharyngeal valving deficit is to correct the basic defect wherever possible.

## CONCLUSION

An attempt has been made to help the beginning student understand that the communication problems associated with clefts and other structural disorders are complex. They can be solved only rarely by the speech-language pathologist working alone or, indeed, by any one specialist. In response to this need for cooperation among disciplines, interdisciplinary treatment teams have sprung up. These teams are usually eager to work closely with community speech-language pathologists and to make them members. This openness works to the advantage of all, especially the patient, who has a coordinated treatment plan.

The close working relationships among specialists treating such patients led to the establishment of the American Cleft Palate Association (ACPA), a professional organization whose membership is open to fully qualified speech-language pathologists with an interest in these structural anomalies. Student memberships are also available. The exchange of information among the many different specialists who make up the association's membership can be a rich and enjoyable experience. *The Cleft Palate Journal,* the official publication of the American Cleft Palate Association, is another way to keep abreast of the field. Students may subscribe to the *Journal* at a reduced rate. The address is 1218 Grandview Avenue, Pittsburgh, Pennsylvania 15211.

# STUDY QUESTIONS

1. If an 8 year old with no history of a palatal cleft demonstrated hypernasality and had reduced intraoral pressure on both fricatives and plosives 1 year following the removal of adenoids, what specific examinations would you as a speech-language pathologist working in a community or school setting want to have before undertaking speech therapy, and how would you go about getting it?

2. Glottal stops as substitions for plosives are usually associated with velopharyngeal incompetence. Describe the circumstances under which a speech-language pathologist might conclude that the valve was competent even in the presence of such speech characteristics.

3. Describe the combination of structural and/or functional conditions that would create nasal turbulence in a speaker.

4. Discuss the implications of ear disease in children with palatal clefts. Include in your answer and carefully identify those factors that we are certain about and those that remain speculative.

5. Devise a plan appropriate to monitor language development in children with clefts and discuss the conditions under which you would recommend intervention.

# SELECTED READINGS

McWilliams, B. J. (Guest Ed.) (1986). Current methods of assessing and treating children with cleft palates. *Seminars in speech and language.* Wm. H. Perkins & J. L. Northern (Eds.) 7.

McWilliams, B. J., Morris, H. L., & Shelton, R. L. (1984). *Cleft palate speech.* Philadelphia and Toronto: B. C. Decker, Inc.

McWilliams, B. J., & Philips, B. J. (1979). *Audio seminar in velopharyngeal incompetence.* Philadelphia: W. B. Saunders.

# CHAPTER TWELVE

# Aphasia and Related Adult Disorders

## AUDREY L. HOLLAND

## CAROL S. SWINDELL

## O. M. REINMUTH

### MYTHS AND REALITIES

- ■ *Myth:* All neurogenic communication disorders acquired in adulthood are the same; they are all aphasias.

- ■ *Reality:* Different communication disorders result from different neuro-logical conditions. Individuals with diffuse brain damage resulting from closed head injury or dementing illnesses often have other cognitive and personality disorders that influence their communication. Individuals with focal brain damage resulting from stroke are the ones that we think of as aphasic.

- ■ *Myth:* Aphasia is a rare disorder that affects only old people.

- *Reality:* Of the one-half million people who will have a stroke each year, 85,000 will be aphasic. Although stroke is more commonly associated with the aged, it can strike at any age—from infancy through adulthood.

- *Myth:* Aphasia always occurs after a severe stroke to the brain.

- *Reality:* Aphasia usually occurs following damage to specific speech/language areas of the left hemisphere. Sometimes the damage is severe, sometimes it is minimal. Other cognitive and behavioral problems are associated with damage to the right hemisphere or to other areas of the left hemisphere.

- *Myth:* There is something wrong with the minds of the people who have had strokes.

- *Reality:* Language disorders and thought disorders are different entities. The "mind" is not affected in aphasia.

- *Myth:* Aphasia is just a speech disorder.

- *Reality:* Aphasia is a multimodality disorder that may affect all aspects of language, including auditory comprehension, reading, writing, naming, gesturing, among others. A language disorder never occurs in a vacuum, however; there are social, medical, and emotional aspects that affect the aphasic individual and her family as well.

- *Myth:* Brain damage is irreversible; therefore, there is little that can be done to help the aphasic individual.

- *Reality:* The brain is a remarkably adaptable organ. We do not know whether all aspects of brain damage are irreversible, but we recognize that it is possible to reduce some of the effects of brain damage.

- *Myth:* The only thing that helps an aphasic individual to regain his language is the natural recovery that follows brain damage. Clinical intervention does not do any good.

- *Reality:* Evidence shows that speech and language intervention are useful in lessening the effects of aphasia.

- *Myth:* Working with stroke patients, and the elderly in general, is depressing and frustrating.

- *Reality:* This work is among the most challenging and interesting in our profession.

STUDENTS often view aphasia as a mysterious disorder. Consequently, their initial encounter with an aphasic individual is often filled with a dreaded anticipation of the unknown. You have just reviewed a series of common myths about aphasia that students helped to compile. Are your impressions of the disorder consistent with the myths or with the realities? This chapter should help to solidify the realities of aphasia. It begins with an illustrative case history, and continues with descriptions of the brain-language connection, aphasia syndromes, diagnostic procedures, and intervention alternatives.

*Ms. J., age 46, was hospitalized following a sudden onset of right-side weakness and loss of speech. Following a complete neurological examination and series of tests, she was diagnosed as having had a thromboembolic stroke involving the left middle cerebral artery.*

*Prior to this, Ms. J. had led an active life working in the public relations department of the Pittsburgh Steelers, raising two teenage sons, and managing the household with the help of her husband. She was an avid potter, and her other interests included professional sports, scuba diving, and reading.*

*One week following her stroke, Ms. J. was transferred to a rehabilitation center where she was engaged in a full-scale rehabilitation program that included physical, occupational, and speech-language therapy. Following three weeks of intensive therapy, Ms. J. was able to walk with the aid of a short leg brace, and had regained some use of her right arm and hand. A formal speech and language evaluation indicated a mild to moderate Broca aphasia. Ms. J.'s spoken output was limited in quantity; she spoke in short phrases that had many grammatical errors. She also had marked word-finding difficulties, which were quite frustrating to her. Ms. J.'s auditory comprehension was considerably better than her spoken language, although she had some problems understanding complex instructions and messages. Reading was affected minimally, but writing content was similar to spoken language. Because of a mild residual muscle weakness in her right arm and hand, Ms. J.'s writing was not as clear as it was prior to her stroke.*

*Ms. J. began to receive 1 hour of daily, individual speech-language therapy. Therapy was designed to increase her functional communication and decrease her anxiety about her faltering speech and language skills. At the onset of treatment, Ms. J. was mildly depressed. But the gains she had made in physical therapy began to lift her spirits, and she worked with determination in speech-language therapy. Her family visited her every other day. Her husband began to attend the family group sessions, run by the rehabilitation center, that prepare families for patients' return to the home. Both the social worker and the clinical psychologist were alerted to Ms. J.'s depression and initiated brief counseling sessions. The social worker centered his activities on realistic appraisal of potential for return to work, while the psychologist focused her sessions on restoring Ms. J.'s self-concept in relation to her problems.*

*Ms. J. was dismissed from the center following 6 weeks of intensive rehabilitation. At that time, she was walking with the assistance of a cane and was able to use her arm and hand to perform most of the activities of daily living, including cooking. She had made many gains in speech-language therapy. Most notable was the improvement in auditory comprehension, which was now near normal. Problems with word finding and writing persisted, however, and it was recommended that speech-language therapy be continued on an outpatient basis. Arrangements were made with the local university clinic for treatment.*

*Ms. J. received 2 hours of individual and group therapy for the ensuing year. Consistent but slow progress was maintained for approximately 10 months, with no apparent progress after that time. At the end of 1 year, Ms. J. agreed to be discharged from treatment. At the time of discharge, Ms. J. demonstrated minimal speech and language problems in most communicative situations. Occasionally, when under pressure, her word-finding problems resurfaced, but she was able to use strategies to overcome these problems.*

*During her time in the clinic, a number of family decisions influenced her treatment. Although Ms. J. was determined to return to work initially, she and her family later decided against this. She did not, however, retire from life. In addition to returning to her major managerial role at home, she undertook a responsible role in the local stroke club. She developed a visitation program for stroke patients by stroke patients. Patients would share information about services available in the community and inspiration about coping with life after stroke.*

*Within the year, Ms. J.'s family resumed its normal functioning. Her teenage children, almost ready for college, felt that they had had a significant learning experience. They were impressed by their mother's courage and strength in pursuing her recovery. Ms. J.'s husband, who felt the major financial and emotional burden of the stroke, was optimistic about the future. "We've learned a lot. We've learned to handle adversity. We've learned what we're made of. I'm terribly sorry it happened. But we've survived—and survived well."*

This chapter is about a communication disorder called **aphasia,** which is usually acquired in adulthood. Aphasia is not simply a speech disturbance. In addition to affecting spoken language, it also produces disturbances in comprehending the speech of others, reading, and writing. *Aphasia* is a general term used to describe a number of related but separate syndromes, as we shall see later. It refers to a breakdown in the ability to formulate, retrieve, or decode the arbitrary symbols of *language*. Aphasia's onset is usually abrupt, occurring without warning to people who have no previous speech or language problems. Although injury to the head, brain tumors, and other neurologic diseases

*Aphasia is an acquired impairment of the abilities to comprehend and express linguistic symbols.*

*This is in contrast to the neurogenic disorders of speech, which are discussed in chapter 14. Recall that these disorders can coexist with aphasia.*

may produce language disturbances, aphasia is most frequently caused by stroke. Aphasia is the most prevalent adult language problem. Most of us know a relative or neighbor who has experienced one or more of its disastrous consequences. Aphasia is a communication problem with which you are likely to have direct personal experience.

The purpose of this chapter is to acquaint you with the mechanisms that produce aphasia, the various forms of the disorder, and treatment for the problem. Aphasia is a fascinating topic, not only to speech-language pathologists, but to neurologists, linguists, and neuropsychologists as well. This is because aphasia affords a unique opportunity to study some of our most perplexing questions about ourselves. These include the nature of brain-behavior relationships, the interaction between thought and language, and the neurologic underpinnings of cognitive activities. As a result, there is much, often contradictory, literature concerning aphasia that has been accumulating for more than a century. We will merely scratch the surface here, but in the process, we hope to share with you our excitement about studying aphasia and working with aphasic adults.

# APHASIA AND THE BRAIN

## Basic Neuroanatomic Considerations

*The* cerebral cortex *is the convoluted layer of grey matter that covers each cerebral hemisphere.*

Although damage to different parts of the brain can also cause some sort of communication problem, the *cortex,* or covering of the cerebrum is of most interest to aphasiologists. This wrinkled and crumpled grey surface appears to be the body's major integrative network for implementing and carrying on our most complex cognitive activities. Speaking, reading, writing, and comprehending are all cognitive activities; therefore, damage to the cortex (*cortical damage*) is most likely to produce aphasia. Damage to some of the structures that lie underneath and are connected with the cortex (*subcortical damage*) also can result in aphasia. Damage just anywhere in the cortex is not sufficient to produce aphasia. Controversy still exists over what particular site of damage produces which form of language problem. No one has more than vague understanding of just how the damage exacts its toll, yet some principles of neurologic function allow us to speculate about cortical damage and aphasia.

To explain, we will begin with a review of the cerebral hemispheres. Like some other organs (the kidneys, for example), the cortex-covered cerebrum appears to be a pair of organs. The cerebrum consists of two halves, called *Hemispheres,* that are roughly similar in size and shape. Most normal brain functioning requires both halves to be operating properly; however, the function of each half of the brain is not reduplicative: each half does different things. We will discuss three broad types of cortical activities—motor, sensory, and cognitive—in terms of their hemispheric control to explain a few of the basics of brain-behavior relationships.

## Movement

Our only means of affecting our environment is through movement. Even our thoughts are inaccessible to the world around us unless we can move our speech musculature to put our thoughts into words, or move our bodies to communicate them nonverbally. Movement seems the most obvious of our abilities, yet movement—how the brain controls the body's muscles—remains at the scientific frontier. The enormous complexity of neuromotor control is not yet satisfactorily explained. For highly skilled motor behavior, nature plays an interesting trick. The left half of the brain (left cerebral hemisphere) controls movement of the right side of the body, and the right half (right cerebral hemisphere) controls the left side of the body. If cortical brain damage results in some motor impairment (and it frequently does), we can often observe a paralysis of the side of the body opposite the brain damage. This condition, called **hemiplegia** or **hemiparesis,** allows us to predict the side of brain damage. If a left hemiplegia is noted, we can infer right hemisphere damage; if a right hemiplegia is noted, we can infer left hemisphere damage. In the case of Ms. J., we could predict from her right-side weakness that she had sustained damage to the left hemisphere. She also experienced a mild degree of sensory loss in her right arm and leg, which further indicates left-side brain damage. Additional sensory changes may also occur after stroke.

Hemiplegia *is the paralysis of one side of the body. Slight or incomplete paralysis is known as* hemiparesis.

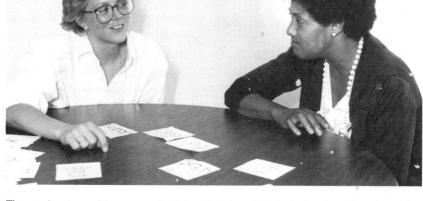

*The evaluation of language in this adult hemiplegic helps to determine corresponding damage to the brain.*

## Sensation

Although all the senses are important in perceiving the world around us, we will limit our discussion to the sensory systems that are most important to language: vision and audition. Let us first consider vision. In organisms with monocular vision, such as pigeons, vision in the left eye is the province of the right hemisphere, and vice versa. But human beings, along with a few other animals, have binocular rather than monocular vision. In humans, the visual pathways are partially (as opposed to totally) crossed. The partial crossing can be described by a do-it-yourself example. Direct both of your eyes to a point in front of you, perhaps to an object directly above the upper edge of this book. Note that both eyes participate in seeing the object. All visual information to the right of that point (the right visual field) is fed by each eye to the left hemisphere. Information to the left of that point (the left visual field) is fed to the right hemisphere. This crossing occurs in the optic chiasm, not far behind the eyeballs. Beyond this crossing point, damage either to the optic tract or to the area of the cortex that receives visual impulses causes a loss of vision of one-half of what is being viewed. This loss is called **hemianopsia.** An interruption of the left optic tract or occipital lobe therefore causes loss of the right half of the visual space. The loss of the *same* visual half field of both eyes is identified by the term *homonymous*—hence, *right homonymous hemianopsia.*

As with vision, there is a peculiarity about the manner in which auditory information is relayed to the cortex. The circuitry involved in hearing, however, is much harder to demonstrate than that of vision. This difficulty is due both to the nature of sound waves and the fact that auditory information is quite generously distributed to both hemispheres. Roughly 70% of the auditory fibers from each ear cross to the opposite hemisphere. Few, if any, effects on hearing sensitivity are caused by purely cortical damage. Deafness in one or the other ear occurs as a result of damage to the ear itself, or the sensory pathways below the level of the cortex. In audition, the cortex serves to *interpret* auditory signals and messages; that is, it makes sense out of the signals received by the ears.

In the case of visual and auditory information, it appears that nature has been careful to protect these two major sources for comprehending the world around us. First, by giving us two eyes and ears, nature has arranged it so that if one member of either pair is damaged, we are not totally cut off from its sensory contributions. Second, nature has protected us by arranging for each member of the pair to have access to both cortical hemispheres. This further ensures access to visual and auditory information, even in cases of unilateral brain damage.

*Hemianopsia is the loss of vision in half of the visual field. Homonymous hemianopsia indicates a loss of the same visual half field of both eyes, and usually results from a single lesion.*

## Cognition

We have seen how sensory input from the eyes and ears is received differentially by the left and right hemispheres. We have also been alerted to the manner in which motor output is controlled differentially by the hemi-spheres. What about the *cognitive* functions of these two halves of the brain? Is there a difference in the hemispheres' respective roles in integrating, processing, and receiving of information?

It has long been recognized that aphasia usually occurs with damage to the left hemisphere, and that people with right brain damage usually escape the traditional language disorders. Thus, language appears to be a function of the left hemisphere. (If the brain-damaged person's lesion also involves the cortical motor areas, you can predict, from what you have just read about motor control, that she will have a right hemiplegia as well. Similarly, she may also have an associated visual problem involving the right visual field, that is, a right homonymous hemianopsia.) And indeed, language sets the tone for the cognitive activities the left hemisphere appears to perform—the logical, sequential aspects of mental operations.

Because language had been demonstrated to be localized to the left hemisphere and because language was so prominent in Western society's beliefs about thinking, the left hemisphere was referred to for many years as the "dominant" hemisphere. There was an added implication that the right hemisphere was a sort of spare part, to be called into thinking only when and if the left was damaged in some way. It was further believed that for left-handed people, this situation was reversed. For these individuals, the right hemisphere was dominant and the left was the cognitive spare part.

Recent advances in neuropsychology have begun to change this view. Far from being the subservient hemisphere, the right is now considered to make its own distinctive contribution to our thinking skills. Briefly, the right hemisphere is thought to have major responsibility for nonverbal aspects of thinking, such as visuospatial problem solving and artistic and creative mental activities. It appears particularly sensitive to music and its apprecia-tion, as another example. If the cognitive operations of the left hemisphere can be characterized as logical, the cognitive operations of the right are, by contrast, probably more intuitive. The dichotomy of function is no longer thought to be related solely to handedness but, rather, characteristic of most people's cognitive organization. Thus, for most of us, neither hemisphere is dominant. Each is different and dominates different types of cognitive activity.

Persons who have damaged right hemispheres have a characteristic set of disturbed behaviors that is too detailed for this chapter. The reader should be aware that speech-language pathologists increasingly are called upon to treat and manage the cognitive problems of such patients.

It is important to caution you at this point. Most of what we know about how the brain functions in normal cognitive activities comes from observing both animal and human behavior under two broad sorts of unnatural conditions—surgical removal or destruction of the cortex, and direct cortical stimulation. Each of these two techniques may yield misinformation. When animals serve as subjects in either stimulation or surgical experiments, a further error source is added. Due to differences in brain structure, the value of animal analogues to human brain function, particularly at high levels of cognition, may be limited.

In studies of humans, cortical stimulation is perhaps most easily exemplified by the considerable contributions of Penfield and his associates (Penfield & Roberts, 1959), who mapped cortical function by direct electrical stimulation of the cortices of patients undergoing surgery to correct brain diseases. There is no doubt that this work is invaluable, yet it is important to remind ourselves that direct cortical stimulation by an experimental electrode is an unusual circumstance. Since Penfield's patients came to be experimental subjects because of neurological problems, the results may not be explicitly generalizable to people with normal function.

Studying what happens to behavior following destruction of part of the brain is possibly the most fruitful source of information about cognitive function and the brain. Unfortunately, it is also the source that is most open to suspicion. Over 100 years ago, Hughlings Jackson, a renowned neurologist, warned that localization of a symptom is not the same thing as localizing a function. What he meant was that, by interrupting an area of the normally working cortex, with its complex, interconnected circuitry, one also disrupts the integrity of the whole brain. The cortex most likely does not physically map cognitive events; that is, there is probably not a tiny spot of cortex that controls nouns, or verbs, or whatever units of language you wish. Yet it would require that sort of mapping for us to conclude that because area $q$, say, was damaged and the patient could no longer produce nouns, that nouns must reside in area $q$. Our best leads are that the brain works in a much more complex and integrated way, and that cognitive activities are probably a product of this general activity. What we see in the cognitive behavior of a brain-damaged person is a result of how the brain adapts to the damage, and how the remaining tissue is affected by the insult, in addition to being a manifestation of the damage itself. We have stressed language here, but language is only one of a store of cognitive events, such as making music, doing arithmetic, reading maps, and remembering events. Jackson's argument applies to all.

## The Left Cerebral Hemisphere and Aphasia

Figure 12.1 shows a lateral (side) view of the left hemisphere. The lobes of the brain are named after the bones of the skull that overlay them, and therefore they are not distinctive anatomically. The regions of the cortex posterior to (behind) the fissure of Rolando and above the Sylvian fissure are primarily responsible for analyzing sensations coming in from the

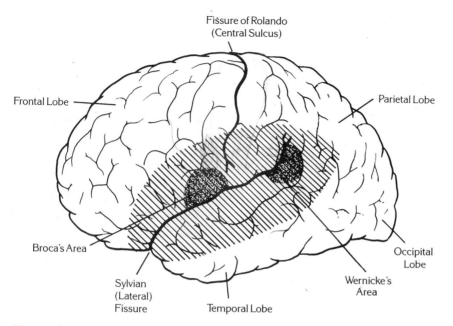

Fissure of Rolando
(Central Sulcus)

Frontal Lobe

Parietal Lobe

Broca's Area

Occipital
Lobe

Sylvian
(Lateral)
Fissure

Wernicke's
Area

Temporal Lobe

**Figure 12.1**   The left cerebral hemisphere

outside world. The occipital lobe is specialized for vision, the parietal for somatic sensory analysis, and the temporal lobe for audition. The area directly anterior to (in front of) the fissure of Rolando initiates movement. The functions of those areas more forward in the frontal lobe are more subtle and harder to describe. Both right and left frontal lobes play an executive role in initiating, planning, and integrating the whole spectrum of behavior, and they receive their inputs from the three other lobes, as well as some structures lying deep within the brain. Their responsibility appears to be for directing individuals as they affect their environment.

Notice on Figure 12.1 that we have shaded the area surrounding the Sylvian fissure. This is the general area of the left hemisphere that is thought to be primarily responsible for speech and language functions. Notice further that in the frontal lobe, there is a portion of the shaded area that is even darker. This is called *Broca's area*. It is the area that was damaged in the case of Ms. J. A similar area, termed *Wernicke's area,* is located in the temporo-parietal lobes. Each was named for the 19th-century researcher who began to delimit that area's special roles in language function: French physician Paul Broca and German neurologist Carl Wernicke, respectively. We will begin our discussion of the ways that speech and language are affected by damage to the general shaded area by discussing the posterior speech areas, including Wernicke's area, first. Then we will discuss anterior speech areas, including Broca's.

## Posterior Speech Areas

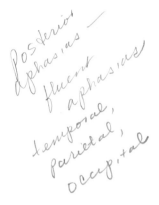

Remember that the posterior cortex is concerned with reception and analysis of stimuli from the outside world. Note that Wernicke's area lies in the temporal lobe (with its relationship to auditory stimuli), and the posterior speech region extends upward into the parietal area (where somatic sensation is integrated). Brain damage in this particular location is associated with the input of language, that is, with understanding language. Damage to Wernicke's area produces difficulties in comprehending speech, and in many instances, difficulties with reading as well. Still further back in the posterior language area is the place of convergence for visual, somatic, and auditory stimuli. It is not surprising to find that difficulties in reading, writing, naming, and so forth, occur as a result of damage here. It should be noted that posterior brain damage does *not* affect the area of the brain responsible for the initiation and production of speech. Thus, patients with posterior damage speak at rather normal rates and intonational contours that are appropriate to the native language. Aphasiologists call the disorders associated with posterior lesions *fluent aphasias.* There are a number of forms of aphasia, depending on the location and extensiveness of the damage that produced them, that constitute the fluent (posterior) aphasias. Each will be discussed later in this chapter. The major points to be emphasized here are that individuals with posterior aphasias speak fluently and have difficulty with the input side of language, such as auditory and reading comprehension, in addition to problems in spoken output.

## Anterior Language Area

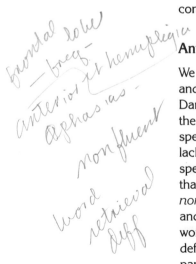

We have indicated that the frontal lobe is responsible for movement (behavior) and its initiation. The anterior language area is thus responsible for speaking. Damage here has much less possibility of interfering with comprehension of the speech of others, but instead disrupts fluent, well-articulated, initiative speech. The speech of a person with Broca's aphasia is slow and labored, lacking the flow and intonation of normal speech. Aphasiologists refer to the speech patterns of anterior aphasias as *nonfluent.* It is important to remember that *nonfluency* in the context of aphasia is somewhat different than the words *nonfluent* and *nonfluency,* as used by experts in stuttering. In addition to slow and labored speech, damage to the anterior language area often results in word retrieval deficits, and the articulatory problems and motor programming deficits that are described in chapter 14. These latter two problems accompany nonfluent aphasias because the anterior language area lies adjacent to the areas of the cortex responsible for motor control of speech. The anterior language area is also near those cortical areas responsible for other motor *aphasia two underlying symptoms auditory probs comp*

436

movement. As in the case of Ms. J., individuals with nonfluent aphasia often have an accompanying right hemiplegia.

# SYNDROMES OF ~~APHASIA~~

## Principles of Typing

We have implied already that a notable array of variations occur in aphasic patients. These variations are often discrete and can be referred to as *syndromes*. The type of aphasic syndrome that a patient manifests is largely related to the location of the damage that produced it. It is also related to the extent of damage, idiosyncracies of a person's age, general health, and cortical topography, in addition to poorly understood neurophysiological, metabolic, and neuropharmacological dynamics that relate both to normal and disturbed brain functioning. Here are some ground rules to keep in mind as you read about the syndromes (or types) of aphasia. First, aphasic symptoms are not bizarre or mysterious—they are extreme variants of everyday occurrences. For example, all of us have misspelled a word we know well; all of us have experienced difficulty in remembering a name or a word, or have heard or read something, even in our own language, that we couldn't understand. It is quite useful to keep these experiences in mind when you explore the world of aphasia.

Second, regardless of the cardinal symptoms, people who have aphasia have some basic underlying problems (often brought to light only through sophisticated testing) with two aspects of language—auditory comprehension and word retrieval. You should know that some authorities emphasize the features that are common to most aphasic patients, while others approach the analysis by identifying distinguishing characteristics of each patient. Each approach may serve a useful function in the attempt to find rules and patterns of organization that help further our imperfect understanding of the mechanisms. These differing approaches may suggest new ways to test, as well as treat, aphasic patients.

Hildred Schuell, a distinguished speech-language pathologist, was a major proponent of the view that aphasic patients' similarities are more important than their differences. Schuell viewed aphasia as a unitary disturbance of language. Her work, which emphasized the role of auditory comprehension in aphasia, is of enormous rehabilitative significance and will be discussed in detail later. While acknowledging the impact and importance of this point of view, we must also acknowledge our preference for a multidimensional view of aphasia; that is, we prefer differentiating symptom complexes as specifically as possible. Even among workers who prefer to describe aphasia multidimensionally, there exists different terminology and differing points of view. Rather than discourage you by these inconsistencies so early in your study of aphasia, we wish only to alert you to the problem. We

*A syndrome is a group of co-occurring symptoms. It is important to note that some of the syndromes that we will describe are inherently more devastating to language than are others. Within each syndrome, there is also a continuum of severity. Thus, you will often find terms such as* mild, moderate, *or* severe *used to qualify the various types of aphasia.*

use the terminology of Geschwind, Benson, and their co-workers because of its currency in the United States. Because aphasia is a language, rather than a speech, disorder, it is appropriate to describe details about other language modalities in addition to spoken language. Therefore, relevant details of speaking, comprehending, reading, writing, and repeating are included in the following discussion of aphasia syndromes.

Finally, as we have seen, lesions involving the posterior portions of the left hemisphere (temporal-parietal-occipital lobes) produce fluent aphasias, and lesions involving the anterior, or frontal, lobe produce nonfluent aphasia. This is not an invariant law, however; some people escape aphasia altogether, even if their damage is in these regions, while others show minor language difficulty in the presence of vast areas of damage. The left hemisphere is usually afflicted when aphasia occurs, even in left-handers, although right hemisphere lesions can produce aphasia in left-handers, and even more rarely in right-handers. Finally, aphasias also occur as a result of subcortical rather than cortical brain damage. Lesions to the left thalamus or the basal ganglia, for example, have been shown to produce aphasic behaviors.

With these ground rules in mind, the following major patterns can be described. These patterns are summarized in Table 12.1.

## Fluent Aphasias

### Wernicke Aphasia

**Jargon** refers to fluent, well-articulated, phonologically correct utterances that makes little or no sense to the listener.

The patient with Wernicke aphasia speaks fluently and often with excessive volubility, sometimes referred to as *press of speech*. The speech of such a patient often lacks content; in the most severe cases, spoken output is composed of incomprehensible and incoherent utterances known as *jargon*. The unsophisticated listener often initially mistakes the fluent output of the Wernicke patient for normal speech. Even for patients whose speech is jargon, the intonational features of the native language are maintained, and, to a large extent, the speaker's jargon observes the sound-combining rules of the native language. She shows reduced ability to comprehend not only the speech of others, but often her own speech as well. In most of the more common types of aphasia, reading and writing abilities are similar to the auditory comprehension and speech patterns on which they are built. The Wernicke aphasic patient is an example: reading, especially reading aloud, is often poor, but occasionally a Wernicke patient may have better preserved reading comprehension than their oral reading might suggest. This feature is a useful cornerstone upon which treatment can be built. The mechanics of handwriting are minimally affected (hemiplegia is usually absent in this type of aphasia), however, the content of writing is disturbed.

Repetition, as we will see, is often a sensitive diagnostic sign regarding the nature of the aphasic syndrome. In the case of the Wernicke patient, her

Table 12.1  Basic Language Characteristics of Some Major Syndromes of Aphasia

| Language Form | Wernicke | Anomic | Conduction | Transcortical Sensory | Broca | Transcortical Motor | Global |
|---|---|---|---|---|---|---|---|
| Conversational speech | Fluent, paraphasic | Fluent, empty | Fluent, paraphasic | Fluent, paraphasic, echolalic | Nonfluent | Nonfluent | Nonfluent |
| Comprehension of speech | Below normal to poor | Relatively good | Relatively good | Poor | Relatively good | Relatively good | Poor |
| Repetition | Predictable from comprehension | Good | Not predictable from comprehension, poor | Not predictable from comprehension, good to excellent | Predictable from comprehension, good | Predictable from comprehension, good to excellent | Predictable from comprehension, poor |
| Confrontation naming | Defective to poor | Defective | Usually defective | Poor | Defective to poor | Defective | Poor |
| Reading comprehension | Defective to poor | Usually moderately good | Usually good | Defective to poor | Not predictable | Not predictable | Poor |
| Writing | Poor, empty | Moderately good; abnormal in substantive word finding | Moderately impaired | Poor | Moderately impaired | Moderately impaired | Poor |

repetition skills are impaired as a result of the comprehension impairment. In fact, one can derive a clue about what a patient with Wernicke aphasia might be hearing by listening to what she says in her repetition attempts.

Here is an example of Wernicke speech from Gardner (1975, p. 68) in response to the question, "What brings you to the hospital?"

> Boy, I'm sweating, I'm awful nervous, you know once in a while I get caught up. I can't mention the tarripoi, a month age, quite a little, I've done a lot well, I impost a lot, while, on the other hand, you know what I mean. I have to run around, look it over, trbbin and all that sort of stuff.

## Anomic Aphasia

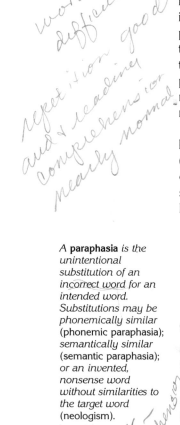

Another fluent aphasia is called *anomic aphasia*. The anomic aphasic patient's otherwise almost normal language is marred by word-retrieval difficulties. Auditory and reading comprehension are usually near normal, but the inability to produce substantive words is evident in writing. When the word the anomic patient is searching for is furnished, she usually recognizes it immediately and can take advantage of it momentarily. Thus, her repetition is usually better than her spontaneously produced speech. Word retrieval problems that typify anomic aphasia are common to all aphasias, but only in these patients are they the salient symptom. Word retrieval problems allow us to speculate about the role of memory in the generation of aphasic problems. Although aphasia can hardly be explained as a language-specific memory loss, memory certainly plays a role in aphasia, and some short-term memory difficulties often coexist.

Here is an example of a patient with anomic aphasia. He is describing a busy scene from a picture in the Boston Diagnostic Aphasia Examination (Goodglass & Kaplan, 1983), in which a little boy and girl are stealing cookies. The boy is standing on a stool about to topple, and their mother is serenely washing dishes, oblivious both to the cookie theft and to the fact that her sink is overflowing.

> This is a boy an' that's a boy an' that's a . . . thing! (Laughs). An' this is goin' off pretty soon (points to toppling stool). This is a . . . a place that this is mostly in (Examiner: "Could you name the room . . . a bathroom?") No . . . kitchen . . . kitchen. An' this is a girl . . . an' that something that they're running an' they've got the water going down here. . . . (p. 86)

## Conduction Aphasia

A **paraphasia** *is the unintentional substitution of an incorrect word for an intended word. Substitutions may be phonemically similar* (phonemic paraphasia); *semantically similar* (semantic paraphasia); *or an invented, nonsense word without similarities to the target word* (neologism).

*Conduction aphasia* is another fluent aphasia syndrome, where comprehension of language is high, but speech is frequently marred by inappropriate words. The majority of these inappropriate words are the result of the speaker's inclusion of incorrect sounds in words; for example, calling someone named Suzie, "Satie," or the individual may incorrectly order the

*phonemic —*
*semantic*
*paraphasia*

sounds in words—calling Suzie, "Seezu." Errors such as these are called *literal* or *phonemic paraphasias.* Other errors include the use of inappropriate words (*table* for *chair*) and are called *verbal* or *semantic paraphasias.* In the rare patient with severe conduction aphasia, these sorts of errors can occur frequently enough to result in spoken output that is incomprehensible to the listener. Since the conduction aphasic patient has high comprehension and is aware of these errors, she makes frequent and often unsuccessful self-correction attempts. The hallmark of the conduction aphasic patient is a disproportionate inability to repeat or make use of verbal cues supplied by others, even though she is quick to recognize the correct word when it is said by others. Reading and writing are usually good in conduction aphasia. Here is an example of a conduction aphasic patient describing the cookie theft picture.

> Well, this um . . . somebody's . . . ah mathher is takin the . . . washin' the dayshes an' the water . . . the water is falling . . . is flowing all over the place, an' the kids sneakin' out in back behind her, takin' the cookies in the . . . out of the top in the . . . what do you call that? (Examiner: "Shelf?") Yes . . . and there's a . . . then the girl . . . not the girl . . . the boy who's getting the cookies is on this ah . . . strool an' startin' to fall off. That's about all I see. (Goodglass & Kaplan, 1983, p. 90)

## Transcortical Sensory Aphasia

*Transcortical sensory aphasia* is the last fluent aphasia we will describe. It is a rare syndrome, usually resulting from brain damage that isolates the language areas from other areas of cortical control. Therefore, there is some question as to whether it should be included among the aphasias. Transcortical sensory aphasia most closely resembles Wernicke aphasia, except for the dramatic preservation of the ability to repeat. In fact, some individuals with this syndrome are almost echolalic.

# Nonfluent Aphasias

## Broca Aphasia

*Broca aphasia* is the more common of the two nonfluent aphasias. It is characterized by paucity of speech, difficulties in word retrieval, and a labored and slow rate of speech. Individuals with this disorder often omit small grammatical elements such as *the, is,* and *on,* and word endings such as *ing, s,* and *ed.* This condition is called **agrammatism.**

Comprehension of spoken and written language is surprisingly better than an individual's spoken output would suggest. Repetition is marred by the fluency problems, and writing mirrors the speech output. The mechanics of writing are also impaired because most patients with Broca aphasia also have right arm and leg paralysis. They must often learn to use the left hand

*In* agrammatism, *content words are produced, but function words and bound morphemes are omitted. The product sounds much like a telegram would read; hence, the speech has been called* **telegraphic.**

for writing. Gardner (1975) provides us with an example, a question and answer sequence with a Broca aphasic man:

Q. What happened to make you lose your speech?
A. Head, fall. Jesus Christ, me no good, str, str ... oh Jesus ... stroke.
Q. I see. Could you tell me what you've been doing in the hospital?
A. Yes, sure, me go er up P. T. nine o'cot, speech two times ... read ... wr
...
ripe, er, rike, er, write ... practice ... getting better. (p. 61)

### Transcortical Motor Aphasia

The remaining nonfluent syndrome is *transcortical motor aphasia.* Like its fluent transcortical counterpart, it has as its hallmark intact repetition. In this case, however, the excellent repetition is embedded in Broca-like symptoms. Patients with this problem typically have trouble initiating speech and writing. Repetition might be the only surviving speaking skill in the extreme case. Because initiation problems are often seen as a consequence of frontal lobe damage, generally there is some question whether or not transcortical motor aphasia is an aphasia per se.

## Mixed and Global Aphasia

It is not unusual for the aphasia-producing lesion to encompass both the anterior and posterior speech areas. The result is likely to be a mixed or global aphasia. The distinction between mixed and global aphasia is a practical one, typically made on the basis of the severity of the presenting problems. *Mixed aphasia* usually refers to aphasia that involves both comprehension and production, but is not more than moderately severe. *Global aphasia* refers to severe comprehension and production deficits. Global aphasia produces the scarcity of speech typical of nonfluent aphasia, and the difficulties with comprehension typical of the Wernicke patient. Often, global aphasic individuals have only a few utterances available to them, and these are used both appropriately and inappropriately. They are called *stereotypes.* We know a global aphasic patient whose entire verbal repertoire was "weema-jeema." Both reading and writing are seriously compromised, and repetition is poor. Global aphasia is generally considered to be the most severely debilitating of the common aphasic syndromes.

**Stereotypes** *may be real or nonsense words and phrases that are produced involuntarily and carry little, if any, meaning.*

## MECHANISMS OF APHASIA

Let us turn now to the manner in which a person might become aphasic. We have been using the term *lesion* frequently in this chapter. A lesion here is an injury that leaves an area of cortical tissue incapable of functioning in its normal way. Tissues may be destroyed directly, as in the case of a wound by a penetrating missile such as a bullet. They may be rendered incapable of functioning because other tissues push on them and distort them in some way, as when a tumor grows into or displaces the brain. And tissue may die as the result of an infectious process, or as the result of being denied the nourishment necessary to its healthy function, usually by interruption of the blood supply.

We mentioned earlier that a stroke is by far the most common cause of aphasia. *Stroke* is the term used by physicians to describe the abnormal neurologic function that occurs when a brain artery is blocked and the area of brain it nourished is destroyed. Figure 12.2 shows the arteries that feed the left cerebral hemisphere. Note especially the area supplied by the middle cerebral artery. Because its territory encompasses the speech areas we have been talking about, it is easy to see that problems with this artery are frequently responsible for aphasia-producing strokes.

*middle cerebral artery blockage risk for freq aphasia prod*

Strokes are of three basic types: (a) thrombotic, (b) embolic, and (c) hemorrhagic. In thrombotic strokes, a buildup of plaque blocks a vessel, which then thromboses (clots). An embolic stroke results when a clot or thrombosis forms elsewhere, as in the heart or the great vessels of the chest or neck, and breaks off to become an embolus that may then be carried to a brain artery. Such an embolus often arises from a location in the carotid artery in the neck—a site predisposed to blockage and embolus formation. Since the basic processes are the same, the term *thromboembolic stroke* is sometimes used to describe these two types. Hemorrhages are different. Arterial walls, weakened by the effects of high blood pressure or losing elasticity due to aging, occasionally burst under pressure. The blood rips into the brain tissue, dissecting it and causing intense inflammation and swelling.

*This condition is called arteriosclerosis, or hardening of the arteries.* *strokes*

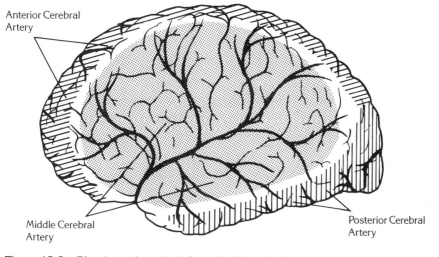

Anterior Cerebral
Artery

Middle Cerebral
Artery

Posterior Cerebral
Artery

**Figure 12.2**  Blood supply to the left cerebral hemisphere

Another cause for hemorrhage that is less common, but that may occur in young adults as well as in older individuals, is the rupture of sacular ("berry") aneurysms. These are blisterlike balloonings of arteries occurring at vessel branch points. They develop through early adult life. When aneurysms rupture, they often bleed into the fluid-filled subarachnoid space surrounding the surfaces of the brain. Although bleeding into this space may damage the brain or even cause death, it is only when the bleeding is directly into the brain tissue itself that characteristic stroke syndromes like aphasia are likely. A well-publicized example of this disorder is the illness suffered by the movie actress Patricial Neal. Even less common, but noteworthy because of the ability to produce hemorrhagic stroke, is bleeding into the brain from abnormal arterial and venous tangles of vessels occasionally present from birth—called an *arteriovenous malformation*.

You may well ask why localized rather than more general damage to the brain occurs in the stroke process. Shouldn't the whole cortex, beyond the point of disruption, be affected by arterial occlusion? You can answer this question by referring again to Figure 12.2. Note the rich intertwining of the vascular tree and the possibilities it affords for developing secondary vascular pathways. The complexity of the vascular network also helps to explain the differences in both extent and severity of damage and the variability of symptoms we find in aphasic patients. Part of this variability is due to the effectiveness with which alternative routes are found for supplying an individual's cortex with its blood supply.

At the beginning of this section, we mentioned other causes for aphasia, including trauma to the head and tumors. While damage to the speech areas by injury can certainly occur, and tumors can grow in such a way as to put pressure directly on the speech areas, it is quite likely in these cases that other cortical areas are also damaged. In the cases of progressive neurologic disorders and infectious disease, more generalized cortical involvement is the most typical result. Thus, while aphasic symptoms are found frequently in these conditions, many other changes in cortical function are almost always present as well. Describing the head-injured or postencephalitic person as aphasic is often likely to be inaccurate; disturbances in language complicated by generalized brain damage often produce far more encompassing and difficult clinical problems than does aphasia occurring as the result of a focal brain lesion.

# THE PERSON WITH APHASIA

We are now in a position to discuss the person who has aphasia. It is possible to learn a lot about language and brain-behavior relationships by studying aphasia, and the literature is mostly about such matters. The literature dealing with the person who becomes aphasic, and the effects of the aphasia on her and her family's life, is sparse by comparison. The result

*agnosia — inability to perceive, integrate, & attach meaning to incoming stimuli*

is hat we know a great deal more about aphasia than we do about people win aphasia.

At the beginning of our courses in aphasia, we often ask students to describe how they would react if injury or illness rendered them aphasic. Frequently, students attempt to advance the problem in time to some future dae when they are older. This suggests that students (like their teachers) have some fear of the problem. When asked to retry the task, the expected descriptions begin to emerge. Students commonly use words like *afraid, frustrated, angry, anxious, depressed, crazy, stupid, useless.* The list goes or, mostly in the same vein, never getting more optimistic than the wistful word *challenged.* We believe students' initial reticence and final descriptions of heir responses to aphasia are representative of what a patient experiences in the aftermath of stroke. Once they have discovered their own survival, the devastating effects of aphasia begin to emerge.

Our own most precious skills, often unappreciated and taken for granted, include our ability to communicate our needs and wants to others, and our power to present ourselves to and affect others by our words. When these skills are suddenly withdrawn or limited, a person becomes less powerful. One's self-concept is threatened and/or seriously compromised. It is important to understand these reactions to a language problem. Even though these reactions may lessen with the passage of time and with learning to make adjustments, they are a formidable aspect of aphasia, and must be dealt with in therapeutic interactions.

In addition to the patient's reaction to the language loss, there are other factors with which to contend in the aftermath of stroke. We have already mentioned the likelihood of sensory and motor problems, hemianopsia and hemiplegia, respectively. Particularly in the case of hemiplegia, a patient's loss of mobility may pose a seemingly unsurmountable deterrent to a return to normal life. Even the patient who escapes aphasia, but must learn to contend with living in a wheelchair; using a cane and a leg brace; or her left hand for eating, dressing, and writing inevitably faces some amount of depression and fear.

Brain damage often subtly changes some aspects of a person's cognition, regardless of the presence of aphasia. Included in these changes are some tendencies to think more concretely—that is, more literally—than previously (reflecting a subtle loss of abstract thinking skills), or engage unintentionally in repetitive behaviors that are vestiges of previous responses (called *perseverations*), be more sensitive to emotional events than previously, lose some initiative, and at the same time to be less inhibited. Other possible effects of brain damage are the possibilities that the aphasic patient may exhibit some **agnosia** (loss of the ability to perceive, integrate, and attach meaning to incoming stimuli) or *apraxia* (loss of ability in programming, planning, sequencing, and initiating motor behaviors). There is much speculation but little hard information concerning the overall effects of

*Perseveration is a common symptom of all types of brain damage, regardless of the lesion location. The repeated responses are involuntary and often unnoticed by patients.*

*Agnosias may be of several types. Patients may lose their ability to recognize the significance of auditory, visual, or tactile stimulation.*

*A special difficulty is apraxia of speech, which is described in chapter 14.*

aphasia on a person's personality. It has been our experience that aphasia does not produce basic personality changes; rather, the disorder tends to emphasize a person's cognitive and social style. Perhaps this is due to the previously mentioned loss of inhibition.

We have been learning to view aphasia as a family's rather than just an individual's problem. The adjectives used to describe the person's reacton may well apply to the family as well. Aphasia takes its toll not only on he patient, but on those around her, primarily because it seriously upsets he family's sense of balance and requires a restructuring of familiar family roles. Financial changes and role reassignments may be the most obvios, but other social roles are affected as well. Webster and Larkins (1979) report four family problems to be paramount. They are (1) the nonaphasic spouse has no time alone, (2) finances, (3) getting used to the new roles that aphasia creates for both spouses, and (4) finding ways to deal with the issue of dependence/ independence for the aphasic spouse. In addiion, research has suggested that guilt for the stricken member's stroke, however irrational that might appear to be, is the most frequent reaction felt by family members. A crucial aspect of rehabilitation involves helping the family to work through their feelings. It is also necessary to mobilize other members of the community to help the family in the restructuring of roles and responsibilities that may be required in the wake of aphasia. Finally, for both the aphasic patient and the family, it is important to remember that aphasia does not occur only to previously well-adjusted people and families. It occurs to people who have the same chances as the rest of us for having unresolved personal, financial, social, and family problems. And aphasia cures none of them. It merely adds another solemn dimension to them.

We have been stressing, up to this point, the darker side of aphasia— there *is* a brighter side. We find work with aphasic patients and their families to be among the most rewarding of clinical speech-language pathology activities. If aphasic patients work through their earliest reactions successfully, they often have an impressive tenacity for solving their own problems. Such patients permit their clinicians to see the basic strength and ability to rise to a challenge that dignifies us all. In many encounters with such patients, it is possible to have an almost constant awareness of the indomitability of the human spirit. Perhaps the best summary of this can be found in the words of the husband of a remarkable aphasic woman:

> When she first got her problem, we (the family) were real scared and we all helped out too much. Then we got angry at her because she needed the help. We finally worked all that out, due to her. I really didn't know who I was married to 'til E. became aphasic. I thought I had a nice, passive housewife on my hands. Instead, I have this tough, gutsy, talented, independent person. It's not at all bad.

Seven years after her stroke, this woman is still experiencing a moderate degree of Broca aphasia. She has minimal use of her right arm and has only recently been able to walk without a leg brace, although she still uses a cane. But she runs her three-child household as well as ever and maintains an active social life. She is a powerful force in the local stroke club. In addition, she has learned to paint with her left hand, and has had numerous, critically successful, one-woman shows. Her rehabilitation is a success story, brought about not only by her, but by the concerted efforts of her family as well.

## THE NATURAL RECOVERY PROCESS IN APHASIA

Immediately following stroke, aphasia, along with other neurological dysfunction, is at its worst. This is related to the severity of the event and to the extent of brain damage incurred. Within a few days, however, the natural recovery process gets underway. Swelling begins to reduce, and, although damaged brain cells never recover completely, some injured cells begin to function more normally again. A clearer picture of the residual damage begins to emerge. Nonetheless, in the early few weeks after damage, it is difficult to predict the course and the degree of a patient's recovery.

Natural recovery is influenced by a number of factors, including a patient's age and general physical condition, the extent and location of brain damage, and, to some extent, the quality of care he receives. Despite these uncertainties, we may be sure that some improvement will occur as the repair process continues for some months. This naturally occurring improvement is called *spontaneous recovery.* It is most rapid soon after onset of brain damage; as time progresses, the rate of change slows down. Spontaneous recovery occurs not only for speech and language, but for other cognitive, motor, and sensory abilities as well.

**Spontaneous recovery** *may last from several weeks to several months poststroke. It reflects the natural resolution of impairments that were brought about as the result of stroke.*

During the period of spontaneous recovery, the whole presenting syndrome may evolve into another, usually milder, form of aphasia. The most likely expectation of evolution is with global aphasia, which may evolve into any of the other types of aphasia that we discussed. For example, at one week poststroke, Ms. J. in the chapter's opening case had a mild to moderate Broca aphasia that evolved into anomic aphasia by one year poststroke. Regardless of the type of aphasia, the greatest gains observed during the period of spontaneous recovery are in auditory comprehension abilities (Kertesz & McCabe, 1977). Although there is some controversy over just how long the period of spontaneous recovery may continue, the latest evidence suggests that the bulk of the changes occur in the first 2 months. The degree to which they continue for a longer period of time is likely to depend on a variety of individual factors.

There is also controversy over the optimal time at which to begin intervention. This particular concern has an impact on the issue of efficacy of treatment. Many authorities have questioned whether speech and language improvement results from intervention or from spontaneous recovery alone. No one knows just how much of a patient's gain is due to treatment and how much is due to the natural healing process. Some argue that until we know more about the contaminating effects of spontaneous recovery on treatment, we should delay intervention. It is hypothesized that such a delay would allow us to separate the factors contributing to a patient's gains to make clearer statements about both unaided and aided recovery. Other authorities, while bowing to the complexity of the problem, suggest that the greatest therapeutic gains can be accomplished when the patient is improving, and that the question of efficacy of treatment must be answered by other means. Therefore, they suggest early intervention. The most recent evidence, a study by Wertz et al. (1984a), suggests that there is little difference between intervention begun at 1 month and therapy begun as late as 6 months post- stroke. It seems logical that a patient's individual condition should determine when to initiate direct treatment. Patients who are responsive to their environments are probably candidates for treatment. Counseling of both patient and family by trained counselors concerning some of the psycho social effects we have just looked at should probably be undertaken as soon as possible following onset.

The bulk of our direct intervention strategies has been designed for working with the *chronically* aphasic patient, that is, the patient whose spontaneous recovery process has reached a plateau. We shall discuss therapy for these patients next.

# THE ASSISTED RECOVERY PROCESS IN APHASIA

Successful rehabilitation of the aphasic patient is essentially an interdisciplinary endeavor, requiring cooperative effort between medical and paramedical specialists. The optimal team includes a neurologist, psychiatrist, physiatrist, physical and occupational therapists, neuropsychologist, social worker, and speech-language pathologist. Although what follows describes language evaluation and treatment, the context for aphasia rehabilitation is one of interdisciplinary interaction.

*A physiatrist is a physician who specializes in rehabilitation by prescribing physical therapy.*

## Evaluation

Before undertaking treatment, the speech-language pathologist should conduct a detailed evaluation. Some aphasic patients, notably those with severe global aphasias or whose aphasias coexist with other problems such as severe confusion or serious medical problems, are not candidates for rehabilitation. The first goal of evaluation, therefore, is to determine if clinical intervention is feasible. The case history is one of the most important features of the evaluation, but more direct assessment of language is also critical. This direct assessment includes detailed analysis of the aphasic

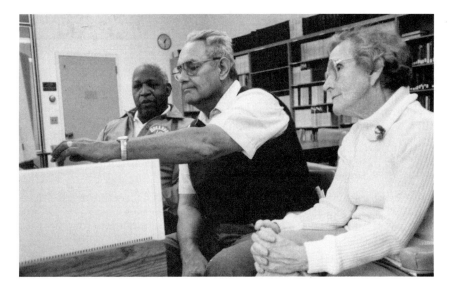

*Victims of stroke undergo therapy for treatment of their resulting aphasia.*

patient's language performance, aimed at defining and describing the type of aphasia the patient has, and measuring the extent of auditory comprehension and/or motor programming deficits. It also includes identification of other disorders, such as apraxia of speech, that can appear along with aphasia.

The formality of the initial evaluation will be directly related to how long after brain damage the evaluation is made. Early evaluation tends to be less structured and more reliant on observation of the patient at bedside. Table 12.2 provides an example of a brief bedside assessment and a guide for determining the type of aphasia and location of lesion. After the aphasic patient's condition has become stabilized, observation is supplemented with formal tests of language ability and comprehension of speech, reading, and writing. Among the more common tests used by speech-language pathologists are the Porch Index of Communicative Abilities (PICA) (Porch, 1967), the Boston Diagnostic Aphasia Examination (BDAE) (Goodglass & Kaplan, 1983), the Minnesota Test of Differential Diagnosis of Aphasia (MTDDA) (Schuell, 1965), and the Western Aphasia Battery (WAB) (Kertesz, 1982), although other tests are available. Darley (1979), for example, reviews 15 tests for aphasia in his handbook.

These tests share a number of features. All sample a range of language behaviors, including reading and writing. All attempt, either by the nature of the stimuli or by the way a response is scored or interpreted, to disentangle what might be causing a particular patient to have difficulty with a given language task. For example, from the syndromes we have described earlier,

**Table 12.2**  A Guide for Evaluating and Labeling Aphasia

Get a sample of each of the following:
1. Ability to comprehend spoken language
    a. Does the patient appear to follow the conversation?
    b. Ask the patient to follow one-, two-, and three-stage commands. For example,
        "Point to the ceiling and then to the door."
        "Put an X on this paper, fold it in half, and give it to me."
    c. Ask the patient a few yes/no questions. For example,
        "Are the lights on in the room?"
        "Do helicopters eat their young?"
2. A conversational speech sample
    a. Check for fluency. Does it sound like normally spoken English, even if it is not comprehensible? If so, the aphasia is fluent. Does it sound slow, labored, amelodic? If so, it is nonfluent.
3. Naming ability
    a. Confrontation naming: "What is this?"
    b. Associative naming: "Table and _____."
    c. Responsive naming: "Where do you buy stamps?"
    d. Using names: "Who is president?" "What is your favorite TV show?"
4. Repetition
    a. "Aluminum."
    b. "Muff, earmuff, muffler, muffintin."
    c. "The dog chewed a bone."
    d. "Three plus six equals nine."
    e. "The Chinese fan had a rare emerald."

Labeling and Localizing
1. Up to 40% of all aphasias are mixed or global. On a probability basis alone, you can guess that the aphasia is one of these. Although any lesion may produce a mixed aphasia, larger lesions affecting anterior and posterior regions are associated with intractible global aphasias.
2. If speech is fluent, you likely have a posterior lesion. If comprehension is good, the type may be anomic. If comprehension is poor, it is Wernicke.
3. If speech is nonfluent, you likely have an anterior lesion. If comprehension is good, you likely have Broca aphasia.
4. If repetition is disproportionately worse than performance on the other three tasks, then the aphasia is conduction. Location of lesion is posterior—possibly in the arcuate fasciculus.
5. If repetition is disproportionately better than performance on the other three tasks, then the aphasia is transcortical sensory or transcortical motor. The lesion is located outside of the perisylvian area.

you can tell that it is important to know if a patient does not supply the appropriate label for a fork because she is unable to retrieve it or because she does not comprehend the question she has been asked. And this is only the most trivial of examples.

Different tests also measure language somewhat differently, and often carry with them a bias about many of the controversies we have discussed earlier. The BDAE, for example, is used not only to gain a detailed description of language behavior, but to profile the various syndromes. Neither the PICA nor the MTDDA makes distinctions as to type of aphasia. The PICA attempts to quantify prediction for recovery, a matter addressed by no other test. Finally, some measures, like the measure of Communicative Ability in Daily Living (CADL) (Holland, 1980) and the Functional Communication Profile (FCP) (Sarno, 1969), do not really address language behavior at all, but how a patient gets along communicatively in her daily life.

The tests a speech-language pathologist decides to use reflect her beliefs about what aspects of the problem must be described. But which tests are selected also influence the subsequent course of treatment. Many of the decisions involved in appropriate treatment depend on the evaluation. It is important to point out, however, that the supportive counseling we have been talking about should be initiated during the first visit with the patient.

## Treatment

Treatment for people with aphasia, as currently practiced in the United States, is a relatively new field. It had its beginning during World War II, with the impetus being the large number of head-injured military survivors. In 1951, Wepman wrote a careful description of these intensive rehabilitation efforts, and his work is still extremely influential. Such early efforts developed the model of treatment for American aphasiology that is still in effect today.

All the evaluation information is brought into play in determining the exact nature of clinical intervention, as well as its goals. Although planning rehabilitation is dictated mostly by the extent of the deficit uncovered by formal evaluation, other aspects of the patient's lifestyle, motivation, medical needs, and so on, are also important. It should be clear that techniques and goals for treatment will differ for a global aphasic patient and for a patient whose residual language deficits are minimal. In even those extreme cases, however, the goals and plans will be influenced by the nonlanguage factors. In the ideal case, goals are made clear, set, and mutually agreed upon by the aphasic patient, his family, and the speech-language pathologist.

There are many approaches to rehabilitating the aphasic adult. Most are outgrowths of the speech-language pathologist's theoretical position regarding how best to effect recovery. One class of techniques stresses that the patient is best served by concentrating clinical activities on underlying processes such as memory or auditory comprehension skills. The techniques for improving memory generally reflect Luria's beliefs about rehabilitation following brain damage (1970), and those for auditory skills come from Schuell's beliefs that auditory skills are the foundation on which aphasia rehabilitation should rest. No one can tell what happens to the brain as it begins to use language again. Nonetheless, Luria hypothesized that, to regain function, it is necessary to lead the cortex into reorganizing itself, to develop new pathways for receiving and acting on stimuli. One way to reorganize the cortex is through practice with a number of cross-modal activities, for example, involving tactile sensation in reading by having the patient trace letters in sand or other rough material. Schuell hypothesized that reauditorization—building sound organization internally—was a key deficit in aphasia, and consistently invoked the auditory modality in clinical activities to retrain the ability to reauditorize. "Deblocking"—that is, using the patient's most intact language modality to trigger her use of others (Weigl, 1970)—is still another example of attempting to reorganize the cortex. Some clinical techniques have been devised to involve the right hemisphere in the language activities we have previously ascribed to the left hemisphere. Melodic intonation therapy (Sparks, Helm, & Albert, 1974) is an excellent example. In this approach, the aphasic patient's usually unimpaired ability to sing or to intone is used. The patient, usually one with Broca aphasia, is taught first to intone words and phrases systematically. The intonation is then gradually faded and supplanted by nonintoned word and phrase production; finally, these words are incorporated into contextual speech. Another right hemispheric technique is the use of visual imagery and training in its application to word finding.

Helm-Estabrooks, Fitzpatrick, and Barresi (1982) have described a technique for use with globally aphasic individuals, called Visual Action Therapy (VAT). VAT is a carefully sequenced series of activities that help the patient to reestablish representational behavior. More specifically, patients are trained to use a gesture to represent an object. Patients profit from this technique not only by learning some symbolic gestures, but by improving auditory comprehension as well. VAT is a silent technique—neither the patient nor clinician talk throughout the various steps of the program. The observation of improved auditory comprehension underscores the notion that training in a basic underlying process (in this case, reestablishing a system of representation) generalizes to other linguistic behaviors.

It is worth repeating that we do not know how the brain capitalizes on the activities our therapy provides to the patient. Some authorities suggest that the damaged brain must relearn what has been lost, and advocate the application of learning principles to treatment regimes. Behaviors, such as using various question forms, are selected as targets for treatment, and carefully controlled, systematic stimulus conditions are provided. In studies designed to evaluate these procedures, the researchers check for indications of how the carefully trained behaviors generalize to other contexts, or to other responses. An excellent example of these approaches to treatment is provided by Thompson and McReynolds (1986).

LaPointe (1985) provides many examples of how different aspects of language behavior can be shaped using behavioral management principles. By using a carefully constructed record-keeping system, called *Base-10 Programming,* he charts the target behaviors, the stimuli used to evoke those behaviors, the reinforcer(s), and the patient's responses to the stimuli on repeated presentations. In this way, both the patient and clinician are

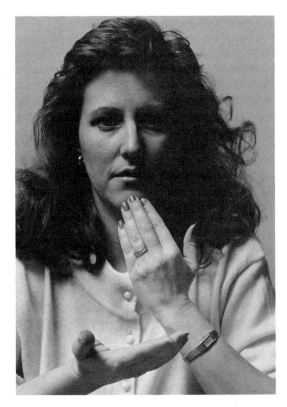

AMERIND
PACE

*Visual Action Therapy (VAT) relies on gestures to represent objects and has proven effective in improving auditory comprehension.*

provided with an ongoing record of progress. LaPointe applies the Base-10 format to a variety of language activities, including writing dictation, generating sentences, reading printed commands, and responding to questions.

A third major approach is built on the premise that aphasia is a product of the interaction of intact and damaged parts of the brain. Treatment, while working within the limitations imposed by the damage, must also compensate for the damage. Patients are taught to rely on both alternative strategies and still intact cerebral mechanisms to solve communicative problems. When speech is most seriously compromised, nonspeech communication systems such as communication boards or AMERIND (American Indian) sign may be used. Another approach is to teach patients alternative communication strategies. These might include training patients to request that others slow down or repeat messages, or training patients to accompany their speech attempts with gestures.

Promoting Aphasic Communication Effectiveness (PACE) (Davis & Wilcox, 1981, 1985) is yet another functional approach to aphasia treatment. Using a situation that is a controlled analog to the give-and-take of natural communication (in which new requests and responses are exchanged), the aphasic patient is required to test the effectiveness of a variety of her communicative attempts, from gesture to writing. Effectiveness in PACE is measured simply by whether or not messages are understood, regardless of the means by which it is accomplished.

Arthur Kopit, in the preface to his remarkable play *Wings* (1978), which explores what the inner world of the aphasic patient might contain, eloquently describes it:

> I had met the older woman while accompanying my father one afternoon on his rounds. When he went down for speech therapy, she was one of the three other patients in the room. I had never observed a speech therapy session before and was nervous. The day, I recall vividly, was warm, humid. The windows of the room were open. A scent of flowers suffused the air. To get the session started, the therapist asked the older woman if she could name the seasons of the year. With much effort, she did, though not in proper order. She seemed annoyed with herself for having any difficulty at all with such a task. The therapist then asked her which of these seasons corresponded to the present. The woman turned at once to the window. She could see the garden, the flowers. Her eyes were clear, alert; there was no question but that she understood what was wanted. I cannot remember having ever witnessed such an intense struggle. At first, she did nothing but sit calmly and wait for the word to arrive on its own. When it didn't, she tried to force the word out by herself, through thinking; as if to assist what clearly was a process of expulsion, she scrunched her face up, squeezed her eyelids shut. But no word emerged. Physically drained, her face drenched with sweat, she tried another trick; she cocked her head and listened to the birds, whose sound was incessant. When this too led to nothing, she sniffed the air. When nothing came of this strategy either, she turned her attention to what she was wearing, a light cotton dress; she even touched the fabric. Finally, something connected. Her lips began to form a word. She shut her eyes. Waited. The word emerged. WINTER.
>
> When informed that it was summer she seemed astonished, how was it possible? . . . a mistake like that . . . obviously she knew what season it was, anyone with eyes could tell at once what season it was! . . . and yet . . . She looked over at where I sat and shook her head in dismay, then laughed and said, "This is really nuts, isn't it!"
>
> I sat there, stunned. I could not believe that anyone making a mistake of such gross proportions and with such catastrophic implications could laugh at it.
>
> So there would be no misunderstanding, the therapist quickly pointed out that this mistake stemmed completely from her stroke; in no way was she demented. The woman smiled (she knew all that) and turned away, stared back out the window at the garden. This is really nuts, isn't it!—I could not get her phrase from my mind. In its intonation, it had conveyed no feeling of anger, resignation, or despair. Rather it conveyed amazement, and in that amazement, a trace (incredible as it seemed) of delight. This is not to suggest that anyone witnessing this incident could, even for an instant,

have imagined that she was in any sense pleased with her condition. The amazement, and its concomitant delight, seemed to me to reflect only an acknowledgement that her condition was extraordinary, and in no way denied or obviated the terror or the horror that were at its core. By some (I supposed) nourishing spring of inner strength and light, of whose source I had no idea, she had come to a station in her life from which she could perceive in what was happening something that bore the aspect of adventure, and it was through this perhaps innate capacity to perceive and appreciate adventure, and perhaps in this sense only, that she found some remaining modicum of delight, which I suspect kept her going.*

## Efficacy of Treatment

We have briefly touched on the issue of the value of aphasia therapy. Perhaps because of the interdisciplinary context in which treatment is conducted, as well as the frequency with which third-party payment is used to finance treatment, the speech-language pathologist who works with aphasic people must take the matter of efficacy of treatment seriously. As a result, the discipline has more literature related to the issue of accountability than we find with most speech problems. It seems worth summarizing here.

The problems inherent in developing a single, thorough, adequately controlled study of the effectiveness of aphasia rehabilitation are great, possibly even insurmountable. They involve statistical issues, such as adequate sample size; ethical questions, such as the justification for withholding treatment; and problems with controlling the multitude of variables presumed to influence recovery from aphasia. These include age, initial severity of the aphasia, the role of spontaneous recovery, and type and frequency of treatment. A *Lancet* editorial recently discussed these problems in assessing recovery from aphasia and concluded that, until more is known about aphasia itself, investigations of treatment should concentrate on small, well-defined studies comparing one mode with another (Editorial: Prognosis, 1977). Of the more than 20 presently available studies regarding the effectiveness of treatment, the clear majority conclude that treatment has a positive effect on recovery from aphasia (Darley, 1972, 1975).

The most impressive evidence for the effectiveness of treatment is the VA cooperative study of Wertz and his colleagues (1984a). This study used extremely carefully selected patients, randomly assigned to one of three treatment groups. The first group received 12 weeks of clinic treatment beginning relatively soon after stroke; the second group received 12 weeks of individually designed treatment administered by a friend or family member. The third group, once entered in the study, sat out the 12 weeks during which the first group was being treated, and *then* began their

*Excerpt from the Preface to *Wings* by Arthur Kopit, pp. ix–xi. Copyright © 1978 by Arthur Kopit. Reprinted by permission of Hill and Wang, a division of Farrar, Straus and Giroux, Inc.

12-week treatment trial. Patients in all three groups were tested at the 12-week point, when it was shown that the treated patients made significantly more language gains as measured by PICA than did the group whose treatment was deferred.

In this way, some of the almost insurmountable problems suggested in this chapter were overcome, and carefully matched patients receiving treatment and not receiving treatment were compared to show that treatment was effective. When the groups were again compared at 24 weeks, after the deferred group was treated, the deferred patients had caught up. This allows us to conclude that deferring treatment at least for this period of time had no ill effects. Finally, the home-treated group was neither better nor worse than the clinic group, so the matter of home treatment remained equivocal. At least, it suggests that treatment designed by therapists to be administered at home might be a possible alternative for patients who live far away from clinics or who can't travel to them.

The thoroughly trained and sensitive speech-language pathologist knows a variety of these techniques, and often applies more than one to the effective treatment of an aphasic patient. In the ideal case, direct treatment is always used in conjunction with patient and family counseling. One important goal of the counseling, in addition to its psychosocial adjustment goals, is to help the family communicate with the patient and further the advances made in the clinic by involving the family in daily practice outside the treatment room.

No one really knows the best schedule for direct aphasia treatment, nor how long it should continue. We believe that the patient's overall condition, his progress in therapy, and his communicated feelings about the usefulness of therapy should all contribute to individual decisions in these matters. We also believe that intensive treatment, that is, frequent clinical sessions, is probably more useful than even the same number of sessions spread over a longer period of time.

In addition to individual sessions, the ideal treatment plan should include group sessions as well. Sometimes these group sessions are used to practice and gain experience with some of the skills developed in individual sessions. These sessions also give the aphasic patient an opportunity to exchange her feelings with other people who are experiencing similar problems, and to help other people in the group with their difficulties—not a small benefit to all the patients' rehabilitation. We have found family groups to be an extremely effective way for working through many of the family adjustment problems we have described earlier.

We have briefly summarized some of the ways speech-language pathologists assist aphasic patients to maximize their potential for language recovery. In the process, it is possible you might conclude that it is a relatively clear-cut and simple matter for the aphasic patient to regain her former language proficiency. This could not be farther from the truth. The treatment of aphasia is, indeed, often successful in helping the aphasic patient to improve her language abilities, but total recovery of language function is rare. It is difficult and often highly emotional work for both professional and patient.

# RELATED DISORDERS

Now that you have a thorough understanding of what aphasia is, let's briefly review what aphasia is not. Up to this point, we have presented aphasia as an adult disorder, but children may also become aphasic in the same ways in which adults become aphasic, although the disorder often differs in the two populations. Differences in cognitive and linguistic symptomology may also be observed in individuals with other types of damage to the central nervous system. For example, like the head-injured child, adults with closed head injury have problems that result from widespread damage to cerebral, cerebellar, and brain stem structures. For this population, linguistic problems are often secondary to changes in personality and other cognitive skills, in addition to a variety of motor speech problems that are described in chapter 14. As with right hemisphere stroke, the mechanisms are the same as those that produce aphasia; however, the cognitive and linguistic consequences are strikingly different. We will review briefly each of these disorders to help you appreciate the similarities and differences each shares with aphasia.

*See chapters 4 and 14.*

## Acquired Aphasia in Children

It may seem unusual to include a discussion of acquired aphasia in children in a chapter that is devoted to adult disorders. Because the terminology is confusing, however, it's important that students understand the similarities and differences between the two disorders. When the term *aphasia* is applied to children, it is almost invariably preceded by a modifier such as *childhood* or *developmental*. The children we will describe briefly here also require a modifier to the term, and in their case, it is *acquired*. We will refer here to children who become aphasic (rather than fail to develop language normally) as having *acquired aphasia*.

Acquired aphasia results from the same causes as aphasia in adults. Unlike the adult population, for whom stroke is the major cause of aphasia, most children become aphasic as the result of head injury or diseases such as encephalitis. It is noteworthy, however, that other cognitive and psychiatric disturbances often accompany the speech and language deficits. When the disorder is truly aphasic, however, there are some striking differences between children and adults. Two of these differences, symptom and recovery patterns, are of particular significance and will be covered next.

### Symptom Pattern

Rather than showing the wide variation in type of language deficits we have described earlier, it appears that some smaller numbers of patterns predominate in children. Typically, once children have recovered consciousness, their former level of ability to comprehend language returns rather rapidly, with their ability to speak lagging far behind. It is not uncommon for a child to remain mute for some time after comprehension of speech appropriate to her age has begun to be reestablished. If the child was a reader before the trauma, level-appropriate reading may also begin to return before speech. Often initial speech attempts are apractic; as this evolves, word-finding difficulties are apparent. Therefore, the pattern we have earlier described as Broca aphasia and anomic aphasia are typical of the problems encountered by children who become aphasic.

## Recovery

The second major difference has to do with recovery rate. Children appear to recover language both more rapidly and more extensively than do adults. Obviously this is affected by the severity of the initial injury, but if it were possible to compare recovery in two identical injuries, one occurring in a child and the other in an adult, it would be a safe prediction that the child would show the greater speed and extent of recovery. The reasons for this difference are not entirely clear, but most authorities believe that the child's brain is more plastic than the adult's—children's brains are less "set in their ways" than are adults' brains; they are more capable of developing alternative routes for transmission of neural messages.

## Diagnosis and Treatment

The diagnosis and treatment of acquired aphasia in children presents one of the strongest examples of cooperative effort in speech-language pathology. The medical and paramedical specialists we have already listed as part of the interdisciplinary team retain their importance in diagnosis and treatment of the child who has acquired aphasia. But some additional disciplines must be involved, including educational specialists and child developmentalists. More striking is the fact that diagnosing and treating children with acquired aphasia requires the *intradisciplinary* cooperation of the specialist in adult language disorders with those fellow professionals who specialize in language acquisition in children. To determine if a child's language "errors" are manifestations of his level of syntactic and lexical development (that is, age-appropriate) or if they represent deviations from the normal brought on by brain damage, you must know a great deal about processes and stages in normal language acquisition. Only a few adult language specialists remain expert enough in child language to accomplish this diagnostic process alone. Similarly, only an occasional child language specialist is well-enough trained in the effects of brain damage occurring after birth to accomplish the same end. Thus, both child and adult language specialists cooperate in diagnosis of acquired aphasia in children.

Because many aphasic children recover rapidly and well, the speech-language pathologist's role may be minimal. It is often the case, however, that children who return to school following head injury have a variety of subtle problems that adversely affect school performance and the learning of new skills. The ideal form of intervention for these children is still not clearly defined or specified, but it is clear that interdisciplinary teamwork, involving learning disability specialists, school psychologists and speech-language pathologists, is necessary for remediation.

For the unfortunate minority of head-injured children who have extensive residual problems, intensive and integrated interdisciplinary rehabilitation centers or special schools become the appropriate placement. In such settings, restitution of linguistic, cognitive, and physical skills is the primary goal.

We must emphasize that little is known about acquired aphasias in children, and that, like everything else in this chapter, we have more questions than answers. Even the two generalizations we mentioned have enough exceptions to make them tentative. For example, some children, particularly those with seizure disorders that only become apparent after the onset of language, have profound and unremitting disorders of auditory comprehension. Even though some children appear to recover language fully, subtle learning deficits, particularly as they relate to language-based skills such as reading, plague these children when they return to school.

# Head Injury in Adults

## Symptom Pattern

Although cerebral trauma may occur at any age, adolescents and young adults are at greatest risk. The mechanism of injury is a blunt blow to the head that most often is associated with a motor vehicle accident. Unlike stroke, closed-head injury is nonfocal. Many areas of the brain may be compromised due to primary (bruises, lacerations) or secondary (swelling, increased pressure) damage. What results is a diverse conglomeration of motor, sensory, and behavioral deficits. Although aphasic syndromes are rare, cognitive-linguistic impairments are common. Attentional problems and difficulties with concentration often result in reduced auditory comprehension. Memory and learning disturbances may be associated with word-finding problems, while poor organizational skills may result in disorganized verbal expression. Decreased inhibition and errors of judgment may also have an effect on the pragmatics of language. For example, individuals may swear or laugh inappropriately, talk excessively, interrupt others while they are talking, or be unable to maintain a topic of conversation.

*See chapter 4.*

### Diagnosis and Treatment

Recovery following closed-head injury is different from stroke recovery. Individuals with closed-head injury evolve through distinctive stages of recovery. Hagen (1981) described an eight-stage recovery scale, the Rancho Los Amigos (RLA) Hospital's Levels of Cognitive Recovery, that is widely used today. During the early stage (RLA 2–3), the individual begins to respond to the environment. Treatment consists of sensorimotor stimulation for the goal of increasing recognition of objects, people, and events. During the middle stage (RLA 4–6), much of the sensorimotor stimulation may have to be eliminated to reduce the individual's agitation. Highly structured therapy sessions should focus on reducing confusion, increasing orientation and goal-directed behavior, and improving memory. To accomplish this, speech-language pathologists work with individuals in the patients' environment to increase the consistency of routines. In therapy, specific language tasks might include listening to increasingly long and complex language samples; following directions; describing objects, events, people, places; defining words; classifying ideas according to a theme; and improving the organization of conversational speech. During the late stage (RLA 7–8 +), the goal is for patients to reach their maximum level of independence. Treatment is designed to help the individual compensate for residual deficits, which may include word-finding difficulties; problems with comprehension of complex materials; shallow reasoning and problem solving; memory disturbances; impulsive and socially awkward behavior; and impairments in goal setting, inhibiting, self-monitoring, and self-evaluation (Ylvisaker & Szekeres, 1986). Treatment may also focus on improving the efficiency of language processing in real-life and stressful situations.

## Right Hemisphere Disorders

### Symptom Pattern

Unlike the characteristics of aphasia, the symptoms of right hemisphere disorders may be difficult to detect during an initial, casual encounter with a patient. One might have the impression that the patient has an optimistic response to stroke, only to discover in subsequent encounters that the patient has an unrealistic appraisal of her deficits. For example, she may minimize or deny the existence of left hemiplegia, and refuse to participate in physical or occupational therapy. She may be disoriented and confused about what has happened. Unlike the aphasic individual, the right-hemisphere–damaged patient does not appear to be concerned about her confusion. Conversely, she may laugh it off or confabulate to fill in the missing gaps.

*Although* **unilateral neglect** *may follow left brain damage, it is a more common symptom of right brain damage. It refers to the inability to attend and/or respond to stimuli on the side opposite the brain damage.*

A variety of attentional and visuospatial disturbances have also been associated with right hemisphere damage. One of the most fascinating is unilateral neglect. Patients with this condition fail to respond to stimuli that are contralateral to the side of brain damage. Although the condition may exist following left brain damage, left side neglect (resulting from right brain damage) is more frequent and more severe. In mild cases, patients may omit or provide little left side detail on drawings; a few examples are provided in Figure 12.3. In more severe cases, patients may ignore people and objects on their left side, and may be unwilling to look in that direction, even with assistance. In addition to unilateral neglect, right-brain–damaged individuals may also demonstrate a host of other visuospatial difficulties. Among the more common are difficulties reading maps, remembering familiar routes, and recognizing familiar faces.

Right-hemisphere–damaged individuals may also have communication problems. Patients will make aphasiclike errors on auditory comprehension, naming, repetition, and reading and writing tasks. As Myers (1986) points out, these deficits are not a major source of their communication impairment. Rather, the pragmatics of their communication is most disturbed. Right-brain–damaged individuals have particular difficulty in appropriately expressing and comprehending the emotional contexts of communication. Their speech lacks the normal prosody that we all use to express sadness, surprise, confusion, elation, and disappointment. Comprehension of these prosodic features, in addition to other representations of emotion (for example, facial expression), is also impaired. Right-hemisphere–damaged patients tend to respond to the more literal or superficial aspects of stimuli, and fail to identify relationships that exist among stimulus items. Thus, their communication may be filled with irrelevant, repetitious detail, yet lack

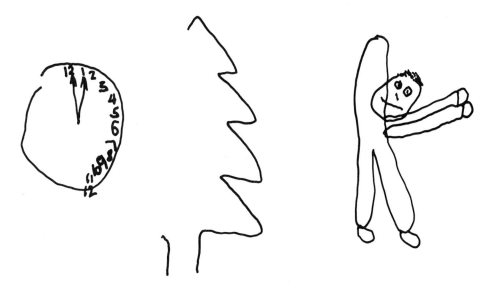

**Figure 12.3**  Clock, tree, and person drawings produced by individuals with right brain damage

organization and an overall theme. The following is an example of speech from a patient with a right hemisphere communication disorder. The patient is describing a picture from the Western Aphasia Battery that shows a family having a picnic at the lake.

> See him flying a kite. Sitting there. Sailboat. See a guy flying a kite. Sitting by a nice big elm tree. Out in the country. A guy in overhauls, he's sitting in a barge in a boat or in a schooner out ready for arrival taking in a boatride headed for down toward the river somebody flying a kite. Man, woman, and child. Two of 'em riding a river down in a boat. Boy might have a place set out to eat.

### Diagnosis and Treatment

The diagnosis of visuospatial deficits is usually under the domain of trained neuropsychologists; however, speech-language pathologists may obtain information through formal testing and informal observations that may help identify individuals with unilateral neglect and other visuospatial disturbances. Standardized aphasia batteries may be used to discover deficits in naming, auditory comprehension, reading, writing, etc. The speech-language pathologists should be cautious about evaluating whether these deficits are secondary to attentional or visuoperceptual deficits. If the deficits are linguistically based, then treatment may be similar to the procedures used for treating the aphasic patient.

The spontaneous speech and picture description subtests of standardized aphasia batteries are perhaps the most effective subtests to discover the other communication problems that we associate with right brain damage. One should augment this assessment with specific tasks designed to measure an individual's comprehension and production of emotional tone. We might ask a patient to point to the face that goes with an angry voice, excited voice, sad voice, etc., and then to produce sentences that convey similar emotions. Treatment will involve similar tasks that help the patient comprehend and express emotional tone.

During the picture description task, we are interested in patients' abilities to utilize contextual cues to provide a well-organized, efficient, coherent description. Sequencing tasks are often effective for assisting the patient with organization of verbal material. Patients may be asked to select the critical items of a picture or story, and then to specify relationships among these items. Limits might be imposed on speaking time to help the individual avoid digression and perseveration.

## CONCLUSION

In this chapter, we have introduced you to the problem of aphasia in both its academic and practical aspects. We have shared what is currently known about this disorder. We hope that you will be challenged by its mysteries and complexities, and sensitized to the problems of people who risk losing part of themselves by losing part of their language.

## STUDY QUESTIONS

1. Describe the central nervous system organization for control of basic motor, sensory, and cognitive/linguistic functions. How does the role of the left cerebral hemisphere differ from the role of the right cerebral hemisphere?

2. How does one become aphasic? Why do we reserve the term for individuals whose communication impairments are the result of stroke, as opposed to other neurogenic disorders?

3. What is spontaneous recovery? What are the factors that influence the manner and degree to which someone's symptoms resolve?

4. List the major syndromes of aphasia and the symptoms that characterize each.

5. What is the purpose of aphasia assessment? What are the components of informal and formal aphasia test batteries?

6. What is meant by the phrase, "Aphasia is a family problem"? Describe the roles of the speech-language pathologist in the treatment of the aphasic individual and her family.

7. How do the communication problems that result from left brain damage differ from the communication problems that result from damage to the right hemisphere?

## SELECTED READINGS

Darley, F. L. (1979). *Evaluation of appraisal techniques in speech and language pathology.* Reading, MA: Addison-Wesley.

Gardner, H. (1975). *The shattered mind.* New York: Knopf.

LaPointe, L. L. (1985). Aphasia therapy: Some principles and strategies for treatment. In D. Johns (Ed.), *Clinical management of neurogenic communicative disorders.* Boston: Little, Brown.

Wepman, J. M. (1951). *Recovery from aphasia.* New York: Ronald Press.

# CHAPTER THIRTEEN

# Neurogenic Disorders of Speech

### LEONARD L. LaPOINTE

## MYTHS AND REALITIES

- *Myth:* Neurogenic disorders of communication result solely from damage to the central nervous system.
- *Reality:* A wide variety of speech disorders result from peripheral nervous system damage, including all those attributed to cranial nerve impairment.
- *Myth:* A standardized and almost universally accepted terminology exists for describing neurogenic speech disorders.
- *Reality:* The literature is filled with a rich variety of descriptive terms, labels, and nomenclature, many of which are inconsistently used for the same conditions.
- *Myth: Broca's aphasia* and *apraxia of speech* are terms for the same condition.
- *Reality:* Most experts recognize that, while Broca's aphasia may entail many of the speech movement or phonologic disturbances seen in apraxia of speech, it encompasses other significant linguistic impairment as well, such as agrammatism or telegraphic sentence production.

- *Myth:* Dysarthria is a disturbance of articulation caused by brain damage.
- *Reality:* The dysarthrias can affect any or all of the speech production processes, including articulation, phonation, resonance, or respiration.
- *Myth:* Motor vehicle accidents account for only a small proportion of traumatic head injury cases.
- *Reality:* In Antarctica maybe. In most developed, industrialized countries, automobile and motorcycle accidents account for as many as 80% of reported traumatic head injury cases.
- *Myth:* If a dysarthric speaker is 100% intelligible, he or she would not be a candidate for speech treatment.
- *Reality:* Dysarthric speech may be compromised not only in understand-ability, but also in the dimension of perceived "bizarreness." Perfectly intelligible speech that fluctuates abnormally in pitch or loudness may require treatment.
- *Myth:* Since speech is an overlaid function, any neurogenic disturbance of the motor act of swallowing will result in disturbed speech.
- *Reality:* Speech and swallowing are not as hierarchically related as many assume. Cases of swallowing disturbance without subsequent speech involvement are well documented in the literature.

As with most topics, the accumulated dust of years of misinformation can give rise to molehills of myth. With the illustrative case study and the information in this chapter, an attempt will be made to sweep away some of the unfounded ideas about neurogenic disorders of speech.

*Jack Dickerson was a 75-year-old gentleman from Booth Bay, Maine, who had presumably suffered a brainstem stroke. He and his wife, desiring a change to a warmer climate and another opinion regarding prognosis and treatment of his speech impairment, sought our services at a Florida Veterans' Administration Medical Center. Presenting signs included paralysis of all limbs, impaired swallowing with no speech output, but intact awareness and intact auditory comprehension.*

*Mr. Dickerson was a tall, muscular gentleman who looked 15 years younger than his age. He was alert, intelligent, and looked the part of one who has spent an active outdoor life engaged in stimulating jobs and adventure. Most of his life had been spent on the sea. He had been a frigate officer in the Coast Guard in World War II, and had worked as a yacht broker, shipyard manager, and marine surveyor, and, in the words of his wife, he "knew tons about sailing, rigging, and navigation and was one of the finest racing helmsmen on the East Coast." In 1958, he ran the Race Committee for the New York Yacht Club for the America's Cup Races. Jack is the type of rugged, knowledgeable, and self-reliant person that you encounter in fiction, but seldom have the opportunity to meet in real life.*

*He was initially treated at a large medical center where he received physical therapy and treatment for his motor speech disorder. He was able to ambulate with the aid of a wheelchair and walker, but he was left with some residual paralysis.*

*We used a standardized protocol to preserve his responses on both audio- and videotape recordings, and evaluated his speech output by careful listening and by observing his responses to a series of speech and non-speech tasks. He showed intact comprehension of both written and spoken language, and at no time did we suspect anything other than completely intact language and mental status. His motor speech system, however, was ravaged. He presented a severe flaccid dysarthria characterized by reduced range, direction, and velocity of movements involving respiration, the velum, the tongue and lips, and, to a lesser extent, the larynx.*

*Jack's speech was unintelligible except for isolated single words. Further evaluation assessed levels of word and sentence intelligibility, as well as the quality of his articulation of vowel and consonant combinations by word position.*

*He and his wife were advised that they should not expect a return to the speech skills he had before his stroke. The best speech treatment could hope to offer would be improvement of some of the parameters of the motor speech system, and perhaps some limited and compensated speech to aid in the expression of daily needs, as well as the possibility of learning to use some nonverbal, alternate methods of communication.*

*Jack's wife is as interesting and self-reliant as her husband. She is a nurse who is knowledgeable, questioning, and tenacious. She proved to be an assertive, independent, and highly motivated spouse who demanded an active role in her husband's rehabilitation. We agreed to a 6-week treatment program of 2 to 3 sessions per week. Throughout the program, Mrs. Dickerson worked with her husband on selected speech tasks that were compatible with our treatment goals.*

*During treatment, careful charting and plotting of base-rate performance and progress on all tasks was documented, and progress was noted on nearly all of the specific treatment objectives. Jack also was provided a Canon Communicator (a pocket-sized, keyboard-operated electronic device with a ticker-tape printout), and was instructed in its use. He expressed the desire to use it only in crisis situations, or when he was unable to convey a message intelligibly. Throughout treatment, his wife maintained an active role, not only in carrying out tasks at home, but frequently by contributing ideas for tasks.*

*Overall intelligibility on words and syllables increased from 4% and 36%, respectively, on April 3 to 12% and 67% on May 16. These gains were modest and the result of an intensive cooperative effort between clinic and spouse, yet they were reported by both Jack and his wife to be worth the effort.*

*At the end of May, they returned to Maine for the summer with the resolve to continue daily work on some of the objectives we had outlined, and with the promise that they would call on us again when the snow flies and the water freezes. Winter indeed returned to Maine, and 8 months later I received another call informing me that Jack and his wife were returning to Florida and wanted to stop in for a week of reevaluation, more specific suggestions for home treatment, and renewal of our acquaintance.*

*Jack's speech had improved remarkably as a result of the direction and persistence of his home program. He had regained enough compensated, functional communication to make his daily needs and wants known, and even communicate by telephone. Word intelligibility was now in the 60% to 80% range.*

Lurking in the dark recesses of the private thoughts of many of us is the fear that if ever we should suffer brain damage, we would end up either insane or mentally retarded. As is evident from previous chapters in this book, sanity and intellectual function are but two of the wonders regulated by the human nervous system. The human nervous system is usually divided into two major parts: the central nervous system (CNS), including the brain and spinal cord; and the peripheral nervous system (PNS), including the cranial nerves and spinal nerves. This division is shown in Figure 13.1. This complex system, the center of which is an unassuming, squishy, three-pound, pinkish-white mass, has evolved into the primary director of human behavior. Unlike that of the striped bass and other lower animals, the human nervous system has added features and functions that allow behaviors far more complex than treading water or devouring a minnow. In addition to centers of language and memory, certain regions are associated with hearing, vision, smell, touch, and taste. Other areas are associated with regulating the vital functions of the body, such as automatic breathing, maintaining blood pressure and heart rate, and digesting food. Still other centers and systems are responsible for movement and patterns of movement, from a simple movement such as pinching the nostrils to indicate reaction to a referee's judgment, to the complex series of moves of a gymnast's full twisting dismount from the parallel bars. Other regions of the brain are responsible for correlating and integrating many tiny bits of information to make plans or programs of action.

Love and Webb (1986) have given a useful synthesis of neurology for the speech-language pathologist. They include a section on the professions of

*See Figure 13.2.*

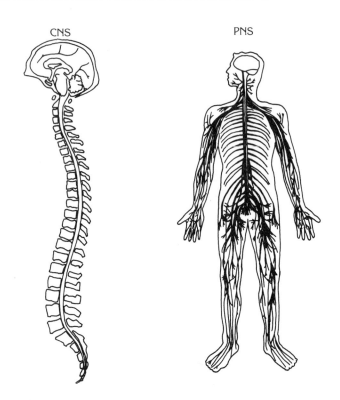

**Figure 13.1**   Central nervous system (CNS) and peripheral nervous system (PNS) of humans

neurology and speech pathology as intersecting specialities, as well as considerable detail on the neural mechanisms of speech, language, and hearing. Particularly well-covered is the intimate relationship between the cranial nerves (a major functional component of the peripheral nervous system) and speech. Included are names, structure, route, testing procedure, and signs of abnormal function.

Impairment of the planning, coordination, and timed execution of the movement patterns that result in the curious act we know as speech is the subject of this chapter. No human movement patterns are as intricate, complex, or intertwined with all the human activities of learning, loving, and living. Far more area of the brain is devoted to the control of the tiny muscular adjustments of the tongue, lips, vocal folds, and other speech articulators than to those muscle groups needed for walking upright. Far more coordination and synchrony is needed for speech than for riding a unicycle, threading a needle, rolling a log, or removing a thorn from the foot. The amazing thing is that the act of speech becomes so automatic that we hardly think about it—until something goes wrong.

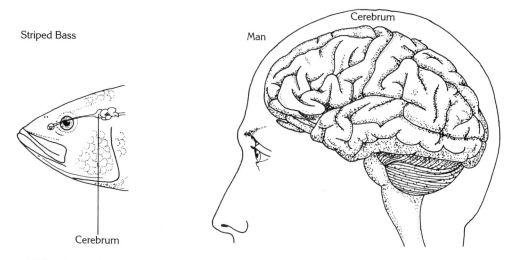

Striped Bass          Man          Cerebrum

Cerebrum

**Figure 13.2** Brain of striped bass and of man

## CLASSIFICATIONS AND DEFINITIONS

The area of neurogenic impairment of speech has been a fertile ground for controversy and desk-pounding argument over the years. Some of this disagreement can be traced to the unbridled proliferation of terms and labels for speech disorders. This growing pool of unclearly defined terms has spawned argument and misunderstanding, particularly in the branch of speech-language pathology that has been so closely related to the medical environment. No standardized terminology or classification system has emerged, and labels have been assigned seemingly at the whim of the labeler. Most labels have been generated to serve the particular interest or specific point of view of a group or a discipline. By contrast, the familiar blind men and the elephant seem remarkably astute. Different goals and different jargon can create barriers to cross-disciplinary cooperation. Fortunately, some of these problems have diminished in recent years.

Neurologically based disturbances in the selection, sequencing, and coordinated production of speech sounds have been labeled *oral apraxia, verbal apraxia, phonemic paraphasia, literal paraphasia, oral-verbal apraxia, anarthria, dysarthria, apraxic-dysarthria, cortical dysarthria, phonetic disintegration,* and a score of other terms. Though we still do not have a standard set of terms, some of the less frequently used and esoteric labels are falling by the wayside, and some labels seem to be gaining acceptance through the frequency of their appearance in the literature. A few writers, notably Darley (1967), have long advocated a more precise and consistent system of terminology. We are far from total agreement, however, on the use of labels and terms, and the reader must be cautioned that the terms

**Neurogenic** *simply means arising from the nervous system.*

preferred in this chapter may not be used by all specialists in this area. Perhaps the future will see the adoption of more precise and reliable systems of describing the dimensions of speech that are apt to go awry after brain damage.

In addition to widely varying use of specific descriptive terms, classification of disturbed oral communication can be problematic. The borderline between speech and language is sometimes unclear, as is the decision about whether or not a specific disturbed speech event is the result of an error in articulatory timing or speech sound selection. Communication is a unitary process in the sense that it is the product of a complex, interrelated system requiring coordination of several components of the body. At the same time, the act of communication loses some of its relevance if the environment and its context are ignored. The damage that disturbs this delicate sequence of sensory-muscular-integrative events therefore can affect the function of the respiratory mechanism, tone-producing mechanism, resonance system, and system of articulation that shapes and molds the air or sound stream into recognizable words.

*See chapters 8, 12, and 14.*

It is wise to bear in mind the holistic nature of communication; it is an act that truly is greater than the sum of its parts. For the sake of understanding, though, we can analyze this integrated system. Disorders of *voice* are adequately covered in other chapters of this book, as will be the syndrome called *cerebral palsy* and its effects on communication, and the linguistic-symbolic disorders of *language* (aphasia). This chapter focuses on the output transmissive disorders of *speech* that are shattered by damage to the nervous system. These include the neurogenic phonological selection and sequencing disorders (apraxia of speech) and the dysarthrias. These disorders can occur in adults or in children, but we will focus on the problem in adults.

## Dysarthria

*Table 13.1 lists some of these colorful, though inexact, perceptual terms gleaned from past writings on dysarthria.*

Current use of the term *dysarthria* is somewhat more precise that earlier concepts of the disorder. If you were to consult a dictionary or several of the dozens of textbooks in the medical field of clinical neurology, you might get the impression that dysarthria is simply a disturbance of articulation caused by nervous system damage. Colorful though not very precise adjectives are used to describe the resultant articulation defect. *Slurred* and *scanning speech* are typical of the speech descriptions of the dysarthric person.

*People with cerebral palsy are more likely to have dysarthria than other neurogenic speech problems; see the next chapter.*

Current definitions are more inclusive than those of the past, and **dysarthria** now refers to a *group* of related speech disorders resulting from disturbed muscular control over the speech mechanism. Clinical research at the Mayo Clinic (Darley, Aronson, & Brown, 1975) has nurtured a concept of the disorder that includes impairment in the coexisting motor processes of respiration, phonation, articulation, resonance, and prosody.

**Table 13.1** Colorful, if Inexact, Early Perceptual Descriptors of Dysarthric Speech

| | | | |
|---|---|---|---|
| Slurred | Unclear | Scanning | Mush mouth |
| Thick | Staccato | Clumsy | Hot potato speech |
| Jerky | Explosive | Cerebral-palsied | Foreign body mouth |
| Indistinct | Squirrel tongue | Slobbery | Wobbly words |

Underlying the condition of dysarthria is a fundamental disturbance of movement or motoric function caused by damage to the nervous system. The motions and synchrony of the components of the speech system may be impaired in range, velocity, direction, force, or timing. Negative signs, such as slowness or inadequate range of movement, are frequently the outcome. In some types of dysarthria, however, depending on the areas of the nervous system affected, the movement disorder is overlaid with positive characteristics, such as excessively fast or involuntary movements, or movement overshoot due to uninhibited activity of intact parts of the nervous system.

Motor impairment of the articulators, including the lips, tongue, jaw, and soft palate, tends to produce a greater effect on the intelligibility of speech than do disturbances of the laryngeal or respiratory systems. The most prominent features that affect intelligibility are those that result from distorted consonant sounds, repeated or prolonged sounds, distorted vowels, or irregular articulatory breakdown.

# Apraxia of Speech

The other disorder to be discussed in this chapter is the neurogenic phonologic selection and sequencing problem that we will call *apraxia of speech*. Arguments over this disorder have existed for a century or more, and the disagreements seemed to have reached a rolling boil in the mid-1970s (LaPointe, 1975). Nearly everyone can find common ground of agreement on some of the speech characteristics exhibited by those who have the disturbance, but there have been objections as to what to call it (Kertesz, 1979; Martin, 1974). The term *apraxia of speech* appears to be gaining favor in the literature, and that is the label we will use.

**Apraxia of speech** is a neurogenic phonologic and/or articulatory disorder resulting from sensorimotor impairment of the capacity to select, program, and/or execute, in coordinated and normally timed sequences, the positioning of the speech muscles for the volitional production of speech sounds. The loss or impairment of the phonologic rules of the native language is not adequate to explain the observed pattern of deviant speech, nor is the disturbance attributable to weakened or slowed actions of specific muscle groups. Prosodic alteration, that is, changes in speech stress, intonation, or rhythm, may be associated with the articulatory problem, either as a primary part of the condition or in compensation for it.

Research in speech motor control laboratories seems to indicate that speech sound distortions may play a more prominent role in apraxia of speech than previously suspected. The detection of this greater prevalence of distorted sound production has been made possible by advances in instrumental speech analysis and narrower phonetic transcription strategies (Kent & Rosenbek, 1983).

One of the remarkable characteristics of the disorder is the demonstration of moments of error-free production during automatic or emotional utterances ("WHY can't I say the word *telephone* when I want to!"), compared to disturbed volitional attempts at uttering the same word or words ("fela ... tef ... Stella! ... felaphone.").

Table 13.2 lists some of the contrasting features of the dysarthrias and apraxia of speech. These differentiating features will vary in usefulness, depending on the severity of the presenting signs and symptoms of each patient, but they can be used as general guidelines for differentiating the dysarthrias from apraxia of speech in most patients.

**Table 13.2**  Characteristic Features of Dysarthria and Speech Apraxia

| Dysarthrias | Apraxia of Speech |
|---|---|
| Very little difference in articulatory accuracy between automatic-reactive and volitional purposive speech (no error-free production). | Articulatory accuracy is better for automatic-reactive speech than for volitional-purposive speech (moments of error-free production). |
| Substitution errors are infrequent. Speech is characterized more by phonetic distortions and omissions. | Substitution errors are more frequent than other error types. |
| Except occasionally in hypokinetic dysarthria, no difficulty with initiation of speech. | Initiation difficulty is frequent; characterized by pauses, restarts, repetition of initial sounds, syllables, or words. |
| Consonant clusters are frequently simplified; speech sound additions are rare. | Consonant clusters may be simplified, but more frequently the intrusive schwa /ə/ is inserted within clusters ("puh-lease" for *please*). |
| Audible and silent groping of the articulators to locate target articulatory placements is rare or nonexistent. | Audible or silent groping and articulatory posturing to locate target articulatory placements is common. |
| Quality of production and error type is consistent when asked to repeat the same utterance; some improvement may be noted under conditions of extreme effort or motivation. | Variability in production of repeated utterances is common. Error type may change or production may vary off and on target, particularly on repeated utterances of polysyllabic words. |

*Movement patterns affected by*
*1 - muscle strength*
*2 - muscle tone*
*timing & synchronization*
*of muscular movement*

**Table 13.3**  Possible Ways to Classify Motor Speech Disorders

| | |
|---|---|
| Age | Congenital, developmental, acquired |
| Cause | Stroke, head trauma, disease, etc. |
| Site of lesion | Brainstem, cerebellar, etc. |
| Level of lesion | Peripheral, central |
| Speech processes | Respiration, phonation, articulation, resonance, prosody |
| Speech valves | 1, 2, 3, 4, 5, 6, 7* |
| Speech events | Neural, muscular, structural, aerodynamic |
| Perceptual features | Pitch, loudness, voice quality, intelligibility, bizarreness |

*See point-place discussion, later in this chapter.

Certain classification systems have come in and out of favor over the years. Today, systems that combine perceptual features with speech processes and the functions of the speech valves seem to be preferred by many clinicians and researchers. This contemporary method of viewing and classifying motor speech disorders will be developed in the following section.

*Table 13.3 lists some of the possible ways of classifying the motor speech disorders.*

# BASIC CONCEPTS

As we mentioned briefly earlier, underlying the speech disturbances of dysarthria and apraxia is motoric impairment, or a fundamental disturbance of movement. What features of movement are necessary for normal speech? Darley et al. (1975) suggest that adequate strength, speed, range, accuracy, steadiness, and muscular tone are necessary.

Against the backdrop of these requisites of movement, the speech production process can be thought of as a chain of events originating in the brain, where the movement plan is conceived, and ending in the formation of acoustic signals that result in sequences of speech sounds (Netsell, 1973). As you can see in Figure 13.3, the genesis of this sequence is in the brain, where the plans of movement are formulated and programmed. Nerve impulses are then generated in the motoric sections of the brain and transmitted along the pathways of the nervous system to the muscles and structures of the speech system. Movements of these muscles and structures (lungs, vocal folds, soft palate, tongue, lips, jaw) create air flows and air pressure that result in the acoustic events we perceive as speech.

*These processes were detailed in chapter 3.*

These basic concepts of motor speech production have been developed further (Netsell & Daniel, 1979) to focus on some of the control variables that influence aspects of movements of speech. Muscle strength, muscular tone, and the timing and synchronization of muscular contraction are three of the variables that can have a strong influence on movement patterns. If one or more of these control variables is defective, movements can be impaired in

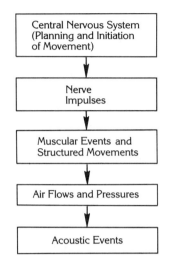

**Figure 13.3**  Levels in the motor speech production process

range (resulting in either an underexcursion or overexcursion), in velocity, or in direction (resulting in missing the mark or the target of an intended movement). Let's look at each of these variables a little more closely.

**Strength** is a concept that is fairly well understood. All of us have experienced or observed differences in strength among individuals. Varying abilities in weight lifting and the experience of having to relinquish the stubborn pickle jar to a person with greater hand strength are reminders of these differences.

**Tone** refers to the relatively constant background state of muscular contraction that is characteristic of normal muscle. Normal posture is partly dependent on adequate muscle tone. Tone may be decreased or increased (rigid), may wax and wane, or vary rhythmically (cogwheel rigidity).

**Timing** refers to the accuracy of onset and termination of muscular contraction. It also can refer to the duration of contraction or the complex coordination required for groups of muscles to work in synchrony.

Another concept related to the organization and execution of movements is *programming* or *planning.* The completion of complex skilled movements requires a preplan or program of the order, duration, and other details of movement sequences. Disturbances at this higher level of the organization of movement, when related to speech, may result in apraxia of speech.

It should be understood, and no doubt has been experienced by most of us, that certain other factors can influence the functioning of the motor speech system. Fatigue, motivation, excitement, and stark fear can have important influences on speech. For instance, most of us have experienced the tongue-slipping, voice-cracking effects of anxiety while speaking in front of large groups.

# COMPONENTS OF THE MOTOR SPEECH SYSTEM

A simplified view of the functional components of the speech production system might conceive of it as a small decision-making computer (the brain) that plans and initiates actions and transmits these orders along pathways (portions of the central and peripheral nervous system) to the muscles and structures of two large bags of air connected to a series of pipes open at one end (the speech apparatus of the respiratory, laryngeal, and upper airway system). Within the system of air containers and pipes are a series of valves that can be opened and closed to varying degrees to regulate the air pressure or flow that is generated or pumped by the lungs.

*If you wish, review chapter 3 on the physiology of speech.*

Figure 13.4 illustrates the functional components of the speech apparatus when this system is viewed as a pump (the respiratory system) and a series of valves. Each of the seven numbered components is a structure or combination of structures that serves to either generate or valve the speech air stream. Number 1 is the pump of the system, the muscles and structures

*The use of the point-place system in assessment is described in detail later in this chapter.*

Point-Place System
(Valves Along the Nile)

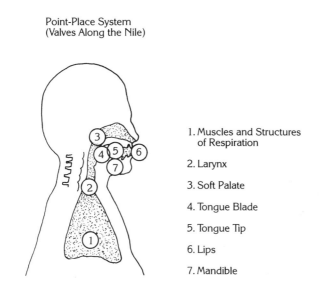

1. Muscles and Structures of Respiration

2. Larynx

3. Soft Palate

4. Tongue Blade

5. Tongue Tip

6. Lips

7. Mandible

**Figure 13.4** Functional components of the motor speech system. *(Note: From "The Dysarthrias: Description, Diagnosis and Treatment" by J. C. Rosenbek and L. L. LaPointe, in D. L. Johns (Ed.),* Clinical Management of Neurogenic Communicative Disorders, *1985. Boston: Little, Brown. Copyright © 1985 by Little, Brown and Company. Adapted by permission.)*

of respiration. Included at this level are the abdomen and diaphragm, the muscles and cartilage of the rib cage, and the lungs. Number 2 refers to the structures and muscles of the larynx, and number 3 includes the soft palate (velum) and the muscles in the velopharyngeal area that can move to separate the oral and nasal cavities. Number 4 refers to the blade of the tongue, while number 5 refers to the muscles that regulate the tongue tip. Number 6 includes all the facial muscles responsible for lip spreading, rounding, opening, and closing. Number 7 refers to the muscles and structures of the jaw. These basic concepts are important for more than academic reasons. Not only can they provide the framework for a model that will allow a better understanding of the complexities of motor speech, but (important for the speech-language pathologist) they can offer valuable guidance for the processes of diagnosis and treatment of people who suffer motor speech dysfunction. Perceptual signs, the interpretation the listener gives to the sound of a person's speech, are still important. But, as we will see, attention to the structures and valves of the speech system can help explain perceptual signs and aid in the planning and execution of treatment. This view is a simplified version of that developed by Netsell (1973), modified by Rosenbek and LaPointe (1978), and elaborated on by Netsell (1984). Amplification of many of these principles can be found in a compendium of work that advocates a neurobiologic view of speech production and the dysarthrias (Netsell, 1986). This collection emphasizes the close relationship of underlying movement physiology or function and the impaired acoustic events of speech.

## CAUSES OF NEUROGENIC SPEECH DISORDERS

Neurological and communication disorders affect 50,000,000 Americans (one out of every five persons), and the dollar cost to the country is $65 billion a year (NIH publication, 1979). What are the causes of these disturbances? What can go wrong with the nervous system to cause these dehumanizing conditions and erode the capacity of a person to enjoy life and interact with other people?

Many conditions can attack the well-being of the brain and create a web of problems for a person, including movement problems related to the production of speech. Stroke is by far the leading cause of neurogenic speech disorders. It is the number three killer in America, and nearly 500,000 Americans are hospitalized with it every year, one out of every 500 people. Stroke killed Franklin Roosevelt, Winston Churchill, Joseph Stalin, and my grandmother. When it doesn't kill, it leaves two thirds of its survivors impaired in speech, movement, or feeling.

Trauma is another major cause of nervous system damage and, as we have seen, has plagued humans since the invention of the rock. Over

420,000 new cases of head injury occur every year. Automobile and motorcycle accidents account for about 80% of the traumatic head injury in this country, while injuries from recreational activities (diving, skiing, javelin, and so on), power equipment, weapons, blows by objects or persons, and self-inflicted injuries account for the remainder. The young are particularly vulnerable to nervous system trauma. More than two thirds of the head and spinal injuries occur in the below-35 age group, typically in far more males than females. The National Head Injury Foundation calls traumatic head injury "the silent epidemic" because its prevalence and devastation have been relatively underrecognized by both the public and the professions (Ylvisaker, 1985).

Trauma also can affect the peripheral nervous system, and occasionally this can lead to speech disturbance if portions of the PNS that control the structures and muscles of speech production are injured. Cuts, burns, crush injuries, and penetrating wounds can cause these underlying injuries.

Another form of trauma the brain can experience is caused by a variety of toxins (poisons). Mercury, pesticides, lead poisoning, and carbon monoxide poisoning are environmental threats to people, but the most prevalent cause of neurotoxicity is alcohol and drug abuse. Other dramatic neural poisons, even if less frequently encountered, are insect, spider, and snake venoms. Our conditioned reaction of avoiding recreational activities with diamondback rattlers and blackwidow spiders is well founded.

Brain tumors (neoplasms) are another source of neuropathology. At any one time, there are approximately 61,000 people in this country with tumors of the nervous system, many of which can affect the speech system. Damage can occur from the robbing of nutritional requirements from surrounding healthy tissue, or the pressing and impinging of a growing mass of cells on surrounding tissue. Some tumors are benign and their growth is self-limited, while others are malignant and can grow and spread their virulent influence to remote regions of the body.

Infections are not the threat to the nervous system they once were, but antibiotics and miracle drugs have not eradicated the problem by any means. Conditions such as bacterial meningitis, viral infections, and chronic fungal infections are often treated successfully or prevented by immunization in this generation, though certain neural infections remain a serious problem.

Finally, inherited or acquired diseases can affect the nervous system. In many, the disease process is one of slow, painful degeneration that progressively involves areas regulating speech production. Myasthenia gravis, multiple sclerosis, amyotrophic lateral sclerosis (ALS), Parkinson's disease, and Huntington's disease are but some of the debilitating progressive conditions that can rob speech, sense, and stability. The baseball player Lou Gehrig, the folk balladeer Woodie Guthrie, and a childhood neighbor named Mabel suffered the ravages of these degenerative diseases.

Active research continues on the understanding, prevention, or amelioration of these neuropathologies, but until fundamental answers are found, we have no course but to treat their outcomes vigorously to the best of our ability.

# CHARACTERISTICS AND TYPES

What does it sound like when someone is unfortunate enough to suffer damage that results in a motor speech disorder? The ear of the beholder is the final arbiter, and a speech difference can only make a difference if listeners perceive it as being unusual or tainted in communicative effectiveness. Motor disorders of speech can vary widely in type or quality. The severity can range from a disturbance that is barely noticeable to one that shackles communication by rendering the speaker completely unintelligible. Type and severity of the disorder are related primarily to the location and extent of the nervous system damage. Generally speaking, large brain lesions result in the most damage; but small areas of destruction, if located in critical brain areas, can produce devastating and severe impairment.

## Dysarthria

Clinical research at the Mayo Clinic by Darley and his associates (1975) has contributed a great deal to our understanding of motor speech disorders. One of the most potent contributions of these researchers was to bring into focus some of the deviant speech dimensions heard in the dysarthrias, and to associate specific clusters of deviant speech with certain neurologic disorders. We have used the work of Darley and his colleagues to organize our listening skills, and perhaps improve our perceptual analysis of dysarthric speakers. The variety of speech features that can go awry in dysarthria sometimes appear overwhelming to the ear if several parameters of the speech production system are involved. The pattern of signs and symptoms that affect voice, articulation, respiration, and prosody sometimes appear so interwoven as to make individual features unidentifiable. If you know what to expect, though, because of a model of motor speech based on a firm understanding of both process and function, the perceptual onslaught can be less confusing. If the parameters of each speech process are attended to systematically, you can discern patterns of behavior and impose order on the seeming chaos.

In our clinic, we use the deviant speech categories presented by the Mayo Clinic research and have adapted them into a checklist to aid us in both sharpening our perceptual skills and pinpointing what is wrong with each patient's speech. This checklist is presented in Table 13.4. What can dysarthric speech sound like? As the checklist shows, the voice may be abnormal along several dimensions.

**Table 13.4**  Checklist of Deviant Speech Dimensions

**Voice**

Pitch characteristics

| | |
|---|---|
| _____ Pitch level overall | _____ Pitch breaks |
| _____ Monopitch | _____ Voice tremor |

Loudness characteristics

| | |
|---|---|
| _____ Loudness level overall | _____ Monoloudness |
| _____ Alternating loudness | _____ Loudness decay |
| _____ Excess loudness variation | |

Quality characteristics

| | |
|---|---|
| _____ Harsh voice | _____ Breathy voice (transient) |
| _____ Breath voice (continuous) | _____ Voice stoppages |
| _____ Strained-strangled voice | _____ Hyponasality |
| _____ Nasal emission | _____ Hypernasality |

**Respiration**

| | |
|---|---|
| _____ Forced expiration-inspiration | _____ Audible inspiration |
| _____ Grunt at end of expiration | |

**Prosody**

| | |
|---|---|
| _____ Rate overall | _____ Short phrases |
| _____ Increased rate overall | _____ Increased rate in segments |
| _____ Variable rate | _____ Reduced stress |
| _____ Intervals prolonged | _____ Inappropriate silences |
| _____ Short rushes of speech | _____ Excess and equal stress |

**Articulation**

| | |
|---|---|
| _____ Imprecise consonants | _____ Phonemes prolonged |
| _____ Phonemes repeated | _____ Vowels distorted |
| **Intelligibility** 1, 2, 3, 4, 5, 6, 7 | **Bizarreness** 1, 2, 3, 4, 5, 6, 7 |

Note: From *Motor Speech Disorders* by F. L. Darley, A. Aronson, and J. Brown, 1975, Philadelphia: W. B. Saunders Co. Adapted by permission.

Pitch level may be too high, too low, monotonous, or may break or squeak. Loudness may be inappropriate. It may decay to inaudible levels, show rapid and disconcerting changes, or be too loud or too soft most of the time. Voice quality may reflect too much nasal resonance, breathy or harsh quality, or the strained-strangled quality characteristic of excessive muscular contraction. Respiration may be audible when it should be silent, too shallow (resulting in not enough breath to finish utterances), or irregular. Articulation may be characterized by distorted and imprecisely formed consonant sounds, repeated sounds, abnormally prolonged vowels and consonants, or irregular breakdown in sound production. Finally, prosody (rate, stress, and melodic line) may be too fast, too slow, inappropriate to sentence meaning, or equalized and reduced without regard for normal syllable or word stress.

Overall, the speech pattern of the dysarthric speaker may be affected along two general dimensions, intelligibility and bizarreness. Speech can be perfectly intelligible and yet be so bizarre that the listener judges it as abnormal. For example, in some of the neurologic diseases that affect control of muscular contraction of the vocal folds, speech may be relatively clearly articulated and easy to understand, but may be characterized by wildly fluctuating pitch or loudness. This can be disconcerting to listen to, and may call undue attention to the speaker along with judgments of a strange or abnormal speech pattern.

## Clusters of Deviant Speech Dimensions

*See Rosenbek and LaPointe (1985) for a summary of distinctive characteristics of the various dysarthria types based on this research. This summary associates each type with its underlying neurologic condition, location of neural damage, deficit in neuromuscular tone or movement, cluster of deviant speech dimension, and most distinctive or characteristic speech deviation.*

Darley, Aronson, and Brown (1975) attempted not only to refine our perceptual skills by directing our attention to precisely defined behavioral aspects of deviant speech, but also to establish ways to distinguish among the varieties of dysarthria by identifying clusters of deviant speech dimensions associated with specific neurologic disorders. Analysis of these clusters led to deductions about the underlying neuromuscular mechanism that was responsible, and led further to the application of an appropriate name for each type of dysarthria. Four distinct types of dysarthria were outlined: (a) flaccid dysarthria (in bulbar palsy or brainstem disorders), (b) spastic dysarthria (in pseudobulbar palsy), (c) ataxic dysarthria (in cerebellar disorders), and (d) hypokinetic dysarthria (in dystonia and chorea). In addition, they describe mixed dysarthrias that result from disorders of multiple motor systems, and are associated with the ravaging diseases of ALS, multiple sclerosis, Wilson's disease, and a variety of other conditions.

While the characteristic cluster of deviant speech that emerges is more dependent on location and extent of brain or cranial nerve damage than on the specific disease involved, certain conditions or diseases many times will produce easily associated speech patterns. For example, Parkinson's disease produces a high prevalence of speech disruption that frequently takes the form of reduced pitch and loudness variability, reduced loudness, reduced speech stress, and short bursts of speech. Another disease process, myesthenia gravis, is characterized by abnormal tiring and weakness of skeletal muscles. This condition results in progressive hypernasality, increased nasal emission during prolonged acts of speech, deterioration of articulation with increasing fatigue, and progressive reduction of loudness level. Description as well as assessment and rehabilitation suggestions for these degenerative disorders and other conditions that result in characteristic speech patterns are covered thoroughly in a work that focuses on clinical management of dysarthric speakers (Yorkston, Beukelman, & Bell, 1988). Though the work on motor speech at the Mayo Clinic has done much to highlight differences among the dysarthrias, in clinical practice these distinctions are rarely clear-cut. In our clinic, many of our evaluations result in judgments of "mixed" dysarthria. Even the most experienced clinician may be unable to classify every dysarthric speaker.

## Apraxia of Speech

"I know what it is, but I can't say it." Anyone who has worked with people with apraxia has heard this affirmation frequently. Patients will report that they have a clear idea of what they intend, but cannot get the speech sequence started or keep it rolling once it is started. There is little doubt that, in many instances, they know well what they intend to say because they can write it, describe it, or give salient features of it. What does the resulting speech attempt sound like? From the definition, we expect the signs to be impaired volitional production of articulation and prosody. These articulation and prosodic disturbances do not result from muscular weakness or slowness, nor do they result from the linguistic disturbances in word meaning or impaired use of grammatical rules that we see in aphasia. This is not to say that apraxia of speech cannot coexist with other disorders. The same brain lesion that disturbs programming of speech movements can impinge on areas that affect language or range of motion of the tongue. Frequently these disorders *do* coexist, thus complicating the sorting-out process and making the speech-language pathologist's judgmental skills all the more important in the decisions about which aspects of deficient speech are the most detrimental to communication, and which ones are amenable to treatment.

*artic*
*& prosody*

*In fact, some authorities consider apraxia to be an integral feature of Broca's aphasia, which is discussed in detail in chapter 12.*

A variety of both speech and nonspeech behaviors have been suggested as being characteristic of apraxia of speech. A small explosion of clinical research interest took place in the 1960s and 1970s, resulting in many attempts to describe and highlight the salient features of the condition. One such description of apraxia of speech is presented by Wertz, LaPointe, and Rosenbek (1984). From their summary, we can see that the person with speech apraxia frequently pauses inordinately, gropes for articulatory position, restarts words and sentences, substitutes speech sounds (sometimes adding complicated clusters of sounds for the intended single sound target), and makes prepositioning or postpositioning errors (just as we sometimes do on the typewriter). Amid all this searching and speech sound groping, she slows down her rate and appears to "tip-toe" through speech in the apparent anticipation of problems stringing sequences together. Remarkable variability on repeated attempts at the same target are often produced. An example of some of these features can be seen in the transcribed dialogue below, as one of our speech-language pathologists elicited words from a patient seen in our clinic. This man was a 48-year-old carpenter from Crystal River, Florida, who suffered a left hemisphere stroke about 2 months before the interview.

*Johns and LaPointe (1976) trace this development in their chapter on neurogenic disorders of output processing.*

**Speech-language pathologist:** All right, say these things after me: pen, knife, hospital.
**Patient:** Pen, knife, hopay, hop, ah, . . . pos, . . . pester, as . . . I can't get all that.
**Speech-language pathologist:** Try it again, hospital.
**Patient:** Hospin-a . . .
**Speech-language pathologist:** I may go fishing on Sunday.

> **Patient:** I may go fishing on Sunday.
> **Speech-language pathologist:** Australia is a small continent.
> **Patient:** Uh . . . Arsale-a is a . . . nah, ah, coneh . . . ah, I can't get that.
> **Speech-language pathologist:** Try it again, Australia is a small continent.
> **Patient:** A las eh . . . I can't get that.
> **Speech-language pathologist:** O.K., we'll go on. You're anxious to get out, huh?
> **Patient:** I gotta get out.
> **Speech-language pathologist:** Are you going to go back to work?
> **Patient:** I sure am. Yessir. Soon as I can.
> **Speech-language pathologist:** What type of work do you do?
> **Patient:** Construction.
> **Speech-language pathologist:** Are you working on a job right now?
> **Patient:** I was, yah. Over in ah, Clivem, ah, ah . . .
> **Speech-language pathologist:** What job?
> **Patient:** A church over in Cri . . . Crystal Riv . . .
> **Speech-language pathologist:** Over where?
> **Patient:** Critchal, ah, Critchal . . . Ril . . . Ril . . . yah.
> **Speech-language pathologist:** Crystal?
> **Patient:** Right. Ridden . . . R-R-Ridden . . .
> **Speech-language pathologist:** That's right, Crystal.
> **Patient:** Criden, criden, Crystal . . . River.
> **Speech-language pathologist:** What kind of work do you do?
> **Patient:** I'm a coffiney . . . eh. A coffiney. ahhh. Carpenter.

This sample illustrates several aspects of speech apraxia. Dozens of features have been catalogued as characteristic of the disorder, but we feel that there are three cardinal behavioral features.

1. *Many sound substitutions and transpositions,* frequently including additive substitutions of more complex consonant clusters for a single sound target. For example, asked to repeat the word *bicycle,* the person may say "tise, tise, sicycle, licycle, sprykle, sprickle, . . . spicyle."

2. *Initiation difficulty,* characterized by stops; restarts; phoneme, syllable, and whole-word repetitions; audible groping for articulatory position; and silent searching and posturing of the articulators. When asked "Where do you live?" one person responded, "[pause] Coneve . . . Goneve . . . Jah . . . Jah . . . Jake. [silent visible tongue movements] . . . L . . . Lake . . . LLLake Geneva . . . whew."

3. *Variability of production pattern* on immediate repeated trials of the same target, including changes in type of error and performance varying on and off target. In imitating the word *refrigerator,* one patient said, "Refrig . . . ridgerator, ridgefrigerator, frigerator, frefridgerator, refrigerator, regrigerator, ridgerator."

Speculation has arisen that types of speech apraxia may exist. Clinical observation seems to confirm the impression that the phonologic impairment in persons with lesions more toward the back portions of the brain is less likely to present the halting, groping, initiation difficulty that seems to characterize patients with brain damage that is more toward the front. This is a rich area for future research and description. Severity of apraxia of speech certainly varies, and sometimes the disorder is so severe that the patient is practically speechless, and the features that are usually used to define the disorder are not apparent. With these severely impaired individuals, we can only infer from the nature of their speech attempts whether or not the disorder seems to resemble one of disturbed programming or neuromuscular sequences. An overview of the research and a few changing ideas about the disorder has been presented by Rosenbek, Kent, and LaPointe (1984).

Much remains to be learned about the precise nature and the underlying mechanisms of all the motor speech disorders. Much also needs to be learned about what to do to correct them. Work from the speech science laboratory and the rehabilitation clinic gives us reason to be hopeful.

# ASSESSMENT

For the speech-language pathologist who works in a hospital or rehabilitation clinic, the usual request for services arrives in the form of a single sheet of paper, often called a "Request for Consultation Services." This form frequently comes from a physician or team of health care providers. It includes a summary of the patient's medical diagnosis, along with a brief statement of the person's medical history. A typical request might read, "This is a 54-year-old man who suffered a left hemisphere CVA 2 weeks ago that left him hemiplegic and without speech. Please evaluate his communicative status and recommend a course of treatment, if appropriate." This request or any other type of referral then serves as the springboard for setting in motion the assessment or evaluation of the individual's communication.

*CVA stands for cerebro-vascular accident, or stroke.*

## Purposes of Evaluation

Why do you undertake the assessment process? The evaluation answers a number of crucial questions and has several purposes.

First of all, the evaluator must decide whether or not a significant problem exists. Occasionally a person is referred and has a dialect of English or a foreign accent that is a long-standing speech pattern, and the person neither requires nor desires intervention. On rare occasions, the referred patient may have a temporary problem easily corrected at bedside, as in the case of a patient referred to me at a Denver hospital with the diagnosis of "muffled speech . . . hard to understand." Upon bedside interview, the patient spoke with imprecise articulation and minimal jaw excursions during conversational speech. Deft questioning and examination of the intraoral cavity revealed the presence of a wad of chewing tobacco the size of a small cornish hen. Upon removal of the tobacco, this man's speech cleared considerably. The patient revealed that he had a long-standing habit of chewing tobacco, and said he wasn't about to stop just because he was hospitalized, even if the doctors had trouble understanding him. In this case, it was determined that no sustaining communication problem existed. A second purpose is to determine the nature of the impairment. If a disorder exists, it is important to determine if it is classifiable by type, and to judge the relative prominence of the deviant speech signs with an eye to determining those that contribute most to the communication handicap.

The next question is how handicapping is the condition. Compared to others with similar problems, is the disorder mild, moderate, or severe? The evaluation will attempt to shed light on these questions of relative severity. Also considered will be the effect of the disorder on functional communication needs for daily living, as well as on any specific vocational or life-style pecularities of the individual.

The establishment of a prognosis is another purpose of the assessment. Information gained from the evaluation will be incorporated with a variety of other variables such as age, time since onset, presence of other medical complications, motivation, and family support. As we have seen, accurate prediction is not a hard science in many areas of speech-language pathology, and here again the speech-language pathologist must be cautious in treading the fine line between dampening hope and igniting unrealistic and unattainable dreams of recovery. Prognosis for what? This is always an important question to answer after assessment is completed, when goals are being established.

Another important function of the evaluation is to find out which functions are intact and which are impaired, and to determine baselines of communication performance. Qualitative and quantitative measurements of performance on clearly defined speech tasks can serve as standards of reference to gauge any future change.

Next, the speech-language pathologist will have to begin somewhere if remediation is attempted. The information gained from the evaluation, along with judgments of the relative severity of components of the speech production system and their relative contribution to effective communication, will be invaluable in deciding on the focus and direction of treatment. This may be one of the single most important reasons for assessment—to answer the questions "What's wrong?" and "What should I attempt to correct?"

Finally, questions about the nature, severity, and outcome of the condition will be asked by family, friends, related medical personnel, and the patient, as well as by the source of the referral. Thus, another function of evaluation is to provide information. It will be comforting to all to be informed that the condition is known, has a label, and has been seen before, and that intervention and amelioration can be tried and may well work.

## Evaluation Strategies

Few published measurement batteries are available for the evaluation of motor speech disorders (unlike aphasia, for which there is a wide choice of commercially available tests). Most of the methods for the assessment of speech apraxia and dysarthria have grown out of the clinical experience of the examiner, or out of principles based on findings in the speech science laboratories. A more systematic approach to evaluation has been developing. This approach combines the principles of perceptual evaluation of the speech process with analysis of function of the components of the speech production system. This strategy is an amalgamation of ideas developed and refined by a host of researchers and clinicians, including some at the University of Iowa, the Mayo Clinic, the Speech Motor Control Laboratory of the University of Wisconsin, The Boys Town Institute for Communicative Disorders, and Veterans' Administration Medical Centers in Madison, Memphis, Martinez, and elsewhere.

The fundamentals of the assessment process are similar to those in other speech-language pathologies. These include arriving at conclusions and decisions by piecing together bits of information from four areas:

1. Personal history (medical, social, educational)
2. Nonspeech function of the structures of speech
3. Conversational and social interactive speech
4. Special speech tasks

Berry and LaPointe (1974) recommend using a standard recording protocol for this evaluation process. This has been supplemented by evaluation of performance on a series of special tasks, based on suggestions by Darley et al. (1975), Hardy (1967), Hixon (1975), Netsell (1973), Rosenbek and LaPointe (1985), and Wertz (1985). Yorkston, Beukelman, and Traynor (1984) is another example. A variety of other instrumental approaches to evaluation of the acoustic and physiological events of speech are described in Rosenbek (1984) and in Baken (1987). The Frenchay Dysarthria Assessment presents a standardized approach to evaluation, and has been validated across five groups of patients with motor speech impairment (Enderby, 1983).

### Nonspeech Movement

Nonspeech function of the structures of speech can be evaluated by requesting a series of movements of the articulators. Careful observation of the symmetry, color, configuration, and general appearance of the lips, tongue, soft palate, teeth, and jaw provides the first clues to judgments of normal structure. A series of systematic tasks designed to test the movements of these structures also can reveal gross abnormalities. For instance, the simple request to pucker the lips may uncover a fundamental problem.

## Swallowing

Frequently individuals who suffer neurologic involvement of the motor speech system also present difficulty in swallowing (dysphagia). It is well documented that a person can experience difficulty in swallowing and eating, and present no discernible impairment of speech, thereby discrediting the assumption that speech and the act of swallowing are inextricably intertwined. Though controversy exists about the role of speech-language professionals in the evaluation and treatment of swallowing disorders, professionals in our field are called on more and more to provide these services. Specific swallowing disorders have been associated with the four stages of swallowing: oral preparatory, oral, pharyngeal, and esophageal. Corresponding disorders at each of these stages, as well as advice on assessment and treatment, are discussed in considerable detail by Logemann (1983).

## The Point-Place System

The point-place model for assessment of the functional components of the motor speech system is a useful strategy for evaluating the integrity of each of the valves in the speech production system. Returning to Figure 13.4, we usually start at the bottom of the system and move sequentially through the numbers. This may be crudely analogous to stopping at evaluative checkpoints along a river that moves from south to north, like the Nile River. Thus, the caption "valves along the Nile" reminds us of the direction and sequence of the assessment process of the functional components of speech.

*Respiration (number 1).* Hixon (1973) has contributed a good deal to our understanding of the normal respiratory process and how to evaluate it. This is the pump or the energy source for speech; if it is impaired, speech can be weak, with reduced loudness, frequent and abnormal inhalation, decreased syllables per breath, short phrases, and reduced duration of phonation.

We have some rather embryonic guidelines for normalcy on some of these special tasks. At the respiratory level, these include the judgment of adequate conversational loudness (including the ability to muster a shout or to talk over noise), enough sustained respiration for speech to produce 10 to 20 syllables on a single breath, the ability to manipulate loudness so that adequate stress for changes in meaning can be produced, and vowel prolongation for a period of 10 to 20 seconds. Tasks specifically designed to evaluate the muscles and structures of respiration include connected, spontaneous speech, and the demonstration of rapid control of the system by the ability to rapidly sniff air up the nose, pant, demonstrate abrupt changes in loudness, imitate patterns of loudness change, and blow into a manometer to observe air pressure matching ability.

*Phonation (number 2).* The precise control of the laryngeal system for the process of phonation is vital to speech production and is interrelated with the process of respiration. It is somewhat artificial to evaluate respiration and phonation segmentally, as it is for all of the individual components of the system, but for convenience and ease of understanding, focus on specific phonatory tasks can be instructive. Impaired range, velocity, or direction of movement within the laryngeal system can result in decreased pitch range, slow pitch change, abnormal voiced-voiceless contrasts, slowed voice onset or offset time, breathiness, strained-strangled voice quality, pitch or loudness bursts, or increased habitual pitch use.

*Resonance (number 3).* The principal feature of resonance that is evaluated at valve number 3 is that of oral-nasal resonance balance. As we have seen, only a few sounds in English (/m, n, ŋ/) require nasal resonance for their production. The production of all other English speech sounds necessitates a closure or nearly complete closure of the velopharyngeal valve, and several muscle groups are responsible for the adequate functioning of this valve. Inadequate movement of this valve is fairly easy to recognize perceptually.

Judgments of appropriateness should always be made with community and dialectal standards in mind. The practiced ear is still the final judge about appropriateness of resonance balance, and when connected speech, the cul-de-sac test, and resonance balance on vowels is deemed adequate and resonance balance is judged to be normal, there is no need for an intervention plan on this particular aspect of speech.

Careful listening to conversation is one of the best strategies for detecting either resonance imbalance or the inappropriate emission of a nasal air stream. Some of the instrumental analysis techniques developed for use with people with cleft palates can be used to trace the velar movement in patients with neurogenic damage as well. These include oral-nasal pressure manometers, high-speed motion picture X rays (cineradiography), and a simple device that is plugged into the nostrils and activates a colorful piece of styrofoam within a sealed tube if excessive nasal air escapes during speech.

*You may wish to review these techniques, which were presented in chapter 11.*

*Articulation (numbers 4, 5, 6, 7).* For many years, the concept of dysarthria was intimately tied to deficient articulation. Deficient range, velocity, or direction of movement with the tongue, lips, and jaw can result in imprecise production of consonant and vowel sounds, and this deficiency can be one of the most noticeable and dramatic barriers to clear speech.

As with all the other functional components of the speech production system, the integrity of the valves of the upper airway is best tested by careful observation of their use in connected speech. Another useful measure is a sentence or single-word test of articulation. This should be organized so that

*See chapter 7.*

it systematically elicits all the sounds of American English in the positions where they are likely to occur.

Other tasks that reveal slowness, timing, or coordination problems at valves 4, 5, 6, and 7 include measures of Sequential Movement Rate (SMR) and Alternating Movement Rate (AMR). This can be measured by rating the quality as well as the number of times per second an individual can produce the sounds "kuh, kuh, kuh . . ." (valve 4), "tuh, tuh, tuh . . ." (valve 5), "puh, puh, puh . . ." (valve 6), and "puh, tuh, kuh . . ." (valves 6, 5, 4).

*Prosody.* As we have seen, *prosody* refers to the aspects of language that convey meaning and melody to the speech act. The meaning imparted by prosody is in addition to that already conveyed by the semantic aspects of the words. If prosodic variables are impaired, both the intelligibility and perception of normalcy of the speaker can be affected. Fine adjustments at all seven levels can alter rate, stress, or speech melody, and the speech evaluation must consider the contribution of each.

## Apraxia of Speech

Many of the measures used to determine the presence and severity of dysarthria can be used to evaluate apraxia of speech. Spontaneous speech and a variety of automatic and imitative utterances can be used to judge the nature of the disturbance, keeping in mind the definitional characteristics that highlight the speech apraxic patient.

Special tasks, many of which have been described earlier, can contribute information on the integrity of both articulation and prosody. These tasks include

1. Repetition of "puh," "tuh," "kuh," and "puh-tuh-kuh"
2. Imitation of single-syllable words
3. Imitation of longer words (three syllables and greater)
4. Sentence imitation
5. Reading aloud standard passages
6. Spontaneous speech

The evaluation of oral, nonverbal movements may also shed light on volitional movement disturbance in the apraxic patient, but the relationship of impaired nonverbal movement ("pucker your lips," "blow," "wiggle your tongue," "pretend you are licking a stamp") to impaired speech remains unclear.

After articulation, prosody, and nonverbal skills have been evaluated, the speech-language pathologist has the basis for deciding whether or not the patient's performance meets the definition of speech apraxia.

## Developmental Apraxia of Speech

The diagnosis of apraxia of speech in children, so-called developmental apraxia of speech, is not nearly as clear-cut as the adult variety that can be associated with an easily documented brain episode. Controversy perists as to whether or not the condition even exists in children, yet many researchers and clinicians maintain that the hard-core articulation disorders that are extremely resistant to remediation might well constitute a special subgroup. Suggestions of high probability indicators to diagnose developmental apraxia of speech include (1) an increasing number of errors on longer responses, (2) an accompanying oral apraxia, (3) groping postures of the speech muscles, and (4) prominent voice/voiceless errors. Details on the symptoms and differential diagnosis of the condition are available in Haynes (1985). Treatment suggestions for the condition are outlined in Blakeley (1983).

## Interpretation of Findings

After all the tests and special tasks have been administered and a stockpile of performance data has accumulated, the speech-language pathologist has the responsibility of making sense of it. Reducing, culling, and organizing the data is no easy job, but it is a crucial one. This is the point when judgments of relative importance of deviant dimensions must be made. The evaluator must decide which deviant aspects of speech contribute most to the nonintelligible or bizarre speech. This is also the time when you can organize hierarchies and priorities of treatment focus. "Relief from the greatest evil" is a guide for organizing a list of priorities. When the lifeboat springs a leak, you do not worry about how soon it can be given a fresh coat of paint. Similarly, we do not begin dysarthria treatment by polishing the precision of word endings if an impaired respiratory system renders the speech signal barely audible. Making sense of the assessment data also includes an attempt to find dimensions that are most easily modified, perhaps by postural adjustment, manipulation of speech rate, or some such change that may have a dramatic effect on speech.

*Chapter 14 discusses some of the ways posture can affect speech.*

Though interpretation of findings can be thought of as the final step in the evaluation process, it is easy to conceive of it as interwoven with the treatment process. In fact, it may well be thought of as the first step in the treatment process. It is to the process of intervention that we now turn.

## TREATMENT

Early attempts at treating people with motor speech disorders ranged from witchcraft to abandonment. Even in relatively recent times, some writers in speech pathology have expressed the view that little can be done to improve the lot of those afflicted with neurologic speech disorders. The tide has turned, though. Not only are people with motor speech disorders no longer neglected, but some exciting advances in clinical management have emerged.

A number of avenues to treatment exist. Some of these are listed in Table 13.5. Most of the time the intervention program chosen by the speech-language pathologist will be behavioral or palliative, or involve the implementation of an alternative communication system, as was attempted with our patient Jack, described in the case history at the beginning of the chapter. Sometimes, though, we must work in cooperation with the family physician, a surgeon, or a specialist in the construction and fitting of prosthedontic devices to implement the best mode of management.

As Darley and colleagues (1975) have outlined, there are some basic principles that undergird our treatment of motor speech. These include

1. *Developing compensatory strategies*—this includes not only working around the physical limitations imposed, but also making maximum use of those strengths that remain.

2. *Automatic to volitional shift*—an inescapable direction to be followed in treatment is that more purposeful control over behaviors that were once automatic and overlearned must be fostered.

3. *Monitoring behavior and change*—skills in patient self-monitoring must be an integral part of treatment. Tape recordings and progress charting are also vital to judgments of change.

4. *Get an early start*—many an indecorous habit can be avoided by early attention to more efficient communication.

5. *Foster motivation*—treatment must include providing information, concern, support, and warm interaction if the patient's motivation for change is to be influenced.

These basic principles provide a firm foundation for any attempt to manipulate communication potential.

**Table 13.5**   Possible Avenues of Treatment

| | |
|---|---|
| Medical | Alleviate cause |
| | Pharmaceutic |
| Surgical | Pharyngeal flap operation |
| Prosthetic | Construct lift for denervated soft palate |
| Behavioral | Modify neuromuscular, aerodynamic events |
| Palliative | "Hold the line" |
| | Lessen effect by acceptance |
| Alternative Mode | Gesture |
| | Communication aid |

Rosenbek and LaPointe (1985) reiterate some of these principles and supplement them with a *behavioral context* for treatment of motor speech disorders. This context is relevant to a variety of communication impairments, as well as speech apraxia and the variety of dysarthrias that may be encountered. The first component is *drill,* a usual mode of behavioral therapy that is useful in the modification of the neuromuscular and aerodynamic events impaired in motor speech disturbance. Drill is systematic practice of specially selected and ordered exercises. *Task continua,* another behavioral technique, reffers to the development of progressively more difficult tasks. The direction and flow of progress can be directed by moving closer and closer to those skills that approximate normal speech, or at least the most efficient means of speech within the limits of the impaired speech production system.

*Knowledge of results* is a fundamental aspect of treatment. It can be accomplished by instruments that provide visual or auditory feedback of performance, the direct remarks of the speech-language pathologist ("Good job!" "Not so hot." "That was almost loud enough, but give it a little more oomph!"), video- or audiotape recordings made periodically during treatment, or the careful recording of baseline performance and session-by-session progress on a percentage graph. Recordings and changes in performance over time were useful in the treatment of Jack, as described in his case history, and provided a means for judging degree of progress. Finally, the *organization of sessions* entails decisions on scheduling, such as the length, frequency, and format of each session.

# SPECIFIC TREATMENT GOALS

As we have seen throughout this book, each plan of therapy must be hand-tailored to fit the peculiar characteristics and desires of the individual. Emphasis and focus of therapy will vary according to the priorities and hierarchies of function and dysfunction established during the interpretation of the evaluation results. Style and specific techniques will vary somewhat from setting to setting, but the underlying principles and the ultimate objectives are fairly constant. We like to use the functional component (point-place) and perceptual speech process approach as a model for our treatment. From this base, we have established a series of rather specific treatment goals (Rosenbek & LaPointe, 1978). A wide variety of specific techniques are possible to attain these goals, and a few of them will be explained in this section.

As you read through these goals, keep in mind that, depending on the presence and severity of individual signs and symptoms, one or more of these goals may be irrelevant to any specific person. Also, the order is not necessarily sequential as listed, and may be rearranged to fit the individual. Some of these specific treatment goals are applicable to people with either dysarthria or apraxia of speech. For example, goal 1 is appropriate to both. Those goals and strategies that are appropriate only to dysarthria or to apraxia of speech are so indicated.

## 1. Help the Person Become a Productive Patient (Appropriate for the Dysarthrias and Apraxia of Speech)

The techniques here are related to patient counseling and family education, and will be discussed in more detail in a following section. To foster productivity, we must be sure that the patient agrees on the necessity and value of treatment. Not everyone wants to return to the maximal levels of speech production, and this should be explored and respected. This was brought to my attention in the case of a 43-year-old former 5th-grade teacher who suffered a stroke and was making an excellent recovery of communication skills. We thought that, with an intensive program of therapy and a lot of diligent homework, we might be able to see him gain enough communication recovery to return to the classroom in about 12 to 14 months and live happily ever after. We assumed too much, though, and forgot to explore *his* desires. After about 6 months of rather intensive treatment, he informed us, "Look, I've got a pretty good disability pension now. My wife works and we have no financial worries. We have a 20-acre farm, and I'm really enjoying puttering around on the tractor and running the farm. Plus, I never could stand those kids in the classroom, and I have no desire to return to teaching. How long does this have to go on?" The astute speech-language pathologist tunes in to these cues of the specific communicative needs and desires of the person. We discharged this gentleman the following week—not only with our blessings but with a bit of envy.

Becoming a more productive patient means a mutual attention to the creation and *order* of specific behavioral goals. At this point, the cooperation of other people who are significant to the person should be enlisted, and they can begin to be educated about the disorder and course of treatment as well.

## 2. Modification of Posture, Tone, Strength (Applicable for the Dysarthrias)

Sometimes braces, slings, girdling, or simple postural adjustments can affect tone and strength, and ultimately provide a firmer foundation for the speech production system. Modifying strength, tone, and posture is a task that should be done in conjunction with other health care team members. The physician, physical therapist, or occupational therapist can offer valuable guidance in accomplishing this goal. Certain cautions must be observed, particularly in girdling a patient, since altering the respiratory system can cause pneumonia. This procedure should *always* be done under the supervision of a physician.

## 3. Modification of Respiration (Appropriate for the Dysarthrias)

Attempting to modify the respiratory system requires simultaneous attention to the phonatory, resonatory, and articulatory valves because they work in finely tuned harmony. Though the old elocution school strategies of breathing exercises are now passé, practice and improvement in developing controlled exhalation is an important objective. Respiration for speech requires predictable production of consistent, low-pressure exhalation over time. This can be facilitated by biofeedback (using the water manometer, with a goal of producing 5 cm of water pressure for a duration of 5 sec) or by other devices that allow visualization of a sustained air stream.

Such exotic instruments as the stopwatch, the tape recorder, and the ear of the speech-language pathologist are mainstays for achieving many of the following specific goals.

## 4. Modification of Phonation (Appropriate for the Dysarthrias)

Specific techniques for modification will vary with the underlying neuromuscular problem and the type of motor speech disturbance. For example, for hyperadduction (too much muscular contraction of the vocal folds, which results in harsh or strained-strangled voice quality), attempts are made to counter the overadduction. Using light, gentle articulation contacts; easy yawn-sigh vocalization; and open-mouth speech with exaggerated jaw excursions sometimes lessens the effects of the hyperadduction and improves quality.

For hypoadduction, with decreased loudness, breathy voice quality, and air wastage, the opposite approach is taken. Increasing the background of muscular effort is accomplished by pushing, lifting, and attempting quicker phonatory onset, and through drills on exaggerated contrastive stress in words and sentences. Any gains in control are expanded to longer, more complex, and more spontaneous speech utterances.

If the phonatory problem results from the abnormal coordination of an ataxic motor problem, the speech will be laced with abnormal pitch and loudness breaks and durational abnormalities because of imprecise timing of turning phonation on and off. These problems sometimes can be influenced by exploring inhibitory postures, drilling on durational control or increase, or what I call the Ethel Merman therapy ("I Got Rhythm") of rate manipulation. Rate can be manipulated by rhythmic pacing, tapping, or squeezing, or the use of external rhythmic sources such as a metronome or amplifying a colleague's heartbeat.

## 5. Modification of Resonance
## (Appropriate for the Dysarthrias)

*For more detail on
dealing with these
problems, refer to
chapter 11 on cleft
palate.*

Problems at valve 3, the velopharyngeal port, usually result in hypernasal voice quality and nasal emission of air. The individual can be made more aware of how this valve contributes to speech by using mirrors, models, and demonstrations. Visual feedback using an instrument that detects air leakage through the nose often aids in highlighting the problem. Contrastive speech drills with nasal-nonnasal words (*meat-Pete, my-pie,* etc.) and drill on correct timing of palatal elevation in words, phrases, and sentences can be useful in reducing the problem.

Occasionally, with a paralyzed soft palate, the services of the prosthodontist can be summoned for the design and fitting of a palatal lift. This is a device that is worn in the mouth, attaches to the teeth, and is designed to improve resonance balance by elevating the poorly innervated velum. The palatal lift is useful, however, only with certain cases.

## 6. Modification of Articulation (Appropriate for the Dysarthrias and Apraxia of Speech)

Lately there seems to be less primary emphasis on treating articulation in the motor speech disorders. In both apraxia of speech and dysarthrias, attention to the interaction of rate, stress, and durational factors in the accuracy of speech sound production is gaining favor.

We attend to the speech sound environment and coarticulating influences on accuracy, and generally treat speech movements in syllables instead of isolated sounds. Our speech targets may be the most involved valves or specific sound manner groups, such as plosives or fricatives. An underlying principle in modifying articulation is that it is paramount to analyze the errors and attempt to determine the reason for them. If faulty range, velocity, or direction of movement are implicated, the focus of attention in modifying articulation becomes clearer. The objective derived from this principle, then, is to attempt to change the range, velocity, direction, coordination, timing, or ordering of the speech movements to produce more acceptable sounds. This can be accomplished by a number of strategies, such as

1. *Integral stimulation*—"Watch me. Listen to me. Do what I do."
2. *Phonetic derivation*—a speech target may be derived from an intact speech gesture, such as producing /n/ by producing /m/, simultaneously lifting the tongue to the position of /l/, and then parting the lips.
3. *Phonetic placement*—points of articulatory contact can be explained and modeled by demonstration, pictures, molding, and hand postures.

Finally, articulatory task continua can be constructed in steps, such as

Step 1. /p/ in final position of vowel-consonant (VC) syllables—*ap*

Step 2. /p/ in final position of CVC syllables—*cap*

Step 3. /p/ in medial position in VCV syllables—*apah*

Step 4. /p/ in initial position, CV—*pay*

Step 5. /p/ in varying positions, words, phrases, sentences, controlled conversation

## 7. Modification of Prosody (Appropriate for the Dysarthrias and Apraxia of Speech)

The three prosodic features of rhythm, stress, and intonation have been neglected too often in the management of neurogenic speech disorders. In both apraxia of speech and dysarthria, attention to varying prosody can have rewarding effects on articulation. We believe that prosody interacts potently with articulation, and that prosodic manipulation is a rich and fruitful strategy for altering speech intelligibility. Contrastive stress drills, rate manipulation (stop strategies, metronome, pacing, tapping), delayed auditory feedback, and gestural reorganization (gestures accompanied by speech) can be excellent approaches to treatment of both apraxia of speech and some of the dysarthrias.

*Details of these techniques are presented in Wertz (1985) and Rosenbek and LaPointe (1985).*

## 8. Providing an Alternate Communication Mode (Appropriate for the Dysarthrias and Apraxia of Speech)

Sometimes, because of the severity of the disorder, the development of speech is out of the question and the decision must be made to provide an alternate mode of communication. Though this is never as desirable as natural speech production, it is much preferred over the alternative of isolation and no communication. A variety of alternatives are becoming available for the nonverbal and nonvocal patient these days, and the state of the art appears to be exploding with technological development. Computers, speech synthesizers, and other sophisticated electronic devices are being adapted to the needs of the speechless.

*See Figure 13.5.*

Other means, including communication and spelling boards, written communication, and gestural systems such as Amer-Ind (based on American Indian sign language), are more traditional. No doubt the future will bring a rich growth of techniques and devices that will make the instruments of the 1980s look quaint. An excellent summary on advances in the development of technology and instrumentation as applied to motor speech disorders has been presented by Rubow (1984).

## COUNSELING

In the motor speech disorders, as in most of the pathologies of communication, the overall objectives of counseling are threefold: to convey informa-

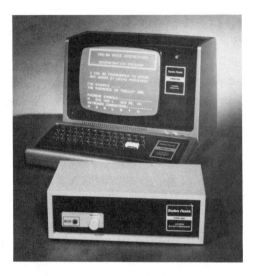

**Figure 13.5** Computers and voice synthesizers adapted to aid nonvocal and nonverbal persons. The TRS-80 voice synthesizer is packaged in a silver-gray cabinet with black front grill, slightly resembling a speaker enclosure. There is a volume control and device select indicator on the front panel next to a speaker. A ribbon cable emerges from the back of the cabinet, with a length sufficient to set the cabinet on top of the TRS-80 video display unit.

tion, to provide reassurance and emotional support, and to improve environmental communication variables. Counseling adults with dysarthria can be viewed as a process of patient and family education (Berry, 1978).

The information aspect of counseling can be carried out easily, and should be accomplished early in the course of management. The most natural questions in the world for anyone afflicted with a health trauma are: "What do I have?" "What is it called?" "What caused it?" "Is it serious?" "Does it threaten my life?" "How long will it last?" "Is it common?" "Can you do anything about it?" These are general questions that are almost reflexive to any medical condition. Specific to motor speech disorders, the patient or family might ask, "How can I make myself more clearly understood?" "What can we do to help?" "Why are eating and swallowing affected?" "Will medication help?" "Should I slow down or speed up my speech?"

Patient and family counseling also are necessary to establish treatment goals and specific treatment tasks. Effective therapy demands that the person with a motor speech disorder know why tasks are selected and the reasons for the employment of particular courses of treatment. The informed patient needs to be counseled on progress as well. The nature of relearning or facilitating speech production tasks must be explained. This means that we must carefully explain the concepts of gradual but consistent change; performance variability as a result of fatigue, illness, or emotional state; and plateauing of behavior.

Since treatment for the neurogenic disorders of speech production relies heavily on structured drill and systematic practice, we must be careful to avoid the suggestion that the therapeutic process is automatized, unswervingly programmed, or rigidly fixed in direction. There is plenty of room in a therapy session for pause, reflection, encouragement ("Way to go!"), humor, some small talk, and the warmth of human interaction. Often the planned activities of the session are best set aside so that more pressing emotional or information issues can be discussed. The quality of interaction, after all, is the core of the therapeutic process; without it, little can be expected in the arduous process of mending shattered communication.

# CONCLUSION

The past 35 years have seen dramatic and awe-inspiring advances in the development of a sophisticated technology in aerospace, electronic microcircuitry, plastics, and a host of other areas that make life more convenient. Some would argue, though, that the advances in fundamental knowledge of normal function of speech and a clearer understanding of the disruptions that occur in communication disorders are equally as impressive as the emergence of the cordless hedge trimmer, cordless Dustbuster™, styling mousse, and frozen yogurt.

These are exciting times for those who have committed and those who will commit their efforts and talents to the study and remediation of neurogenic speech impairment. Perhaps many of the current ideas we have about the nature and causes of neurologic speech disorders will be regarded as tentative working hypotheses in the future. There is no doubt, however, that we have a firm foundation for continued observation and systematic clinical research that will refine our abilities to help people afflicted with these disorders. The communication barriers created by neurologic disorders can be isolating, dehumanizing, and identity wrenching. Efforts to dissolve these barriers and restore efficient communicative interaction can be one of the noblest contributions to the restoration of human dignity.

# STUDY QUESTIONS

1. Review the section of this chapter that discusses the neurogenic disorders of speech. Compare and contrast the causes of neurogenic disorders of speech and of aphasia in adults discussed in Chapter 12. Make a listing of the causes that are shared and the causes that differ.

2. Dysarthria is associated with disorders of voice, prosody, and articulation as outlined in Table 13.4. Review Chapter 12 on aphasia in adults and identify which of the major aphasia types shares the characteristics listed for dysarthria. Make a list of the characteristics presented for each aphasia type to assist in the process.

3. Review the section of this chapter that covers the point-place model for evaluation. Compare this evaluation model with the model for evaluating voice disorders described in Chapter 8. Identify techniques and procedures which overlap in the two models.

4. Review the section covering specific treatment goals. Make a table which summarizes goals that are shared and goals that differ for treating dysarthria and speech apraxia.

5. Read the example of a dialogue with an adult with speech apraxia. Compare the features of this sample with features of the speech samples and with descriptions of the characteristics of the major aphasia types provided in Chapter 12. Identify which aphasia type the sample resembles the most.

# SELECTED READINGS

Johns, D., & LaPointe, L. L. (1976). Neurogenic disorders of output processing: Apraxia of speech. In H. Avakian-Whitaker & H. A. Whitaker (Eds.), *Current trends in neurolinguistics.* New York: Academic Press.

LaPointe, L. L. (1975). Neurologic abnormalities affecting speech. In D. B. Tower (Ed.), *The nervous system: Vol. 3. Human communication and its disorders.* New York: Raven Press.

Netsell, R. (1973). Speech physiology. In F. D. Minifie, T. J. Hixon, & F. Williams (Eds.), *Normal aspects of speech, hearing, and language.* Englewood Cliffs, NJ: Prentice-Hall.

Netsell, R., & Daniel, B. (1979). Dysarthria in adults: Physiologic approach to rehabilitation. *Archives of Physical Medicine and Rehabilitation, 60,* 502–508.

Rosenbek, J. C. (1978). Treating apraxia of speech. In D. F. Johns (Ed.), *Clinical management of neurogenic communicative disorders.* Boston: Little, Brown.

Rosenbek, J. C. (1984). Advances in the evaluation of speech apraxia. In F. C. Rose (Ed.), *Advances in neurology: Vol. 42. Progress in aphasiology.* New York: Raven Press.

Rosenbek, J. C., Kent, R., & LaPointe, L. (1984). Apraxia of speech: An overview and some perspectives. In J. Rosenbek, M. McNeil, & A. Aronson (Eds.), *Apraxia of speech: Physiology, acoustics, linguistics, management.* San Diego: College-Hill Press.

Rosenbek, J. C., & LaPointe, L. L. (1985). The dysarthrias: Description, diagnosis and treatment. In D. F. Johns (Ed.), *Clinical management of neurogenic communicative disorders* (2nd ed.). Boston: Little, Brown.

Wertz, R. T. (1985). Neuropathologies of speech and language: An introduction to patient management. In D. F. Johns (Ed.), *Clinical management of neurogenic communicative disorders* (2nd ed.). Boston: Little, Brown.

# CHAPTER FOURTEEN

# Cerebral Palsy

EDWARD D. MYSAK

## MYTHS AND REALITIES

- *Myth:* Because of advances in obstetrics, there should be fewer children born with cerebral palsy.

- *Reality:* Advances in obstetrics have resulted in many more fetuses surviving negative prenatal conditions, and many more babies surviving premature and difficult deliveries and early postnatal disorders; therefore, if anything, an increase in the number of infants with neurological disorders may be expected.

- *Myth:* All cases of cerebral palsy are due to some form of prenatal, natal, or early postnatal trauma.

- *Reality:* There is a small percentage of cases of cerebral palsy that appear related to familial or inherited factors.

- *Myth:* Cerebral palsy is primarily a neuromotor problem.

- *Reality:* In many cases of cerebral palsy, the most debilitating component is the sensory-perceptual-conceptual one.

- *Myth:* Children with cerebral palsy are mentally retarded.

- *Reality:* It is likely that half or more of these children have normal learning potential, and some show intelligence up to the gifted level.

**497**

- *Myth:* Speech and language disorders among children with cerebral palsy are pretty much alike.

- *Reality:* Cerebral palsy speech and language disorders may range from almost no discernible symptoms to profound involvement. There is no single cerebral palsy speech pattern.

- *Myth:* Children with cerebral palsy usually do not have hearing problems.

- *Reality:* As many as 20% or more of the children with cerebral palsy may have problems with hearing, including middle-ear, inner-ear, and central involvements.

- *Myth:* Since cerebral palsy is a medical problem, evaluations of such children should be coordinated by physicians.

- *Reality:* Cerebral palsy is a complex disorder with motor, perceptual, cognitive, socioemotional, and communicative components. Evaluations, therefore, must be conducted by a team of experts, including physicians, physical and occupational therapists, psychologists, special educators, and speech-language pathologists and audiologists.

- *Myth:* Since children with cerebral palsy are brain damaged, little or no improvement may be expected through therapy.

- *Reality:* Early intervention with a team approach to management may result in significant changes in motor, perceptual, cognitive, socioemotional, and communicative behaviors.

$\text{A}$s with so many afflictions (such as stuttering, mental retardation, emotional problems, and epilepsy) that have plagued humankind for a long time, myths frequently develop and accumulate. The condition known as cerebral palsy is no exception, and many myths have grown around it as well. The next section provides a case history that includes background and information frequently encountered in cases of cerebral palsy, such as problems during pregnancy; cesarean section delivery; low birthweight; and delays in motor, speech, social, and cognitive developments.

*Because Sally was in a breech position, she was delivered by cesarean section. She weighed 5 pounds at birth and was placed in an incubator. She remained in the hospital for about 2 weeks.*

*Sally's early development was slow. She did not sit alone until she was about 15 months old, did not crawl until she was about 2½ years old, and did not walk until she was almost 4 years old. At 4 years of age, toilet training was still a problem and she had not developed speech. She also had recurring ear infections.*

*When Sally was 4 years 5 months old, she was given a complete speech and hearing evaluation at a university speech and hearing center. The impression was that Sally exhibited a severe delay in speech, language, and cognitive abilities related to her neurological involvement. More specifically, auditory awareness was poor, and vocalization appeared confined to infrequent monosyllabic babbling.*

*At 4 years 11 months of age, an educational evaluation stated that Sally was functioning far below expectations in all areas of development. She was described as a child who was not toilet trained, did not ask for food, and did not make eye contact. A psychological evaluation estimated that Sally was functioning in the severely retarded range, her poorest performance was on expressive language tasks, and she was most advanced in the area of gross motor functioning. A social history report indicated that Sally was attending a normal nursery school and received special occupational and speech therapy. It stated that Sally's mother was concerned about Sally's educational needs and about obtaining an appropriate school placement for her. The social worker recommended that the mother receive some supportive help as well.*

*A total therapy program was recommended. It included facilitation of cognitive development, stabilization of speech posture, stimulation of listening movements and behavior, and stimulation of imitative vocalization and expressive communication. A home program involving the mother was also developed.*

*After about 1½ years of therapy, modest gains can be reported. Improvement was noted in language comprehension. Sally's monosyllabic vocalizations include plosives, nasals, and fricatives. Some multisyllabic utterances marked by intonation, stress, and prosody features have also been heard. One or two true words appear to be emerging.*

*Although Sally has made some progress, a lot more needs to be done. More family participation in the habilitation program will be requested. Increased emphasis will be placed on stimulating listening behavior, developing compensatory communication, and stimulating speech communication.*

**Cerebral palsy** is a general term for a brain injury resulting in a display of certain kinds of neurological symptoms. It is not a disease; it does not have a single specific cause or lead to specific symptoms. In fact, cerebral palsy can be so slight that it is hard to detect, or so severe that the person may never be able to be completely independent of support services. It is usually associated with the period of childhood, thought of as chronic and crippling, and commonly accompanied by significant speech problems. Many people with cerebral palsy are noticeable because of their motor and postural problems, which also affect their speech. Yet these same people, who may be confined to wheelchairs, may have average or above-average intelligence.

The symptoms associated with cerebral palsy may affect most of the important human functions, including the neurosensory, neuromotor, perceptual, cognitive, behavioral, and speech functions, as is true of Sally in the case history. To more fully understand the communication problems associated with cerebral palsy, we will first examine the general problem, and then follow with a discussion of the speech and language problem and its management.

## CHARACTERISTICS OF CEREBRAL PALSY

*See general texts (such as Connor, Williamson, & Siepp, 1978; Cruikshank, 1976; Marks, 1974; and Scherzer & Tscharnuter, 1982) for more information on the management of cerebral palsy.*

Because of the natural of cerebral palsy, much has been written about the various problems (including medical, intellectual, personality, visual, and dental) that occur among these children, and about the various types of management they need (including medical, psychological, special educational, occupational and physical therapy, social work, and vocational guidance). The professional organization devoted to the understanding and care of cerebral palsy is the American Academy for Cerebral Palsy and Developmental Medicine; the official journal of the academy is *Developmental Medicine and Child Neurology.*

### History

Prenatal, infantile and early childhood brain injury and consequent brain dysfunction have no doubt been a bane of humans from the earliest of times. Descriptions of crippled individuals appear in ancient Hebrew and Greek writings and in the Bible, and there is no reason to believe that some of the people referred to did not have neurological symptoms that today would be called cerebral palsy.

During the second half of the 15th century, pediatric textbooks began to describe symptoms of brain dysfunction: however, the classic paper on the connection between abnormal birth histories and childhood brain dysfunctions did not appear until 1861. It was written by an English physician by the name of Dr. Little. In the United States, concern for helping these children grew rapidly in the early 1940s. Dr. Winthrop Phelps (1940) organized one of the earliest systematic programs of management for children with cerebral palsy.

### Definition

*Cerebral palsy* is an umbrella term for a variety of congenital and early neurological disorders. Cerebral palsy, as we use it here, includes the full range of chronic brain syndromes from isolated articulation problems—which may only be heard and seen during the speech act—to severe and generalized sensorimotor involvement—in which the child is unable to walk, stand, sit, or even hold up his head, and where reaching, eating, and speaking movements are severely restricted. More specifically, cerebral palsies are complexes that result from damage to various parts of the brain; occur between conception and 2 years of age or so; and appear in various forms and combinations of sensorimotor, perceptual, behavioral, and speech disorders.

## Causes

Like many other conditions we have looked at, it is hard to pinpoint a specific cause for most cases of cerebral palsy. In general, we can say that the causes may be divided into two categories, familial and environmental.

### Familial

Certain cranial malformations, degenerative diseases, and static conditions such as familial tremor contribute a relatively small number of cases to the congenital cerebral palsies. Cranial malformations and degenerative diseases are usually excluded from the more restrictive definition of childhood cerebral palsy as a chronic and static disease.

*Recall that a congenital disorder is present at birth.*

### Environmental

Lesions acquired during the period from conception to about 1 month following birth account for the large majority of conditions that are eventually diagnosed as cerebral palsy. Prenatal causes, or all those factors that may contribute to brain injury before birth, include infections in the mother, such as mumps, rubella, and influenza; blood incompatibility in the mother, such as the Rh-negative factor; anesthesia, irradiation, and accidents; and placental and cord anomalies and disturbances. Central nervous system (CNS) malformations in the embryo and fetus can also be prenatal causes of cerebral palsy.

*The term placental anomalies describes abnormalities in the organ of metabolic interchange between fetus and mother.*

Natal factors, or all those factors that may contribute to brain injury during the birth period, include precipitate (less than 2 hours) or prolonged (more than 24 hours) deliveries, premature deliveries, breech or cesarean deliveries, irregular implantation of the placenta, and forceps manipulation and trauma.

Postnatal factors, or all those factors that may contribute to brain injury during approximately the first month of life, include infections, such as meningitis, encephalitis, roseola, measles, and whooping cough; lead poisoning; trauma; anoxia; and neoplasms or growths of the brain.

This long list of possible environmental causes of cerebral palsy suggests that, in any one case, more than one factor may be operative. In addition, the many disease processes represented may be related to lesions in different parts of the brain, which helps explain the variety of symptoms found in any one case of cerebral palsy.

## Incidence

*For a review of studies of incidence, see Cruickshank (1976), chapter 1.*

The true incidence of cerebral palsy is difficult to determine for many reasons. Not all specialists agree on the definition of the disorder with respect to the time of occurrence; location of the lesion; and type, severity, and predominance of the symptoms. Consistency, or lack of it, in reporting the disorder is another factor. Reported rates of occurrence of cerebral palsy range from 1 to 6 per 1,000.

## Types

We recognize a number of types of cerebral palsy. The types are named basically for clinical findings because of the lack of consistency between presenting symptoms and their severity and the location, cause, and size of the lesion. *Spasticity, athetosis, ataxia, rigidity, tremor,* and *atonia* are traditional terms used to describe various forms of cerebral palsy. Pure forms of tremor or atonia are rare, and are more likely to appear as part of other forms of cerebral palsy; on the other hand, mixed types are common, but usually children are classified according to their predominant symptoms. The speech-language pathologist may find it useful to include congenital isolated dysarthria and other manifestations of limited involvement of the brain under the category of subclinical forms of cerebral palsy.

### Spastic

Movements of children with **spastic** cerebral palsy are described as labored, stiff, or jerky. They show increased muscle tone and consistent limitations in direction and range of movement of body parts. The standing spastic child may demonstrate flexor spasms and inward rotation of the upper limbs or shoulder, elbow, and wrist, and extensor spasms and inward rotation of the lower limbs or thigh, knee, and foot. The walking spastic child may exhibit toe-walking because his lower limbs are hyperextended, and "scissors gait" or leg crossover because of the overadduction and inward rotation of the thighs.

*When a muscle flexes, it contracts and tightens; when it extends, it stretches.*

Traditionally, spastic symptoms are thought to be caused by involvement of the pyramidal tract in the cortical or subcortical areas of the brain. The neurodynamics of the condition may be described as a lack of automatic inhibition by the cerebrum of various levels of the CNS, from which basic muscle tone is controlled. Neurological signs of this interference with higher center regulation over lower centers include exaggerated stretch reflexes (uncontrolled counteraction to the muscle being stretched), Babinski's reflex

*These portions of the central nervous system are described in chapter 3.*

*Figure 14.1 shows a child with a spastic posture.*

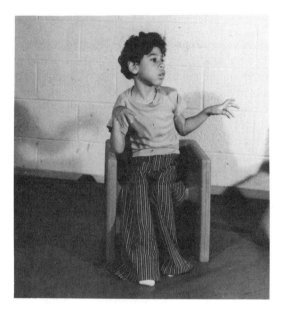 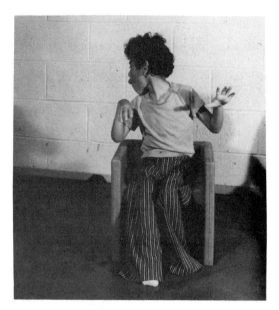

**Figure 14.1**   Two views of a child displaying a spastic posture

(fanning of toes in response to a stimulus applied to the sole of the foot), and ankle clonus (alternating contraction and relaxation of the foot in response to sudden flexion of the ankle).

## Athetotic

Movements of children with **athetotic** cerebral palsy are described as involuntary and wormlike or writhing. They are characterized by variability in muscle tone, and by inconsistency in movements in appropriate directions and of appropriate ranges. The child with athetosis who is at rest and relaxed may make few of these involuntary movements; however, when she is required to reach for something or to speak, she may have a burst of involuntary, writing movements. Attempts at voluntary movements during periods of emotion or excitement usually intensify the problem.

*Athetotic means without a fixed base.*

Traditionally, athetotic symptoms are ascribed to involvement of the basal nuclei and their connections, or to involvement of the extrapyramidal system. The neurodynamics of the condition may be described in at least two ways: (a) interference of the regulating or smoothening influence of the extrapyramidal system over the pyramidal system; or (b) a lack of control by the higher, voluntary movement centers of the extrapyramidal system. The neurological signs of this impairment in the relationship between pyramidal and extrapyramidal systems are pre-emptive movements (involuntary movements preceding voluntary ones), writhing movements, and variable muscle tone.

## Ataxic

**Ataxic** *means lack of order.*

Movements of children with ataxic cerebral palsy are described as awkward, clumsy, and uncoordinated. They are characterized by reduced muscle tone (hypotonia) and problems in the guidance of movements in appropriate directions. Because of his problems in maintaining balance, the standing ataxic child may display a wide-based stance. When walking, he may display a birdlike posture of a forward placed head and backward placed arms, in addition to a gait that accelerates involuntarily.

Traditionally, ataxic symptoms are ascribed to involvement of the cerebellum. The neurodynamics of the condition may be described as a failure of the CNS to receive appropriate feedback concerning the progress of movements due to disturbance in general proprioception (muscle, joint, tendon sense) and special proprioception (balance sense from the ears). The cerebellum appears to compare the intended movements of the voluntary motor center with the actual movements, as reflected by the position and movement feedback it receives. If there are discrepancies, the cerebellum automatically relays adjustment signals to the voluntary motor center until there is a match between intended and actual movements. Neurological signs of cerebellar dysfunction include:

- Problems in coordination of multimuscle groups, as may be used in returning a ping-pong ball, for example
- Undershooting or overshooting a fork on the table with a reaching hand, for example
- Difficulty in maintaining a serial repetitive movement, such as repetitive eyebrow raising, panting, or uttering /pʌ/ rapidly and rhythmically
- A tremor that appears only during a voluntary movement
- Ocular and head **nystagmus** (an involuntary slow movement in one direction followed by a rapid movement in the opposite direction)

## Rigidity

*Figure 14.2 shows a child with a rigidity posture.*

Children with cerebral palsy of the rigidity type show extremely limited or almost no movements. They appear stiff and inflexible. In the extreme form, a child with rigidity who is lying on the back may exhibit a "bridging" posture, where her head and feet are in contact with the surface and the rest of her body is arched upward from the surface.

Traditionally, rigidity symptoms are ascribed to widespread involvement of inhibitory centers of the brain. In rigidity, in contrast to spastic symptoms, the resistance to slow passive motion is greater than that to rapid passive motion, antagonists to antigravity muscles are more involved, and clonus and stretch reflexes are absent.

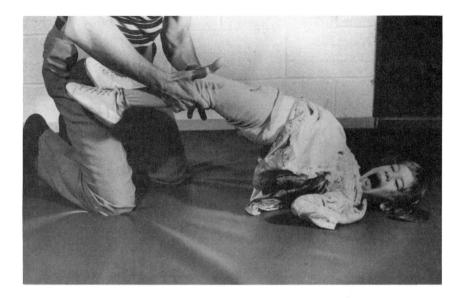

**Figure 14.2**   Child displaying a rigidity posture in supine position

## Tremor and Atonia

Pure tremor or atonia types of cerebral palsy are rare, and usually appear as part of the symptom complexes of other forms of cerebral palsy. *Tremor* means trembling or shaking; unlike the writhing movements found in athetosis, tremor is characterized by regular and symmetrical movements produced by the alternating contraction of muscles and their antagonists. Tremor appears in two forms: intention and nonintention. Intention tremor, or that tremor triggered by a voluntary movement, is traditionally attributed to cerebellar involvement; nonintention tremor, or the tremor that appears when the individual is at rest, is traditionally attributed to basal nuclei involvement.

*Atonia* describes a condition where the muscles are overrelaxed or flaccid. The atonic infant may be described as a floppy baby. Traditionally, the condition is attributed to involvement of the cerebellum—the center responsible for maintaining normal muscle tension.

## Subclinical

The term *subclinical* refers to those children who do not show obvious sensorimotor problems, but who nevertheless have central nervous system (CNS) involvement. Children with neurogenic learning disabilities including dyslexia or those with perceptual problems, for example, may be viewed as having minimal brain dysfunction or "subclinical cerebral palsy." These

*These problems were discussed in depth in chapters 5 and 6.*

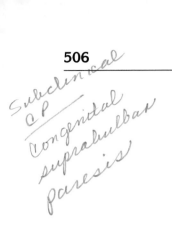

children may display uneven intellectual profiles, hyperactivity, and delayed onset of speech. The potential value of viewing these minimally involved children as having subclinical cerebral palsy is that many may benefit from some of the management techniques developed for children with obvious cerebral palsy.

One condition that may be considered a specific form of subclinical cerebral palsy is congenital suprabulbar paresis (Worster-Drought, 1968). At least two forms of the condition are recognized: the complete syndrome, characterized by paralysis of the lips, tongue, velum, and larynx and by swallowing difficulty; and the incomplete syndrome, characterized by an isolated paresis of the velum or tongue.

### Neurophysiological Age

*See, for example, Bobath and Bobath (1967) and Rood (1954).*

Before leaving this section of the chapter, we should describe a nontraditional basis for classifying cerebal palsy—the neurophysiological basis—that is growing in use. A number of workers have developed orientations and management approaches to cerebral palsy that are based less on the traditional types and more on what might be called the "neurophysiological age" of the child. I myself take this approach; see Mysak, 1980. As Twitchell (1965) said, "[F]rom the neurophysiological view, the separation of patients into various categories—such as spasticity, rigidity, athetosis, tremor—is wholly artificial." Regardless of classification, the same physiological substrata for the different cerebral palsies can be demonstrated in all children. "Strict adherence to the various classifications of cerebral palsy are artificial and based on unphysiologic tenets" (Twitchell, 1965).

*For more information on the concept of neurophysiological age, see Mysak (1980), chapter 6, and Mysak (1987a).*

In short, a classification system based on neurophysiological age entails an analysis of the child's development and functional level; that is, does the child exhibit the reflexes and reactions that allow for head balance, rolling over, body support on elbows, and sitting and standing? This approach also entails neuroanalyses of hand movements, basic speech reflexes, and skilled speech movements. Later in the chapter, we will see the implications of this orientation for speech diagnosis and speech therapy.

## Component Problems

Along with the characteristic neuromotor symptoms, cerebral palsy often carries many other components. Among these component problems are convulsions, mental retardation, emotional problems, sensory disturbances, and perceptual problems. There is no clear-cut relationship between the severity of the neuromotor problem and the number or severity of the component problems. A severely spastic child may show normal intelligence, normal vision, and normal hearing, while another with mild athetosis may be moderately retarded and hearing impaired.

## Convulsions

Since cerebral palsy results from various types of brain injury, and since brain injury predisposes people to seizure disorders, it is not surprising that these children show a higher than normal incidence of convulsive disorders. The incidence of convulsive disorders among cerebral palsied children varies depending on the source. As we have seen before, incidence figures are influenced by the reporter's definitions and by the accuracy of diagnosis of the wide range of possible symptoms. Among athetotics, figures of about 2, 10, and 30% have been reported, while among spastics, figures as high as 50, 60, and 80% have been reported. Almost every possible variety of seizure has been reported. Speech-language pathologists who deal with children with seizure disorders should become familiar with the types of seizures, procedures for handling a seizure, and the medications often prescribed to prevent them.

*Sources of reliable information are the Epilepsy Foundation of America, 1828 L Street, N.W., Washington, D.C. 20036, and Gummit (1983).*

## Mental Retardation

Intellectual development and achievement among children with cerebral palsy varies considerably. Some people with cerebral palsy are profoundly retarded; others are gifted. Primary factors that contribute to this variability include the different locations and sizes of the offending brain lesions, and the degree of specific linguistic involvement. In addition, many children with cerebral palsy have fewer than normal sensory-perceptual experiences, both because their mobility is limited and because of the overprotectiveness of their parents and other caretakers. Cerebral palsy is frequently associated with relatively severe retardation, and these children may have drastically limited communication skills, as well as reduced environmental stimulation and social interactions.

It is difficult to assess accurately the intelligence of these children because of their motor, sensory, perceptual, and communication limitations. Therefore, incidence figures on mental retardation in this population must be interpreted with caution. Figures range from 30% up to about 70%, with most around 50%.

## Emotional Problems

Given the complex of sensorimotor, perceptual, and communication problems of children with cerebral palsy, it is easy to understand how their socioemotional development may be affected. Complicating the situation are not infrequent parental reactions of guilt, rejection, and overprotection. The reactions of other people to a child who drools, makes facial grimaces, or walks strangely further compound the problem. Emotional immaturity and instability, introversion, and depression are findings that are likely to appear in psychological studies of these children.

### Sensory-Perceptual Problems

Because the motor problems of children with cerebral palsy are so obvious, their many sensory-perceptual involvements may go relatively unnoticed. Adding to the problem of undetected or unnoticed sensory problems is the difficulty in testing the various senses, especially when the child's ability to communicate is limited or nonexistent.

Sensory problems found among these children include problems in tactile sensation, two-point discrimination, position sense, and pain and temperature sense. Visual acuity problems have been observed in over 50% of these children, and visual field defects in about 25%. To further complicate matters, many people with cerebral palsy are hearing impaired. Tactile, auditory, and visual perception problems may also be found among children with cerebral palsy. Difficulty in perceiving objects grasped or placed in their hands, such as small toys, figures, or coins, and in perceiving plastic forms representing various shapes placed in their mouths may be observed. Hearing the difference between certain sounds, synthesizing combinations of sounds, and memory span for sounds may also be a problem. Problems in seeing the whole pattern of a letter, the word pattern of a group of letters, or discriminating a visual figure on a background of other visual stimuli are also found. Complicating these visual perceptual problems are problems of binocular balance (**strabismus**) and ocular nystagmus. Oculomotor imbalances have been observed in over half of these children.

Among the problems exhibited by Sally in the case history were possible sensory-perceptual problems, and problems in cognitive and socioemotional development.

## SPEECH AND LANGUAGE DISORDERS

All or any one of the component problems we have just discussed—convulsions, mental retardation, emotional problems, sensory-perceptual problems—can contribute to an individual's speech and language difficulties. The speech-language pathologist should expect to find a large variety of factors underlying any one communication disorder, and a large variety of patterns of communication disorders. One child may have no speech at all; another may show little (if any) difference from children without cerebral palsy. But the reported incidence of communication problems among people with cerebral palsy ranges from 70% (Wolfe, 1950) to 86% (Achilles, 1955).

*See chapter 12.*

At least two types of symptoms may be found in developmental cerebral palsies: those of immaturity, and those of paralysis or pathology. Whenever a brain lesion develops before birth or in infancy, it may contribute to general delay, retardation, or arrest of certain functions (immaturity); also, depending on the location of the lesion, it may cause some specific defect of function (paralysis or pathology symptom). For example, a lesion in the frontal lobe of the brain may contribute to general symptoms of immaturity in a child, such as persisting infantile feeding reflexes; but because it is near the primary motor area that supplies muscles of the tongue, the child may also show specific difficulty in raising the tongue tip.

# Characteristics of Communication Deficits

Because the communication disorders in cerebral palsy are so complex, we cannot describe a typical case. A more useful approach is to attempt to identify the possible components of any one case. The job of the speech-language pathologist is to study each child for all the components that appear to be present, as well as to identify the immaturity and paralysis features of each component. Let us now look at several conditions that may underlie the communication disorders associated with cerebral palsy: disorders of posture, listening, breathing, voice, articulation, and language. As we discuss each one, we will also discuss diagnostic considerations. In addition, you may wish to refer to the section on assessment in the chapters relating to each specific type of disorder.

# Speech Posture Disorders

An important feature of the progression of motor control in the human being is that postural control of a part of the body always precedes movement control of that part. The importance of the relationship between postural control and movement control has not been well developed in speech-language pathology, but we do have some information available. To listen for speech, a child should be able to assume trunk and head positions that facilitate the reception of the speech signal. In other words, if a child is able to quickly orient his upper trunk and head toward the source of speech signals, listening for speech is facilitated. In speaking, coordinated movements of respiratory, phonatory, resonatory, and articulatory mechanisms depend to a great degree on postural control of the trunk, neck, and head. This postural control may be observed when a child speaks while lying on his back, lying on his elbows, sitting in various positions, and standing. Since problems in trunk, neck, and head balance and control are a common part of cerebral palsy, their possible role in a presenting speech disorder should be appreciated and assessed. Figure 14.3 shows a person who has difficulty in assuming and maintaining sit and stand speech postures.

*For more information on speech postures, see Mysak (1980, 1987b).*

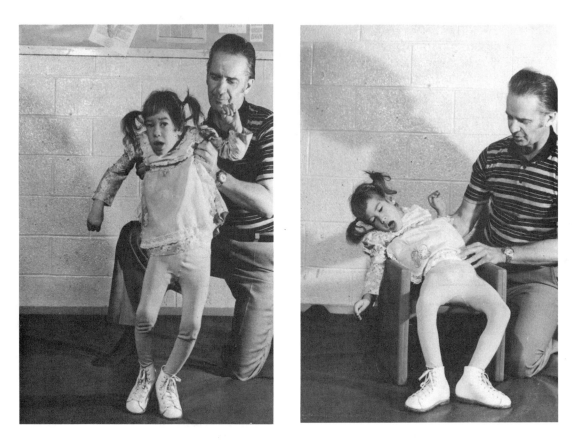

**Figure 14.3**   Child who has problems in sit and stand speech postures

## Listening Disorders

We use the word *listening* rather than *hearing* to describe the auditory disorders that may be found in children with cerebral palsy. Here, listening denotes not only hearing for speech, but also the body position and preparation designed to facilitate hearing.

### Immaturity

*A **Moro reflex** is an extensor startle pattern in response to sound.*

Symptoms of listening immaturity in the cerebral palsied child may include the inability of the child to assume automatically the head and trunk positions that facilitate hearing speech, and the persistence of the auditory Moro and cry reflexes in response to sound. Underdeveloped postural control and persistent startle reflexes are likely to interfere with processing speech signals. Also, the child may show a delay or retardation in the ability to localize speech, for example, the localization of the primary caretaker's voice (which normally appears around age 6 months).

## Pathology

Almost every type of hearing loss has been found among people with cerebral palsy. Defects have been found in the external, middle, and inner ears, and in the central auditory tracts and cortices. Estimates of the incidence of hearing loss among people with cerebral palsy range from 6% to 41%, but in general the incidence appears to be about 20% (Nober, 1976).

Susceptibility to middle-ear disease has also been observed in cerebral palsy, especially among spastics. Sources of inner-ear problems include hereditary deafness, viral infections, and toxemia. Some athetotics have been suspected of showing central deafness, or involvement of retrocochlear mechanisms.

*You may wish to review chapter 10.*

## Diagnosis

Among the factors that a speech-language pathologist must keep in mind when evaluating the listening behavior of the cerebral palsied person are the high rate of involvement, the wide range in types of involvement, and the difficulty of audiometric testing and interpreting findings. These factors all suggest that testing by an audiologist is essential.

*The special difficulties of audiometric testing with the multiply handicapped were discussed in chapter 10.*

## Breathing Disorders

There are at least two forms of breathing: vegetative breathing and speech breathing. Vegetative breathing is characterized by nasal breathing with approximately even inspiratory and expiratory phases; speech breathing is characterized by oral breathing with a rapid inspiratory phase followed by a long expiratory phase. Automatic and rapid shifting from vegetative breathing (vb) to speech breathing (sb) is a prerequisite of efficient speech. This automatic vb-sb shifting requires intact central mechanisms for respiratory regulation, and these, unfortunately, are frequently involved in cerebral palsy. Reported breathing problems among the different types of cerebral palsy range from 40% to 80%.

## Immaturity

All sorts of breathing differences among cerebral palsied children have been reported by researchers and clinicians. Most of these differences appear related to immaturity of the CNS centers involved with the regulation of breathing. Some children may show a delay in the vb-sb shift, while others may not be able to effect the shift at all. Breaths per minute may remain high, and the depth of the breathing cycle may remain shallow.

## Paralysis

Some of the breathing problems among people with cerebral palsy appear to be related to irregular innervation of the muscles that are directly or indirectly involved with respiration, rather than to immaturity of neuroregulatory centers. Among the paralytic symptoms may be weak thoracic and abdominal muscles, respiration accompanied by retracted abdominal muscles and little movement of the diaphragm, and air stream obstruction due to irregular movements of the vocal folds.

### Diagnosis

When evaluating the breathing mechanisms, the speech-language pathologist must again be alert to the high rate of involvement and the wide range in types of involvement. When attempting to relate breathing dysfunctions to possible speech symptoms, the following possible relationships should be considered: (a) problems in vb-sb shifting and delay in voluntary phonation, producing only one or two syllables per expiration, and slow and irregular rate; (b) poor thoracic-abdominal muscle coordination and weak voice, forced voice, difficulty in sustaining voice, interrupted voice, and inspiratory voice; and (c) poor respiratory-laryngeal coordination and inspiratory voice, forced voice, sudden arrest of voice, and uncontrolled loudness.

## Voice Disorders

Efficient voicing (including resonation) results from the coordination of inspiratory and expiratory movements with laryngeal and velopharyngeal movements, and from primary monitoring of the consequent phonation by the ear. Given the high rate of hearing and breathing disorders alone, voice problems among people with cerebral palsy are not surprising.

### Immaturity

*These problems may be similar to those caused by cleft palates and related disorders. See chapters 8 and 11.*

Voicing inefficiency may be related to the immaturity of various reflexes. The glottic-opening reflex, which allows for inspiration, and the glottic-closing reflex, which allows for buildup of intrathoracic pressure, for example, may be unregulated and cause phonatory problems. The velar opening reflex, which allows nasal inspiration, and the velar closing reflex, which allows for the creation of negative or positive oral pressure, may also be unregulated and cause problems in speech resonance.

### Paralysis

In addition to unregulated glottic and velar reflexes influencing voicing and resonation, voice problems may also stem from difficulties with the voluntary use of laryngeal muscles. Possible reflections of this difficulty are flaccid or weak vocal folds, as well as spasms and arrhythmic activity of the folds.

## Diagnosis

To properly diagnose voice problems among the cerebral palsied, the speech-language pathologist should be concerned about differentiating symptoms of immaturity from paralysis, and should also attempt to identify whether the source of the problem is respiratory, laryngeal, or the coordination of the two. The following possible relationships should be considered: (a) involuntary open-close activity of the glottis (unregulated glottic reflexes) and inspiratory voice, sudden loss of voice, intermittent voice, uncontrolled loudness, and forced voice; (b) involuntary open-close activity of the velum (unregulated velar reflexes) and reduced nasality, increased nasality, and mixed and intermittent imbalance in nasality; (c) flaccid paralysis of the folds and breathy voice; and (d) hypertonic vocal folds, and difficulty in initiating voice and hoarseness.

# Articulation Disorders

Problems with articulation are usually the most obvious component of the communication disorder. In the context of cerebral palsy, these disorders are referred to as *developmental dysarthrias* and *developmental dyspraxias.* In some cases of cerebral palsy, the dysarthria may be the major observable symptom; articulation may be almost normal, with major symptoms in other areas; or it may appear in severe form with only minor symptoms in other areas. Reports of the incidence of some degree of articulation disorder among the cerebral palsied range as high as 80% and higher.

*Also see chapter 13 for an in-depth discussion of dysarthria and apraxia.*

## Immaturity

Some of the articulation problems in cerebral palsy may be attributed to the persistence of infantile feeding reflexes such as rooting, lip, mouth-opening, biting, and suckling reflexes. These conditions affect speech only when particular speech efforts also elicit certain reflexive movements; for example, when movement for tongue-tip sounds stimulates the suckle reflex and the tongue moves too far forward and into an interdental position; when efforts at producing /r/ or /l/ sounds stimulate the lip reflex, and there is simultaneous lip rounding accompanying the tongue-tip elevation; or when efforts at producing an open-mouth sound like /a/ stimulate the mouth-opening reflex, and there is an exaggeration of the open-mouth posture.

*The rooting reflex is characterized by the orientation of the infant's head and mouth toward the stimulus or source of nourishment.*

## Paralysis

Various forms of paralytic involvement of the articulators complicate articulation disorders among people with cerebral palsy. The paralytic involvement may be spastic, athetotic, or ataxic. The nonparalytic movement disorder is called *articulatory dyspraxia.*

In spasticity, the articulators may move in a labored fashion and be either hypertonic or flaccid. In athetosis, the articulators may move involuntarily before the voluntary speech movement is attempted. The movements may be slow and irregular. Movements of the articulators in ataxia may be slow, clumsy, and inaccurate. Finally, in articulatory dyspraxia, the person may have no difficulty in moving the articulators spontaneously, but great difficulty in moving them voluntarily to speak.

### Diagnosis

In evaluating cerebral palsy articulation disorders, the speech-language pathologist must first assess the possible roles of listening disorders and of mental retardation. Separating immaturity symptoms from paralytic symptoms should also be attempted. The following possible relationships should be considered: (a) speech-elicited rooting reflex and lateralization of sibilants, lip reflex and bilabialized /r/ and /l/, mouth-opening reflex and vowel distortion, and suckle reflex and forward placed tongue-tip sounds; (b) slow, clumsy movements characterized by consistent limitations in direction and range of movement and spastic dysarthria (especially with tongue-tip sounds); (c) involuntary movements characterized by inconsistency in moving in appropriate directions with appropriate ranges and athetotic dysarthria (all sounds may be involved during athetotic episodes); (d) clumsy, uncoordinated movements characterized by uncertainty and inconsistency in the direction and range of movement and ataxic dysarthria; and (e) difficulty in voluntarily reproducing certain movements that can be made spontaneously and articulatory dyspraxia.

## Language Disorders

Children develop language as they develop other cognitive skills. In particular, spoken language develops as a function of general motor maturation up to standing, which allows the child to move around and experience the world; perceptual maturation, which allows the child to develop perceptual representations of the world; and central speech mechanism maturation, which allows the child to learn oral symbols and associate them with their referents. Since children with cerebral palsy may show involvement with all these aspects of spoken language development, many of them also are delayed in developing language.

### Immaturity

Oral language immaturity is reflected in delay in the onset of speech, as well as delay in the development of vocabulary and grammar. The oral language of some children with cerebral palsy is characterized by a predominance of social gesture speech, such as *hi* and *bye*; memorized speech, such as counting and nursery rhymes; and emotional utterances. The child may communicate only to express her wants and needs. Frequently, conversation and narration forms of speech are minimal or nonexistent. In short, the form and function of speech is infantile.

You may recall that Sally, in the case history at the beginning of the chapter, was limited in oral communication to monosyllabic, babbling vocalization.

## Pathology

Complicating language disorders among people with cerebral palsy may be symptoms that appear more directly related to involvement of the central neural mechanisms devoted to the function of spoken language. Symptoms may be observed that are similar to those found among otherwise normal children and adults who have language disorders due to some form of brain lesion. Among these symptoms may be perseveration, echolalia, confusion between similar-sounding words, syllable reversals, grammatical confusions, word-finding difficulty, and telegraphic speech.

## Diagnosis

In the analysis of the child with a language disorder, the speech-language pathologist needs to determine the relative influence of factors such as listening disorder, speech mechanism paralysis, mental retardation, and reduction in general mobility and sensory-perceptual stimulation. Differentiating simple language retardation from specific language pathology is another important task.

# SPEECH AND LANGUAGE THERAPY

How well a therapy program for any particular child with cerebral palsy may work depends on many factors, including how accurately the speech-language pathologist has identified the components of the child's problem and formulated an individualized therapy regimen. Because the disorder in any given case may have begun at birth or before, have various causes, and present itself in various forms, we must take a wide-spectrum approach to management.

Incorporated within the concept of a wide-spectrum approach are the principles of holistic and early intervention. By *holistic intervention,* we mean that the speech-language pathologist must not only be concerned with the child's speech and language development, but also with how that development relates to and depends on the child's overall motor, perceptual, cognitive, and socioemotional development. By *early intervention,* we mean the earliest possible intervention after the diagnosis of cerebral palsy has been made. Early intervention should help minimize secondary communication problems. Wide-spectrum management includes the consideration of primary and secondary preventive measures, as well as causal, symptom, compensatory, and supportive therapies. In the case history, such considerations were made when planning the therapy program for Sally. Because the area of speech therapy for the cerebral palsied is so large and complex, we will present only a philosophy of therapy and some basic principles and methods.

*If you have a special interest in therapy, you might wish to read further; see for example, Hardy (1983), Lencione (1976), Mysak (1980, 1987a).*

## Primary Preventive Measures

Prevention should be a password in every profession, and we should spend major amounts of energy and resources on it. Alas, like many other fields, the field of speech-language pathology and audiology has not done too well in this area. With respect to communication problems in cerebral palsy, the best way to prevent them is to prevent cerebral palsy. And one important way to help prevent cerebral palsy is through public education conducted by all concerned agencies and specialists. Mothers-to-be should be informed that various infections may cause cerebral palsy, and should guard against them. Prenatal causal factors include mumps, rubella, influenza, Rh-negative factor, and toxemia. Similarly, mothers should guard their infants against infections such as meningitis, encephalitis, and measles, as well as against trauma and lead poisoning.

In those cases of existing cerebral palsy where speech and hearing mechanisms seem to be intact, certain primary preventive measures may also be carried out. Certainly, parents must obtain immediate medical attention for any ear infections in their child. Frequent audiometric screening is also recommended to identify and treat undetected problems, and to ensure against the development of future speech and language problems.

*Ideas on the role of the family in facilitating communication may be found in O'Brian and Andreses (1983).*

Facilitating the development of normal speech and hearing processes may also be viewed as a primary preventive measure. Parents may be advised to keep their child near talkative children and adults, speak a lot when the child is experiencing positive feelings (for instance, during feeding, bathing, playing), expand and enrich the child's social and perceptual spheres by exposure to speakers and places outside the home, and reward all efforts on the part of the child to perceive and produce speech.

## Secondary Preventive Measures

The aim of secondary preventive measures for the cerebral palsied child is to ensure that the child's personal reaction to existing communication problems and the reactions of those around her do not add to her problems. Helpful suggestions may be given to parents by the speech-language pathologist. The parents should be informed that, in general, a therapeutic environment is one in which the child is regularly exposed to situations where carefully measured challenge always exceeds carefully measured assistance. Accordingly, she should be allowed to spend as much time as possible in positions in which she can support herself; for example, on elbows or in various floor-sit positions (tailor position, side-sit, or long-sit positions). She should be given *every* opportunity to move from point to point, using whatever mode of body progression is available to her. The child should be allowed to nurse and be exposed to solid foods as soon as possible (depending on circumstances, supplementary feeding may also be necessary). Whether it be supporting a particular body posture (perhaps sitting), moving through space, or eating, the child must be encouraged and allowed to do as much as possible for herself, and to begin doing whatever she can for others. This may mean that everything the child needs to do will take a little longer to accomplish, but for the child, it is time well spent.

*For ideas on physically handling the young cerebral palsied child at home, parents may refer to Finnie (1975).*

The parents should also use the ideas we mentioned to facilitate the development of normal speech and hearing processes. In general, the parents should be sure to provide an atmosphere rich with adult and child speakers, create situations that require the child to communicate orally, and reward all attempts to communicate and any growth in communication skills.

## Causal Therapy

Causal therapy includes all those techniques aimed at what the speech-language pathologist thinks is directly responsible for the presenting speech and language problem. Techniques designed to counteract disorders of speech posture, listening, breathing-voicing, and articulation are described here.

### Speech Posture

Postural control of the trunk, neck, and head contributes substantially to movement control of the speech mechanism. Helping the child with cerebral palsy to develop balance in a back-pattern, on-elbows, or a sit-pattern speech posture is, therefore, an important goal of speech therapy. Physicians, physical therapists, occupational therapists, and parents all share this goal, and hence their efforts can contribute to reaching it. To apply specific techniques for developing speech postures, a good deal of background information is required that cannot be given here. In many cases, the speech-language pathologist will want to work closely with a physical therapist to choose and develop postures that facilitate speech.

### Listening

Developing head balance and control in speech postures also serves the listening function of allowing the child to orient his hearing mechanism toward the source of speech signals. Whenever a hearing loss is detected, appropriate listening enhancement techniques should be applied as early as possible. This includes fitting a personal hearing aid, decreasing the distance between the child and speakers, having speakers raise their loudness level, and making sure that the child is in a position to see the speaker's face.

Localizing exercises involving speech and nonspeech stimuli should be done with the child in back-pattern, elbow-pattern, and sit-pattern speech postures whenever possible. Head localization should be stimulated, first to the right and then the left, and first upward, then downward. Interesting, novel, and changing stimuli should be used inside and outside the home. Distances from the stimuli should be progressively increased, and loudness levels progressively decreased. When the child does not spontaneously move his head, a therapy partner should initiate and guide these movements until the child develops some degree of independent localization.

### Breathing-Voicing

Improving vegetative breathing and speech breathing are both important goals, and of course, breathing is also essential to voicing. Goals in vegetative breathing are to deepen breathing cycles, normalize breaths per minute, and stimulate thoracic participation. The goal in speech breathing is to effect a rapid vb-sb shift, which includes a shift from nasal to oral inspiration and a shift from a ratio of 40% time spent in the inspiratory phase (as compared to the expiratory phase of breathing) to one of about 15%. There are many maneuvers available for facilitating inspiration. Only one will be described here.

The "leg-roll technique" is done with the child lying on a mat, for example, with the speech-language pathologist at the child's feet or at her side. The clinician grasps the child's shins, flexes and abducts the legs, and presses them toward the child's armpits, thereby displacing the internal organs upward, stretching the diaphragm, and facilitating expiration. Following the expiratory phase, the speech-language pathologist quickly extends and brings the legs downward, returning them to their original position and facilitating inspiration.

In applying breathing techniques, a rhythm similar to normal vegetative breathing should be imposed first. Next, the expiratory phase is lengthened, and the speech-language pathologist stimulates voicing, either sustained vowels or syllable strings, during the maneuver. At the same time, the inspiratory phase is quickened so that it lasts for approximately 10% to 15% of the entire breathing cycle.

### Articulation

The major goals of articulation techniques are to increase the kinds, range, accuracy, and speed of movements of the mandible, lips, and tongue, and to coordinate those movements with the breathing-voicing mechanism. Work on vegetative movements of the articulators, as well as direct work on speech movements and their coordination, should serve these goals.

Many experts believe that improvement of early eating movements like suckling, chewing, and swallowing contribute to the development of articulatory movements. Among the early advocates of eating therapy to improve speech movements were Meader (1940), Palmer (1947), and Westlake (1951); there has been a continued interest and development of this therapy by many new workers. Methods and techniques in eating therapy have grown to such a degree that a discussion of them is not possible here. In general, the speech-language pathologist should instruct parents and other family members in eating therapy, and should not become a main provider of it.

*See, for example, Alexander (1987), Davis (1978), Morris (1977), and Mueller (1972).*

Causal therapy for speech movements and their coordination includes work in moving a body part in isolation from other body parts, in performing specific movements, and in performing speeded movements. The first goal here is for the child to be able to move one articulator in isolation from other articulators and from all other body parts. It is done through a technique appropriately called an *isolation maneuver.* First, the speech-language pathologist holds or stabilizes all body parts, sometimes with the aid of an assistant, except for the part to be differentiated. The child is then asked to move the isolated part. If the child cannot do so, the movement of the part is assisted by the professional. Progress is measured by the reduction in the amount of stabilization imposed by the speech-language pathologist, and by the increase in the amount of voluntary movement shown by the child. The sequence in the differentiation process is as follows: head from trunk; larynx (while producing vowels or strings of syllables) from the head; mandible from the head; lips from the head; tongue from the head; and finally mandible, lips, and tongue from each other.

The ability to move specific articulators is improved through stimulating-feedback and movement-facilitation maneuvers. Stimulating-feedback maneuvers impose particular articulatory patterns on the child's mechanism, with the expectation that the imposed feedback will encourage the target movement to develop. Therapeutic feedback is provided, therefore, by bringing the child's articulators through the movements and points of contact associated with production of bilabial, labiodental, linguadental, lingua-alveolar, and linguavelar articulatory patterns. Maneuvers should be carried out along with appropriately timed audiovisual stimulation from the speech-language pathologist so that the child receives all the important sensory information associated with a particular sound.

*Because these techniques require some background information and knowledge of neurofacilitatory techniques, they cannot be discussed in detail here. See Mysak (1980).*

Movement-facilitation maneuvers are used when the child shows certain limitations in direction and range of articulatory movements. Among the maneuvers that could be used are the resisted-movement, associated-movement, countermovement, reversed-movement, and reflex-movement maneuvers.

## Symptom Therapy

Symptom therapy is aimed directly at improving the child's use of oral language and speech production skills. Its goal is to capitalize on all the potential for speech production that emerges from the effort spent in secondary preventive measures and causal therapy. There are at least two reasons why any one child may not be speaking at maximum potential: the child learned sounds at a time when her articulatory system was not as efficient as it may now be, and the child did not automatically make use of any new potential resulting from preventive and causal therapy.

### Articulation

*For information on these approaches, look back at chapter 7.*

If a particular child is not articulating certain sounds, either because he learned the sounds prior to being able to make certain articulatory movements, or because he has not put to use new movements that have resulted from causal therapy, various traditional approaches to articulation therapy may be applied.

### Language

*Information on language intervention work is found in chapters 5 and 6.*

Some general principles for language stimulation may be applied by all individuals who come into contact with the child. Basic goals are to provide large amounts of speech stimulation when the child is experiencing pleasant sensations, reward the child for all listening attitudes and efforts at communication, ask the child to name first silently and then aloud whatever her eyes fix upon in the environment, and ask the child to accompany her activities with a running description of them. Also, those around the child may describe aloud the child's activities or objects in the child's visual field whenever the child is not speaking. They can also describe aloud (simply and appropriately) their own activities whenever the child is nearby, watching and listening.

## Compensatory Therapy

Compensatory therapy techniques are used to facilitate the development of spoken language and to supplement or replace spoken language when its development is proceeding slowly, is limited, or is unlikely to be achieved. Both modified speech forms and nonspeech forms are available.

### Modified Speech

Forms of modified speech include spell and topic talk, electronically treated speech, and synthetic speech. Spell and topic talk are ways to improve communication in instances of questionable intelligibility. Children should be willing and ready to spell aloud words that they believe listeners are having trouble understanding, and should identify the topic of what they intend to talk about before they begin to communicate.

Electronically treated speech requires the child to wear a device designed to increase understandability. Two such devices have been developed: the electronic speaking aid (National Institute for Rehabilitation Engineering, Pompton Lakes, New Jersey) and the Auditory Feedback Mechanism, or AFM (Berko, 1965). The electronic speaking aid amplifies and filters the child's speech, and transmits the treated signal into a loudspeaker. The AFM also amplifies and filters the child's speech, but then the treated speech is fed back to a headset worn by the child.

Synthetic speech may also be viewed as a form of modified speech. Portable models of speech synthesizers that can "speak" for the child are now commercially available (Phonic Mirror, H. C. Electronics, Inc.). High cost and a particular child's physical and mental abilities limit the use of these synthesizers.

## Nonspeech Communication

The nonspeech forms of compensatory therapy include the use of signals and code, symbols, communication boards, and computer-assisted communication aids. These modes of communication are used with more severely involved children. Mental abilities, motivation, and voluntary movements available to the child are considerations in the selection of an alternate mode of communication. Also important is the cooperation of the child's parents, family, friends, teachers, and therapists. The use of nonspeech communication should not preclude speech therapy, since a number of studies have shown that an increase in speech attempts and intelligibility accompany their use.

*See, for example, Beukelman and Yorkston (1977), McDonald and Schutz (1973), and Vanderheiden (1978).*

Signal and code forms of communication include the use of a simple yes-no system, audio-signalling, and Morse code. Yes or no signals may be given by the child via some sort of hand, head, face, or eye movement. A portable audio-oscillator that emits a loud tone has been used to teach cerebral palsied children four simple signals: I need help, Yes, No, See the list (Hagen, Porter, & Brink, 1973). Morse code has also been used as a means of communication for severely involved children (Clement, 1961).

Symbol forms of communication involve the use of special symbols that represent sounds or words. Two-symbol systems have been used frequently with cerebral palsied children. First, Blissymbol communication has been used effectively with certain severely involved children with cerebral palsy (Vanderheiden & Harris-Vanderheiden, 1976). Blissymbols represent concepts rather than specific words. Depending on the child's ability, Blissymbol vocabularies of up to 400 items may be learned. Second, an electronic conversation board called the "Expressor" was designed to facilitate the use of the Initial Teaching Alphabet (ITA) (Shane, 1972). In this system, one symbol represents one sound; if the child learns the 44 symbols, he would be capable of producing any English word.

Communication boards may be nonelectronic or electronic. Nonelectronic boards have been used with the cerebral palsied for some time (McDonald & Chance, 1964; Westlake & Rutherford, 1964). Boards should be developed on an individual basis, in accordance with each child's needs and physical and intellectual abilities. More organized forms of communication boards have also been developed (McDonald & Schultz, 1973). These boards may display numbers, letters, words, pictures, and sentences. They may also display Blissymbols, the ITA, or other symbol systems. The vocabulary should reflect the child's own priorities and interests. An electronic communication board called the Auto-Monitoring Communication Board, or Auto-Com, has also been used with a severely involved cerebral palsied child (Bullock, Dalrymple, & Danca, 1975). Some of the features of the Auto-Com include a capacity to print out letter, words, phrases, and sentences; a television read-out component; and interfacing with a typewriter. Finally, Ferrier and Shane 1987 have reviewed selection procedures and available software for computer-based communication aids for the non-speaking child.

## Supportive Therapy

In certain cases of cerebral palsy, the speech-language pathologist may find that there is little hope for any progress in verbal or nonverbal communication. Such cases are appearing with increasing frequency in the caseload of the speech-language pathologist who now, more than in the past, may be working in state developmental centers. In such cases, the clinician has at least two goals: (a) to ensure that parents and others who relate to the child comprehend any body, hand, facial, or sound communication that the child may be able to use; and (b) to help the parents and others who relate to the child to understand and accept the child's severe limitations in the use of any form of verbal or nonverbal communication.

## CONCLUSION

After reading this chapter, you should have little doubt that the analysis of the communication problem in cerebral palsy, formulation of an individualized therapy plan, and effective execution of that plan should be regarded as some of the greatest challenges to the speech-language pathologist. Some of the greatest rewards await those who accept and meet those challenges.

## STUDY QUESTIONS

1. Define cerebral palsy, and differentiate among spastic, athetotic, and ataxic varieties.

2. Discuss causation of cerebral palsy in terms of familial and environmental factors.

3. Identify the various problems that are frequently associated with the condition of cerebral palsy, and how each may contribute to the cerebral palsy speech complex.

4. Describe the full range of speech-language-hearing symptoms that may comprise the communication disorder in cerebral palsy.

5. Differentiate between symptoms of immaturity and paralysis (or pathology) relative to the possible symptoms in the cerebral palsy speech complex.

6. Define wide-spectrum intervention in cerebral palsy.

7. Define and give examples of the full range of measures and therapies available to the speech-language pathologist in treating the cerebral palsy speech complex.

## SELECTED READINGS

Connor, F. P., Williamson, G. G., & Siepp, J. M. (Eds.). (1978). *Program guide for infants and toddlers with neuromotor and other developmental disabilities.* New York: Teachers College Press, Teachers College, Columbia University.

Cruickshank, W. M. (Ed.). (1976). *Cerebral palsy: Its individual and community problems.* Syracuse: Syracuse University Press.

Hardy, J. C. (1983). *Cerebral palsy.* Englewood Cliffs, NJ: Prentice-Hall, Inc.

Lencione, R. M. (1976). The development of communication skills. In W. J. Cruickshank (Ed.), *Cerebral palsy: A developmental disability.* Syracuse: Syracuse University Press.

McDonald, E. T., & Schultz, A. (1973). Communication boards for cerebral palsied children. *Journal of Speech and Hearing Disorders, 38,* 73–88.

Mueller, H. (1972). Facilitating feeding and prespeech. In P. H. Pearson & C. E. Williams (Eds.), *Physical therapy services in the developmental disabilities.* Springfield, IL: Charles C Thomas.

Mysak. E. D. (1980). *Neurospeech therapy for the cerebral palsied.* New York: Teachers College Press, Teachers College, Columbia University.

Nober, E. H. (1976). Auditory processing. In W. J. Cruickshank (Ed.), *Cerebral palsy. A developmental disability.* Syracuse: Syracuse University Press.

Westlake, H. & Rutherford. D. (1964). *Speech therapy for the cerebral palsied.* Chicago: National Society for Crippled Children and Adults.

# Requirements for the
# Certificates of Clinical Competence
(Revised April 1, 1985)[*]

The American Speech-Language-Hearing Association issues Certificates of Clinical Competence to
individuals who present satisfactory evidence of their
ability to provide independent clinical services to
persons who have disorders of communication
(speech, language and/or hearing). An individual who
meets these requirements may be awarded a Certificate in Speech-Language Pathology or in Audiology,
depending upon the emphasis of preparation; a person who meets the requirements in both professional
areas may be awarded both Certificates.

## I. STANDARDS

The individual who is awarded either or both of the
Certificates of Clinical Competence must hold a
master's degree or equivalent[1] with major emphasis
in speech-language pathology, audiology, or speech-
language and hearing science. The individual must
also meet the following qualifications.

[*]© 1985, The American Speech-Language-Hearing Association, Rockville, MD.

[1]Equivalent is defined as holding a bachelor's degree from
an accredited college or university, and at least 42 post
baccalaureate semester hours acceptable toward a master's degree, of which at least 30 semester hours must be
in the areas of speech-language pathology, audiology, or
speech-language and hearing science. At least 21 of these
42 semester hours must be obtained from a single college
or university, none may have been completed more than
10 years prior to the date of application and no more than
six semester hours may be credit offered for clinical
practicum.

524

## I,A. General Background Education

As stipulated below, applicants for a certificate should
have completed specialized academic training and
preparatory professional experience that provides an
in-depth knowledge of normal communication processes, development and disorders thereof, evaluation
procedures to assess the bases of such disorders, and
clinical techniques that have been shown to improve
or eradicate them. It is expected that the applicant will
have obtained a broad general education to serve as
a background prior to such study and experience and
demonstrates adequate oral and written communication skills. The specific content of this general background education is left to the discretion of the applicant and to the training program attended. However,
it is highly desirable that it include study in the areas
of human psychology, sociology, psychological and
physical development, the physical sciences (especially those that pertain to acoustic and biological phenomena) and human anatomy and physiology, including neuroanatomy and neurophysiology.

## I,B. Required Education

A total of 60 semester hours[2] of academic credit
must have been accumulated from accredited colleges or universities that demonstrate that the applicant has obtained a well-integrated program of

[2]In evaluation of credits, one quarter hour will be considered
the equivalent of two-thirds of a semester hour. Transcripts
that do not report credit in terms of semester or quarter-
hours should be submitted for special evaluation.

course study dealing with the normal aspects of human communication, development thereof, disorders thereof, and clinical techniques for evaluation and management of such disorders.

Twelve (12) of these 60 semester hours must be obtained in courses that provide information that pertains to normal development and use in speech, language and hearing.

Thirty (30) of these 60 semester hours must be obtained in courses that provide (1) information relative to communication disorders, and (2) information about and training in evaluation and management of speech, language and hearing disorders. At least 24 of these 30 semester hours must be in courses in the professional area (speech-language pathology or audiology) for which the certificate is requested, and at least six (6) must be in audiology for the certificate in speech-language pathology or in speech-language pathology for the certificate in audiology. Moreover, no more than six (6) semester hours may be in courses that provide credit for clinical practicum obtained during academic training.

Credit for study of information pertaining to related fields that augment the work of the clinical practitioner of speech-language pathology and/or audiology may also apply toward the total 60 semester hours.

Thirty (30) of the total 60 semester hours that are required for a certificate must be in courses that are acceptable toward a graduate degree by the college or university in which they are taken.[3] Moreover, 21 of these 30 semester hours must be within the 24 semester hours required in the professional area (speech-language pathology or audiology) for which the certificate is requested or within the six (6) semester hours required in the other area.

### I,C. Academic Clinical Practicum

The applicant must have completed a minimum of 300 clock hours of supervised clinical experience with individuals who present a variety of communication disorders, and this experience must have been obtained within the training institution or in one of its cooperating programs.

[3]This requirement may be met by courses completed as an undergraduate, providing the college or university in which they are taken specifies that these courses would be acceptable toward a graduate degree if they were taken at the graduate level.

### I,D. The Clinical Fellowship Year

The applicant must have obtained the equivalent of nine (9) months of full-time professional experience (the Clinical Fellowship Year) in which bona fide clinical work has been accomplished in the major professional area (speech-language pathology or audiology) in which the certificate is being sought. The Clinical Fellowship Year must have begun after completion of the academic and clinical practicum experiences specified in Standards, I,A., I,B., and I,C. above.

### I,E. The National Examinations in Speech-Language Pathology and Audiology

The applicant must have passed one of the National Examinations in Speech-Language Pathology and Audiology, either the National Examination in Speech-Language Pathology or the National Examination in Audiology.

## II. EXPLANATORY NOTES

### II,A. General Background Education

While the broadest possible general educational background for the practitioner of speech-language pathology and/or audiology is encouraged, the nature of the clinician's professional endeavors suggests the necessity for some emphasis in general education. For example, elementary courses in general psychology and sociology are desirable as are studies in mathematics, general physics, zoology, as well as human anatomy and physiology. Those areas of introductory study that do not deal specifically with communication processes are not to be credited to the minimum 60 semester hours of education specified in Standard I,B.

### II,B. Required Education

**II,B.1. Basic Communication Processes Area.** The 12 semester hours in courses that provide information applicable to the normal development and use of speech, language, and hearing should be selected with emphasis on the normal aspects of human communication in order that the applicant has a wide exposure to the diverse kinds of information suggested by the content areas given under the three broad categories that follow: (1) anatomic and physiological bases for the normal development and use of speech, language, and hearing such as anatomy, neurology, and physiology of speech, language and hearing mechanisms; (2) physical bases and processes or the production and perception of speech, language, and hearing, such as (a) acoustics or physics of sound, (b) phonology, (c) physiologic and acoustic phonetics, (d) perceptual processes, and (e) psychoacoustics, and (3) linguistic and psycholinguistic variables related to normal development and use of speech, language and hearing, such as (a) linguistics (historical, descriptive, sociolinguistics, urban language), (b) psychology of language, (c) psycholinguistics, (d) language and speech acquisition, and (e) verbal learning or verbal behavior.

It is emphasized that the three broad categories of required education given above, and the examples of areas of study within these classifications, are not meant to be analogous to, or imply, specific course titles. Neither are the examples of areas of study within these categories meant to be exhaustive.

At least two (2) semester hours of credit must be earned in each of the three categories.

Obviously, some of these 12 semester hours may be obtained in courses that are taught in departments other than those offering speech-language pathology and audiology programs. Courses designed to improve the speaking and writing ability of the student will not be credited.

**II,B.2. Major Professional Area, Certificate in Speech-Language Pathology.** The 24 semester hours of professional education required for the Certificate of Clinical Competence in Speech-Language Pathology should include information pertaining to speech and language disorders as follows: (1) understanding of speech and language disorders, such as (a) various types of disorders of communication, (b) their manifestations, and (c) their classifications and causes; (2) evaluation skills such as procedures, techniques, and instrumentation used to assess (a) the speech and language status of children and adults, and (b) the bases of disorders of speech and language and (3) management procedures, such as principles in remedial methods used in habilitation and rehabilitation for children and adults with various disorders of communication.

Within these categories at least six (6) semester hours must deal with speech disorders and at least six (6) semester hours must deal with language disorders.

**II,B.3. Minor Professional Area, Certificate in Speech-Language Pathology.** For the individual to obtain the Certificate in Speech-Language Pathology, at least six (6) semester hours of academic credit in audiology are required. Where only the minimum requirement of six (6) semester hours is met, three (3) semester hours must be in habilitative/rehabilitative procedures with speech and language problems associated with hearing impairment, and three (3) semester hours must be in study of the pathologies of the auditory system and assessment of auditory disorders. However, when more than the minimum six (6) semester hours is met, study of habilitative/rehabilitative procedures may be counted in the Major Professional Area for the Certificate in Speech-Language Pathology (See Section II,B.8).

**II,B.4. Major Professional Area, Certificate in Audiology.** The 24 semester hours of professional education required for the Certificate of Clinical Competence in Audiology should be in the broad, but not necessarily exclusive, categories of study as follows: (1) auditory disorders, such as (a) pathologies of the auditory system, and (b) assessment of auditory disorders and their effect on communication; (2) habilitative/rehabilitative procedures, such as (a) selection and use of appropriate amplification instrumentation for the hearing impaired, both wearable and group, (b) evaluation of speech and language problems of the hearing impaired, and (c) management procedures for speech and language habilitation and/or rehabilitation of the hearing impaired (that may include manual communication), (3) conservation of hearing, such as (a) environmental noise control, and (b) identification audiometry (school, military, industry); and (4) instrumentation, such as (a) electronics, (b) calibration techniques, and (c) characteristics of amplifying systems.

Not less than six (6) semester hours must be in the auditory pathology category, and no less than six (6) semester hours must be in the habilitation/rehabilitation category.

**II,B.5. Minor Professional Area, Certificate in Audiology.** For the individual to obtain the Certificate in Audiology, at least six (6) semester hours must be in the area of speech-language pathology. Of these, three (3) hours must be in the area of speech pathology and three (3) hours in the area of language pathology. It is suggested that where only this minimum requirement of six (6) semester hours is met, such study be in the areas of evaluation procedures and management of speech and language problems that are not associated with hearing impairment.

**II,B.6. Related Areas.** In addition to the 12 semester hours of course study in the Basic Communication Processes area, the 24 semester hours in the Major Professional Area and the six (6) semester hours in the Minor Professional Area, the applicant may receive credit toward the minimum requirement of 60 semester hours of required education through advanced study in a variety of related areas. Such study should pertain to the understanding of human behavior, both normal and abnormal, as well as services available from related professions, and, in general should augment the background for a professional career. Examples of such areas of study are as follows: (a) theories of learning and behavior, (b) services available from related professions that also deal with persons who have disorders of communication and (c) information from these professions about the sensory, physical, emotional, social, and/or intellectual status of a child or an adult.

Academic credit that is obtained from practice teaching or practicum work in other professions will not be counted toward the minimum requirements.

In order that the future applicant for one of the certificates will be capable of critically reviewing scientific matters dealing with clinical issues relative to speech-language pathology and audiology, credit for study in the area of statistics, beyond an introductory course, will be allowed to a maximum of three (3) semester hours. Academic study of the administrative organization of speech-language pathology and audiology programs also may be applied to a maximum of three (3) semester hours.

**II,B.7. Education Applicable to All Areas.** Certain types of course work may be acceptable among more than one of the areas of study specified above, depending upon the emphasis. For example, courses that provide an overview of research, e.g., introduction to graduate study or introduction to research, that consist primarily of a critical review of research in communication sciences, disorders, or management thereof, and/or a more general presentation of

research procedures and techniques that will permit the clinician to read and evaluate literature critically will be acceptable to a maximum of three (3) semester hours. Such courses may be credited to the Basic Communication Processes Area, or one of the Professional Areas or the Related Area, if substantive content of the course(s) covers material in those areas. Academic credit for a thesis or dissertation may be acceptable to a maximum of three (3) semester hours in the appropriate area. An abstract of the study must be submitted with the application if such credit is requested. In order to be acceptable, the thesis or dissertation must have been an experiment or descriptive investigation in the areas of speech, language, and hearing science, speech-language pathology or audiology; that is, credit will not be allowed if the project was a survey of opinions, a study of professional issues, an annotated bibliography, biography, or a study of curricular design.

As implied by the above, the academic credit hours obtained from one course or one enrollment may, and should be in some instances, divided among the Basic Communication Processes Area, one of the Professional Areas, and/or the Related Area. In such cases, a description of the content of that course should accompany the application. This description should be extensive enough to provide the Clinical Certification Board with information necessary to evaluate the validity of the request to apply the content to more than one of the areas.

**II,B.8. Major Professional Education Applicable to Both Certificates.** Study in the area of understanding, evaluation, and management of speech and language disorders associated with hearing impairment may apply to the 24 semester hours in the Major Professional Area required for either certificate (speech-language pathology or audiology). However, no more than six (6) semester hours of that study will be allowed in that manner for the certificate in speech-language pathology.

### II,C. Academic Clinical Practicum

It is highly desirable that students who anticipate applying for one of the Certificates of Clinical Competence have the opportunity, relatively early in their training, to observe the various procedures involved in a clinical program in speech-language pathology and audiology, but this passive participation is not to be construed as direct clinical practicum during academic training. The student should participate in supervised direct clinical experience during that training only after the student has had sufficient course work to qualify for work as a student clinician and only after the student has sufficient background to undertake clinical practice under direct supervision. A minimum of 150 clock hours of the supervised clinical experience must be obtained during graduate study. Once this experience is undertaken, a substantial period of time may be spent in writing reports, in preparation for clinical sessions, in conferences with supervisors, and in class attendance to discuss clinical procedures and experiences; such time may not be credited toward the 300 minimum clock hours of supervised clinical experience required.

All student clinicians are expected to obtain direct clinical experience with both children and adults, and it is recommended that some of their direct clinical experience be conducted with groups. Although the student clinician should have experience with both speech-language and hearing disorders, at least 200 clock hours of this supervised experience must be obtained in the major professional area (speech-language pathology or audiology) in which certification is sought, and at least 35 clock hours must be obtained in the minor area. At least 50 supervised clock hours of the required 300 hours of clinical experience must be obtained in each of two distinctly different clinical settings. (The two separate clinical settings may be within the organizational structure of the same institution and may include the academic program's clinic and affiliated medical facilities, community clinics, public schools, etc.)

For certification in speech-language pathology, the student clinician is expected to have experience in both the evaluation and management of a variety of speech and language problems. The student must have at least 50 clock hours of experience in evaluation of speech and language problems. The applicant must also have at least 75 clock hours of experience in management of language disorders of children and adults, and at least 25 clock hours each of experience in management of children and adults with whom disorders of (1) voice, (2) articulation, and (3) fluency

are significant aspects of the communication handicap.[4]

Where only the minimum 35 clock hours of clinical practicum in audiology is met that is required for the person seeking certification in speech-language pathology, that practicum must include 15 clock hours in assessment and/or management of speech and language problems associated with hearing impairment, and 15 clock hours must be in the assessment of auditory disorders. However, where more than this minimum requirement is met, clinical practicum in assessment and/or management of speech and language problems associated with hearing impairment may be counted toward the minimum clock hours obtained with language and/or speech disorders.

For the student clinician who is preparing for certification in audiology, 50 clock hours of direct supervised experience must be obtained in identification and evaluation of hearing impairment, and 50 clock hours must be obtained in habilitation or rehabilitation of the communication handicaps of the hearing impaired. It is suggested that the 35 clock hours of clinical practicum in speech-language pathology required for certification in audiology be in the evaluation and management of speech and language problems that are not related to hearing impairment.

Supervisors of clinical practicum must be competent professional workers who hold a Certificate of Clinical Competence in the professional area (speech-language pathology or audiology) in which supervision is provided. This supervision must entail the personal and direct involvement of the supervisor in any and all ways that will permit the supervisor to attest to the adequacy of the student's performance in the clinical training experience. At least 25% of the therapy sessions conducted by a student clinician must be directly supervised, with such supervision being appropriately scheduled throughout the training period. (Direct supervision is defined as on-site

[4]Work with multiple problems may be credited among these types of disorders. For example, a child with an articulation problem may also have a voice disorder. The clock hours of work with that child may be credited to experience with either articulation or voice disorders, whichever is most appropriate.

observation or closed-circuit TV monitoring of the student clinician.) At least one-half of each diagnostic evaluation conducted by a student clinician must be directly supervised. (The amount of direct supervision beyond these minima should be adjusted upward depending on the student's level of competence.) The first 25 hours of a student's clinical practicum must be supervised by a qualified clinical supervisor who is a member of the program's professional staff (i.e., a primary employee of the training program). In addition to the required direct supervision, supervisors may use a variety of other ways to obtain knowledge of the student's clinical work such as conferences, audio- and videotape recordings, written reports, staffings, and discussions with other persons who have participated in the student's clinical training.

## II,D. The Clinical Fellowship Year

Upon completion of professional and clinical practicum education, the applicant must complete a Clinical Fellowship Year under the supervision of one who holds the Certificate of Clinical Competence in the professional area (speech-language pathology or audiology) in which that applicant is working (and seeking certification).

Professional experience is construed to mean direct clinical work with patients, consultations, record keeping, or any other duties relevant to a bona fide program of clinical work. It is expected, however, that a significant amount of clinical experience will be in direct clinical contact with persons who have communication handicaps. Time spent in supervision of students, academic teaching, and research, as well as administrative activity that does not deal directly with management programs of specific patients or clients will not be counted as professional experience in this context.

The Clinical Fellowship Year is defined as no less than nine months of full-time professional employment, with full-time employment defined as a minimum of 30 clock hours of work a week. This requirement also may be fulfilled by part-time employment as follows: (1) work of 15–19 hours per week over 18 months, (2) work of 20–24 hours per week over 15 months, or (3) work of 25–29 hours per week over 12 months. In the event that part-time employment is used to fulfill a part of the Clinical Fellowship Year, 100% of the minimum hours of the part-time work

per week requirement must be spent in direct professional experience as defined above. The Clinical Fellowship Year must be completed within a maximum period of 36 consecutive months. Professional employment of less than 15 hours per week will not fulfill any part of this requirement. If the CFY is not initiated within two years of the date the academic and practicum education is completed, the applicant must meet the academic and practicum requirements current when the CFY is begun. Whether or not the Clinical Fellow (CF) is a member of ASHA, the CF must understand and abide by the ASHA Code of Ethics.

CFY supervision must entail the personal and direct involvement of the supervisor in any and all ways that will permit the CFY supervisor to monitor, improve, and evaluate the CF's performance in professional employment. The CFY supervisor must base the total evaluation on no less than 36 supervisory activities during the CFY. The supervisor must include 18 on-site observations of the CF (1 hour = one on-site observation; up to 6 hours may be accrued in one day; at least 6 on-site observations must be accrued during each third of the experience). The CFY supervisor must complete 18 other monitoring activities (at least one per month). These other monitoring activities may be executed by correspondence and include conferences with the CF, evaluation of written reports, evaluations by professional colleagues, etc. If multiple sites are utilized in the CFY experience, at least one on-site observation must be conducted at each site of the same provider type[5] during two of the three (1/3) segments. (NOTE: Requests for utilizing alternative mechanisms for meeting the CFY requirements stated in this paragraph must be submitted in writing to the Clinical Certification Board for prior approval.)

Should any supervisor suspect at any time during the Clinical Fellowship Year that the CF under supervision will not meet requirements, the CFY supervisor must counsel the CF both orally and in writing and maintain careful written records of all contacts and conferences in the ensuing months.

[5]Provider type: defined as one or more physical settings in which the client populations are similar (e.g., nursing homes, hospitals, schools, industrial locations, hearing aid provider offices, etc.).

## II,E. The National Examinations in Speech-Language Pathology and Audiology

The National Examinations in Speech-Language Pathology and Audiology are designed to assess, in a comprehensive fashion, the applicant's mastery of professional concepts as outlined above to which the applicant has been exposed throughout professional education and clinical practicum. The applicant must pass the National Examination, in either Speech-Language Pathology or Audiology, which is appropriate to the certificate being sought. An applicant will be declared eligible for the National Examination on notification of the acceptable completion of the education and clinical practicum requirements. The Examination must be passed within three years after the first administration for which an applicant is notified of eligibility.

In the event the applicant fails the examination, it may be retaken. If the examination is not successfully completed within the above mentioned three years, the person's application for certification will lapse. If the examination is passed at a later date, the person may reapply for clinical certification.[6]

### II,F. Applicants Educated in Other Countries

In the case of an applicant who has received all or most of his/her professional education in another country, and who has qualified under the standards of another country as an independent practitioner in speech-language pathology and/or audiology, the Clinical Certification Board has the discretion to waive all or part of Standards I,A through I,D provided that the Board is satisfied that the applicant has received fairly equivalent professional preparation. In all such cases, however, Standard I,E shall not be waived. (Note:

Standard I,A—General Background Education
Standard I,B—Required Education
Standard I,C—Academic Clinical Practicum
Standard I,D—The Clinical Fellowship Year
Standard I,E—The National Examinations in Speech-Language Pathology and Audiology.)

---

[6]Upon such reapplication, the individual's application will be reviewed and current requirements will be applied. Appropriate fees will be charged for this review.

## III. PROCEDURES FOR OBTAINING THE CERTIFICATES

### III,A.

The applicant must submit to the Clinical Certification Board a description of professional education and academic clinical practicum on the form provided for that purpose. The applicant should recognize that it is highly desirable to list upon this application form the entire professional education and academic clinical practicum training.

No credit may be allowed for courses listed on the application unless satisfactory completion is verified by an official transcript. *Satisfactory completion* is defined as the applicant's having received academic-credit (i.e., semester hours, quarter hours, or other unit of credit) with a passing grade as defined by the training institution. If the majority of an applicant's professional training is received at a program accredited by the Educational Standards Board (ESB) of the American Speech-Language-Hearing Association (ASHA), approval of education and academic clinical practicum requirements will be automatic.

The applicant must request that the director of the training program where the majority of graduate training was obtained sign the application. In the case where the training program is not accredited by ESB of ASHA that director (1) certifies that the applicant has met the educational and clinical practicum requirements, and (2) recommends that the applicant receive the certificate upon completion of all the requirements.

In the event that the applicant cannot obtain the signature of the director of the training program, the applicant should send with the application a letter giving in detail the reasons for the inability to do so. In such an instance, letters of recommendation from other faculty members may be submitted.

Application for approval of education requirements and academic clinical practicum experiences should be made (1) as soon as possible after completion of these experiences, and (2) either before or shortly after the Clinical Fellowship Year is begun.

### III,B.

Upon completion of education and academic clinical practicum training, the applicant should proceed to obtain professional employment and a supervisor for the Clinical Fellowship Year. A Clinical Fellowship Year Registration must be filed within 30 days of initiating the Clinical Fellowship Year experience. Although the filing of a CFY Plan is not required, applicants may submit such a plan to the Clinical Certification Board (CCB) if they wish prior approval of the planned professional experience.

Within one month following completion of the Clinical Fellowship Year, the CF and the CFY supervisor must submit a CFY Report to the Clinical Certification Board. If the CFY was completed in a program accredited by the Professional Services Board (PSB) of ASHA, approval of the CFY will be automatic. In such instance, the director of the PSB program must sign the CFY Report verifying compliance with requirements.

## III,C.

Upon notification by the Clinical Certification Board of approval of the academic course work and clinical practicum requirements the applicant will be sent registration material for the National Examinations in Speech-Language Pathology and Audiology. Upon approval of the Clinical Fellowship Year, achieving a passing score on the National Examination, and payment of all fees the applicant will become certified.

## III,D.

As mentioned in Footnote 6, a schedule of fees for certification may be obtained, and payment of these fees is requisite for the   obtaining a certificate. Check  able to the American Speech-La  sociation.

## III,E.

After certification has been awarded, an A  tification Fee (ACF) is payable in advance eac  by January first. A certificate holder whose ACF  arrears on April 1 will be dropped from the registry  certificate holders.

## IV. APPEALS

In the event that at any stage the Clinical Certification Board informs the applicant that the application has been rejected, the applicant has the right of formal appeal. In order to initiate such an appeal, the applicant must write to the Chair of the Clinical Certification Board and specifically request a formal review of the application. If that review results, again, in rejection, the applicant has the right to appeal the case to the Council on Professional Standards in Speech-Language Pathology and Audiology (the Standards Council) by writing to the Chair of the Standards Council at the National Office of the American Speech-Language-Hearing Association. The applicant must submit a letter of intent to appeal within 30 days and a memorandum specifying the grounds of the appeal within 60 days from the date of the rejection letter. The decision of the Standards Council will be final.

# APPENDIX B

## Code of Ethics of the American ...ge-Hearing Association—1987

(Revised January 1, 1986)*

### PREAMBLE

The preservation of the highest standards of integrity and ethical principles is vital to the successful discharge of the professional responsibilities of all speech-language pathologists and audiologists. This Code of Ethics has been promulgated by the Association in an effort to stress the fundamental rules considered essential to this basic purpose. Any action that is in violation of the spirit and purpose of this Code shall be considered unethical. Failure to specify any particular responsibility or practice in this Code of Ethics should not be construed as denial of the existence of other responsibilities or practices.

The fundamental rules of ethical conduct are described in three categories: Principles of Ethics, Ethical Proscriptions, Matters of Professional Propriety.

1. *Principles of Ethics.* Six Principles serve as a basis for the ethical evaluation of professional conduct and form the underlying moral basis for the Code of Ethics. Individuals[1] subscribing to this Code shall observe these principles as affirmative obligations under all conditions of professional activity.

2. *Ethical Proscriptions.* Ethical Proscriptions are formal statements of prohibitions that are derived from the Principles of Ethics.

*© 1985, the American Speech-Language-Hearing Association, Rockville, MD.

[1]"Individuals" refers to all members of the American Speech-Language-Hearing Association and non-members who hold a Certificate of Clinical Competence from this Association.

3. *Matters of Professional Propriety.* Matters of Professional Propriety represent guidelines of conduct designed to promote the public interest and thereby better inform the public and particularly the persons in need of speech-language pathology and audiology services as to the availability and the rules regarding the delivery of those services.

### PRINCIPLE OF ETHICS I

Individuals shall hold paramount the welfare of persons served professionally.

A. Individuals shall use every resource available, including referral to other specialists as needed, to provide the best service possible.

B. Individuals shall fully inform persons served of the nature and possible effects of the services.

C. Individuals shall fully inform subjects participating in research or teaching activities of the nature and possible effects of these activities.

D. Individuals' fees shall be commensurate with services rendered.

E. Individuals shall provide appropriate access to records of persons served professionally.

F. Individuals shall take all reasonable precautions to avoid injuring persons in the delivery of professional services.

G. Individuals shall evaluate services rendered to determine effectiveness.

**Ethical Proscriptions**

1. Individuals must not exploit persons in the delivery of professional services, including accepting persons for treatment when benefit cannot reasonably be expected or continuing treatment unnecessarily.

2. Individuals must not guarantee the results of any therapeutic procedures, directly or by implication. A reasonable statement of prognosis may be made, but caution must be exercised not to mislead persons served professionally to expect results that cannot be predicted from sound evidence.

3. Individuals must not use persons for teaching or research in a manner that constitutes invasion of privacy or fails to afford informed free choice to participate.

4. Individuals must not evaluate or treat speech, language, or hearing disorders except in a professional relationship. They must not evaluate or treat solely by correspondence. This does not preclude follow-up correspondence with persons previously seen, nor providing them with general information of an educational nature.

5. Individuals must not reveal to unauthorized persons any professional or personal information obtained from the person served professionally, unless required by law or unless necessary to protect the welfare of the person or the community.

6. Individuals must not discriminate in the delivery of professional services on any basis that is unjustifiable or irrelevant to the need for and potential benefit from such services, such as race, sex, age, or religion.

7. Individuals must not charge for services not rendered.

## PRINCIPLE OF ETHICS II

Individuals shall maintain high standards of professional competence.

A. Individuals engaging in clinical practice or supervision thereof shall hold the appropriate Certificate(s) of Clinical Competence for the area(s) in which they are providing or supervising professional services.

B. Individuals shall continue their professional development throughout their careers.

C. Individuals shall identify competent, dependable referral sources for persons served professionally.

D. Individuals shall maintain adequate records of professional services rendered.

**Ethical Proscriptions**

1. Individuals must neither provide services nor supervision of services for which they have not been properly prepared, nor permit services to be provided by any of their staff who are not properly prepared.

2. Individuals must not provide clinical services by prescription of anyone who does not hold the Certificate of Clinical Competence.

3. Individuals must not delegate any service requiring the professional competence of a certified clinician to anyone unqualified.

4. Individuals must not offer clinical services by supportive personnel for whom they do not provide appropriate supervision and assume full responsibility.

5. Individuals must not require anyone under their supervision to engage in any practice that is a violation of the Code of Ethics.

## PRINCIPLE OF ETHICS III

Individuals' statements to persons served professionally and to the public shall provide accurate information about the nature and management of communicative disorders, and about the profession and services rendered by its practitioners.

**Ethical Proscriptions**

1. Individuals must not misrepresent their training or competence.

2. Individuals' public statements providing information about professional services and products must not contain representations or claims that are false, deceptive, or misleading.

3. Individuals must not use professional or commercial affiliations in any way that would mislead or limit services to persons served professionally.

## Matters of Professional Propriety

1. Individuals should announce services in a manner consonant with highest professional standards in the community.

## PRINCIPLE OF ETHICS IV

Individuals shall maintain objectivity in all matters concerning the welfare of persons served professionally.

A. Individuals who dispense products to persons served professionally shall observe the following standards:

(1) Products associated with professional practice must be dispensed to the person served as a part of a program of comprehensive habilitative care.

(2) Fees established for professional services must be independent of whether a product is dispensed.

(3) Persons served must be provided freedom of choice for the source of services and products.

(4) Price information about professional services rendered and products dispensed must be disclosed by providing to or posting for persons served a complete schedule of fees and charges in advance of rendering services, which schedule differentiates between fees for professional services and charges for products dispensed.

(5) Products dispensed to the person served must be evaluated to determine effectiveness.

## Ethical Proscriptions

1. Individuals must not participate in activities that constitute a conflict of professional interest.

## Matters of Professional Propriety

1. Individuals should not accept compensation for supervision or sponsorship from the clinical fellow being supervised or sponsored beyond reasonable reimbursement for direct expenses.

2. Individuals should present products they have developed to their colleagues in a manner consonant with highest professional standards.

## PRINCIPLE OF ETHICS V

Individuals shall honor their responsibilities to the public, their profession, and their relationships with colleagues and members of allied professions.

## Matters of Professional Propriety

1. Individuals should seek to provide and expand services to persons with speech, language, and hearing handicaps as well as to assist in establishing high professional standards for such programs.

2. Individuals should educate the public about speech, language, and hearing processes; speech, language, and hearing problems; and matters related to professional competence.

3. Individuals should strive to increase knowledge within the profession and share research with colleagues.

4. Individuals should establish harmonious relations with colleagues and members of other professions, and endeavor to inform members of related professions of services provided by speech-language pathologists and audiologists, as well as seek information from them.

5. Individuals should assign credit to those who have contributed to a publication in proportion to their contribution.

## PRINCIPLE OF ETHICS VI

Individuals shall uphold the dignity of the profession and freely accept the profession's self-imposed standards.

A. Individuals shall inform the Ethical Practice Board when they have reason to believe that a member or certificate holder may have violated the Code of Ethics.

B. Individuals shall cooperate fully with the Ethical Practice Board concerning matters of professional conduct related to this Code of Ethics.

## Ethical Proscriptions

1. Individuals shall not engage in violations of the Principles of Ethics or in an attempt to circumvent any of them.

2. Individuals shall not engage in dishonesty, fraud, deceit, misrepresentation, or other forms of illegal conduct that adversely reflect on the profession or the individuals' fitness for membership in the profession.

# ETHICAL PRACTICE BOARD STATEMENT OF PRACTICES AND PROCEDURES
### (Effective February 15, 1986)

The Ethical Practice Board (EPB) is charged by the Bylaws of the American Speech-Language-Hearing Association with the responsibility to interpret, administer, and enforce the Code of Ethics of the Association. Accordingly, the EPB hereby adopts the following practices and procedures to be followed in administering and enforcing that Code.

A fundamental precept that guides the EPB in the discharge of its responsibility is that an effective Code of Ethics requires an orderly and fair administration and enforcement of its terms and requires full compliance by all members of the Association and all holders of Certificates of Clinical Competence. The EPB recognizes that each case must be judged on an individual basis, and that no two cases are likely to be identical. Thus, the EPB has the responsibility to exercise its judgment on the merits of each case and on its interpretation of the Code.

## A. Definition of Terms

| | |
|---|---|
| 1. *EPB:* | Ethical Practice Board |
| 2. *Association:* | American Speech-Language-Hearing Association |
| 3. *Code:* | Code of Ethics of the Association |
| 4. *Certificate(s):* | Certificate(s) of Clinical Competence |
| 5. *Respondent:* | The alleged offender |
| 6. *Complainant(s):* | The person(s) alleging that a violation occurred |
| 7. *Initial Determination:* | Initial Determination by the EPB, subject to Further Consideration and appeal, of the (a) finding, (b) proposed sanction, and (c) extent of disclosure |
| 8. *Sanction(s):* | Penalties imposed by the EPB |
| 9. *Disclosure:* | Announcement of the final EPB Decision to other than Respondent |
| 10. *Further Consideration:* | Further Consideration by the EPB of its initial Determination |
| 11. *EPB Decision:* | Final decision of the EPB after: 1) Further Consideration, or 2) 30 days from the date of notice of the Initial Determination by the EPB if no request for Further Consideration is received |
| 12. *Appeal:* | Written request from Respondent to EPB alleging error in the EPB Decision and asking that it be reversed in whole or in part by the Executive Board |

## B. Investigative Procedures

1. Alleged violations shall be reviewed by the EPB in such manner as the EPB may, in its discretion, deem necessary and proper. If, after review, the EPB elects to investigate the allegation, the EPB shall notify Respondent of the alleged offense in writing and shall advise Respondent that Respondent's answer to the allegation shall be in writing and must be received by the EPB no later than 45 days after the date of the EPB notice to Respondent. Voluntary resignation of membership and/or voluntary surrender of the Certificate(s) shall not preclude the EPB from continuing to process the alleged violation to conclusion, and the notice from the EPB to Respondent requesting an answer shall so advise Respondent.

2. At the discretion of the EPB, the Director of the Professional Affairs Department of the Association's National Office may be informed that Respondent is under investigation by the EPB for alleged violation of the Code and may be instructed that no change in membership and/or certification status shall be permitted without approval of the EPB.

3. The EPB shall consider all information secured from its investigation, including Respondent's answer to the allegation, and shall base its Initial Determination on that information.

4. If the EPB finds that there is not sufficient evidence to warrant further proceedings, Respondent and Complainant(s) shall be so advised and the investigation shall be terminated.

5. If the EPB finds that there is sufficient evidence to warrant further proceedings, the EPB shall make an Initial Determination, which includes (a) the finding of violation, (b) the proposed sanction, and (c) the proposed extent of disclosure. In this regard, the final decision of any State, Federal, regulatory, or judicial body may be considered sufficient evidence that the Code was violated.

6. The EPB may, as part of its Initial Determination, order that the Respondent cease and desist from any practice found to be a violation of the Code. Failure to comply with such a Cease and Desist Order is, itself, a violation of the Code, and shall normally result in Revocation of Membership and/or Revocation of the Certificate(s).

7. The EPB shall give Respondent notice of its Initial Determination, with copy to Complainant(s). The notice shall also advise Respondent of the right to request Further Consideration by the EPB and of the right, *after Further Consideration,* to request an appeal to the Executive Board. The procedures to be followed in exercising those rights are described in Sections F and G of this statement.

## C. Notices and Answers

All notices and answers shall be in writing and considered to be given or furnished (1) to Respondent when *sent*—Certified Mail, Addressee Only, Return Receipt Requested—to the address then listed in the ASHA membership records, and (2) to the EPB when *received* by the EPB.

## D. Sanctions

Sanctions shall consist of one or more of the following: Reprimand; Censure; Withhold, Suspend, or Revoke Membership; Withhold, Suspend, or Revoke the Certificate(s); or other measures determined by the EPB at its discretion.

## E. Disclosure

1. The EPB Decision, upon becoming final, shall be published in the Journal *Asha* unless the sanction is Reprimand. In the case of Reprimand, the EPB Decision normally shall be disclosed only to Respondent, Respondent's counsel, Complainant(s), witnesses at the EPB Further Consideration Hearing and/or at the Executive Board Hearing, staff, Association counsel, and the Coordinator of the Professional Ethics Section of the Association's National Office, each of whom shall be advised that the decision is strictly confidential and that any breach of that confidentiality by any party who is a member and/or certificate holder of the Association is, itself, a violation of the Code.

2. In appropriate cases, including when the sanction is Reprimand, the EPB may also determine that its Decision shall be disclosed to aggrieved parties and/or other appropriate individuals, bodies, or agencies.

## F. Further Consideration by the EPB of the Initial Determination

1. When the notice of Initial Determination from the EPB states that Respondent has violated the Code and announces a proposed sanction and extent of disclosure, Respondent may request that the EPB give Further Consideration to the Initial Determination.

2. Respondent's request for Further Consideration shall be in writing and must be *received* by the EPB Chair no later than 30 days after the date of notice of Initial Determination. *The request for Further Consideration must specify in what respects the Initial Determination was allegedly wrong and why.* In the absence of a timely request for Further Consideration, the Initial Determination shall be the EPB Decision, which decision shall be final; there shall be no further right of appeal to the Executive Board.

3. If Respondent submits a timely request for Further Consideration by the EPB, the EPB shall schedule a hearing and notify Respondent. At the hearing, Respondent shall be entitled to submit a written brief or to appear personally to present evidence and to be accompanied by counsel. The proceed-

ing shall be informal; strict adherence to the rules of evidence shall not be observed, but all evidence shall be accorded such weight as it deserves. As an alternative to personal appearance at the hearing, the EPB shall afford Respondent the opportunity to make a presentation to the EPB and to respond to questions from the EPB via a conference telephone call placed to Respondent by the EPB. All personal costs in connection with the Further Consideration hearing, including travel and lodging costs incurred by Respondent, Respondent's counsel and witnesses, and counsel and other fees, shall be Respondent's sole responsibility. The hearing shall be transcribed in full and, upon request, a copy of the transcript shall be made available to Respondent at Respondent's sole expense.

4. After the Further Consideration Hearing, the EPB shall render its decision and notify Respondent. If evidence presented at the hearing warrants, the EPB may modify the finding, increase or decrease the severity of the sanction, and/or modify the extent of disclosure that was announced to Respondent in the notice of Initial Determination. This decision shall be the EPB Decision, and in the absence of a timely appeal to the Executive Board, the EPB Decision shall be final.

## G. Appeal of EPB Decision to Executive Board

1. Respondent may appeal the EPB Decision to the Executive Board. The request for appeal shall be in writing and must be *received* by the EPB Chair no later than 30 days after the date of notice of the EPB Decision. *The request for appeal shall specify in what respects the EPB Decision was allegedly wrong and why.*

2. The procedures for a hearing before the Executive Board are described in the *Executive Board Statement of Practices and Procedures for Appeals of Decisions of the Ethical Practice Board.*

## H. Reinstatement

Persons whose membership or certification has been revoked may, upon application therefore, be reinstated after one year upon a two-thirds vote of the EPB. The applicant bears the burden of demonstrating that the reason(s) for revocation no longer exist and that, upon reinstatement, applicant will abide by the Code.

## I. Amendment

This *Statement of Practices and Procedures* may be amended upon recommendation of the EPB and a vote of the Executive Board. All such changes will be given appropriate publicity.

# GLOSSARY

**Abdomen** That portion of the body lying between the thorax and pelvis.

**Abduct** To draw away from the midline.

**Acoustic Immittance** Measurements of the compliance of the eardrum made on an electroacoustic device.

**Acquired Language Disorder** Loss or reduction of language ability, usually as the result of brain damage, after the acquisition of a first language.

**Acquisition** (As related to phonology) Learning to produce a target sound in restricted contexts.

**Acting Out** A receptive language task in which the child responds by manipulating toys or objects.

**Adduct** To move toward the midline.

**Agnosia** Loss of the ability to perceive, integrate, and attach meaning to sensory stimuli.

**Agrammatism** Omission of small grammatical words and word endings.

**Air Conduction** The propagation of sound, beginning at the opening of the external ear.

**Alexia** Acquired inability to perform some or all of the tasks involved in reading; caused by brain damage.

**Allophone** A speech sound that is accepted as a variant of a phoneme, but is not used to differentiate two words in a language.

**Alveolar Ridge** The upper dental arch with its sockets, in which the teeth rest, and the overlying soft tissues, sometimes called the gums.

**Alveolus** A small hallow or pit.

**Ambiguity** Referring to an expression capable of eliciting more than one meaning, as in the sentence, *He drew the gun.*

**Ambiguous** Having multiple meanings.

**Anacusis** Total hearing loss.

**Ankylosis** Impairment of arytenoid movement resulting from stiffness or fixation of the cricoarytenoid joint.

**Anomia** Acquired word-finding difficulty; caused by brain damage.

**Anoxia** Lack of oxygen.

**Antagonist** Muscle that acts in opposition to another muscle.

**Antecedent Event** Event that occurs before a target response.

**Anterior** Toward the front; away from the back.

**Anterior Commissure** Where the vocal folds attach to the thryroid cartilage and are in contact with each other.

**Aphasia** Acquired language disorder caused by brain damage and resulting in partial or complete impairment of language comprehension, formulation, and use for communication.

**Aphonia** Complete loss of voice.

**Apraxia of Speech** Disturbance in the selection and sequencing of speech sounds due to brain damage. Neurologic, phonologic disorder resulting from sensorimotor impairment of the capacity to select, program, or execute, in coordinated and normally timed sequences, the positioning of the speech muscles for the volitional production of speech sounds; involuntary movements remain intact. Sometimes considered a form of aphasia.

**Arbitrary** Word that derives meaning from a random choice rather than from a similarity, logical reason, resemblance, or need.

**Articulation** Using the articulators (teeth, tongue, etc.) to produce speech sounds.

**Articulators** Those structures responsible for the modification of the vocal tract: tongue, lips, soft and hard palates, and teeth.

**Artificial Larynx** An electronic or pneumatic sound source that substitutes for the larynx after it has been surgically removed.

**Assimilation** The process of making a sound or a word more like another by assuming features of it.

**Ataxic** (1) Lack of order; (2) type of cerebral palsy characterized by poor sense of body position and balance, and by lack of coordination of voluntary muscles.

**Athetosic** (1) Without a fixed base; (2) type of cerebral palsy characterized by large, irregular, uncontrollable twisting actions; muscles may have too much or too little tone.

**Audiogram** A graph depicting hearing sensitivity, measured in decibels, as a function of different frequencies.

**Auditory-Evoked Potentials** The measurement of electrical responses in the brain to acoustic signals.

**Auditory Nerve** The VIIIth cranial nerve that carries impulses from the inner ear to the brain. It conveys information about the body's balance and hearing functions.

**Auditory Training** Training in the maximal use of residual hearing.

**Autism** A condition characterized by a failure to develop normal verbal and nonverbal communication behaviors and responsivity to other persons, a failure to use objects appropriately, and a generalized overreaction to certain sensory stimuli or a notable lack of response to other sensory stimuli.

**Automatic** Production of a speech sound without conscious effort.

**Autonomous Phonemic** Traditional study of the sounds of a language, independent of changes that may occur between or within words.

**Auxiliary** A helping verb that can indicate time, the manner in which the verb action is experienced or viewed (aspects), and moods or attitudes.

**Babbling** Long strings of sounds that children begin to produce at 4 months of age.

**Baseline** The pretreatment level of a target behavior, which, when quantified, can be used as a basis against which to measure progress.

**Behavior Modification** Systematic application of behavioral learning principles to increase or decrease a target response.

**Bernoulli Effect** A drawing inward of the walls of a narrowed section of a flexible tube, such as at the vocal folds in the larynx, when the velocity of the airflow is increased.

**Bidialectical** Having linguistic competence in two or more variations of a langue and the ability to code-switch appropriately for use of each.

**Bifid Uvula** A uvula that has been divided vertically; the condition is usually congenital.

**Biopsy** Surgical removal of a small sample of tissue that is then examined microscopically.

**Black English** The collective varieties of English spoken by people of African descent throughout the world, including American Black English (the collective varieties of English spoken by blacks in the United States).

**Black English Vernacular** The varieties of Black English spoken by people of African descent in formal situations throughout the world, including American Black English Vernacular.

**Block** An instance of stuttering usually characterized by a complete or partial interruption of the smooth flow of speech.

**Bone Conduction** Measurement made with a special vibrator that checks hearing sensitivity by vibrating the skull. It theoretically bypasses the outer and middle ears and sends vibrations directly to the inner ear.

**Bronch-, Broncho-** Referring to the windpipe.

**Bronchiole** The smallest division of the bronchial tree.

**Carcinoma** A malignant tumor that develops from epithelium.

**Carrier Phrase Task** An expressive language task in which the child completes a sentence initiated by the examiner.

**Cartilage** A nonvascular connective tissue, softer and more flexible than bone.

**Central Nervous System (CNS)** Portion of the nervous system that includes the brain and spinal cord.

**Cerebral Palsy** A group of irreversible, nondeteriorating disorders caused by an irregularity in the central nervous system, primarily at motor centers; damage may be caused at any time before muscular coordination is attained. Characteristics may include too much or too little muscle tone, abnormal positioning, and general lack of coordination. Intellect, speech, hearing, vision, and emotional control may be affected.

**Circumlocution** A roundabout way of referring to or describing an object, action, or event when a speaker cannot find the exact or intended word.

**Classical Conditioning** Process in which two stimuli are repeatedly paired to give one (the conditioned stimulus) the power to elicit the unconditioned response (reflex) already elicited by the other (unconditioned) stimulus.

**Cleft** A fissure or elongated opening, especially one resulting from the failure of parts to fuse in embryonic life, as in cleft lip and palate.

**Closed-Head Injury** Cerebral trauma in which one or more cognitive functions are temporarily or permanently disturbed.

**Cluttering** Rapid, often unintelligible speech characterized by omission of speech sounds or entire words.

**Coarticulation** Movement of the articulators to a target sound before the sound is produced.

**Code Switching** The act of shifting from one language or one dialect of a language to another, usually under the control of the social situation or context.

**Cognates** Pair of constant phonemes with the same place and manner of articulation and differing only in voicing.

**Communication** Process of encoding, transmitting, and decoding signals to exchange information and ideas between the participants.

**Communication Competence** Knowledge that users of a language must have to understand and produce an infinite number of acceptable grammatical structures.

**Communicative Competence** Knowledge required by members of a speech community to communicate effectively and appropriately.

**Complement** A noun or adjective, phrase or clause that has a function similar to that of a noun phrase.

**Comprehension-Based Approach** A treatment approach in which the child is taught to understand particular linguistic features prior to instruction on their production.

**Conch** A shell-like organ or structure, pronounced "khongk."

**Conductive Hearing Loss** Loss of hearing sensitivity produced by abnormalities of the outer ear and/or middle ear.

**Congenital** Present at birth.

**Conjoining** The process of joining or combining two or more clauses into larger units or sentences.

**Conjunction** A word used to join or combine two or more clauses into larger units or sentences.

**Connotative Meaning** A meaning of a word, in addition to the primary meaning, that results from evaluative or affective reactions.

**Consequence** Contingent event following a response that functions to increase or decrease the probability that the response will occur again.

**Contingent Query** A conditional request form such as "Who?" that can ask for repetition or elaboration of a prior statement.

**Continuity** Continuous development of speech from infant vocalizations to language.

**Contrastive Elements** Speech sounds that serve to distinguish meanings, as /p/ and /b/ in *pig* and *big*.

**Cortical** Referring to the outer layer of the brain, consisting primarily of cell bodies of neurons.

**Counterconditioning and Reciprocal Inhibition** Learning a response that competes with an undesirable response.

**Creole** A language formed on the basis of the phonology and grammar of a dominant language, but using vocabulary of a nondominant language.

**Criterion-Referenced Probes** A form of assessment focusing on the child's comprehension or production of linguistic features known to be acquired by the majority of children at a particular age or stage of development.

**Criterion-Referenced Test** Test that compares an individual's scores to a standard, rather than to scores of other subjects, for mastery.

**Cul-de-Sac Resonance** Resonance created by a faulty velopharyngeal valve and nasal passages that are obstructed.

**Culture** The set of values, perceptions, beliefs, institutions, technologies, and survival systems used by members of a specified group to ensure the acquisition and perpetuation of what *they* consider to be a high quality of life.

**Cut-Off Score** A score below which a child's performance is considered to be significantly lower than that expected for her age level.

**Deaf** Having a hearing loss of at least 70 dB HL, which precludes comprehending speech aurally.

**Decibel (dB)** A logarithmic unit for expressing a ratio between two sound pressures or two sound powers.

**Deciduous** Temporary; falling off and shedding at maturity.

**Declarative** A sentence form that expresses a statement or assertion.

**Decode** The act of interpreting spoken and written symbols.

**Decoding** Process of deducing a thought or message from oral or written language.

**Deep Structure** Basic meaning of a sentence.

**Delayed Imitation Task** An expressive language task in which the child repeats an utterance provided by the examiner after a brief period that may or may not have contained other verbal information.

**Derivation** The process of adding an ending to a base word form, thereby changing its grammatical class relationship to allow it to function in different syntactic constructions.

**Descriptive Test** A test whose results are reported in terms of the items passed or failed. The items may be associated with a particular level of development, as reported by other sources.

**Developmental** (Related to phonology) Gradual acquisition of speech sounds as age increases.

**Developmental Disfluency** A normally occurring increase in the effortless repetitions of syllables and words; usually appears for a short time between the ages of 2½ to 3½ years, then disappears.

**Dialect** A variety within a specific language.

**Diaphragm** (1) A partition separating two cavities; (2) muscle tht separates thorax from abdomen.

**Diphthong** Blend of two vowels within the same syllable.

**Discourse** The systematic conjoining of utterances in either monologue or dialogue to achieve a specific communicative purpose.

**Disfluencies** Properties in speech that interrupt the smooth, forward flow of an utterance; usually refers to pauses, hesitations, interjections, prolongations, and repetitions.

**Distinctive Feature** The articulatory and/or acoustic characteristics of speech sounds.

**Distortion** Producing a speech sound in a substandard manner.

**Distributed Practice** Practice sessions that are separated by rest periods.

**Down's Syndrome** Specific syndrome caused by chromosomal abnormality, occurring in approximately 1 in 700 births. It is often characterized by wideset, Oriental-looking eyes; mild to moderate mental retardation; a Simian or single crease across the palm; and a wide range of other birth defects.

**Dysarthria** A group of motor speech disorders caused by central or peripheral nervous system damage that may include disruptions of respiration, phonation, articulation, resonance, or prosody.

**Dyslexia** Failure to master reading at the expected age level in the absence of a major debilitating disorder.

**Dysnomia** Developmental word-finding difficulty that interferes with accuracy in finding intended words. *See also* Anomia.

**Dysphagia** Disturbance in the normal act of swallowing or deglutition.

**Dysphemia** Theory about stuttering that claims it is a biological breakdown occurring under emotional or physical stress. Related to biochemical theory, which states that the breakdown is specifically biochemical.

**Dysphonia** Poor or unpleasant voice quality.

**Echolalia** An involuntary, parrotlike imitation of words and phrases spoken by others, often accompanied by twitching of muscles; frequently seen in autism and schizophrenia.

**Elaboration** The process or result of expanding an utterance by adding details or modifying words or phrases.

**Elicited Imitation Task** An expressive language task in which the child repeats utterances produced by the examiner.

**Embedding** The process or result of placing a word, phrase, or clause in an existing sentence.

**Endematous** Filled with fluid; swollen.

**Endocrinologist** A medical doctor who specializes in the treatment of diseases of the endocrine glandular system.

**Epigastrium** The upper, anterior wall of the abdomen that lies over the stomach.

**Erythema** Abnormal redness.

**Esophageal Speech** Speech produced with the sound generated by vibration of the tissues at the upper end of the esophagus; caused by expulsion of air from the esophagus; used primarily by laryngectomized persons.

**Ethnography of Communication** The study of communication rules, including rules for verbal and nonverbal communication, in a cultural context.

**Etiology** Cause or causes of a disorder.

**Extinguish** To eradicate an undesirable behavior completely.

**Extrinsic** Originating outside the part.

**Facial Grimace** A ticlike movement of the nostrils or adjacent facial muscles, used in an attempt to reduce nasal air flow.

**Facilitative** The enhancing influence of a preceding speech sound on a target sound.

**Figurative Language** Expressions that use words or phrases to represent an abstract concept. Such expressions cannot be interpreted literally. For example, *My father hit the roof* cannot be explained at a syntactic level. Types of figurative language include idioms, metaphors, similes, and proverbs.

**Fissure**   A cleft or split.

**Fistula**   An abnormal channel in the body connecting two spaces, or extending from a space or abcess in the body.

**Fluency**   The smooth, effortless, uninterrupted flow of an utterance.

**Focused Stimulation Approach**   A treatment approach in which the child is provided with concentrated exposure to a particular linguistic feature.

**Formant (Bands)**   Regions of prominent energy distribution in a speech sound.

**Frequency**   The number of back and forth vibrations of an oscillating body in a given amount of time.

**Functional**   An articulation disorder of unknown etiology.

**Generalization**   Producing a target sound, word, or structure in contexts and situations in which no training is provided.

**Gerund**   A verbal noun ending in *-ing* that expresses the meaning of the verb, but functions as a noun.

**Glissando**   Gliding up or down a musical scale.

**Glottal Fry**   A grating or popping sound that occurs most often toward the end of sentences or phrases, where the pitch and breath pressure customarily drop.

**Glottal or Laryngeal Tone**   The tone generated by the vibrating vocal folds; distinguished from the tone produced by the oscillation or ringing of the vocal tract.

**Glottal Stop**   A plosive sound produced when air held beneath the glottis is suddenly released.

**Glottis**   The space between the vocal folds.

**Gross Motor**   Referring to movements that involve major body parts or muscle groups for activities such as walking and running.

**Gyrus**   A fold in the cerebral cortex; a convolution.

**Hard-of-Hearing**   A person with a hearing loss of 35 to 69 dB HL, which makes comprehension of speech by hearing alone difficult, but not impossible.

**Hard Palate**   The hard, front part of the roof of the mouth and the floor of the nose, composed of bone and covered by mucous membrane.

**Hearing-Impaired**   Suffering from any degree of hearing loss.

**Hematoma**   A tumor filled with blood, such as a blood blister.

**Hemianopsia (Hemianopia)**   Defective vision in one half of the visual field of one eye. Homonymous hemianopsia indicates a corresponding visual field loss in both eyes.

**Hemiparesis**   Weakness of one lateral half of the body.

**Hemiplegia**   Paralysis of one lateral half of the body.

**Hertz (Hz)**   The number of cycles per second exhibited by a vibrating body.

**Homonymous**   Having the same meaning.

**Hypernasal**   Speech that is too greatly resonated in the nasal cavities.

**Hypernasality**   Excessive nasal resonance.

**Hyponasality**   Speech that varies from the norm because it has little or no nasal resonance.

**Iconic**   Word that bears a resemblance to its reference, as a picture, gesture, or sound.

**Ideation**   Organization of ideas into concepts that can be communicated.

**Identification**   Ability to point differentially to two words that contrast minimally.

**Identification Task**   A receptive language task in which the child responds by pointing or otherwise indicating the correct item from among a set of alternative items.

**Illocutionary**   Referring to the intent or intention of an utterance.

**Imitation-Based Approach**   A treatment approach in which the child repeats utterances produced by the speech-language pathologist to increase his ability with the features contained in these utterances.

**Imperative**   A statement or exclamation that commands action, as in *Be quiet.*

**Inconsistent Error**   An error sound produced correctly in some contexts and incorrectly in others.

**Indirect Request**   A request for action that is stated indirectly, as in *Shouldn't someone check the cookies?* to indicate they are burning and should be taken out of the oven.

**Inflection**   The process or outcome of adding a word ending to a noun or verb to indicate number, gender, case, or time.

**Inner Ear**   The portion of the hearing apparatus that converts sound impulses from the middle ear into an electrochemical signal sent to the brain. It also sends signals to the balance centers in the brain about the body's orientation in space.

**Intelligibility** The degree to which speech is understood by others.

**Intensity** Sound energy per unit volume of air.

**Internal Discrimination Testing** A child's evaluation of her own speech sound error production.

**Interrogative** A sentence that asks for information (for example, wh- question) or serves to control others (for example, yes/no question).

**Intrinsic** Rising from the nature or constitution of a thing; inherent, situated within.

**Jargon** Fluent, well-articulated, phonologically correct utterances that make little sense.

**Judgment Task** A receptive language task requiring the child to make a formal assessment of the suitability of the utterance presented by the examiner.

**Kinesics** The study of bodily movement, particularly in relation to communication.

**Kinesthetic Feedback** Knowledge of the location of muscles and body parts, or whether they are moving, derived from sensory end-organs in the muscles, tendons, joints, and sometimes inner ears.

**Language** A socially shared code or conventional system for representing concepts through the use of arbitrary symbols and rule-governed combinations of those symbols.

**Language-Learning Disability** The developmental language disability associated with a diagnosed learning disability.

**Language Retardation** Developmental delay in language acquisition associated with mental retardation.

**Laryngeal Web** A membrane extending from one vocal fold to the other, and varying in extent from small to complete obstruction of the glottis. Webs may also occur above or below the glottis.

**Laryngectomee** An individual who has had the larynx removed.

**Laryngectomy** Surgery to remove the larynx.

**Laryngologist** A medical doctor who specializes in the treatment of diseases of the larynx and associated structures.

**Larynx** Anatomical structure located above the trachea and below the hyoid bone and tongue root; consists of cartilage and muscle and, due to its vocal folds, is the primary organ of phonation.

**Learning** Acquisition of a behavior through a structured teaching approach.

**Lexicon** The inventory of words stored in memory and available for use in communication.

**Ligament** A band of fibrous tissue that connects bones or holds organs in place.

**Linguistic Competence** A native speaker's underlying knowledge of the rules for generating and understanding conventional linguistic forms.

**Linguistic Performance** Language use. Performance reflects linguistic competence and the communication constraints.

**Mainstreaming** Education of handicapped children in the least restrictive environment possible by placing them with nonhandicapped children.

**Maintenance** Continued production of a target sound after training has been completed.

**Main Verb** A verb that indicates the predication in a proposition (sentence). Also referred to as a *lexical verb*.

**Mandible** Lower jaw.

**Mandibular Arch** Lower dental arch.

**Manometer** Instrument for measuring the pressure of liquids or gases.

**Marked Word** Word in an antonym pair with negative, nonpreferred, or unusual reference, for example *hate* (love).

**Masking** Process of presenting a sound to the nontest ear to remove it from an audiological test procedure.

**Massed Practice** Continuous practice sessions that are not separated by rest periods.

**Maxilla** Upper jaw.

**Maxillary Arch** Upper dental arch.

**Meatus** An opening to a passageway in the body.

**Medial** Toward the axis; near the midline.

**Membrane** A thin layer of tissue that binds structures, divides spaces or organs, and lines cavities.

**Mental Retardation** A condition characterized by subaverage overall intellectual functioning, and personal independence and social responsibility below age and cultural expectations.

**Metacommunication** Nonverbal aspects of communication.

**Metalinguistics** Linguistic intuitions on the acceptability of communication.

**Metastasis** The transfer or migration of a disease from one location to another, and the establishment of the disease in a new location.

**Middle Ear**   A small cavity behind the eardrum membrane that houses three small bones carrying sound vibrations to the inner ear.

**Middle Ear Effusion**   Accumulation of fluid behind the tympanic membrane.

**Mixed Hearing Loss**   The loss of sound sensitivity produced by damage to the conductive apparatus (outer or middle ear) and the sensorineural apparatus (inner ear or auditory nerve).

**Modal**   An auxiliary verb used to express moods or attitudes, such as ability (can), intent (will), possibility (may), or obligation (must).

**Modeling Approach**   A treatment approach that focuses on the language rule or pattern reflected in utterance examples provided by a model.

**Modifier**   A word, phrase, or clause that qualifies the meaning of a previous or following word, phrase, or clause.

**Mongolism**   Vernacular term for Down's syndrome.

**Moro Reflex**   Extensor startle pattern in response to sound; exhibited by most newborns.

**Morpheme**   Smallest unit of meaning. Morphemes (for example, *dog*) are indivisible without violating the meaning of the morpheme or producing meaningless units (for example, *do, g*). There are two types of morphemes, free and bound.

**Morphology**   Aspect of language concerned with rules governing change in meaning at the intraword level.

**Motor Schema**   An internalized rule for sound production.

**Multiview Videofluoroscopy**   A moving X-ray image recorded on videotape during speech.

**Myasthenia**   Overall condition of muscular weakness.

**Myringotomy**   A small surgical incision in the tympanic membrane.

**Narrative**   A dimension of discourse involving translating experiences into stories. A recital of facts, or a composition or talk that confines itself to fact.

**Narrow-Band Noise**   Filtered noise presented in certain frequencies at near equal intensities.

**Nasopharynx**   The upper part of the pharynx associated with the back of the nasal space.

**Negative**   A sentence form that invalidates a statement or an assertion, usually using the word *not* to signify the negative function.

**Neurogenic**   Arising from the nervous system.

**Neurologist**   A medical doctor who specializes in the treatment of the nervous system and its diseases.

**Noise**   Any complex sound composed of irregular vibrations to which a pure pitch cannot be assigned.

**Nonlinguistics**   Coding devices that contribute to communication but are not a part of speech. Examples include gestures, body posture, eye contact, head and body movement, facial expression (kinesics), and physical distance (proxemics).

**Nonverbal Communication**   Reciprocal interaction between two or more individuals without the use of oral or written symbols.

**Normal**   A trait property or behavior that occurs naturally in a given population.

**Normative Data**   Performance scores, in the form of raw scores, percentile levels, or standard scores, that allow an examiner to compare a child's scores to those obtained by her peers in the standardization sample.

**Norm-Referenced Standardized Test**   A test that allows an examiner to compare a child's performance to that of his peers in the standardization sample.

**Norms**   Descriptions of the articulation, speech sound repertoires, or language of children at different age levels.

**Nystagmus**   An involuntary slow movement in one direction followed by a rapid movement in the opposite direction.

**Objective case**   A form of personal pronouns that function as objects, prepositional complements, and sometimes as subject complements in sentences.

**Object Permanence**   The recognition that objects, animals, or people continue to exist, even if they are not directly visible.

**Obligatory**   Referring to a required, rather than optional, structural form of sentences or intents.

**Omission**   Not producing one or more sounds in a word.

**Operant Conditioning**   Use of reinforcement principles for modifying behavior.

**Optimum Pitch**   That vocal pitch at which the voice is produced with maximum efficiency. It is usually about five musical tones above the low end of the individual's range.

**Oral Peripheral**   The structures used in the production of speech.

**Organic**   Having a physical cause or source.

**Origin**   The place of attachment of a muscle, remaining relatively fixed during contraction.

**Otitis Media**   Infection of the middle ear space.

**Outer Ear**   The outermost portion of the hearing apparatus that contains the pinna (to funnel sound), the external auditory canal, and the eardrum membrane.

**Papilloma**   (Plural is papillomata.) A benign tumor that develops on the skin (such as warts) or on the mucous membrane.

**Paradigmatic**   Referring to relationships among words that share semantic attributes and form a semantic class or category, as for the words *cat* and *dog*.

**Paralanguage**   The study of prosodic variation; sounds produced in speech that are not part of the phonetic code.

**Paralinguistics**   Vocal and nonvocal codes that are superimposed on a linguistic code to signal the speaker's attitude or emotion, or to clarify or provide additional meaning.

**Parallel Sentence Production Task**   An expressive language task in which the child responds to a stimulus, using as a basis the example provided by the examiner for a different stimulus.

**Paramedian**   Near the midline; almost at its normal median position.

**Paraphasia**   The unintentional substitution of an incorrect word for an intended word.

**Partial Tones**   Components of a complex sound. When partials are integral multiples of the fundamental, they are also overtones; however, a partial need not be harmoniously related to the fundamental.

**Patterns**   (As related to phonology) An articulation error that affects classes of sound, not just single sounds.

**Percentile Scores or Ranks**   Scores that represent the percentage of children, at a particular age level, who scored below a given raw score in the standardization sample.

**Perfect**   An aspect of the verb associated with a time-orientation in relation to the past, indicating a period of time in the past (present perfect—" ... has lived in Paris ... ") or a past-in-the-past (past perfect—" ... had lived in Paris ... ").

**Peripheral Nervous System (PNS)**   Portion of the nervous system that includes the cranial and spinal nerves.

**Perseveration**   Responses that are involuntary repetitions of previous responses.

**Pharyngeal Flap**   A flap elevated from the posterior wall and attached to the soft palate to correct velopharyngeal incompetence.

**Pharyngeo-Esophageal Segment (P-E Segment)**   The junction between the lower part of the pharynx and the upper section of the esophagus. It is the location of the sound generator for esophageal speech and for speech with the tracheoesophageal fistula.

**Pharynx**   The membranous-muscular tube connecting the mouth and posterior nares with the esophagus and larynx.

**Phonation**   The production of sound by the vibration of the vocal folds.

**Phone**   Any speech sound.

**Phoneme**   Smallest meaningful unit of speech sound. Each phoneme consists of a set of distinctive features.

**Phonological Conditioning**   Process by which the choice of inflectional word ending is governed by the sound immediately preceding it.

**Phonological Disorder**   A problem in the organization of the child's or adult's phonological system.

**Phonology**   (1) Aspect of language concerned with the rules governing the structure, distribution, and sequencing of speech sounds in a language; (2) science of speech sounds and sound patterns.

**Phrase Structure Rules**   Chomskyan concept; rules that delineate basic relationships underlying sentence organization. Chomsky found the phrase structure rules to be universal, and thus concluded that they were innate.

**Pitch**   Quality of sound caused by its frequency; proceeding on a scale from low to high.

**Pleura**   The serous membranes lining the thoracic cavity and investing the surfaces of the lungs.

**Polarity**   The possession of two meanings with contrary or opposing qualities, as in antonyms (for example, hot–cold).

**Polyp**   A benign tumor that projects outward from surface membranes. Polyps are found frequently in the larynx, nose, and elsewhere in the respiratory and alimentary tracts.

**Position Generalization**   The ability to use a feature of language in an utterance position that is different from the position in which the feature was originally learned.

**Posterior**   Toward the back; away from the front.

**Postlingual Hearing Loss**   Loss of hearing that develops after the individual has begun development of speech and language.

**Pragmatics**   Aspect of language concerned with the use of language in a communication context.

**Prefix**   A unit of meaning, word, or syllable placed before another word to modify meaning or to form a new meaning.

**Prelingual Hearing Loss**   Loss of hearing that develops before the individual has begun development of speech and language.

**Processes (Phonological)**   Children's simplifications of difficult-to-produce adult sounds.

**Prognosis**   Indication of how rapid and complete recovery from a disorder will be.

**Prosodic**   Referring to the stress pattern (voice, pitch, loudness, duration) of an utterance.

**Prosody**   Aspects of language that convey meaning and mood, and give melody to the speech act by changes in rate, rhythm, or stress.

**Proxemics**   The study of bodily position and spatial relations, in particular with respect to communication.

**Pseudoglottis**   An artificial glottis.

**Psychiatrist**   A medical doctor who specializes in the treatment of mental, emotional, behavioral and personality disorders.

**Psycholinguistic Theory**   Study of the psychological aspects of language, especially as they apply to the psychological processes involved in learning, processing, and using language.

**Punishment**   Presenting a negative consequence to decrease the frequency of the behavior it follows.

**Reactive Language Stimulation Approach**   A treatment approach in which the child controls the topic, and the speech-language pathologist responds in a nonpunitive manner to the child's utterances.

**Reauditorization**   The process of reconstructing spoken and heard words, phrases, sentences, or digits to oneself, in "one's head" or "one's mind's ear."

**Reciprocal Inhibition**   *See* Counterconditioning and Reciprocal Inhibition.

**Reduplication**   The process or outcome of repeating a sound or syllable within a word.

**Referent**   The event or object to which a symbol refers.

**Reflex**   An involuntary, relatively invariable, adaptive response to a stimulus.

**Register**   Range of word, phrase, sentence, and utterance choices and language styles available to a speaker to meet the needs or expectations of a given listener.

**Reinforcement**   Consequent positive event that increases the probability that the behavior it follows will occur again.

**Relapse**   Return to pretherapy state. It may also refer to substitution of new undersirable behaviors for the old ones.

**Relative Clause**   Subordinate clause joined to a main clause with a pronoun that may be omitted, as in *Sue told me about a movie [that] she had seen.*

**Relaxation Pressure**   Intrapulmonic pressure due to tissue elasticity, torque, and gravity, that tends to expel air from the lungs.

**Residual Hearing**   Amount of hearing present along with some loss.

**Residual Volume**   Quantity of air that cannot be expelled from the lungs; usually expressed in $cm^3$.

**Resonance**   (1) An acoustical phenomenon; the vibratory response of a body or air-filled cavity to a frequency imposed on it. (2) As related to voice, the process of increasing the prominence of certain tones or overtones by adjusting the cavities of the respiratory tract to respond to the frequency of particular partials (to resonate). (3) The selective absorption and radiation of acoustic energy at specific wavelengths or frequencies.

**Resonant Frequency**   The rate at which any given object can most easily be made to vibrate.

**Resource Room**   An educational setting in which students with moderate special needs can receive instruction or tutoring.

**Respiration**   The interchange of gases between living organisms and their environment.

**Respiratory Tract**   The nares, nasal cavities, pharynx, oral cavity, larynx, trachea, and bronchial tubes.

**Retrieval**   The process of recalling information stored in memory.

**Rugae**   The ridges on the dental arch behind the teeth.

**Schwa**   The ultimate reduced vowel /ə/, which is unstressed, lax or short, and midcentral. It can achieve the minimal duration for a vowel sound.

**Screening** A brief assessment of an individual's articulation, language, or other communication ability.

**Secondary Behaviors** Behaviors associated with instances of stuttering, such as eye blinking, head shaking, and facial grimaces, that stutterers think releases them from stuttering blocks.

**Segmentation** Process of dividing a stream of speech into discrete sounds, words, and sentences.

**Semantics** Aspect of language concerned with rules governing the meaning or content of words, and grammatical rules.

**Semivowels** Sounds that are neither completely vowel nor consonant, but fall between them in articulation and perception.

**Sensorineural Hearing Loss** The loss of sound sensitivity produced by damage to the inner ear or auditory nerve.

**Shaping** The act of modifying a response or behavior through gradually closer approximations of target.

**Shunt** As used in this book, a surgically created tracheo-esophageal fistula or channel extending from the back wall of the trachea to the esophagus. Produced in laryngectomized persons to divert pulmonary air to the esophagus for voice production.

**Sociolinguistics** Study of the sociological influence, especially cultural and situational variables, on language learning and use, including dialects, bilingualism, and parent-child interactions.

**Sociolinguistic Variables** Nonlinguistic factors that may change an act of communication, for example, audience, topic, or setting.

**Sonogram** Graph of a sound or sounds produced by a special electromechanical device.

**Sound Discrimination** Ability to differentiate between two sounds auditorally.

**Southern White Nonstandard English** Dialect of American English spoken by working class Southern whites.

**Spastic** (1) Characterized by muscle contractions that are involuntary and jerky; (2) a type of cerebral palsy characterized by spastic movements and too much muscle tone.

**Spatial** Referring to aspects of location, space, orientation, or relationship in space.

**Specific Language Impairment** A significant deficit in linguistic functioning that does not appear to be accompanied by deficits of hearing, intelligence, or motor functioning.

**Speech** Dynamic neuromuscular process of producing speech sounds for communication. A verbal means of communicating or conveying meaning.

**Speech Community** A group of individuals sharing a common set of linguistic and communication rules, values, and experiences.

**Spirometer** An instrument for measuring vital capacity or volume of inspired and exhaled air.

**Spontaneous Recovery** The period that reflects the natural resolution of impairments that were incurred as the result of stroke.

**Standard Black English** Varieties of English spoken by formally educated people of African descent throughout the world; used especially in formal situations.

**Standard Dialect** The primary language spoken by groups with the highest social, economic, or educational prestige or power within the society.

**Standardized Test** A test that has been given to a large number of individuals who are representative of the age levels, cultural groups, and the like, of students for whom the test is to be used.

**Standard Scores** Converted raw scores that have been weighted by computing the group mean and variability of scores at an age level.

**Stent** A splint or mold that fits into the larynx and supports fractured laryngeal cartilages while they are healing.

**Stereotypes** Real or nonsense words and phrases that are produced involuntarily and carry little, if any, meaning.

**Stimulability** Ability of a child to imitate a target sound when presented with a model.

**Stimulus Control** An antecedent stimulus that appears to consistently evoke a response because the response has been reinforced when the stimulus has occurred.

**Stimulus Generalization** The ability to use a feature of language in a physical or communicative context that is different from the context in which the feature was originally learned.

**Stoma** As related to laryngectomy or obstructed airway, a surgically created opening in the lower front part of the neck to which the trachea is attached and through which the individual breathes.

**Storage**   The process or outcome of transferring information to long-term memory for later use.

**Strabismus**   Inability to focus the eye; caused by unbalanced muscular strength or control in one eye.

**Strength**   Component of movement that contributes to differential ability in the velocity or amount of muscle contractability and load shift.

**Stridor**   A harsh or wheezing vocal sound that is symptomatic of a partial obstruction in the airway. The sound may be generated during inhalation, exhalation, or both. The condition may be congenital.

**Structural Ambiguity**   Characteristic of a sentence structure that allows it to be interpreted in more than one way.

**Subcortical**   Referring to the areas of the brain lying beneath the cerebral cortex.

**Subjective Case**   Personal pronouns that function as subjects or sometimes as subject complements.

**Submucous Cleft Palate**   A cleft in underlying muscle, and often of the bony palate, with a thin mucous covering that may obscure the condition.

**Subordinating**   Functioning as a link between two joined clauses, one of which is of lesser importance than the other.

**Substitution**   The process of replacing one speech sound (phoneme), word, phrase, or clause with another.

**Suffix**   A sound, syllable, or syllable sequence that, when added to an existing word, can change or modify its meaning.

**Sulcus**   A groove, trench, or furrow. The labial sulcus is the space between the lip and mandible or maxilla. Furrows or grooves are also found in other locations, especially in the brain.

**Suprasegmental**   Characteristics greater than the linguistic segments of an utterance, relating to junctural or prosodic features.

**Surface Structure**   The actual form of spoken sentences.

**Symbol**   A unit in oral or written expression that is used to represent an object, event, or idea.

**Syndrome**   A cluster or set of usually co-occuring characteristics or symptoms that form a pattern. In genetics, a combination of phenotypic manifestations.

**Syntagmatic**   Referring to relationships among individual words that reflect their functions (noun, verb, etc.) in sentences.

**Syntagmatic-Paradigmatic Shift**   Change in word association behavior from a syntactic to a semantic basis. This occurs during the school-age years.

**Syntax**   Organizational rules for ordering words in a sentence, specifying word order, sentence organization, and word relationships.

**System**   As related to articulation, the way in which a child organizes her phonology.

**Systematic Phonemic**   A system in the study of sounds that tries to classify and explain changes in sounds as words are used in different ways.

**Telegraphic Speech**   Communication that sounds like a spoken telegram due to the omission of grammatical words and word endings.

**Temporal**   Referring to aspects of time and time relationships.

**Tendon**   A nonelastic band of connective tissue that attaches a muscle to bone or cartilage.

**Tensor Veli Palatini Muscles**   Muscles responsible for opening the eustachian tube.

**Tetrahedral**   Having the form of a tetrahedron, which is a solid connected by four triangular plane faces (a triangular pyramid).

**Thalamus**   A subcortical region that receives, synthesizes, and relays all sensory stimuli, with the exception of olfactory stimuli, to specific cortical areas.

**Thoraco-**   Pertaining to the chest.

**Tidal Volume**   The quantity of air exchanged during a cycle of quiet normal breathing; usually expressed in $cm^3$.

**Timing**   Accuracy in the onset and termination of muscular contraction.

**Tone**   Relatively constant background state of muscular contraction characteristic of normal muscle.

**Trachea**   The tube extending from the larynx to the bronchi.

**Tranformation**   Operation in which elements in the base structure of an utterance are substituted, deleted, or rearranged into an appropriate surface structure.

**Transformational Rules**   Chomskyan concept. Rules that operate on "strings" of symbols, rearranging phrase structure elements to form an acceptable sentence for output. There are rules for negatives, interrogatives, and so on.

**Trauma**   An injury from a blow, wound, or, in the case of vocal folds, excessive vocal abuse.

**Tympanometry** Measurement, on an acoustic immitance meter, of the movement of the eardrum caused by various degrees of positive and negative air pressure.

**Tympanostomy Tubes** Minute tubes inserted through the tympanic membrane to ensure aeration of the middle ear.

**Underlying Representation** The form of a lexical item as it is stored in a child's memory.

**Unilateral Neglect** Inability to attend and/or respond to stimuli on the side opposite the brain damage.

**Universal** Referring to a pattern, usually of development, that occurs regardless of a child or speaker's language or cultural or dialectical background.

**Unmarked Word** Word in an antonym pair with positive, preferred, or usual reference, for example, *love* (hate).

**Unvoiced** Consonant sound produced with no vibration of the larynx.

**Utterance Form Generalization** The ability to use utterances that conform to a pattern or rule that was taught, but are not identical to any of the utterances used during the instruction period.

**Velar Eminence** The point of highest elevation of the soft palate during function of the levator palatini muscles.

**Velum** Thin, veil-like structure; the muscular portion of the soft palate.

**Ventricular Folds** Also called *false vocal cords* or *folds*. They are folds of tissue that lie above and approximately parallel to the vocal folds. The space between the true and ventricular folds is the laryngeal ventricle.

**Vernacular** Common mode of expression in a speech community; especially used for informal exchanges among members of that community.

**Vital Capacity** The maximum amount of air that can be exhaled after a maximum inhalation.

**Vocable** Recognizable, repeatable, consistent sound patterns that demonstrate sound-meaning relationships, and thus function as words for the prelinguistic infant.

**Vocal Nodules** Polyplike benign protrusions on the free borders of the vocal folds. They are usually bilateral, and located opposite each other approximately at the middle area of the membranous portion of the folds.

**Voiced** Sound produced with vibration of the vocal folds; includes some consonants and all vowels.

# REFERENCES

Abbott, J. A. (1947). Repressed hostility as a factor in adult stuttering. *Journal of Speech Disorders, 12,* 428–430.

Achilles, R. F. (1955). Communicative anomalies of individuals with cerebral palsy: I. Analysis of communicative processes in 151 cases of cerebral palsy. *Cerebral Palsy Review, 16,* 15–24.

Adams, M. (1980). The young stutterer: Diagnosis, treatment and assessment of progress. In W. Perkins (Ed.), *Seminars in speech-language-hearing: Strategies in stuttering therapy* (pp. 289–299). New York: Thieme-Stratton, Inc.

Adams, M. R. (1978). Further analysis of stuttering as a phonetic transition defect. *Journal of Fluency Disorders, 3*(4), 265–271.

Adlam, D. S. (1977). *Code in context.* London: Routledge & Kegan Paul.

Adler, S. (1973). The reliability and validity of test data from culturally different children. *Journal of Learning Disabilities, 6*(7), 429–434.

Ainsworth, M., Bell, S., & Slayton, D. (1974). Infant-mother attachment and social development: "Socialization" as a product of reciprocal responsiveness to signals. In M. Richards (Ed.), *The integration of a child into a social world.* New York: Cambridge University Press.

Ainsworth, S. (1945). Integrating theories of stuttering. *Journal of Speech Disorders, 10,* 205–210.

Alexander, R. (1987). Oral-motor treatment for infants and young children with cerebral palsy. In E. D. Mysak (Ed.), *Communication disorders of the cerebral palsied: Assessment and treatment.* New York: Thieme Medical Publishers.

Allen, R. R., & Brown, K. L. (1977). *Developing communication competence in children.* Skokie, IL: National Textbook.

*American College Dictionary.* (1951). New York: Random House.

American National Standards Institute. (1970). *Specifications for audiometers.* ANSI S3.6-1969. New York: author.

American Speech and Hearing Association. (1974). Guidelines for audiometric symbols. *Asha,* 260–264.

American Speech and Hearing Association, Committee on the Mid-Century White House Conference. *Journal of Speech and Hearing Disorders,* (1952). *17*(1), 129–137.

American Speech-Language-Hearing Association, Committee on the Status of Racial Minorities. Position Paper: Social Dialects. Asha, 25(9), 23–24.

American Speech-Language-Hearing Association. (1985). Code of Ethics of the American Speech-Language-Hearing Association 1985. *Asha, 27*(1), 67–69.

Anderson, E. *Learning to speak with style.* (1977). Paper presented at the Stanford Child Language Research Forum, Stanford University, Stanford, CA.

Aram, D. M., & Kamhi, A. G. (1982). Perspectives on the relationship between phonological and language disorders. In J. M. Panagos (Ed.), *Seminars in Speech Language and Hearing, 3*(2), 101–114.

Aronson, A. E. (1980). *Clinical voice disorders.* New York: Brian C. Decker.

Backus, O., & Beasley, J. (1951). *Speech therapy with children.* Boston: Houghton Mifflin.

Baken, R. J. (1987). *Clinical measurement of speech and voice.* Boston: College-Hill Press.

Baldie, B. (1976). The acquisition of the passive voice. *Journal of Child Roman Language, 3,* 331–348.

Bangs, T. E. (1975). *Vocabulary comprehension scale.* Boston: Teaching Resources.

Bankson, N. W. (1977). *Bankson language screening test.* Austin, TX: ProEd.

Barbara, D. (1954). *Stuttering: A psychodynamic approach to its understanding and treatment.* New York: Julian Press.

Bartlett, C. (1982). Learning to write: Some cognitive and linguistic components. In R. Shuy (Ed.), *Linguistics and literacy series, No. 2.* Washington, DC: Center of Applied Linguistics.

Bashir, A. S., Wiig, E. H., & Abrams, J. C. (1987). Language disorders in childhood and adolescence: Implications for learning and socialization. *Pediatric Annals, 16,* 145–156.

Bates, E. (1976). *Language and context: The acquisition of pragmatics.* New York: Academic Press.

Bates, E., Benigni, L., Bretherton, I., Camaioni, L., & Volterra, V. (1979). *The emergence of symbols: Cognition and communication in infancy.* New York: Academic Press.

Bateson, M. (1979). The epigenesis of conversational interaction: A personal account of research development. In M. Bullow (Ed.), *Before speech.* New York: Cambridge University Press.

Baynes, R. A. (1966). An incidence study of chronic hoarseness among children. *Journal of Speech and Hearing Disorders, 31,* 172–174.

Beilin, H., & Spontak, G. (1969). *Active-passive transformations and operational reversibility.* Paper presented at meeting of Society for Research in Child Development.

Bell, K. (1968). A reinterpretation of the direction of effects in studies of socialization. *Psychological Review, 75,* 81–95.

Bell, R. T. (1976). *Sociolinguistics: Goals, approaches and problems.* London: B. T. Batsford.

Bell, S., & Ainsworth, M. (1972). Infant crying and maternal responsiveness. *Child Development, 43,* 1171–1190.

Bennett, A. T. (1982). Discourses of power, the dialects of understanding the power of literacy. *Journal of Education, 165,* 53–74.

Bennett, M. J. (1979). Trials with the auditory response cradle. I: Neonatal responses to auditory stimuli. *British Journal of Audiology, 14,* 1–6.

Bennett-Kaster, T. (1986). Cohesion and predication in child narrative. *Journal of Child Language, 13,* 353–370.

Benson, D. F. (1979). *Aphasia, alexia, apraxia.* New York: Churchill Livingstone.

Benson, D. R., & Geschwind, N. (1976). The aphasias and related disturbances. In A. B. Baker & L. H. Baker (Eds.), *Clinical neurology* (Vol. 1). Hagerstown, MD: Harper & Row.

Berko, F. (1965). *Amelioration of athetoid speech by manipulation of auditory feedback.* Unpublished doctoral dissertation, Cornell University, New York.

Berko, J. (1958). The child's learning of English morphology. *Word, 14,* 150–177.

Bernstein, B. (1971). Socialization: With some reference to educability. In B. Bernstein (Ed.), *Class, codes and control: Theoretical studies towards a sociology of language.* London: Routledge & Kegan Paul.

Bernstein-Ellis, E., Wertz, R. T., Dronkers, N. F., & Milton, S. B. (1985). PICA performance by traumatically brain injured and left hemisphere CVA patients. In R. H. Brookshire (Ed.), *Clinical aphasiology: Conference proceedings, 1985,* (pp. 97–106). Minneapolis: BRK Publishers.

Bernthal, J. E., & Bankson, N. W. (1988). *Articulation disorders* (2nd ed.). Englewood Cliffs, NJ: Prentice-Hall.

Bernthal, J. E., & Beukelman, D. R. (1977). The effect of changes in velopharyngeal oriface area on vowel intensity. *Cleft Palate Journal, 14,* 63–77.

Berry, W. R. (1978). *Adults with dysarthria: Patient / family education.* Paper presented at Conference on Treatment of Motor Speech Disorders, Mayo Clinic, Rochester, MN.

Berry, W. R., & LaPointe, L. L. (1974). *The adult dysarthric patient: Part I. Evaluation* [Videocassette]. Washington, DC: Medical Media Service, Veterans' Administration.

Beukelman, D., & Yorkston, K. (1977). A communication system for the severely dysarthric speaker with an intact language system. *Journal of Speech and Hearing Disorders, 42,* 256–270.

Bigler, E. D. (1987a). Acquired cerebral trauma: An introduction to the special series. *Journal of Learning Disabilities, 20,* 454–457.

Bigler, E. D. (1987b). Neuropathology of acquired cerebral trauma. *Journal of Learning Disabilities, 20,* 458–473.

Birch, J., & Matthews, J. (1951). The hearing of mental defectives: Its measurement and characteristics. *American Journal of Mental Deficiency,* 55, 384–393.

Blache, S. E. (1982). Minimal word-pairs and distinctive feature training. In M. Crary (Ed.), *Phonological intervention: Concepts and procedures* (pp. 61–96). San Diego, CA: College-Hill Press.

Blagden, C. M., & McConnell, N. L. (1983). *Interpersonal language skills assessment.* Moline, IL: LinguiSystems.

Blakeley, R. W. (1983). Treatment of developmental apraxia of speech. In W. H. Perkins (Ed.), *Dysarthria and apraxia* (pp. 25–33). New York: Thieme-Stratton, Inc.

Blakeley, R. W., & Porter, D. R. (1971). Unexpected reduction and removal of an obturator in a patient with palate paralysis. *British Journal of Communication, 6,* 33–36.

Blehar, M., Lieberman, A., & Ainsworth, M. (1977). Early face-to-face interaction and its relation to later mother-infant attachment. *Child Development, 48,* 182–194.

Bless, D., Ewanowski, S. J., & Dibbell, D. G. (1980). Clinical note: A technique for temporary obturation of fistulae. *Cleft Palate Journal, 16,* 297–300.

Bloodstein, O. (1958). Stuttering as an anticipatory struggle reaction. In J. Eisenson (Ed.), *Stuttering: A symposium.* New York: Harper and Row.

Bloodstein, O. (1960a). The development of stuttering: 1. Changes in nine basic features. *Journal of Speech and Hearing Disorders, 25,* 219–237.

Bloodstein, O. (1960b). The development of stuttering: 11. Development phases. *Journal of Speech and Hearing Disorders, 25,* 366–376.

Bloodstein, O. (1975). *A handbook on stuttering.* Chicago: National Easter Seal Society for Crippled Children and Adults.

Bloodstein, O. (1986). Semantics and beliefs. In G. H. Shames & Rubin, H. (Eds.), *Stuttering, then and now.* Columbus, OH: Merrill.

Bloodstein, O. (1987). *A handbook on stuttering.* Chicago: National Easter Seal Society for Crippled Children and Adults.

Bloom, L. (1970). *Language development: Form and function of merging grammars.* Cambridge, MA: MIT Press.

Bloom, L. (1973). *One word at a time: The use of single-word utterances before syntax.* The Hague, Netherlands: Mouton.

Bloom, L. (1974). Talking, understanding and thinking. In R. Schiefelbusch & L. Lloyd (Eds.), *Language perspectives: Acquisition, retardation and intervention.* Baltimore, MD: University Park Press.

Bloom, L., & Lahey, M. (1978). *Language development and language disorders.* New York: John Wiley.

Bloom, L., Lahey, P., Hood, L., Lifter, K., & Fiess, K. (1980). Complex sentences: Acquisition of syntactic connectors and the semantic relations they encode. *Journal of Child Language, 7,* 235–262.

Bloom, L., Rocissano, L., & Hood, L. (1976). Adult-child discourse: Development interaction between information processing and linguistic interaction. *Cognitive Psychology, 8,* 521–552.

Bluestone, C. D., Musgrave, R. H., & McWilliams, B. J. (1968). Teflon injection pharyngoplasty—Status 1968. *The Laryngoscope, 78,* 558–564.

Bluestone, C. D., Musgrave, R. H., McWilliams, B. J., & Crozier, P.A. (1968). Teflon injection pharyngoplasty. *Cleft Palate Journal, 5,* 19–22.

Bobath, K., & Bobath, B. (1967). The neurodevelopmental treatment of cerebral palsy. *Journal of American Physical Therapy Association, 47,* 1039–1041.

Boberg, E., Howie, P., & Woods, L. (1979). Maintenance of fluency: A review. *Journal of Fluency Disorders, 4,* 93–116.

Bogen, J. (1977). Unpublished address, Academy of Aphasia.

Bolinger, D. (1975). *Aspects of language.* New York: Harcourt Brace Jovanovich.

Boone, D. R. (1983). *The voice and voice therapy* (3rd ed.). Englewood Cliffs, NJ: Prentice-Hall.

Bowerman, M. (1973). *Learning to talk: A cross-linguistic comparison of early syntactic development with special reference to Finnish.* London: Cambridge University Press.

Bowerman, M. (1974). Discussion summary— Development of concepts underlying language. In R. Schiefelbusch & L. Lloyd (Eds.), *Language perspectives: Acquisition, retardation and intervention.* Baltimore, MD: University Park Press.

Bransford, J., & Johnson, M. (1972). Contextual prerequisites for understanding some investigations of comprehension and recall. *Journal of Verbal Learning and Verbal Behavior, 11,* 717–726.

Bray, C. M., & Wiig, E. H. (1987). *Let's talk inventory for children.* San Antonio, TX: Psychological Corporation.

Bridges, A. (1980). SVD comprehension strategies reconsidered: The evidence of individual patterns of response. *Journal of Child Language, 7,* 89–104.

Broen, R. (1972). The verbal environment of the language-learning child. *Monograph of the American Speech and Hearing Association, 17.*

Brookshire, B. L., Lynch, J. I., & Fox, D. R. (1980). *A parent-child cleft palate curriculum, developing speech and language.* Tigard, OR: C. C. Publications.

Brown, A. (1978). Knowing when, where, and how to remember: A problem in metacognition. In R. Glaser (Ed.), *Advances in instructional psychology.* Hillsdale, NJ: Erlbaum.

Brown, B., & Leonard, L. (1986). Lexical influences on children's early positional patterns. *Journal of Child Language, 13,* 219–229.

Brown, R. (1958). How shall a thing be called? *Psychological Review, 65,* 18–21.

Brown, R. (1965). *Social psychology.* New York: Free Press.

Brown, R. (1973). *A first language: The early stages.* Cambridge, MA: Harvard University Press.

Brown, R., & Bellugi, U. (1964). Three processes in the child's acquisition of syntax. *Harvard Educational Review, 34,* 133–151.

Brown, R., & Berko, J. (1960). Word associations and the acquisition of grammars. *Child Development, 31,* 1–14.

Bruner, J. (1975). The ontogenesis of speech acts. *Journal of Child Language, 2,* 1–19.

Bruner, J. (1977). Early social interaction and language acquisition. In H. Schaffer (Ed.), *Studies in mother-infant interaction.* New York: Academic Press.

Bruner, J. (1978). Learning the mother tongue. *Human Nature,* 42–49.

Brutten, E. J., & Shoemaker, D. J. (1967). *The modification of stuttering.* Englewood Cliffs, NJ: Prentice-Hall.

Bryan, T. H. (1978). Social relationships and verbal interactions of learning disabled children. *Journal of Learning Disabilities, 11,* 107–115.

Bryngelson, B. (1935). Sidedness as an etiological factor in stuttering. *Journal of Genetic Psychology, 47,* 204–217.

Bryngelson, B. (1939). A study of laterality of stutterers and normal speakers. *Journal of Speech Disorders, 4,* 231–234.

Bryngelson, B. (1955). Voluntary stuttering. In C. Van Riper (Ed.), *Speech therapy: A book of readings.* Englewood Cliffs, NJ: Prentice-Hall.

Bullock, A., Dalrymple, G. F., & Danca, J. M. (1975). Communication and the nonverbal, multihandicapped child. *American Journal of Occupational Therapy, 29,* 150–152.

Bullow, M. (1979). *Before speech.* New York: Cambridge University Press.

Bunce, B., & Ruder, K. (1981). Articulation therapy using distinctive feature analysis to structure the training program: Two case studies. *Journal of Speech and Hearing Disorders, 46,* 59–65.

Bzoch, K. R. (1959). A study of the speech of a group of preschool cleft palate children. *Cleft Palate Bulletin, 9,* 2–3.

Calvert, D. (1982). Articulation and hearing impairment. In N. Lass, L. V. McReynolds, J. Northern, & D. Yoder (Eds.), *Speech, language, and hearing* (Vol II). Philadelphia: W. B. Saunders.

Calvin, W. H., & Ojemann, G. A. (1980). *Inside the brain.* New York: New American Library.

Cantwell, D. P., & Carlson, G. A. (1983). *Affective disorders in childhood and adolescence.* New York: Spectrum Publications.

Capozzi, M., & Mineo, B. (1984). Nonspeech language and communication systems. In A. Holland (Ed.), *Language disorders in children.* San Diego: College-Hill Press.

Carey, S., & Bartlett, E. (1978). Acquiring a single new word. In *Papers and Reports on Child Language Development* (Stanford University), *15,* 17–29.

Carrow, E. (1973a). *Test of auditory comprehension of language.* Austin, TX: Urban Research Group.

Carrow, E. (1973b). *Test of auditory comprehension of language, English/Spanish.* Boston: Teaching Resources.

Carrow, E. (1974). *Elicited language inventory.* Hingham, MA: Teaching Resources Corporation.

Carter, E. T., & Buck, M. G. (1958). Prognostic testing for functional articulation disorders among children in the first grade. *Journal of Speech and Hearing Disorders, 23,* 124–133.

Case, J. L. (1984). *Clinical management of voice disorders.* Rockville, MD: Aspen Systems Corp.

Charlesworth, W., & Kreutzer, M. (1973). Facial expressions of infants and children. In P. Ekman (Ed.), *Darwin and facial expression.* New York: Academic Press.

Cheng, L. (1987). Cross-cultural and linguistic considerations in working with Asian populations. *Asha, 29*(6), 33–37.

Cherry, J., & Margulies, S. (1968). Contact ulcer of the larynx. *Laryngoscope, 78,* 1937–1940.

Chodosh, P. L. (1977). Gastro-esophago-pharyngeal reflux. *Laryngoscope, 87,* 418–427.

Chomsky, N., & Halle, M. (1968). *The sound pattern of English.* New York: Harper & Row.

Christiansen, R. L., & Evan, C. A. (1975). Habilitation of severe craniofacial anomalies—The challenge of new surgical procedures: An NIDR workshop. *Cleft Palate Journal, 12,* 167–176.

Clark, E. (1971). On the acquisition of the meaning of "before" and "after." *Journal of Verbal Learning and Verbal Behavior, 10,* 266–275.

Clark, E. (1973). Non-linguistic strategies and the acquisition of word meanings. *Cognition, 2,* 161–182.

Clark, E. (1978). From gesture to word: On the natural history of deixis in language acquisition. In J. Bruner & A. Garton (Eds.), *Human growth and development.* Oxford: Oxford University Press.

Clark, H. H., & Clark, E. V. (1977). *Psychology and language: An introduction to psycholinguistics.* New York: Harcourt Brace Jovanovich.

Clement, M. (1961). Morse code method of communication for the severely handicapped cerebral palsied child. *Cerebral Palsy Review, 22,* 15–16.

Cohen, M. M., Jr. (1978). Syndromes with cleft lip and cleft palate. *Cleft Palate Journal, 15,* 306–328.

Cole, L. (1984). Computer assisted sociolinguistic analysis. Scientific exhibit at the American Speech-Language-Hearing Association Convention, San Francisco, CA.

Coleman, R. F., Mabis, J. H., & Hinson, J. K. (1977). Fundamental frequency—Sound pressure level profiles of adult male and female voices. *Journal of Speech and Hearing Research, 20,* 197–204.

Colick, M. (1976). Language disorders in children: A linguistic investigation. Doctoral dissertation, McGill University.

Collis, G. (1977). Visual co-orientation and maternal speech. In H. Schaffer (Ed.), *Studies in mother-infant interaction.* New York: Academic Press.

*Computer managed articulation treatment.* (1985). [Computer program]. Tucson, AZ: Communication Skill Builders.

Condon, W., & Sanders, L. (1974). Neonate movement is synchronized with adult speech: Interactional participation and language acquisition. *Science, 83,* 99–101.

Connell, P. (1987). An effect of modeling and imitation teaching procedures on children with and without specific language impairment. *Journal of Speech and Hearing Research, 30,* 105–113.

Connor, F. P., Williamson, G. G., & Siepp, J. M. (Eds.). (1978). *Program guide for infants and toddlers with neuromotor and other developmental disabilities.* New York: Teachers College Press, Teachers College, Columbia University.

Conture, E. G., McCall, G., & Brewer, D. W. (1977). Laryngeal behavior during stuttering. *Journal of Speech and Hearing Research, 20,* 661–668.

Cooper, E. B. (1984). Personalized fluency control therapy: A status report. In M. A. Peins (Ed.), *Contemporary approaches in stuttering therapy* (pp. 1–37). Boston, MA: Little, Brown.

Costello, J. (1977). Programmed instruction. *Journal of Speech and Hearing Disorders, 42,* 3–28.

Costello, J., & Onstine, J. (1976). The modification of multiple articulation errors based on distinctive feature theory. *Journal of Speech and Hearing Disorders, 41,* 199–215.

Cruickshank, W. M. (Ed.). (1976). *Cerebral palsy: Its individual and community problems.* Syracuse, NY: Syracuse University Press.

Curlee, R. F. (1980). A case selection strategy for young disfluent children. In W. Perkins, (Ed.), *Seminars in speech-language-hearing: Strategies in stuttering therapy* (pp. 277–287). New York: Thieme-Stratton, Inc.

Curlee, R. F., & Perkins, W. H. (1969). Conversational rate control therapy for stuttering. *Journal of Speech and Hearing Disorders, 34,* 245–250.

Damsté, P. H., & Lerman, J. W. (1975). *An introduction to voice pathology.* Springfield, IL: Charles C. Thomas.

Daniloff, R. (1973). Normal articulation processes. In F. Minifie, T. Hixon, & F. Williams (Eds.), *Normal aspects of speech, hearing, and language.* Englewood Cliffs, NJ: Prentice-Hall

Daniloff, R., & Moll, K. (1968). Coarticulation of lip rounding. *Journal of Speech and Hearing Research, 11,* 707–721.

Daniloff, R. G., & Hammarberg, R. E. (1973). On defining coarticulation. *Journal of Phonetics, 1,* 239–248.

Darley, F. (1972). Efficacy of language rehabilitation in aphasia. *Journal of Speech and Hearing Disorders, 37,* 3–21.

Darley, F. (1975). Treatment of acquired aphasia. In W. Friedlander (Ed.), *Advances in neurology. Vol. 6: Current review of higher nervous system dysfunction.* New York: Raven Press.

Darley, F., Aronson, A., & Brown, J. (1975). *Motor speech disorders.* Philadelphia: W. B. Saunders.

Darley, F. L. (1967). Lacunae and research approaches to them. IV. In C. Milliken & F. L. Darley (Eds.), *Brain mechanisms underlying speech and language.* New York: Grune & Stratton.

Darley, F. L. (1979). *Evaluation of appraisal techniques in speech and language pathology.* Reading, MA: Addison-Wesley.

Darley, F. L., Aronson, A. R., & Brown, J. R. (1975). *Motor speech disorders.* Philadelphia: W. B. Saunders.

Davis, A., & Wilcox, J. (1981). Incorporating parameters of natural conversation in aphasia treatment. In R. Chapey (Ed.), *Language intervention strategies in adult aphasia.* Baltimore, MD: Williams and Williams.

Davis, D. M. (1939). The relation of repetitions in the speech of young children to certain measures of language maturity and situational factors. Part 1. *Journal of Speech and Hearing Disorders, 4,* 303–318.

Davis, D. M. (1940). The relation of repetitions in the speech of young children to certain measures of language maturity and situational factors. Parts II and III. *Journal of Speech and Hearing Disorders, 5,* 235–246.

Davis, G. A., & Wilcox, M. J. (1985). *Adult aphasia rehabilitation.* San Diego: College Hill Press.

Davis, L. F. (1978). Pre-speech. In F. P. Connor, G. F. Williamson, & J. J. Siepp (Eds.), *Program guide for infants and toddlers with neuromotor and other developmental disabilities.* New York: Teachers College Press, Teachers College, Columbia University.

DeCamp, D. (1971). The study of pidgin and creole languages. In D. Hymes (Ed.), *Pidginization and creolization of language.* London: Cambridge University Press.

Deese, J. (1965). *The structure of associations in language and thought.* Baltimore, MD: Johns Hopkins Press.

DeFries, J. C., Ashton, G. C., Johnson, R. C., Kuse, A. R., McClearn, G. E., Mi, M. P., Rashad, M. N., Vandenberg, S. G., & Wilson, J. R. (1976). Parent-offspring resemblance for specific cognitive abilities in two ethnic groups. *Nature, 261,* 131–133.

DeHart, G., & Maratsos, M. (1984). Children's acquisition of presuppositional usages. In R. Schiefelbusch & J. Pickar (Eds.), *The acquisition of communication process.* Baltimore, MD: University Park Press.

Delahunty, J. E., & Cherry, J. (1968). Experimentally produced vocal cord granulomas. *Laryngoscope, 78,* 1941–1947.

Denckla, M. B., (1978). Retrospective study of dyslexic children. In A. L. Benton & D. Pearl (Eds.), *Dyslexia: An appraisal of current knowledge.* New York: Oxford University Press.

Denckla, M. B., & Rudel, R. G. (1976). Naming of object-drawings by dyslexic and other learning disabled children. *Brain and Language, 3,* 1–15.

Denes, P. B., & Pinson, E. N. (1963). *The speech chain.* New York: Bell Telephone Laboratories.

DePompei, R., & Blosser, J. (1987). Strategies for helping head-injured children successfuly return to school. *Language, Speech, and Hearing Services in Schools, 18,* 292–300.

Dever, R. (1978). *Talk: Teaching the American language to kids.* Columbus, OH: Merrill.

de Villiers, J., & de Villiers, P. (1973). Development of the use of word order in comprehension. *Journal of Psycholinguistic Research, 2,* 331–341.

de Villiers, J., & de Villiers, P. (1979). *Early language.* Cambridge, MA: Harvard University Press.

Diedrich, W. M. (1983). Stimulability and articulation disorders. In J. Locke (Ed.), *Seminars in Speech and Language, 4*(4), 297–312.

Diedrich, W. M. (1984). Consistency and context. In R. G. Daniloff (Ed.), *Articulation assessment and treatment issues.* San Diego: College Hill Press.

Diedrich, W. M., & Youngstrom, K. A. (1966). *Alaryngeal speech.* Springfield, IL: Charles C. Thomas.

Dollaghan, C. (1985). Child meets word: "Fast mapping" in preschool children. *Journal of Speech and Hearing Research, 28,* 449–454.

Donahue, M. (1985). Communicative style in learning disabled children: Some implications for classroom discourse. In D. N. Ripich & F. M. Spinelle (Eds.), *School discourse problems* (pp.97–124). San Diego: College Hill Press.

Dore, J. (1974). A pragmatic description of early language development. *Journal of Psycholinguistic Research, 3,* 343–350.

Downs, M. P., & Sterritt, G. M. (1967). A guide to newborn and infant screening programs. *Archives of Otolaryngology, 85,* 15–22.

Driscoll, M., & Driscoll, S. (1984). Distinctive feature analysis on an Apple computer. Paper presented at the American Speech-Language-Hearing Association Convention, San Francisco, CA.

Dunlap, K. (1932). *Habits: Their making and unmaking.* New York: Liveright.

Dunn, L. M. (1965). *Peabody picture vocabulary test.* Circle Pines, MN: American Guidance Service.

Dunn, L. M. (1980). *Peabody picture vocabulary test—revised.* Circle Pines, MN: American Guidance Service.

Dunn-Engel, E. (1988). A quality-oriented solo private practice. *Asha, 30*(1), 33.

Editorial: Prognosis in aphasia. (1977). *Lancet, 2,* 24.

Edwards, A. D. (1976). *Language in culture and class.* London: Heinemann Educational Books.

Edwards, M. L., & Shriberg, L. (1983). *Phonology: Applications in communicative disorders.* San Diego: College Hill Press.

Eimas, P. (1974). Linguistic processing of speech by young infants. In R. Schiefelbusch & L. Lloyd (Eds.), *Language perspectives: Acquisition, retardation and intervention.* Baltimore, MD: University Park Press.

Eisenberg, R. (1976). *Auditory competence in early life: The roots of communicative behavior.* Baltimore, MD: University Park Press.

Elbert, M. (1988). Generalization in treatment of articulation disorders. In L. McReynolds & J. Spradlin (Eds.), *Generalization strategies in the treatment of communication disorders.* Toronto: B. C. Decker Inc.

Elbert M., Dinnsen, D. A., & Weismer, G. (1984). *Phonological theory and the misarticulating child. ASHA Monograph, 22.* Rockville, MD: American Speech-Language-Hearing Association.

Elbert, M., & Gierut, J. (1986). *Handbook of clinical phonology.* San Diego: College-Hill Press.

Elbert, M., & McReynolds, L. V. (1975). Transfer of /r/ across contexts. *Journal of Speech and Hearing Disorders, 40,* 380–387.

Elbert, M., & McReynolds, L. V. (1978). An experimental analysis of misarticulating children's generalization. *Journal of Speech and Hearing Research, 21,* 136–150.

Elkind, D. (1970). *Children and adolescents.* New York: Oxford University Press.

Emerick, J., & Hamre, C. (1972). *An analysis of stuttering: Selected readings.* Danville, IL: Interstate Printers and Publishers.

Emerson, H., & Gekoski, W. (1976). Interactive and categorical grouping strategies and the syntagmatic-paradigmatic shift. *Child Development, 47,* 1116–1125.

Enderby, P. M. (1983). *Frenchay dysarthria assessment.* San Diego: College-Hill Press.

Erenberg, G., Mattis, S., & French, J. H. (1976). Four hundred children referred to an urban ghetto developmental disabilities clinic: Computer assisted analysis of demographic, psychological, social, and medical data. Unpublished manuscript.

Erickson, J. G., & Omark, D. R. (1981). *Communication assessment of the bilingual, bicultural child.* Baltimore, MD: University Park Press.

Ervin, S. (1961). Changes with age in the verbal determinants of word-association. *American Journal of Psychology, 74,* 361–372.

Ervin, S. (1963). Correlates of associative frequency. *Journal of Verbal Learning and Verbal Behavior, 1,* 422–431.

Ervin-Tripp, S. (1973). Some strategies for the first two years. In T. Moore (Ed.), *Cognitive development and the acquisition of language.* New York: Academic Press.

Ervin-Tripp, S. (1977). Wait for me, roller skate! In S. Ervin-Tripp & C. Mitchell-Kernan (Eds.), *Child discourse.* New York: Academic Press.

Ervin-Tripp, S. (1980). Lecture, University of Minnesota.

Ervin-Tripp, S., & Mitchel-Kernan, E. (Eds.). (1977). *Child discourse.* New York: Academic Press.

Faircloth, M. A., & Blasdell, R. C. (1979). Conversational speech behaviors. In N. Lass (Ed.), *Speech and language: Advances in basic research and practice* (Vol. 2). New York: Academic Press.

Farb, P. (1973). *Word play: What happens when people talk.* New York: Alfred A. Knopf.

Farber, S. (1981). *Identical twins reared apart: A re-analysis.* New York: Basic Books.

Fasold (1984). The sociolingiustics of society. London: Basil Blackwell.

Fawcus, B. (1986). Persistent puberphonia. In Margaret Fawcus (Ed.), *Voice disorders and their management.* Loundon-Sydney-Dover, NH: Croom Helm.

Feigenbaum, I. (1970). The use of Nonstandard English in teaching standard: Contrast and comparison. In R. W. Fasold & R. W. Shuy (Eds.), *Teaching Standard English in the inner city.* Washington, DC: Center for Applied Linguistics.

Feldman, A. S. (1988). Some observations about us and private practice. *Asha, 30*(1), 29–30.

Ferguson, C. (1964). Baby talk in six languages. *American Anthropologist, 66,* 103–114.

Ferguson, C. (1978). Learning to pronounce: The earliest stages of phonological development in the child. In F. Minifie & L. Lloyd (Eds.), *Communicative and cognitive abilities: Early behavior assessment.* Baltimore, MD: University Park Press.

Ferguson, C. (1979). Phonology as an individual access system: Some data from language acquisition. In C. J. Fillmore, D. Kempler, & W. S. Y. Wang (Eds.), *Individual differences in language ability and language behavior.* New York: Academic Press.

Ferguson, C., & Farwell, C. (1975). Words and sounds in early language acquisition: English initial consonants in the first words. *Language, 51,* 419–439.

Ferguson, C., & Garnica, O. (1975). Theories of phonological development. In E. Lenneberg & E. Lenneberg (Eds.), *Foundations of language development* (Vol. 2). New York: Academic Press.

Ferguson, C., & Macken, M. (1983). The role of play in phonological development. In K. E. Nelson (Ed.), *Children's language* (Vol. 4) (pp. 231–254). Hillsdale, NJ: Erlbaum.

Ferreiro, E., & Teberosky, A. (1982). *Literacy before schooling.* Exeter, NH: Heinemann.

Ferrier, L. J., & Shane, H. C. (1987). Computer-based communication aids for the nonspeaking child with cerebral palsy. In E. D. Mysak (Ed.), *Communication disorders of the cerebral palsied: Assessment and treatment.* New York: Thieme Medical Publishers.

Fey, M. (1986). *Language intervention with young children.* San Diego: College-Hill Press.

Finnie, N. R. (1975). *Handling the young cerebral palsied child at home.* New York: E. P. Dutton-Sunrise.

Finucci, J. M., Guthrie, J. T., Childs, A. L., Abbey, H., & Childs, B. (1976). The genetics of specific reading disability. *Annals of Human Genetics, 40,* 1–23.

Fischer, S. (1982). Sign language and manual communication. In D. G. Sims, G. G. Walter, & R. L. Whitehead (Eds.), *Deafness and communication: Assessment and training* (pp. 90–106). Baltimore, MD: Williams & Wilkins.

Fisher, H. B. (1966). *Improving voice and articulation.* Boston: Houghton Mifflin.

Fisher, H. B., & Logemann, J. A. (1971). *The Fisher-Logemann test of articulation competence.* Boston: Houghton Mifflin.

Fitch, J. L. (1985a). *Computer managed articulation diagnosis* [Computer program]. Tuscon, AZ: Communication Skill Builders.

Fitch, J. L. (1985b). *Computer managed articulation treatment* [Computer program]. Tuscon, AZ: Communication Skill Builders.

Fitch, J. L., Flanagan, B., Goldiamond, I., & Azrin, N. (1958). Operant stuttering: The control of stuttering behavior through response-contingent consequences. *Journal of the Experimental Analysis of Behavior, 1,* 173–177.

Flanagan, B., Goldiamond, I., & Azrin, N. (1958). Operant stuttering: The control of stuttering behavior through response-contingent consequences. *Journal of the Experimental Analysis of Behavior, 1,* 173–177.

Flavell, J. (1977). *Cognitive development.* Englewood Cliffs, NJ: Prentice-Hall.

Flavell, J., & Wellman, H. (1977). Metamemory. In R. Kail & J. Hagen (Eds.), *Perspectives on the development of memory and cognition.* Hillsdale, NJ: Erlbaum.

Flavell, J. H. (1976). Metacognitive aspects of problem solving. In L. B. Resnick (Ed.), *The nature of intelligence.* Hillsdale, NJ: Erlbaum.

Fletcher, S. G. (1978). *Diagnosing speech disorders from cleft palate.* New York: Grune & Stratton.

Florance, C. L., & Shames, G. H. (1981). Stuttering treatment: Issues in transfer and maintenance. In J. Northern (Ed.) and W. Perkins (Guest Ed.), *Seminars, speech language hearing, strategies in stuttering therapy.* New York: Grune & Stratton.

Fordham, S. (1988). Racelessness as a factor in black students' school success: Pragmatic strategy or pyrrhic victory? *Harvard Educational Review.*

Fourcin, A. (1978). Acoustic patterns and speech acquisition. In N. Waterson & C. Snow (Eds.), *The development of communication.* New York: John Wiley.

Fox, D., & Johns, D. (1970). Predicting velopharyngeal closure with a modified tongue-anchor technique. *Journal of Speech and Hearing Disorders, 35,* 248–251.

Fox, D. R. (1980). Competency and commitment. *Asha, 22*(5), 383–384.

Francis, H. (1972). Toward an explanation of the syntagmatic-paradigmatic shift. *Child Development, 43,* 949–958.

Freeman, F., & Ushijima, T. (1978). Laryngeal muscle activity during stuttering. *Journal of Speech and Hearing Research, 21,* 538–562.

French, L., & Brown, A. (1977). Comprehension of "before" and "after" in logical and arbitrary sequences. *Journal of Child Language, 4,* 247–256.

Fried-Oken, M. B. (1983). The development of naming skills in normal and language deficient children. Doctoral dissertation, Boston University, Graduate School.

Fristoe, M., & Lloyd, L. (1979). Non-speech communication. In N. Ellis (Ed.), *Handbook of mental deficiency.* New York: Erlbaum.

Froeschels, E. (1952). Chewing method as therapy. *Archives of Otolaryngology, 56,* 427–434.

Froeschels, E., Kastein, S., & Weiss, D. A. (1955). A method of therapy for paralytic conditions of the mechanisms of phonation, respiration and glutination. *Journal of Speech and Hearing Disorders, 20,* 365–370.

Fudala, J. (1974). *Arizona articulation proficiency scale.* Los Angeles: Western Psychological Services.

Galaburda, A. M., & Kemper, T. L. (1979). Cytoarchitectonic abnormalities in developmental dyslexia: A case study. *Annals of Neurology, 6,* 94.

Gallagher, T. (1977). Revision behaviors in the speech of normal children developing language. *Journal of Speech and Hearing Research, 20,* 303–318.

Gallagher, T. (1983). Pre-assessment: A procedure for accommodating language use variables. In T. M. Gallagher & C. A. Prutting (Eds.), *Pragmatic assessment and intervention issues in language.* San Diego: College Hill.

Gallagher, T., & Prutting, C. (1983). *Pragmatic assessment and intervention issues in language.* San Diego: College-Hill Press.

Gardner, H. (1975). *The shattered mind.* New York: Knopf.

Gardner, H., Kirchner, M., Winner, E., & Perkins, D. (1975). Children's metaphoric productions and preferences. *Journal of Child Language, 2,* 125–141.

Garnica, O. (1977). Some prosodic and paralinguistic features of speech to young children. In C. Snow & C. Ferguson (Eds.), *Talking to children: Language input and acquisition.* New York: Cambridge University Press.

Garrett, E. R. (1973). Programmed articulation therapy. In W. D. Wolfe & D. J. Goulding (Eds.), *Articulation and learning.* Springfield, IL: Charles C. Thomas.

Garvey, C. (1975). Requests and responses in children's speech. *Journal of Child Language, 2,* 41–63.

Gerber, A. (1977). Programming for articulation modification. *Journal of Speech and Hearing Disorders, 42,* 29–43.

Gerkin, K. P. (1984). The high risk register for deafness. *Asha, 23,* 17–23.

German, D. J. N. (1982). Word-finding substitutions in children with learning disabilities. *Language, Speech, and Hearing Services in Schools, 13,* 223–230.

Giolas, T. G. (1982). *Hearing-handicapped adults.* Englewood Cliffs, NJ: Prentice-Hall.

Glauber, I. P. (1958). The psychoanalysis of stuttering. In J. Eisenson (Ed.), *Stuttering: A symposium.* New York: Harper and Row.

Gleason, J. B. (1973). Code switching in children's language. In T. E. Moore (Ed.), *Cognitive development and the acquisition of language.* New York: Academic Press.

Glucksberg, S., Krauss, R. M., & Weisberg, R. (1966). Referential communication in school children:

Method and some preliminary findings. *Journal of Experimental Child Psychology, 3,* 333–342.

Goldiamond, I. (1965). Stuttering and fluency as manipulable operant response classes. In L. Krasner & L. P. Ullman (Eds.), *Research 7, in behavior modification.* New York: Holt, Rinehart and Winston.

Goldman, R. (1967). Cultural influences on the sex ratio in the incidence of stuttering. *American Anthropologist, 69,* 78–81.

Goldman, R., & Fristoe, M. (1969, 1972). *Goldman-Fristoe test of articulation.* Circle Pines, MN: American Guidance Service, Inc.

Goldman, R., Fristoe, M., & Woodcock, R. (1970). *Goldman-Fristoe-Woodcock test of auditory discrimination.* Circle Pines, MN: American Guidance Service, Inc.

Goldstein, K., & Blackman, S. (1978). *Cognitive styles: Five approaches and relevant research.* New York: John Wiley and Sons.

Golick, M. (1976). *Language disorders in children: A linguistic investigation.* Doctoral dissertation, McGill University, Montreal.

Goodglass, H., & Kaplan, E. (1972). *Boston diagnostic aphasia examination.* Philadelphia: Lea & Febiger.

Goodglass, H., & Kaplan, E. (1983). *The assessment of aphasia and related disorders* (2nd ed.). Philadelphia: Lea & Febiger.

Goodstein, L. D. (1958). Functional speech disorders and personality: A survey of the research. *Journal of Speech and Hearing Research, 1,* 359–516.

Gordon, D., and Ervin-Tripp, S. (1984). The structure of children's requests. In R. Schiefelbusch and J. Pickar (Eds.), *The acquisition of communicative competence.* Baltimore, MD: University Park Press.

Greenberg, J., & Kuczaj, S. (1982). Towards a theory of substantive word-meaning acquisition. In S. Kuczaj (Ed.), *Language development Vol. 1: Syntax and semantics.* Hillside, NJ: Erlbaum.

Greenberg, J. H. (1966). Language universals. In T. Sebeok (Ed.), *Current trends in linguistics: Theoretical foundations* (Vol. 3). Hawthorne, NY: Mouton.

Greenfield, P. (1978). Informativeness, presupposition, and semantic choice in single word utterances. In N. Waterson & C. Snow (Eds.), *The development of communication.* New York: John Wiley.

Greenfield, P., & Smith, J. (1976). *The structure of communication in early language development.* New York: Academic Press.

Greenlee, M. (1974). Interacting processes in the child's acquisition of stop-liquid clusters. *Papers and Reports on Child Language Development, 7,* 85–100.

Gregory, H. (1986). Environmental manipulation and family counseling. In G. Shames and H. Rubin (Eds.), *Stuttering then and now* (pp. 273–291). Columbus, OH: Merrill.

Grimm, H. (1975). *Analysis of short-term dialogues in 5–7 year olds: Encoding of intentions and modifications of speech acts as a function of negative feedback loops.* Paper presented at Third International Child Language Symposium.

Grossman, H. J. (Ed.). (1983). *Manual on terminology and classification in mental retardation.* Washington, DC: Association on Mental Deficiency.

Gruenewald, L. (1980). Language and learning disabilities ad hoc develops position statement. *Asha, 22,* 628–636.

Grummit, R. J. (1983). *The epilepsy handbook: The practical management of seizures.* New York: Raven Press.

Grunwell, P. (1982). *Clinical phonology.* Rockville, MD: Aspen System.

Gumperz, J. J., & Hymes, D. (Eds.). (1972). *Directions in sociolinguistics: The ethnography of communication.* New York: Holt, Rinehart & Winston.

Haas, A. (1979). The acquisition of genderlect. *Annals of the New York Academy of Sciences, 327,* 101–113.

Hagen, C. (1981). Language disorders secondary to closed head injury: Diagnosis and treatment. *Topics in Language Disorders, 1,* 73–87.

Hagen, C. (1982). Language-cognitive disorganization following closed head injury: A conceptualization. In L. E. Trexler (Ed.), *Cognitive rehabilitation: Conceptualization and intervention.* New York: Plenum Press.

Hagen, C. (1984). Language disorders in head trauma. In A. Holland (Ed.), *Language disorders in adults.* San Diego: College-Hill.

Hagen, C., Porter, W., & Brink, J. (1973). Nonverbal communication: An alternative mode of communication of the child with severe cerebral palsy.

*Journal of Speech and Hearing Disorders, 38,* 448–455.

Hahn, E. (1961). Indications for direct, nondirect, and indirect methods in speech correction. *Journal of Speech and Hearing Disorders, 26,* 230–236.

Hahn, E. (1979). Directed home programs for infants with cleft lip and palate. In K. R. Bzoch (Ed.), *Communicative disorders related to cleft lip and palate* (pp. 311–317). Boston: Little, Brown.

Hakes, D. T. (1980). *The development of metalinguistic abilities in children.* Berlin: Springer Verlag.

Hallgren, B. (1950). Specific dyslexia ("congenital word blindness"): A clinical study. *Acta Psychiatrica et Neurologica Scandinavica,* Supp. No. 65.

Halliday, M. (1975a). Learning how to mean. In E. Lenneberg & E. Lenneberg (Eds.), *Foundations of language development: A multidisciplinary approach.* New York: Academic Press.

Halliday, M. (1975b). *Learning how to mean: Explorations in the development of language.* New York: Edward Arnold.

Halliday, M. A. K. (1978). *Language as social semiotic.* Baltimore, MD: University Park Press.

Hammill, D. D., Brown, V., Larsen, S., & Wiederholt, J. (1980). *Test of adolescent language: A multidimensional approach to assessment.* Austin, TX: ProEd.

Hammill, D. D., Leigh, J. E., McNutt, G., & Larsen, S. C. (1981). A new definition of learning disabilities. *Learning Disabilities Quarterly, 4,* 336–342.

Hanson, M. (1983). *Articulation.* Philadelphia: W. B. Saunders.

Hardy, J. C. (1967). Suggestions for physiological research in dysarthria. *Cortex, 3,* 128–156.

Hardy, J. C. (1983). *Cerebral palsy.* Englewood Cliffs, NJ: Prentice-Hall, Inc.

Hatch, E. (1971). The young child's comprehension of time connectives. *Child Development, 42,* 2111–2113.

Haynes, S. (1985). Developmental apraxia of speech: Symptoms and treatment. In S. Johns (Ed.), *Clinical management of neurogenic communicative disorders* (2nd ed.). Boston: Little, Brown.

Heath, S. B. (1982). What no bedtime story means: Narrative skills at home and school. *Language in Society, 11,* 49–76.

Heilman, K. M., Safron, A., & Geschwind, N. (1971). Closed head trauma and aphasia. *Journal of Neurology, Neurosurgery, and Psychiatry, 34,* 265–269.

Helm-Estabrooks, N., Fitzpatrick, P. F., & Barresi, B. A. (1982). Visual action therapy for global aphasia. *Journal of Speech and Hearing Disorders, 47,* 385–389.

Henja, R. (1968). *Developmental articulation test.* Madison, WI: Wisconsin College Typing.

Hermann, K. (1959). *Reading disability: A medical study of work-blindness and related handicaps.* Copenhagen: Munksgaard.

Hill, H. (1944a). Stuttering: I. A critical review and evaluation of biochemical investigations. *Journal of Speech Disorders, 9,* 245–261.

Hill, H. (1944b). Stuttering: II. A review and integration of physiological data. *Journal of Speech Disorders, 9,* 289–324.

Hirano, M. (1981). Clinical examination of voice. In G. E. Arnold, F. Winckel, & B. D. Wyke (Eds.), *Disorders of human communication* (Vol. 5). New York: Springer-Verlag.

Hirschman, R., & Katkin, E. (1974). Psychophysiological functioning, arousal, attention, and learning during the first year of life. In H. Reese (Ed.), *Advances in child development and behavior.* New York: Academic Press.

Hixon, T. J. (1973). Respiratory function in speech. In F. D. Minifie, T. J. Hixon, & F. Williams (Eds.), *Normal aspects of speech, hearing, and language.* Englewood Cliffs, NJ: Prentice-Hall.

Hixon, T. J. (1975). *Respiratory-laryngeal evaluation.* Paper presented at VA Workshop on Motor Speech Disorders, Madison, WI.

Hoch, L., Golding-Kushner, K., Siegel-Sadewitz, V. L., & Shprintzen, R. J. (1986). Speech therapy. In B. J. McWilliams (Guest Ed.), *Seminars in Speech and Language* (pp. 313–326). New York: Thieme.

Hodson, B. W. (1984). Facilitating phonological development in children with severe speech disorders. In H. Winitz (Ed.), *Treating articulation disorders: For clinicians by clinicians.* Baltimore, MD: University Park Press.

Hodson, B. W. (1986). *The assessment of phonological processes* (rev. ed.). Danville, IL: Interstate Printers & Publishers.

Hoffman, P. (1983). Interallophonic generalization of /r/ training. *Journal of Speech and Hearing Disorders, 48,* 215–221.

Holdgrafer, G., & Sorenson, P. (1984). Informativeness and lexical learning. *Psychological Reports, 54,* 75–80.

Holland, A. (1980). *Communicative abilities in daily living: A test of functional communication for aphasic adults.* Baltimore, MD: University Park Press.

Holland, A. L. (1982). When is aphasia aphasia?: The problem of closed head injury. In R. H. Brookshire (Ed.), *Clinical aphasiology: Conference proceedings* (pp. 345–349). Minneapolis: BRK Publishers.

Hollingshead, A. B. (1965). *Two factor index of social position.* Cambridge: Yale University Press.

Hood, J. R. (1984). *Articulation error analysis* [Computer program]. Tucson, AZ: Communication Skill Builders.

Hood, L., & Bloom, L. (1979). What, when, and how about why: A longitudinal study of early expressions of causality. *Monographs of the Society for Research in Child Development, 44.*

Horgan, D. (1978). The development of the full passive. *Journal of Child Language, 5,* 65–80.

Hubbard, T. W., Paradise, J. L., McWilliam, B. J., Elster, B. A., & Taylor, F. H. (1985). Consequences of unremitting middle-ear disease in early life: Otologic, audiologic, and developmental findings in children with cleft palate. *The New England Journal of Medicine, 312,* 1529–1534.

Hymes, D. (1966). On communicative competence. Paper presented at the Research Planning Conference on Language Development Among Disadvantaged Children, Yeshiva University, New York.

Hymes, D. (1974). *Foundations of sociolinguistics: An ethnographic approach.* Philadelphia, PA: University of Pennsylvania Press.

Hymes, D. (1981). "In vain I tried to tell you." *Essays in Native American ethnopoetics,* Philadelphia: University of Pennsylvania Press.

Ingham, R., Gow, M., & Costello, J. (1985). Stuttering and speech naturalness: Some additional data. *JSHD, 50,* 217–219.

Ingham, R., Martin, R., Haroldson, S., Onslow, M., & Leney, M. (1985). Modification of listener-judged naturalness in the speech of stutterers. *JSHR, 28,* 494–504.

Ingham, R., & Onslow, M. (1985). Measurement and modification of speech naturalness during stuttering therapy. *JSHD, 50,* 261–281.

Ingham, R. J. (1975a). Operant methodology in stuttering. In J. Eisenson (Ed.), *Stuttering: A second symposium.* New York: Harper and Row.

Ingham, R. J. (1975b). A comparison of covert and overt assessment procedures in stuttering therapy outcome evaluation. *JSHR, 18,* 346–354.

Ingham, R. J. (1984). Paper presented at the convention of the New York State Speech, Language and Hearing Association, New York.

Ingham, R. J., & Andrews, G. (1973). An analysis of a token economy in stuttering therapy. *Journal of Applied Behavior Analysis, 6,* 219–229.

Ingram, D. (1974a). Phonological rules in young children. *Journal of Child Language, 1,* 49–64.

Ingram, D. (1974b). The relationship between comprehension and production. In R. Schiefelbusch & L. Lloyd (Eds.), *Language perspectives: Acquisition, retardation, and intervention.* Baltimore, MD: University Park Press.

Ingram, D. (1976). *Phonological disability in children.* New York: Elsevier.

Ingram, D. (1981). *Procedures for the phonological analysis of children's language.* Baltimore, MD: University Park Press.

Ingram, D. (1983). The analysis and treatment of phonological disorders. In J. Locke (Ed.), *Seminars in speech and language, 4*(4), 375–388.

Ingram, D., & Terselic, B. (1983). Final ingression: A case of deviant child phonology. *Topics in Language Disorders, 3,* 45–50.

Ingram, T. T. S. (1970). The nature of dyslexia. In F. A. Young & D. B. Lindsey (Eds.), *Early experience and visual information in perceptual and reading disorders.* Washington, DC: National Academy of Sciences.

Inhelder, B., & Piaget, J. (1969). *The early growth of logic in the child.* New York: W. W. Norton.

Irwin, E. C., & McWilliams, B. J. (1974). Play therapy for children with cleft palates. *Children Today, 3,* 18–22.

Irwin, J. V., & Weston, A. J. (1975). The paired stimuli monograph. *Acta Symbolica, 4,* 1–76.

Irwin, O. (1972). Integrated articulation test. In Orvis C. Irwin, *Communication variables of cerebral palsied and mentally retarded children.* Springfield, IL: Charles C. Thomas.

Jackson, C., & Jackson, C. L. (1937). *The larynx and its diseases.* Philadelphia: W. B. Saunders.

Jacobson, E. (1976). *You must relax* (5th ed.). New York: McGraw-Hill.

Jakobson, R., (1968). *Child language, aphasia and phonological universals.* (A. R. Keiler, Trans.). The Hague, Netherlands: Mouton. (Original work published 1941)

Jakobson, R., Fant, C., & Halle, M. (1951). *Preliminaries to speech analysis.* Cambridge, MA: MIT Press.

James, S., & Seebach, M. (1982). The pragmatic function of children's questions. *Journal of Speech and Hearing Research, 25,* 2–11.

Jenkins, J., & Palermo, D. (1964). Mediation processes and the acquisition of linguistic structure. In U. Bellugi & R. Brown (Eds.), *Monographs of the Society for Research in Child Development, 29.*

Jerger, J. (1970). Clinical experience with impedance audiometry. *Archives of Otolaryngology, 92,* 311–324.

Johns, D., & LaPointe, L. L. (1976). Neurogenic disorders of output processing: Apraxia of speech. In H. Avakian-Whitaker & H. A. Whitaker (Eds.), *Current trends in neurolinguistics.* New York: Academic Press.

Johnson, D. J., & Myklebust, H. R. (1967). *Learning disabilities: Educational principles and practices.* New York: Grune & Stratton.

Johnson, H. (1975). The meaning of before and after for preschool children. *Journal of Exceptional Child Psychology, 19,* 88–99.

Johnson, L. (1980). Facilitating parental involvement in therapy of the disfluent child. *Seminars in speech-language-hearing strategies in stuttering therapy.* New York: Thieme-Stratton, Inc.

Johnson, S. W., & Morasky, R. L. (1977). *Learning disabilities.* Boston: Allyn & Bacon.

Johnson, T. S. (1983). In W. H. Perkins (Ed.), *Current therapy of communication disorders: Voice disorders.* New York: Thieme-Stratton, Inc.

Johnson, T. S. (1985). *Vocal abuse reduction program.* San Diego, CA: College-Hill Press, Inc.

Johnson, W. (1933). An interpretation of stuttering. *Quarterly Journal of Speech, 19,* 70–76.

Johnson, W. (1938). The role of evaluation in stuttering behavior. *Journal of Speech Disorders, 3,* 85–89.

Johnson, W. (1942). A study of the onset and development of stuttering. *Journal of Speech Disorders, 7,* 251–257.

Johnson, W. (1944). The Indians have no word for it. 1. Stuttering in children. *Quarterly Journal of Speech, 30,* 330–337.

Johnson, W. (1961). *Stuttering and what you can do about it.* Minneapolis: University of Minnesota Press.

Joint Committee on Dentistry and Speech Pathology-Audiology. (1975). Position statement on tongue thrust. *Asha, 17,* 331–340.

Joint Committee on Infant Hearing Screening. (1982). *Asha,* Position Statement, *24,* 1017–1018.

Kahn, J. (1975). Relationship of Piaget's sensorimotor period to language acquisition of profoundly retarded children. *American Journal of Mental Deficiency, 79,* 640–643.

Kahn, L., & Lewis, N. (1986). *Kahn-Lewis phonological analysis.* Circle Pines, MN: American Guidance Service.

Kaplan, E. N., Jobe, R. P., & Chase, R. A. (1969). Flexibility in surgical planning for velopharyngeal incompetence. *Cleft Palate Journal, 6,* 166–174.

Kasprisin-Burrelli, A., Egolf, D. B., & Shames, G. H. (1972). A comparison of parental verbal behavior with stuttering and nonstuttering children. *Journal of Communication Disorders, 5,* 335–346.

Katz, J. (1966). *The philosophy of language.* New York: Harper & Row.

Kearsley, R. (1973). The newborn's response to auditory stimulation: A demonstration of orienting and defense behavior. *Child Development, 44,* 582–590.

Kellum, G. D., Wylde, M. A., Dickerson, M. V., & Ulrich, S. L. (1987). Legislative councilors and ASHA members demographic comparisons. *Asha, 29*(12), 41–42.

Kent, R. D. (1982). Contextual facilitation of correct sound production. *Language, Speech and Hearing Services in Schools, 13,* 66–76.

Kent, R. D., & Rosenbek, J. C. (1983). Acoustic patterns of apraxia of speech. *Journal of Speech and Hearing Research, 26,* 231–249.

Keogh, B. K., Tchir, C., & Windeguth-Behn, A. (1974). A teacher's perception of educationally high risk children. *Journal of Learning Disabilities, 7,* 367–374.

Kernahan, D. A., & Stark, R. B. (1958). A new classification for cleft lip and palate. *Plastic and Reconstructive Surgery, 22,* 435–441.

Kertesz, A. (1979). *Aphasia and associated disorders: Taxonomy, localization and recovery.* New York: Grune & Stratton.

Kertesz, A. (1982). *The western aphasia battery.* New York: Grune & Stratton.

Kertesz, A., & McCabe, P. (1977). Recovery patterns and prognosis in aphasia. *Archives of Neurology, 34,* 590–601.

Kidd, K. K. (1977). A genetic perspective on stuttering. *Journal of Fluency Disorders, 2,* 259–269.

Kiparsky, P., & Menn, L. (1977). On the acquisition of phonology. In J. MacNamara (Ed.), *Language learning and thought* (pp. 47–78). New York: Academic Press.

Klee, T. (1985). Role of inversion in children's question development. *Journal of Speech and Hearing Research, 28,* 225–232.

Klein, H. (1978). *The relationship between perceptual strategies and productive strategies in learning the phonology of early lexical items.* Unpublished doctoral dissertation, Columbia University, New York.

Kochman, T. (1970). Toward an ethnography of black American speech behavior. In N. E. Witten & J. F. Szweo (Eds.), *Afro-American Anthropology.* New York: Free Press.

Kochman, T. (1971). *Rappin and stylin out in the black community.* Champaign: University of Illinois Press.

Kochman, T. (1981). *Black and white: Styles in conflict.* Chicago: University of Chicago Press.

Kopit, A. (1978). *Wings.* New York: Hill & Wang.

Labov, W. (1972). Rules for ritual insults. In D. Sudnow (Ed.), *Studies in social interaction.* New York: Free Press.

Lakoff, G. (1972). Language in context. *Language, 48,* 97–927.

Lakoff, R. (1973). Language and woman's place. *Language of Sociology, 2,* 75–80.

Lakoff, R. (1975). *Language and woman's place.* New York: Harper Colophon Books.

Lanyon, R. J. (1969). Behavior change in stuttering through systematic desensitization. *Journal of Speech and Hearing Disorders, 34,* 253–259.

LaPointe, L. L. (1975). Neurologic abnormalities affecting speech. In D. B. Tower (Ed.), *The nervous system: Vol. 3. Human communication and its disorders.* New York: Raven Press.

LaPointe, L. L. (1978). Aphasia therapy: Some principles and strategies for treatment. In D. Johns (Ed.), *Clinical management of neurogenic communicative disorders.* (2nd ed.) Boston: Little, Brown.

LaPointe, L. L. (1985). Aphasia therapy: Some principles and strategies for treatment. In D. Johns (Ed.), *Clinical management of neurogenic communicative disorders.* (2nd ed.) Boston: Little, Brown.

Laufer, M., & Horii, Y. (1977). Fundamental frequency characteristics of infant nondistress vocalization during the first twenty-four weeks. *Journal of Child Language, 4,* 171–184.

Lee, L. (1971). *Northwestern syntax screening test.* Evanston, IL: Northwestern University Press.

Lee, L., Koenigsknecht, R., & Mulhern, S. (1975). *Interactive language development teaching.* Evanston, IL: Northwestern University Press.

Leith, W. R., & Mims, H. A. (1975). Cultural influences in the development and treatment of stuttering: A preliminary report on the black stutterer. *Journal of Speech and Hearing Research, 40*(4), 459–466.

Lencione, R. M. (1976). The development of communication skills. In W. J. Cruickshank (Ed.), *Cerebral palsy: A developmental disability.* Syracuse, NY: Syracuse University Press.

Lenneberg, E. H. (1967). *Biological foundations of language.* New York: John Wiley.

Leonard, L. B., Nippold, M. A., Kail, R., & Hale, C. A. (1983). Picture naming in language-impaired children: Differentiating lexical storage from retrieval. *Journal of Speech and Hearing Research, 26,* 609–615.

Levine, M. D. (1984). Persistent inattention and unintention. In M. D. Levine & P. Satz (Eds.), *Middle childhood: Development and dysfunction.* Baltimore, MD: University Park Press.

Levine, M. D. (1987). *Developmental variation and learning disorders.* Boston: Educators Publishing Service.

Levine, M. D., & Zallan, B. G. (1984). The learning disorders of adolescence: Organic and nonorganic failure to strive. *Pediatric Clinics of North America, 31,* 345–369.

Limber, J. (1973). The genesis of complex sentences. In T. Moore (Ed.), *Cognitive development and the acquisition of language.* New York: Academic Press.

Linde, C., & Labov, W. (1975). Spatial networks as a site for the study of language and thought. *Language, 51,* 924–939.

Little, W. J. (1861). On the influence of abnormal parturition, difficult labor, premature birth, and asphyxia neonatorum in the mental and physical condition of the child, especially in relation to deformities. *Transcriptions of the Obstetrical Society of London, 3,* 293.

Locke, J. L. (1983). Clinical phonology: The explanation and treatment of speech sound disorders. *Journal of Speech and Hearing Disorders, 48,* 339–341.

Logemann, J. (1983). *Evaluation and treatment of swallowing disorders.* San Diego: College-Hill Press.

Loman, B. (1967). *Conversations in a Negro American dialect.* Washington, DC: Center for Applied Linguistics.

Long, S. (1987). 'Computerized profiling' of clinical language samples. *Clinical Linguistics and Phonetics, 1,* 97–105.

Lord Larson, V., & McKinley, N. L. (1987). *Communication assessment and intervention strategies for adolescents.* Eau Claire, WI: Thinking Publications.

Love, R. J., & Webb, W. G. (1986). *Neurology for the speech-language pathologist.* Boston: Butterworths.

Luria, A. (1970). *Traumatic aphasia.* The Hague, Netherlands: Mouton.

Lust, B., & Mervis, C. (1980). Development of coordination in the natural speech of young children. *Journal of Child Language, 7,* 279–304.

Luterman, D. M. (1987). Counseling parents of hearing-impaired children. In F. N. Martin (Ed.), *Hearing disorders in children* (pp. 303–319). Austin, TX: Pro-Ed.

Lynch, J. I. (1986). Language of cleft infants: Lessening the risk of delay through programming. In B. J. McWilliams (Guest Ed.), *Seminars in speech and language* (pp. 255–268). New York: Thieme Inc.

Macken, M. A., & Ferguson, C. A. (1983). Cognitive aspects of phonological development: Model, evidence, and issues. In K. E. Nelson (Ed.), *Children's language* (Vol. 4) (pp. 255–282). Hillsdale, NJ: Erlbaum.

MacNeilage, P. (1970). Motor control of serial ordering in speech. *Psychological Review, 77,* 182–196.

Mahoney, G. (1975). An ethological approach to delayed language acquisition. *American Journal of Mental Deficiency, 80,* 139–148.

Marks, N. C. (1974). *Cerebral palsied and learning disabled children.* Springfield, IL: Charles C. Thomas.

Marsh, J. L. (1986). Long-term results of craniofacial surgery. *Cleft Palate Journal, 23,* Supplement No. 1.

Martin, A. D. (1974). Some objections to the term "apraxia of speech." *Journal of Speech and Hearing Disorders, 39,* 53–64.

Martin, F. N. (1986). *Introduction to audiology* (3rd ed.). Englewood Cliffs, NJ: Prentice-Hall.

Martin, F. N., George, K. A., O'Neal, J., & Daly, J. A. (1986). Audiologists' and parents' attitudes regarding counseling of families of hearing-impaired children. *Asha, 29,* 27–33.

Martin, R. R., Haroldson, S. K., & Triden, K. A. (1984). Stuttering and speech naturalness. *JSHD, 49,* 53–58.

Mason, A. W. (1976). Specific (developmental) dyslexia. *Developmental Medicine and Child Neurology, 9,* 183–190.

Mason, R. M., & Proffit, W. R. (1974). The tongue thrust controversy: Background and recommendations. *Journal of Speech and Hearing Disorders, 39,* 115–132.

Matthews, J. (1964). Communicology and individual responsibility. *Asha, 6*(1).

Matthews, J. (1971). Personal and professional responsibility related to current social problems. *Asha, 13*(6).

Matthews, J. (1974). Speech and language development. In J. J. Gallagher (Ed.), *Windows on Russia.* Washington, DC: U.S. Government Printing Office.

Matthews, J. (1982). Disorders of language. In C. Bluestone & S. Stool (Eds.), *Pediatric Otolaryngology.* Philadelphia: W. B. Saunders.

Mattis, S., French, J. H., & Rapin, I. (1975). Dyslexia in children and young adults: Three independent neuropsychological syndromes. *Developmental Medicine and Child Neurology, 17,* 150–163.

McCarthy, D. (1954). Language disorders and parent-child relationships. *Journal of Speech and Hearing Disorders, 19*(4), 514–523.

McCormack, W. C., & Wurm, S. A. (Eds.). (1976). *Language and man: Anthropological issues.* The Hague, Netherlands: Mouton.

McDonald, E. T. (1964). *Articulation testing and treatment: A sensory-motor approach.* Pittsburgh, PA: Stanwix House.

McDonald, E. T., & Chance, B. (1964). *Cerebral palsy.* Englewood Cliffs, NJ: Prentice-Hall.

McDonald, E. T., & Koepp-Baker, H. (1951). Cleft palate speech: An integration of research and clinical observation. *Journal of Speech and Hearing Disorders, 16,* 9–20.

McDonald, E. T., & Schultz, A. (1973). Communication boards for cerebral palsied children. *Journal of Speech and Hearing Disorders, 38,* 73–88.

McFall, R. M. Parameters of self monitoring. (1977). In R. Stewart (Ed.), *Behavioral self management, strategies, techniques and outcomes.* New York: Brunner/Mazel.

McLean, J., & Snyder-McLean, L. (1978). *A transactional approach to early language training.* Columbus, OH: Merrill.

McNeill, D. (1966). Developmental psycholinguistics. In F. Smith & G. Miller (Eds.), *The genesis of language.* Cambridge, MA: MIT Press.

McReynolds, L. V. (1981). Generalization in articulation training. *Analysis and intervention in developmental disabilities, 1,* 245–258.

McReynolds, L. V. (1987). A perspective on articulation generalization. In R. Ingham (Ed.), *Seminars in Speech and Language, 8*(3), 217–240.

McReynolds, L. V. (1988a). Articulation disorders of unknown etiology. In N. Lass, L. McReynolds, J. Northern, & D. Yoder (Eds.), *Handbook of speech-language pathology and audiology.* Toronto: B. C. Decker, Inc.

McReynolds, L. V. (1988b). Perspectives on generalization. In L. McReynolds & J. Spradlin (Eds.), *Generalization strategies in the treatment of communication disorders.* Toronto: B. C. Decker, Inc.

McReynolds, L. V., & Bennett, S. (1972). Distinctive feature generalization in articulation training. *Journal of Speech and Hearing Disorders, 37,* 462–470.

McReynolds, L. V., & Elbert, M. (1981a). Criteria for phonological process analysis. *Journal of Speech and Hearing Disorders, 46,* 197–204.

McReynolds, L. V., & Elbert, M. (1981b). Generalization of correct articulation in clusters. *Applied Psycholinguistics, 2,* 119–132.

McReynolds, L. V., & Elbert, M. (1984). Phonological processes in articulation intervention. In M. Elbert, D. A. Dinnsen, & G. Weismer (Eds.), *Phonological theory and the misarticulating child. Asha Monograph, 22,* 53–58. Rockville, MD: American Speech-Language-Hearing Association.

McReynolds, L. V., & Engmann, D. L. (1975). *Distinctive feature analysis of misarticulations.* Baltimore, MD: University Park Press.

McReynolds, L. V., & Kearns, K. (1983). *Single subject experimental designs in communication disorders.* Baltimore, MD: University Park Press.

McReynolds, L. V., & Spradlin, J. E. (1988). *Generalization strategies in the treatment of communication disorders.* Toronto: B. C. Decker Inc.

McWilliams, B. J. (1980). Communication problems associated with cleft palate. In R. J. Van Hattum (Ed.), *Communication disorders* (pp. 379–432). New York: Macmillan.

McWilliams, B. J. (1982). Social and psychological problems associated with cleft palate. In F. C. Macgregor (Guest Ed.), *Clinics in plastic surgery* (pp. 317–326). Philadelphia: W. B. Saunders.

McWilliams, B. J. (1984). Speech problems associated with craniofacial anomalies. In J. M. Costello (Ed.), *Speech disorders in children: Recent advances* (pp. 187–223). San Diego: College Hill Press.

McWilliams, B. J., Bluestone, C. D., & Musgrave, R. H. (1969). Diagnostic implications of vocal cord nodules in children with cleft palate. *The Laryngoscope, 79,* 2072–2080.

McWilliams, B. J., & Girdany, B. R. (1964). The use of televex in cleft palate research. *Cleft Palate Journal, 1,* 398–401.

McWilliams, B. J., Glaser, E. R., Philips, B. J., Lawrence, C., Lavorato, A. S., Berry, Q. C., & Skolnick, M. L. (1981). A comparative study of four methods of evaluating velopharyngeal adequacy. *Plastic and Reconstructive Surgery, 68,* 1–9.

McWilliams, B. J., Lavorato, A. S., & Bluestone, C. D. (1973). Vocal cord abnormalities in children with velopharyngeal valving problems. *The Laryngoscope, 83,* 1745–1753.

McWilliams, B. J., & Matthews, H. P. (1979). A comparison of intelligence and social maturity in children with unilateral complete clefts and those with isolated cleft palates. *Cleft Palate Journal, 16,* 363–372.

McWilliams, B. J., Morris, H. L., & Shelton, R. L. (1984). *Cleft palate speech*. Philadelphia & Toronto: B. C. Decker, Inc.

McWilliams, B. J., Musgrave, R. H., & Crozier, P. A. (1968). The influence of head position upon velopharyngeal closure. *Cleft Palate Journal, 5,* 117–124.

McWilliams, B. J., & Philips, B. J. (1979). *Audio seminar in velopharyngeal incompetence*. Philadelphia: W. B. Saunders.

Meader, M. H. (1940). The effect of disturbances in the developmental processes upon emergent specificity of function. *Journal of Speech Disorders, 5,* 211–219.

Menn, L. (1976). Evidence for an interactionist-discovery theory of child phonology. *Papers and Reports on Child Language Development, 12,* 169–177.

Menn, L. (1983). Development of articulatory, phonetic, and phonological capabilities. In B. Butterworth (Ed.), *Language production* (Vol. 2). New York: Academic Press.

Menyuk, P. (1964). Syntactic rules used by children from preschool through first grade. *Child Development, 35,* 533–546.

Menyuk, P. (1965). *A further evaluation of grammatical capacity in children*. Paper presented at the Society for Research in Child Development.

Menyuk, P. (1969). *Sentences children use*. Cambridge, MA: MIT Press.

Menyuk, P. (1977). *Language and maturation*. Cambridge, MA: MIT Press.

Menyuk, P. (1983). Language development and reading. In T. M. Gallagher & C. A. Prutting (Eds.), *Pragmatic assessment and intervention issues in language* (pp. 151–170). San Diego: College Hill.

Michaels, S. (1981). 'Sharing time': Children's narrative styles and differential access to literacy. *Language in Society, 10,* 423–442.

Michaels, S., & Collins, J. (1984). Oral discourse styles: Classroom interaction and the acquisition of literacy. In D. Tannen (Ed.), *Coherence in Spoken and Written Discourse*. Norwood, NJ: Ablex.

Milisen, R. (1954). A rationale for articulation disorders. *Journal of Speech and Hearing Disorders.* Monograph Supplement No. 4, 6–17.

Milisen, R. (1971). The incidence of speech disorders. In L. E. Travis (Ed.), *Handbook of speech pathology and audiology*. New York: Appleton-Century-Crofts.

Miller, G. A., & Gildea, P. M. (1987). How children learn words. *Scientific American, 257,* 94–99.

Miller, J. (1981). *Assessing language production in children: Experimental procedures*. Baltimore, MD: University Park Press.

Miller, J., & Chapman, R. (1981). The relation between age and mean length of utterance in morphemes. *Journal of Speech and Hearing Research, 24,* 154–161.

Miller, J., & Chapman, R. (1983). *Systematic analysis of language transcriptions*. Madison, WI: University of Wisconsin.

Miller, N. (1984). *Bilingualism and language disability: Assessment and remediation*. San Diego: College-Hill Press.

Mitchell, C. (1969). *Language behavior and the black urban community*. Unpublished doctoral dissertation, University of California, Berkeley.

Mitchell-Kernan, C., & Kernan, K. T. (1977). Pragmatics of directive choice among children. In S. Ervin-Tripp & C. Mitchell-Kernan (Eds.), *Child discourse*. New York: Academic Press.

Moerk, E. (1972). Principles of dyadic interaction in language learning. *Merrill-Palmer Quarterly, 18,* 229–257.

Moerk, E. L. (1974). Changes in verbal child-mother interaction with increasing language skills of the child. *Journal of Psycholinguistic Research, 3,* 101–116.

Moffitt, A. (1971). Consonant cue perception by twenty to twenty-four week old infants. *Child Development, 42,* 717–731.

Moncur, J. P., & Brackett, I. P. (1974). *Modifying vocal behavior*. New York: Harper & Row.

Monnin, L. M. (1984). Speech sound discrimination testing and training: Why? Why not? In H. Winitz (Ed.), *Treating articulation disorders: For clinicians by clinicians*. Baltimore, MD: University Park Press.

Moog, J., & Geers, A. (1979). *CID grammatical analysis of elicited language*. St. Louis, MO: Central Institute for the Deaf.

Morley, M. (1967). *Cleft palate and speech* (6th ed.). Baltimore, MD: Williams and Wilkins.

Morris, H. L. (1968). Etiological basis for speech problems. In D. C. Spriestersbach & D. Sherman (Eds.), *Cleft palate and communication*. New York: Academic Press.

Morris, S. E. (1977). *Program guidelines for children with feeding problems*. Edison: Childcraft Education Corp.

Moskowitz, B. (1978). The acquisition of language. *Scientific American, 239,* 93–108.

Mowrer, D. E. (1973). Behavioral application to modification of articulation. In D. Wolfe & D. Goulding (Eds.), *Articulation and learning*. Springfield, IL: Charles C. Thomas.

Mowrer, D. E. (1978). *Methods of modifying speech behaviors*. Columbus, OH: Merrill.

Mueller, H. (1972). Facilitating feeding and prespeech. In P. H. Pearson & C. E. Williams (Eds.), *Physical therapy services in the developmental disabilities*. Springfield, IL: Charles C. Thomas.

Muma, J. (1978). *Language handbook*. Englewood Cliffs, NJ: Prentice-Hall.

Muma, J., & Zwycewicz-Emory, C. (1979). Contextual priority: Verbal shift at seven? *Journal of Child Language, 6,* 301–311.

Mumm, M., Secord, W., & Dykstra, K. (1980). *Merrill language screening test*. San Antonio, TX: Psychological Corporation.

Musgrave, R. H., McWilliams, B. J., & Matthews, H. P. (1975). A review of the results of two different surgical procedures for the repair of clefts of the soft palate only. *Cleft Palate Journal, 12,* 281–290.

Myers, P. S. (1986). Right hemisphere communication impairment. In R. Chapey (Ed.), *Language intervention strategies in adult aphasia* (pp. 444–461). Baltimore, MD: Williams & Wilkins.

Myerson, R. (1975). *A developmental study of children's knowledge of complex derived words of English*. Paper presented at the International Reading Association.

Mysak, E. (Ed.). (1987a). Communication disorders of the cerebral palsied: Assessment and treatment. *Seminars in Speech and Language*. New York: Thieme Medical Publishers.

Mysak, E. (1987b). Assessment of speech movement readiness in cerebral palsy. In E. D. Mysak (Ed.), *Communication disorders of the cerebral palsied: Assessment and treatment*. New York: Thieme Medical Publishers.

Mysak, E. D. (1980). *Neurospeech therapy for the cerebral palsied*. New York: Teachers College Press, Teachers College, Columbia University.

National Institutes of Health. (1979). *National research strategy for neurological and communicative disorders* (No. 79-1910). Washington, DC: National Institutes of Health.

Nelson, K. (1973). Some evidence for the cognitive primacy of categorization and its functional basis. *Merrill-Palmer Quarterly, 19,* 21–39.

Nelson, K. (1974). Concept, word and sentence: Interrelations in acquisition and development. *Psychological Review, 81,* 267–285.

Netsell, R. (1973). Speech physiology. In F. D. Minifie, T. J. Hixon, & F. Williams (Eds.), *Normal aspects of speech, hearing, and language*. Englewood Cliffs, NJ: Prentice-Hall.

Netsell, R. (1984). Physiological studies of dysarthria and their relevance to management. In J. Rosenbek (Ed.), *Current views of dysarthria: Seminars in speech and language, 5*(4), 279–291.

Netsell, R. (1986). *A neurobiologic view of speech production and the dysarthrias*. San Diego: College-Hill Press.

Netsell, R., & Daniel, B. (1979). Dysarthria in adults: Physiologic approach to rehabilitation. *Archives of Physical Medicine and Rehabilitation, 60,* 502–508.

Newcomer, P. L., & Hammill, D. D. (1977). *Test of language development*. Austin, TX: Pro-Ed.

Newport, E. L. (1976). Motherese: The speech of mothers to young children. In N. J. Castellan, D. B. Pisoni, & G. R. Potts (Eds.), *Cognitive theory* (Vol. 2). Hillsdale, NJ: Erlbaum.

Nicolosi, L., Harryman, E., & Kresheck, J. (1978). *Terminology of communication disorders*. Baltimore, MD: Williams and Wilkins.

Nippold, M. A. (1985). Comprehension of figurative language in youth. *Topics in Language Disorders, 5,* 1–20.

Nist, J. (1966). *A structural history of English*. New York: St. Martin's Press.

Nober, E. H. (1976). Auditory processing. In W. J. Cruickshank (Ed.), *Cerebral palsy: A developmental disability*. Syracuse, NY: Syracuse University Press.

Northern, J. L., & Downs, M. P. (1984). *Hearing in children* (3rd ed.). Baltimore, MD: Williams and Wilkins.

Obler, L. (1985). Language through the life-span. In J. Berko Gleason (Ed.), *The development of language*. Columbus, OH: Merrill.

Obler, L. K., & Albert, M. L. (1981). Language and aging: A neurobehavioral analysis. In D. Beasley & G. Davis (Eds.), *Aging: Communication processes and disorders.* New York: Grune and Stratton.

O'Brian, L., & Andreses, J. (1983). A family matter: Stimulating communication in the young cerebral palsied child. *Teaching Exceptional Children, 16,* 47–50.

Ojemann, G., & Mateer, C. (1979). Human language cortex: Localization of memory, syntax, and sequential motor-phoneme identification systems. *Science, 205,* 1401–1403.

Oller, D. (1974). Simplification as the goal of phonological processes in child speech. *Language Learning, 24,* 299–303.

Oller, D. (1978). Infant vocalization and the development of speech. *Allied Health and Behavior Sciences, 1,* 523–549.

Oller, D., Wieman, L., Doyle, W., & Ross, C. (1976). Infant babbling and speech. *Journal of Child Language, 3,* 1–12.

Olmsted, D. (1971). *Out of the mouth of babes.* The Hague, Netherlands: Mouton.

Olson, D. (1970). Language and thought: Aspects of a cognitive theory of semantics. *Psychological Review, 77,* 257–273.

Olson, G. (1973). Developmental changes in memory and the acquisition of language. In T. Moore (Ed.), *Cognitive development and the acquisition of language.* New York: Academic Press.

Orton, S., & Travis, L. E. (1929). Studies in stuttering: IV. Studies of action currents in stutterers. *Archives of Neurology and Psychiatry, 21,* 61–68.

Owen, F. W., Adams, P. A., Forrest, T., Stolz, L. M., & Fisher, S. (1971). Learning disorders in children: Sibling studies. *Monographs of the Society for Research in Child Development, 36* (4, Serial No. 144).

Owens, R. (1978). *Speech acts in the early language of non-delayed and retarded children: A taxonomy and distributional study.* Unpublished doctoral dissertation, The Ohio State University, Columbus.

Owens, R. (1988). *Language development: An introduction* (2nd ed.). Columbus, OH: Merrill.

Paden, E. P. (1970). *A history of the American Speech and Hearing Association, 1925–1958.*

Washington, DC: American Speech and Hearing Association.

Palmer, M. (1947). Studies in clinical techniques. II: Normalization of chewing, sucking, and swallowing reflexes in cerebral palsy: A home program. *Journal of Speech and Hearing Disorders, 12,* 415–418.

Panagos, J. M. (1982). The case against the autonomy of phonological disorders in children. In J. M. Panagos (Ed.), *Seminars in Speech Language and Hearing, 3*(2), 172–182.

Paradise, J. L., Bluestone, C. D., & Felder, H. (1969). The universality of otitis media in 50 infants with cleft palate. *Pediatrics, 44,* 35–42.

Paradise, J. L., McWilliams, B. J. (1974). Simplified feeder for infants with cleft palate. *Pediatrics, 53,* 566–568.

Parker, F. (1986). *Linguistics for nonlinguists.* San Diego, CA: College-Hill Publications.

Peñalosa, F. (1981). *An Introduction to the sociology of language.* Rowley, MA: Newbury House.

Peñalosa, F. (1983). *Chicano sociolinguistics.* Rowley, MA: Newbury House.

Pendergast, K., Dickey, S., Selmar, J., & Sodor, A. (1984). *Photo articulation test* (2nd ed.). Interstate Printers and Publishers, Inc.

Penfield, W., & Roberts, L. (1959). *Speech and brain mechanisms.* Princeton, NJ: Princeton University Press.

Perkins, W. H. (1971). *Speech pathology: An applied behavioral science.* St. Louis, MO: C. V. Mosby.

Perkins, W. H. (1973a). Replacement of stuttering with normal speech. I. Rationale. *Journal of Speech and Hearing Disorders, 38,* 283–294.

Perkins, W. H. (1973b). Replacement of stuttering with normal speech. II. Clinical procedures. *Journal of Speech and Hearing Disorders, 38,* 295–308.

Perkins, W. H. (1978). *Human perspectives in speech and language disorders.* St. Louis, MO: C. V. Mosby.

Perkins, W. M. (1983). *Current therapy of communication disorders: Phonologic-articulatory disorders.* New York: Thieme-Stratton, Inc.

Perkins, W., Ruder, J., Johnson, L., & Michael, W. (1976). Stuttering: Discoordination of phonation with articulation and respiration. *Journal of Speech and Hearing Research, 19,* 509–522.

Peterson-Falzone, S. J. (1973). *Speech pathology in craniofacial malformations other than cleft lip and palate.* Asha Reports No. 8. Washington, DC: American Speech and Hearing Association.

Peterson-Falzone, S. J. (1986). Speech characteristics: Updating clinical decisions. In B. J. McWilliams (Guest Ed.), *Seminars in speech and language* (pp. 269–295). New York: Thieme Inc.

Peterson-Falzone, S. J. (1988). Speech disorders related to craniofacial structural defects: Parts 1 and 2. In N. J. Lass, L. V. McReynolds, J. L. Northern, and D. E. Yoder, *Handbook of speech-language pathology and audiology.* Toronto: B. C. Decker, Inc.

Phelps, W. M. (1940). The treatment of cerebral palsies. *Journal of Bone Joint Surgery, 22,* 1004–1012.

Philips, B. J. (1986). Speech assessment. In B. J. McWilliams (Guest Ed.), *Seminars in speech and language* (pp. 297–311). New York: Thieme Inc.

Philips, B. J., & Harrison, R. J. (1969). Articulation patterns of preschool cleft palate children. *Cleft Palate Journal, 6,* 245–253.

Philips, B. J., & Kent, R. D. (1984). Acoustic-phonetic descriptions of speech production in speakers with cleft palate and other velopharyngeal disorders. In N. J. Lass (Ed.), *Speech and language: Advances in basic research and practice* (Vol. 11) (pp.113–168), New York: Academic Press.

Piaget, J. (1952). *The origins of intelligence in children.* New York: International Universities Press.

Piaget, J., & Inhelder, B. (1969). *The psychology of the child.* New York: Basic Books.

Poole, I. (1934). Genetic development of articulation of consonant sounds in speech. *Elementary English Review, 11,* 159–161.

Porch, B. E. (1967). *Porch index of communicative ability.* Palo Alto, CA: Consulting Psychologists Press.

Powell, T., & Elbert, M. (1984). Generalization following the remediation of early-and-late developing consonant clusters. *Journal of Speech and Hearing Disorders, 49,* 211–218.

Prather, E., Beecher, S., Stafford, M., & Wallace, E. (1980). *Screening test of adolescent language.* Seattle, WA: University of Washington Press.

Prather, E., Hendrick, D., & Kern, C. (1975). Articulation development in children aged two to four years. *Journal of Speech and Hearing Disorders, 40,* 179–191.

Prather, E., Minor, A., Addicott, M., & Sunderland, L. (1971). *Washington speech sound discrimination test.* Interstate Printers & Publishers.

Prinz, P. M. (1985). Language and communication development, assessment and intervention in hearing-impaired individuals. In J. Katz (Ed.), *Handbook of clinical audiology* (3rd ed.) (pp. 788–814). Baltimore: Williams & Wilkins.

Prizant, B., & Rydell, P. (1984). Analysis of functions of delayed echolalia in autistic children. *Journal of Speech and Hearing Research, 27,* 183–192.

Pronovost, W. (1953). *The Boston University speech sound discrimination test.* Go-Mo Products.

Prutting, C. A., & Kirchner, D. M. (1983). Applied pragmatics. In T. M. Gallagher & C. A. Prutting (Eds.), *Pragmatic assessment and intervention issues in language* (pp. 29–64). San Diego: College Hill.

Prutting, C. A. & Kirchner, D. M. (1987). A clinical appraisal of the pragmatic aspects of language. *Journal of Speech and Hearing Disorders, 52,* 105–119.

Punch, J. (1983). Characteristics of ASHA members. *Asha, 25*(1), 31.

Read, C. (1981). Writing is not the inverse of reading for young children. In C. Frederiksen and J. Dominic (Eds.), *Writing: The nature, development, and teaching of written communication.* Hillsdale, NJ: Erlbaum.

Reed, C. E. (1981). Teaching teachers about teaching writing to students from varied linguistic, social and cultural groups. In M. F. Whiteman (Ed.), *Writing: The nature, development and teaching of written communication.* Hillsdale, NJ: Erlbaum.

Rees, N., & Wollner, S. (1981). *An outline of children's pragmatic abilities.* Paper presented at American Speech-Language-Hearing Association Convention, Detroit, Michigan.

Reich, P. (1986). *Language development.* Englewood Cliffs, NJ: Prentice-Hall.

Rice, M. (1980). *Cognition to language: Categories, word meanings, and training.* Baltimore, MD: University Park Press.

Rice, M. (1983). Contemporary accounts of the cognition/language relationship: Implication for speech-language clinicians. *Journal of Speech and Hearing Disorders, 48,* 347–359.

Rice, M. (1984). Cognitive aspects of communicative development. In R. Schiefelbusch and J. Pickar (Eds.), *The acquisition of communicative competence*. Baltimore, MD: University Park Press.

Richards, M. (1974). *The integration of a child into a social world*. New York: Cambridge University Press.

Richman, L. C. (1976). Behavior and achievement of cleft palate children. *Cleft Palate Journal, 13,* 4–10.

Richman, L. C. (1978). The effect of facial disfigurement on teacher's perception of ability in cleft palate children. *Cleft Palate Journal, 15,* 155–160.

Richman, L. C., & Eliason, M. J. (1986). Development in children with cleft lip and/or palate: Intellectual, cognitive, personality, and parental factors. In B. J. McWilliams (Guest Ed.), *Seminars in speech and language* (pp. 225–239). New York: Thieme Inc.

Riley, G., & Riley, J. (1984). A component model for treating stuttering in children. In M. A. Peins (Ed.), *Contemporary approaches in stuttering therapy* (pp. 123–172). Boston, MA: Little, Brown.

Roberts, K., & Horowitz, F. (1986). Basic level categorization in seven- and nine-month-old infants. *Journal of Child Language, 13,* 191–208.

Robertson, S. (1975). *The cognitive organization of action events: A developmental perspective.* Paper presented at American Psychological Association.

Rockman, B., & Elbert, M. (1984). Generalization in articulation training. In H. Winitz (Ed.), *Treating articulation disorders: For clinicians by clinicians*. Baltimore, MD: University Park Press.

Rodgon, M., Jankowski, W., & Alenskas, L. (1977). A multifunctional approach to single word usage. *Journal of Child Language, 4,* 23–45.

Rood, M. S. (1954). Neurophysiological reactions as a basis for physical therapy. *Physical Therapy Review, 34,* 444–448.

Rosch, E. (1979). Style variables in referential language: A study of social class difference and its effect on dyadic communication. In R. O. Freedle (Ed.), *Advances in discourse processes*. Norwood, NJ: Ablex.

Rosenbek, J. C. (1978). Treating apraxia of speech. In D. F. Johns (Ed.), *Clinical management of neurogenic communicative disorders*. Boston, MA: Little, Brown.

Rosenbek, J. C. (1984). Current views of dysarthria. *Seminars in Speech and Language, 5*(4).

Rosenbek, J. C., Kent, R., & LaPointe, L. L. (1984). Apraxia of speech: An overview and some perspectives. In J. Rosenbek, M. McNeil, & A. Aronson (Eds.), *Apraxia of speech: Physiology, acoustics, linguistics, management.* San Diego: College-Hill Press.

Rosenbek, J. C., & LaPointe, L. L. (1978). The dysarthrias: Description, diagnosis and treatment. In D. F. Johns (Ed.), *Clinical management of neurogenic communicative disorders*. Boston: Little, Brown.

Rosenbek, J. C., & LaPointe, L. L. (1985). The dysarthrias: Description, diagnosis and treatment. In D. F. Johns (Ed.), *Clinical management of neurogenic communicative disorders* (2nd ed.). Boston: Little, Brown.

Rourke, B. P. (1975). Brain-behavior relationship in children with learning disabilities. *American Psychologist, 30,* 911–920.

Rubin, H., & Culatta, R. (1971). A point of view about fluency. *Journal of the American Speech and Hearing Association, 13,* 380–387.

Rubow, R. (1984). A clinical guide to the technology of treatment in dysarthria. In J. Rosenbek (Ed.), *Current views of dysarthria: Seminars in speech and language, 5*(4), 315–335.

Ruscello, D. M. (1984). Motor learning as a model for articulation training. In J. Costello (Ed.), *Speech disorders in children* (pp. 129–156). San Diego, CA: College-Hill Press.

Ryan, B. P., & Van Kirk, B. (1974). The establishment, transfer and maintenance of fluent speech in 50 stutterers using DAF and operant procedures. *Journal of Speech and Hearing Disorders, 38,* 3–10.

Sachs, J., & Devin, J. (1976). Young children's use of age-appropriate speech styles in social interaction and role-playing. *Journal of Child Language, 3,* 81–98.

Salmon, S. J., & Goldstein, L. P. (Eds.). (1978). *The artificial larynx handbook*. New York: Grune and Stratton.

Sander, E. (1972). When are speech sounds learned? *Journal of Speech and Hearing Disorders, 37,* 55–63.

Sarno, M. (1980). The nature of verbal impairment after closed head injury. *Journal of Nervous and Mental Disease, 168,* 685–692.

Sarno, M. (1984). Verbal impairment after closed head injury: Report of a replication study. *Journal of Nervous and Mental Disease, 172,* 475–479.

Sarno, M. T. (1969). *The functional communication profile.* New York: New York University Medical Center, Institute of Rehabilitation Medicine.

Sauchelli, K. R. (1979). *The incidence of hoarseness among school-aged children in a pollution-free community.* Unpublished master's thesis, University of Florida, Gainesville, FL.

Saville-Troike, M. (1978). *A guide to culture in the classroom.* Rosslyn, VA: National Clearinghouse for Bilingual Education.

Saville-Troike, M. (1986). Anthropological considerations in the study of communication. In O. Taylor (Ed.), *Nature of communication disorders in culturally and linguistically diverse populations.* San Diego: College-Hill Press.

Saywitz, K., & Cherry-Wilkinson, L. (1982). Age-related differences in metalinguistic awareness. In S. Kaczaj (Ed.), *Language development* (Vol. 2). Hillsdale, NJ: Erlbaum.

Schank, R. (1972). Conceptual dependency: A theory of natural language understanding. *Cognitive Psychology, 3,* 552–631.

Scherzer, A. L., & Tscharnuter, I. (1982). *Early diagnosis and therapy in cerebral palsy.* New York: Marcel Dekker, Inc.

Schlesinger, I. (1971). Production of utterances and language acquisition. In D. Slobin (Ed.), *The ontogenesis of grammar.* New York: Academic Press.

Schmidt, M. (1984). Intelligibility and the child with multiple articulation deviations. In H. Winitz (Ed.), *Treating articulation disorders: For clinicians by clinicians.* Baltimore, MD: University Park Press.

Schuell, H. M. (1965). *The Minnesota test for differential diagnosis of aphasia.* Minneapolis: University of Minnesota Press.

Schutte, H. K. (1980). *The efficiency of voice production.* Druk: Kemper, Groningen.

Schwartz, M. (1974). The core of the stuttering block. *Journal of Speech and Hearing Disorders, 39,* 169–177.

Scollon, R., & Scollon, S. (1979). The literate two-year old: The fictionalization of self. *Working Papers in Sociolinguistics.* Austin, TX: Southwest Regional Laboratory.

Scollon, R., & Scollon, S. (1981). *Narrative, literacy, and face in interethnic communication.* Norwood, NJ: Ablex.

Scoville, R., (1983). Development of the intention to communicate. The eye of the beholder. In L. Feagans, C. Garvey, & R. Golinkoff (Eds.), *The origins of growth and communication.* Norwood, NJ: Ablex.

Semel, E. M., Wiig, E. H., & Secord, W. S. (1987). *Clinical evaluation of language fundamentals* (rev. ed.). San Antonio, TX: Psychological Corporation.

Semel, E. M., Wiig, E. H., & Secord, W. S. (in press). *CELF screening test* (rev. ed.). San Antonio, TX: Psychological Corporation.

Senturia, B. H., & Wilson, F. B. (1968). Otorhinolaryngic findings in children with voice deviations. *Annals of Otolog, Rhinology, and Laryngology, 77,* 1027–1042.

Seymour, H., & Miller-Jones, D. (1981). Language and cognitive assessment of black children. *Speech and language: Advances in basic research and practice.* New York: Academic Press.

Seymour, H. N., & Seymour, C. M. (1977). A therapeutic model for communicative disorders among children who speak Black English Vernacular. *Journal of Speech and Hearing Disorders, 42*(2), 247–256.

Shames, G. H. (1968). *Pediatric clinics of North America.* Philadelphia: W. B. Saunders.

Shames, G. H. (1979). *Relapse in stuttering.* Paper presented at Banff International Conference on Maintenance of Fluency, Banff, Canada.

Shames, G. H. (1981). Relapse in stuttering. In E. Boberg (Ed.), *Maintenance of fluence.* New York: Elsevier, North Holland, Inc.

Shames, G. H. (1987). Vibrotactile feedback of phonation in therapy for stuttering. Unpublished paper presented at Research Symposium, University of Pittsburgh, PA.

Shames, G. H., & Egolf, D. B. (1971). *Experimental therapy for school-age children and their parents* (Final Report, Project No. 482130, Grant No.

OEG-0-8-080080). Washington, DC: Department of Health, Education and Welfare, U.S. Office of Education.

Shames, G. H., & Egolf, D. B. (1976). *Operant conditioning: The management of stuttering.* Englewood Cliffs, NJ: Prentice-Hall.

Shames, G. H., Egolf, D. B., & Rhodes, R. C. (1969). Experimental programs in stuttering therapy. *Journal of Speech and Hearing Disorders, 34,* 38–47.

Shames, G. H., & Florance, C. L. (1980). *Stutter-free speech: A goal for therapy.* Columbus, OH: Merrill.

Shames, G. H., & Rubin, H. (1971). Psycholinguistic measures of language and speech. In W. C. Grabb, S. W. Rosenstein, & K. R. Bzoch (Eds.), *Cleft lip and palate.* Boston, MA: Little, Brown.

Shames, G. H., & Rubin, H. (Eds.). (1986). *Stuttering then and now.* Columbus, OH: Merrill.

Shames, G. H., & Sherrick, C. E., Jr. (1963). A discussion of nonfluency and stuttering as operant behavior. *Journal of Speech and Hearing Disorders, 28,* 3–18.

Shane, H. (1972). *A device and program for aphonic communication.* Unpublished master's thesis, University of Massachusetts, Amherst, MA.

Sharf, D. J., & Ohde, R. N. (1981). Physiological, acoustic, and perceptual aspects of coarticulation: Implications for remediation of articulatory disorders. In N. J. Lass (Ed.), *Speech and language: Advances in basic research and practice* (Vol. 5). New York: Academic Press.

Shatz, M., & Gelman, R. (1973). The development of communication skills: Modification in the speech of young children as a function of the listener. *Monographs of the Society for Research in Child Development, 38*(5, Serial No. 152).

Sheehan, J. G. (1953). Theory and treatment of stuttering as an approach-avoidance conflict. *Journal of Psychology, 36,* 27–49.

Sheehan, J. G. (1958a). Conflict theory of stuttering. In J. Eisenson (Ed.), *Stuttering: A symposium.* New York: Harper and Row.

Sheehan, J. G. (1958b). Prospective studies of stuttering. *Journal of Speech and Hearing Disorders, 23,* 18–25.

Sheehan, J. G. (1975). Conflict theory and avoidance reduction therapy. In J. Eisenson (Ed.), *Stuttering: A second symposium.* New York: Harper and Row.

Sheehan, J. G., and Martyn, M. M. (1966). Spontaneous recovery from stuttering. *Journal of Speech and Hearing Research, 9,* 121–35.

Shelton, R. L. (1978). Disorders of articulation. In D. H. Skinner & R. L. Shelton (Eds.), *Speech, language & hearing.* Reading MA: Addison-Wesley.

Shelton, R. L., Chisum, L., Youngstrom, K. A., Arndt, W. B., & Elbert, M. (1969). Effects of articulation therapy on palatopharyngeal closure, movement of the pharyngeal wall, and tongue posture. *Cleft Palate Journal, 6,* 440–448.

Shelton, R. L., & McReynolds, L. V. (1979). Functional articulation disorders: Preliminaries to treatment. In N. Lass (Ed.), *Speech and language: Advances in basic research and practice* (Vol. 2). New York: Academic Press.

Shelton, R. L., Morris, H. L., & McWilliams, B. J. (1973). Anatomical and physiological requirements for speech. In B. J. McWilliams (Ed.), *Asha Report No. 9.* Washington, DC: American Speech and Hearing Association.

Sherzer, J. (1983). *Kuna ways of speaking: An ethnographic perspective.* Austin: University of Texas Press.

Shewan, C. M. (1987). ASHA members: You are a changin'! Part II. *Asha, 29*(11) 41.

Shewan, C. M. (1988). ASHA members at work. *Asha, 30*(1) 74.

Shine, R. (1984). Assessment and fluency training with the young stutterer. In M. A. Peins (Ed.), *Contemporary approaches in stuttering therapy* (pp. 173–216). Boston, MA: Little, Brown.

Shprintzen, R. J. (1982). Palatal and pharyngeal anomalies in craniofacial syndromes. *Birth Defects Original Article Series, 18,* 53–78.

Shriberg, L., & Kwiatkowski, J. (1980). *Natural process analysis.* New York: Wiley.

Shriberg, L. D. (1980). Developmental phonological disorders. In T. J. Hixon, J. H. Saxman, & L. D. Shriberg (Eds.), *Introduction to communication disorders.* Englewood Cliffs, NJ: Prentice-Hall.

Shriberg, L. D. (1982). Programming for the language component in the developmental phonological disorders. In J. M. Panagos (Ed.), *Seminars in Speech, Language & Hearing 3*(2), 115–127.

Siegel, G. M. (1970). Punishment, stuttering and disfluency. *Journal of Speech and Hearing Research, 13,* 677–714.

Siegel-Sadewitz, V. L., & Shprintzen, R. J. (1982). The relationship of communication disorders to syndrome identification. *Journal of Speech and Hearing Disorders, 47,* 338–354.

Signer, M. B. (1988). Great rewards from a smaller practice. *Asha, 30*(1) 34.

Silliman, E. R. (1984). Interactional competencies in the instructional context: The role of teaching discourse in learning. In G. Wallach & K. Butler (Eds.), *Language learning disabilities in school-age children.* Baltimore, MD: Williams & Wilkins.

Silverman, E. M., & Zimmer, C. H. (1975). Incidence of chronic hoarseness among school-age children. *Journal of Speech and Hearing Disorders, 40,* 211–215.

Simmons, F. B. (1976). Automated hearing screening test for newborns: The Crib-O-Gram. In G. Mencher (Ed.), *Proceedings of the Nova Scotia Conference on Early Identification of Hearing Loss* (pp. 171–180). Basel, Switzerland: S. Karger.

Simmons, F. B., & Russ, F. (1974). Automated newborn hearing screening: Crib-O-Gram. *Archives of Otolaryngology, 100,* 1–7.

Simon, C. S. (1985). The language-learning disabled student: Description and theory implications. In C. S. Simon (Ed.), *Communication skills and classroom success* (pp. 1–56). San Diego, College Hill.

Sinclair-DeZwart, H. (1973). Language acquisition and cognitive development. In T. Moore (Ed.), *Cognitive development and the acquisition of language.* New York: Academic Press.

Singer, M. I., & Blom, E. D. (1980). An endoscopic technique for restoration of voice after laryngectomy. *Annals of Otology, Rhinology and Laryngology, 89*(6), 529–533.

Singh, S., & Frank, D. (1972). A distinctive feature analysis of the consonantal substitution pattern. *Language and Speech, 15,* 209–218.

Singh, S., Woods, D., & Becker, G. (1972). Perceptual structure of 22 prevocalic English consonants. *Journal of the Acoustical Society of America, 52,* 1698–1713.

Skolnick, M. L. (1970). Videofluoroscopic examination of the velopharyngeal portal during phonation in lateral and base projections: A new technique for studying the mechanics of closure. *Cleft Palate Journal, 7,* 803–816.

Slobin, D. (1973). Cognitive prerequisites for the development of grammar. In C. Ferguson & D. Slobin (Eds.), *Studies of child language development.* New York: Holt, Rinehart & Winston.

Smit, A. B. (1986). Ages of speech sound acquisition: Comparisons and critiques of several normative studies. *Language Speech and Hearing Services in Schools, 17,* 175–186.

Smitherman, G. (1978). *Talkin' and testifyin': The language of black Americans.* Boston, MA: Houghton Mifflin.

Smitherman, G. (1988). Discriminatory discourse on Afro-American speech. In G. Smitherman and T. Van Dijk (Eds.), *Discourse and discrimination.* Detroit, MI: Wayne State University Press.

Smitherman, G., & Van Dijk, T. (Eds.). (1988). *Discourse and discrimination.* Detroit, MI: Wayne State University Press.

Snidecor, J. C. (1962). *Speech rehabilitation of the laryngectomized.* Springfield, IL: Thomas.

Snidecor, J. C. (1971). Speech without a larynx. In L. E. Travis (Ed.), *Handbook of speech pathology and audiology.* New York: Appleton-Century-Crofts.

Snow, C. (1972). Mother's speech to children learning language. *Child Development, 43,* 549–566.

Snow, C. (1977a). The development of conversation between mothers and babies. *Journal of Child Language, 4,* 1–22.

Snow, C. (1977b). Mother's speech research: From input to interaction. In C. Snow & C. Ferguson (Eds.), *Talking to children: Language input and acquisition.* New York: Cambridge University Press.

Sommers, R. K. (1983). *Articulation disorders.* Englewood Cliffs, NJ: Prentice-Hall.

Sparks, R., Helm, N., & Albert, M. (1974). Aphasia rehabilitation resulting from melodic intonation therapy. *Cortex, 10,* 303–310.

Sparks, S. N. (1984). *Birth defects and speech-language disorders.* Boston, MA: College-Hill Press.

St. Louis, K. O., Hinzman, A. R., & Hull, F. H. (1985). Studies of cluttering: Disfluency and language measures in young possible clutterers and stutterers. *Journal of Fluency Disorders, 10,* 151–172.

Stanback, M. (1985). Language and black women's place: Evidence from black middle-class. In P.

Treichler, C. Kramarae, and B. Stafford (Eds.), *Alma mater: Theory and practice in feminist scholars* (pp. 177–193). Urbana: University of Illinois Press.

Stark, R. (1978). Features of infant sounds: The emergence of cooing. *Journal of Child Language, 5,* 1–12.

Stark, R. (1979). Prespeech segmental feature development. In P. Fletcher & M. Garman (Eds.), *Language acquisition.* New York: Cambridge University Press.

Starkweather, W. (1982). Stuttering and laryngeal behavior: A review. *Asha Monographs,* No. 21.

Starr, S. (1975). The relationship of single words to two-word sentences. *Child Development, 46,* 701–708.

*Stedman's Medical Dictionary* (23rd ed.). (1976). Baltimore, MD: Williams and Wilkins.

Stemple, J. C. (1984). *Clinical voice pathology.* Columbus, OH: Merrill.

Stephens, M. I. (1977). *Stephens oral language screening test.* Peninsula, OH: Interim Publishers.

Stern, D. (1977). *The first relationship.* Cambridge: Harvard University Press.

Stevenson, M. H., Daly, J., & Martin, F. N. (1986). A survey of hearing-impaired adults' initial diagnostic experiences in Texas. *Texas, 12,* 19–23.

Stewart, R. (1977). Self help group approach to self management. In R. Stewart (Ed.), *Behavioral self management, strategies, techniques and outcomes.* New York: Brunner/Mazel.

Stoel-Gammon, C., & Dunn, C. (1985). *Normal and disordered phonology in children.* Baltimore, MD: University Park Press.

Stool, S. E., & Randall, P. (1967). Unexpected ear disease in infants with cleft palate. *Cleft Palate Journal, 4,* 99–103.

Strominger, A. (1982). A follow-up of reading and linguistic abilities in language delayed children. Doctoral dissertation, Boston University, Sargent College.

Strupp, H. (1962). Patient-doctor relationship: Psychotherapist in the therapeutic process. In W. J. Bachrach (Ed.), *Experimental foundations of clinical psychology.* New York: Basic Books.

Strupp, H. (1972). On the technology of psychotherapy. *Archives of General Psychiatry, 26,* 270–278.

Stubbs, M. (1983). *Discourse analysis: The sociolinguistic analysis of natural language.* Chicago: University of Chicago Press.

Subtelny, J., & Subtelny, J. D. (1959). Intelligibility and associated physiological factors of cleft palate speakers. *Journal of Speech and Hearing Research, 2,* 353–360.

Tallal, P. (1987). The neuropsychology of developmental language disorders. *Proceedings of the First International Symposium on Specific Language Disorders in Children* (pp. 36–47). England: University of Reading Press.

Tannen, D. (1981). Implications of the oral/literate continuum for cross-cultural communication. In J. Alatis (Ed.), *Current issues in bilingualism: Georgetown University roundtable on languages and linguistics, 1980.* Washington, DC: Georgetown University Press.

Tannen, D. (1982). Oral and literate strategies in spoken and written narratives. *Language, 58,* 1–21.

Taylor, J. S. (1980). Public school speech-language certification standards: Are they standard? *Asha, 22*(3), 159–165.

Taylor, O. (in press). Clinical practice as a social occasion. In L. Cole & V. Deal (Eds.), *Communication disorders in multicultural populations.* Rockville, MD: American Speech-Language-Hearing Association.

Taylor O., & Lee, D. (1987). Standardized tests and African Americans: Communication and language issues. *Negro Education Review, 38,* 67–80.

Taylor, O., & Matsuda, M. (1988). Narratives as a source of discrimination in the classroom. In G. Smitherman & T. Van Dijk (Eds.), *Discourse and discrimination.* Detroit, MI: Wayne State University Press.

Taylor, O. L. (1973). Teachers' attitudes toward Black and Nonstandard English as measured by the Language Attitude Scale. In R. Shery & R. Fasold (Eds.), *Language attitudes: Current trends and prospects.* Washington, DC: Georgetown University Press.

Taylor, O. L. (1978). Language issues and testing. *Journal of Non-White Concerns, 6*(3), 125–133.

Taylor, O. L. (1983). Black English: An agenda for the 1980s. In J. Chambers (Ed.), *Black English: Educational equity and the law.* Ann Arbor, MI: Karoma Press.

Taylor, O. L., & Payne, K. (1983). Culturally valid testing: A proactive approach. *Topics in Language Disorders, 3*(7) 8–20.

Templin, M. (1957). *Certain language skills in children.* Minneapolis, MN: University Park Press.

Templin, M. C. (1957). Templin speech-sound discrimination test. In M. C. Templin, *Certain language skills in children.* Minneapolis: University of Minnesota Press.

Templin, M. C., & Darley, F. L. (1969). *The Templin-Darley test of articulation* (2nd ed.). Iowa City: University of Iowa, Bureau of Educational Research and Service, Division of Extension and University Services.

Tessier, P. (1971). The definitive plastic surgical treatment of the severe facial deformities of craniofacial dysostosis. *Plastic and Reconstructive Surgery, 48,* 419.

Thompson, C. K., & McReynolds, L. V. (1986). Wh-interrogative production in agrammatic aphasia: An experimental analysis of auditory visual stimulation and direct-production treatment. *Journal of Speech and Hearing Research, 29,* 193–205.

Thompson, R. J., Jr. (1986). *Behavior problems in children with developmental and learning disabilities.* International Academy for Research on Learning Disabilities. Monograph Series No. 3. Ann Arbor, MI: University of Michigan Press.

Travis, L. E. (1957). The unspeakable feeling of people with special reference to stuttering. In L. E. Travis (Ed.), *Handbook of speech pathology.* New York: Appleton-Century-Crofts.

Trudgill, P. (1974). *Sociolinguistics: An introduction.* New York: Penguin Books.

Turnure, C. (1971). Response to voice of mother and stranger by babies in the first year. *Developmental Psychology, 4,* 182–190.

Twitchell, T. E. (1965). Variations and abnormalities of motor development. *Journal of American Physical Therapy Association, 45,* 424–430.

Vallino, L. D. (1987). The effects of orthognathic surgery on speech, velopharyngeal function, and hearing. Doctoral dissertation, University of Pittsburgh.

Van Bergeijk, W. A., Pierce, J. R., & David, E. E. (1960). *Waves and the ear.* New York: Doubleday.

Van Demark, D. R. (1966). A factor analysis of the speech of children with cleft palate. *Cleft Palate Journal, 3,* 159–170.

Van Demark, D. R., & Hardin, M. A. (1986). Effectiveness of intensive articulation therapy for children with cleft palate. *Cleft Palate Journal, 23,* 215–224.

Van Demark, D. R., Morris, H. L., & Vandehaar, C. (1979). Patterns of articulation abilities of speakers with cleft palate. *Cleft Palate Journal, 16,* 230–239.

Vanderheiden, G. C. (Ed.) (1978). Non-vocal communication resource book. Baltimore, MD: University Park Press.

Vanderheiden, G. C., & Harris-Vanderheiden, D. (1976). Communication techniques and aids. In L. Lloyd (Ed.), *Communication assessment and intervention strategies.* Baltimore, MD: University Park Press.

Van Riper, C. (1954). *Speech correction: Principles and methods* (3rd ed.). Englewood Cliffs, NJ: Prentice-Hall.

Van Riper, C. (1971). *The nature of stuttering.* Englewood Cliffs, NJ: Prentice-Hall.

Van Riper, C. (1972). *Speech correction: Principles and Methods* (5th ed.). Englewood Cliffs, N. J.: Prentice-Hall.

Van Riper, C. (1978). *Speech correction: Principles and methods* (6th ed.). Englewood Cliffs, NJ: Prentice-Hall.

Van Riper, C. (1979). *A career in speech pathology.* Englewood Cliffs, NJ: Prentice-Hall.

Van Riper, C., & Erickson, R. L. (1969). *The predictive screening test of articulation.* Kalamazoo: Western Michigan University.

Van Riper, C., & Irwin, J. V. (1958). *Voice and articulation.* Englewood Cliffs, NJ: Prentice-Hall.

Vaughn-Cooke, F. B. (1983). Improving language assessment in minority children. *Asha, 25,* 29–34.

Vihman, M., Macken, M., Miller, R., Simmons, H., & Miller, J. (1985). From babbling to speech: A reassessment of the continuity issue. *Language, 61,* 397–445.

Vogel, S. A. (1977). Morphological ability in normal and dyslexic children. *Journal of Learning Disabilities, 10,* 35–43.

Wallach, G., & Butler, K. G. (1984). *Language learning disabilities in school-age children.* Baltimore, MD: Williams & Wilkins.

Wardhaugh, R. (1976). *The contexts of language.* Rowley, MA: Newberry House.

Warren, D. W. (1979). Perci: A method for rating palatal efficiency. *Cleft Palate Journal, 16,* 279–285.

Warren, D. W. (1986). Compensatory speech behaviors in cleft palate: A regulation/control phenomenon? *Cleft Palate Journal, 23,* 251–260.

Warren, D. W., & Dubois, A. B. (1964). A pressure-flow technique for measuring velopharyngeal orifice area during continuous speech. *Cleft Palate Journal, 1,* 52–71.

Warren, S., & Kaiser, A. (1986). Incidental language teaching: A critical review. *Journal of Speech and Hearing Disorders, 51,* 291–299.

Waterhouse, L., & Fein, D. (1982). Language skills in developmentally disabled children. *Brain and Language, 15,* 307–333.

Webb, M. W., & Irving, R. W. (1964). Psychologic and anamnestic patterns characteristic of laryngectomies: Relation to speech rehabilitation. *Journal of American Geriatric Society, 12,* 303–322.

Webster, E., & Larkins, P. (1979). *Counseling aphasic families* [Videotape lecture].

Webster, R. L. (1980). Evolution of a target-based behavioral therapy for stuttering. *Journal of Fluency Disorders, 5,* 303–320.

Wechsler D. (1974). *Wechsler intelligence scale for children* (rev. ed.). San Antonio, TX: Psychological Corporation.

Wehren, A., De Lisi, R., & Arnold, M. (1981). The development of noun definition. *Journal of Child Language, 8,* 165–175.

Weigl, E. (1970). Neuropsychological studies of structure and dynamics of semantic fields with the deblocking methods. In A. T. Greimes et al. (Eds.), *Sign, language, culture.* The Hague, Netherlands: Mouton.

Weiner, F. F. (1979). *Phonological process analysis.* Austin, TX: Pro-Ed, Inc.

Weiner, F. F. (1981). Treatment of phonological disability using the method of meaningful minimal contrast. *Journal of Speech and Hearing Disorders, 46,* 97–103.

Weiner, F. F. (1984a). *Process analysis by computer* [Computer program]. State College, PA: Parrot Software.

Weiner, F. F. (1984b). *Minimal contrast therapy* [Computer program]. State College, PA: Parrot Software.

Weiner, F. F. (1985). *Phonological tutor* [Computer program]. State College, PA: Parrot Software.

Weiner, P. (1985). The value of follow-up studies. *Topics in Language Disorders, 5,* 78–92.

Weiss, C. E. (1971). Success of an obturator reduction program. *Cleft Palate Journal, 8,* 291–297.

Weiss, C. E., Lillywhite, H. S., & Gordon, M. D. (1980). *Clinical management of articulation disorders.* St. Louis, MO: The C.V. Mosby Company.

Weiss, D. A. (1964). *Cluttering.* Englewood Cliffs, NJ: Prentice-Hall.

Weiss, R. (1981). INREAL intervention for language handicapped and bilingual children. *Journal of the Division for Early Childhood, 4,* 40–51.

Wellman, B. L., Case, I. M., Mengert, I. G., & Bradbury, D. E. (1931). Speech sounds of young children. *University of Iowa Studies in Child Welfare, 5*(2).

Wells, G. (1974). Learning to code experience through language. *Journal of Child Language, 1,* 243–269.

Wepman, J. M. (1951). *Recovery from aphasia.* New York: Ronald Press.

Wepman, J. M. (1973). *Auditory discrimination test.* Chicago: Language Research Associates, Inc.

Wertz, R. T. (1985). Neuropathologies of speech and language: An introduction to patient management. In D. F. Johns (Ed.), *Clinical management of neurogenic communicative disorders* (2nd ed.). Boston: Little, Brown.

Wertz, R. T., Aten, J. L., LaPointe, L. L., Holland, A. L., Brookshire, R. H., Weiss, D., Kurtske, J., & Garcia, L. (1984a). *Veterans' Administration cooperative study on aphasia: Comparison of clinic, home and deferred treatment.* Miniseminar presented at the American Speech-Hearing-Language Association Annual Convention, San Francisco, California.

Wertz, R. T., LaPointe, L. L., & Rosenbek, J. C. (1984b). *Apraxia of speech: The disorder and its management.* Orlando: Grune & Stratton.

West, R. (1958). An agnostic's speculations about stuttering. In J. Eisenson (Ed.), *Stuttering: A symposium.* New York: Harper and Row.

Westlake, H. (1951). Muscle training for cerebral palsied speech cases. *Journal of Speech and Hearing Disorders, 16,* 103–109.

Westlake, H., & Rutherford, D. (1964). *Speech therapy for the cerebral palsied.* Chicago: National Society for Crippled Children and Adults.

White, B. (1975). Critical influences in the origins of competence. *Merrill-Palmer Quarterly, 2,* 243–266.

White, E. J. (1979). Dysonomia in the adolescent dyslexic and developmentally delayed adolescent. Doctoral dissertation, Boston University. Graduate School.

Wiig, E. H. (1982). *Let's talk inventory for adolescents.* San Antonio, TX: Psychological Corporation.

Wiig, E. H. (1989). *Steps to language competence: Developing metalinguistic strategies.* San Antonio, TX: Psychological Corporation.

Wiig, E. H., Alexander, E. W., & Secord, W. (1987). Linguistic competence and level of cognitive functioning in adults with traumatic closed head injury. In H. A. Whitaker (Ed.), *Neuropsychological studies of non-focal brain damage: Dementia and trauma* (pp.187–201). New York: Springer Verlag.

Wiig, E. H., Bray, C. M., Colquhoun, A. E., Posnick, B., Vines, S., & Watkins, A. (1983). Elicited speech acts: Developmental and diagnostic patterns. Miniseminar. *ASHA Annual Convention,* Cincinnati, Ohio.

Wiig, E. H., & Secord, W. S. (1985). *Test of language competence.* San Antonio, TX: Psychological Corporation.

Wiig, E. H., & Secord, W. S. (1988). *Test of language competence—expanded.* San Antonio, TX: Psychological Corporation.

Wiig, E. H., & Semel, E. M. (1976). *Language disabilities in children and adolescents.* Columbus, OH: Merrill.

Wiig, E. H., & Semel, E. M. (1984). *Language assessment and intervention for the learning disabled* (2nd ed.). Columbus, OH: Merrill.

Wiig, E. H., Semel, E. M., & Abele, E. (1981). Perception and interpretation of ambiguous sentences by learning disabled twelve-year-olds. *Learning Disabilities Quarterly, 4,* 3–12.

Wiig, E. H., Semel, E. M., & Crouse, M. A. B. (1973). The use of morphology by high-risk and learning disabled children. *Journal of Learning Disabilities, 6,* 457–465.

Wilkinson, L., Calculator, S., & Dollaghan, C. (1982). Ya wanna trade—just for awhile: Children's requests and responses to peers. *Discourse Processes, 5,* 161–176.

Williams, D. E. (1957). A point of view about stuttering. *Journal of Speech and Hearing Disorders, 22,* 390–397.

Williams, D. E. (1979). A perspective on approaches to stuttering therapy. In H. Gregory (Ed.), *Controversies about stuttering therapy.* Baltimore, MD: University Park Press.

Williams, R., & Wolfram, W. (1977). *Social differences vs. disorders.* Washington, DC: American Speech and Hearing Association.

Wingate, M. (1959). Calling attention to stuttering. *Journal of Speech and Hearing Research, 2,* 326–335.

Wingate, M. (1964). A standard definition of stuttering. *Journal of Speech and Hearing Disorders, 29,* 484–489.

Wingate, M. (1969). Stuttering as phonetic transition defect. *Journal of Speech and Hearing Disorders, 34,* 107–108.

Winitz, H. (1961). Repetitions in the vocalizations and speech of children in the first two years of life. *Journal of Speech and Hearing Disorders,* Monograph Supplement 7, 55–62.

Winitz, H. (1969). *Articulatory acquisition and behavior.* New York: Appleton-Century-Crofts.

Winitz, H. (1973). Problem solving and the delaying of speech as strategies in the teaching of language. *Asha, 15,* 583–586.

Winitz, H. (1975). *From syllable to conversation.* Baltimore, MD: University Park Press.

Winitz, H. (1984). Auditory considerations in articulation training. In H. Winitz (Ed.), *Treating articulation disorders: For clinicians by clinicians.* Baltimore, MD: University Park Press.

Winograd, T. (1972). Understanding natural language. *Cognitive Psychology, 3,* 1–19.

Wischner, G. J. (1950). Stuttering behavior and learning: A preliminary theoretical formulation. *Journal of Speech and Hearing Disorders, 15,* 324–335.

Wischner, G. J. (1952a). Anxiety reduction as reinforcement in maladaptive behavior: Evidence in stutterers' representations of the moment of difficulty. *Journal of Abnormal Social Psychology, 47,* 566–571.

Wischner, G. J. (1952b). An experimental approach to expectancy and anxiety in stuttering behavior. *Journal of Speech and Hearing Disorders, 17,* 139–154.

Wisniewski, A. T., & Shewan, C. M. (1987). There is joy in Mudville career satisfaction. *Asha, 29*(10), 30–31.

Wolfe, W. G. (1950). A comprehensive evaluation of fifty cases of cerebral palsy. *Journal of Speech and Hearing Disorders, 15,* 234–251.

Wolfram, W. (1970). Souslinguistic implications for educational sequencing. In R. Fasold and R. Shery, *Teaching Standard English in the inner city.* Washington, DC: Center for Applied Linguistics.

Wolfram, W. (1986). Language variation in the United States. In O. Taylor (Ed.), *Nature and treatment of communication disorders in culturally and linguistically diverse populations.* San Diego: College-Hill Press.

Wolfram, W., & Fasold, R. W. (1974). *The study of social dialects in American English.* Englewood Cliffs, NJ: Prentice-Hall.

Wolpe, J. (1958). *Psychotherapy by reciprocal inhibition.* Stanford: Stanford University Press.

Wood, K. S. (1971). Terminology and nomenclature. In L. E. Travis (Ed.), *Handbook of speech pathology and audiology.* New York: Appleton-Century-Crofts.

Work, R. S. (1987). Microcomputer applications for speech-language services in the schools. *Asha, 29*(11), 50.

Worster-Drought, C. (1968). Speech disorders in children. *Developmental Medicine and Neurology, 10,* 427–440.

Ylvisaker, M. (1985). *Head injury rehabilitation: Children and adolescents.* San Diego: College-Hill Press.

Ylvisaker, M., & Szekeres, S. F. (1986). Management of the patient with closed head injury. In R. Chapey (Ed.), *Language intervention in adult aphasia* (pp. 474–490). Baltimore, MD: William & Wilkins.

Yorkston, K. M., Beukelman, D. R., & Bell, K. R. (1988). *Clinical management of dysarthric speakers.* Boston: College-Hill Press.

Yorkston, K. M., Beukelman, D. R., & Traynor, C. (1984). *Computerized assessment of intelligibility of dysarthric speech.* Austin: TX: Pro-Ed.

**George H. Shames**, Professor in Communication Disorders and Psychology at the University of Pittsburgh, has had a dual interest in stuttering and training of speech-language pathologists for many years. He has been guest lecturer at universities and colleges throughout the United States and Canada, and in Australia, in addition to presenting many miniseminars, short courses, and workshops on the management of stuttering. A member of the American Speech-Hearing-Language Association, American Psychological Association, and American Association for the Advancement of Science, Shames holds a CCC in Speech and is a Licensed Clinical Psychologist. He is an active leader of ASHA, and has served as a site visitor for and on the Educational and Training Board of the American Board of Examiners in Speech Pathology and Audiology. He has been a consultant in research and training. His research grants and wide range of clinical experiences have produced an even longer list of papers, articles, international presentations, and books, including *Stutter-Free Speech: A Goal for Therapy* (with C. L. Florance), *Stuttering Then and Now* (with H. Rubin), and *Operant Conditioning and the Management of Stuttering* (with D. Egolf).

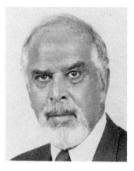

A native of Denmark, where she received her B.S., **Elisabeth H. Wiig** completed her professional schooling in the United States with a Ph.D. from Case Western Reserve University. She served as Professor in the Communication Disorders Department at Boston University from 1970 until 1987, and chaired the program for several years. She is currently Professor Emerita at Boston University and Adjunct Professor at Texas Christian University in Fort Worth. In addition to holding a CCC in Speech-Language Pathology and Audiology, Wiig is a member and Fellow of the American Speech-Language-Hearing Association. She is also a member of the Texas Speech-Language-Hearing Association, Council for Exceptional Children, Council on Learning Disabilities, International Academy of Research on Learning Disabilities, and International Neuropsychology Society. She has published more than 30 articles in refereed journals, and made numerous conference presentations dealing primarily with language-learning disabilities. Her current work focuses on the language disorders associated with learning disabilities in children, adolescents, and young adults. This focus is reflected in texts, diagnostic tests, and language intervention programs, among them the *Clinical Evaluation of Language Fundamentals—Revised* (with E. M. Semel and W. Secord), *Test of Language Competence—Expanded* (with W. Secord), and *Let's Talk Communication Skills* series (with C. M. Bray).

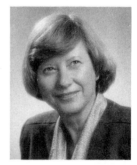

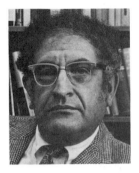

**Jack Matthews,** who is Professor Emeritus in the Communication Department at the University of Pittsburgh, has been a leader in the fields of speech pathology and psychology for more than 25 years. He currently serves as Vice President of Western Pennsylvania School for the Deaf. A past president of the Pennsylvania Speech Association, American Cleft Palate Association, and the American Speech and Hearing Association, he has also served as assistant editor or on the editorial board of many of the field's most highly respected journals. He has been and continues to act as a Consultant for many private and government agencies, including the National Advisory Committee on Handicapped Children; U.S. Office of Education; National Institutes of Health; Veterans Administration; Department of Health, Education and Welfare; and United Cerebral Palsy. His many interests range from teaching communication skills to program evaluation of intervention strategies.

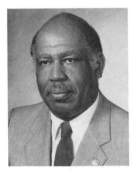

**Orlando L. Taylor** is presently Dean of the School of Communications at Howard University in Washington, D.C. He is also a Graduate Professor of Communication Sciences at the same institution. Taylor received his bachelor's degree from Hampton University, master's from Indiana University, and Ph.D. from the University of Michigan. He has published over 75 articles, monographs, and book chapters in the fields of communication disorders and language sciences, combining the theories of sociolinguistics and speech pathology to develop new approaches to the study of communication disorders and language learning that focus on the needs of culturally and linguistically diverse populations. He has also developed an approach to teaching Standard English to Nonstandard English speakers that utilizes the indigenous language and culture of the learner.

In 1984, Taylor was awarded the Distinguished Scholar/Teacher Award from Howard University. He is a Fellow of the American Speech-Language-Hearing Association, has served as founding president of the National Communication Association and vice president of the American Speech and Hearing Foundation, and is listed among *American Men and Women of Science.* He was the leading organizer of four World Congresses on Communication and Development in Africa and the African Diaspora.

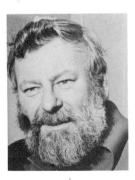

A professor of Speech and Hearing Science and School of Basic Medical Sciences at the University of Illinois, **Willard R. Zemlin** has had a career-long interest in the anatomy and physiology of speech and hearing. He is a member of the American Speech-Language-Hearing Association (of which he is a Fellow), the Acoustic Society of America, and the American Association of Phonetic Sciences. Zemlin has written numerous books and articles, and presented dozens of papers on speech and hearing science and the related physiological mechanisms in humans and animals (from dalmations to guinea pigs). He is also actively involved in directing graduate student research. His many honors include winning the 1972–73 Swedish Medical Research Council Fellowship.

**Leija V. McReynolds** is a Professor of Hearing and Speech at the University of Kansas Medical Center, and a Research Associate at the Bureau of Child Research Laboratory and at the Kansas Center for Mental Retardation and Human Development. A member of several professional organizations, she has also served in editorial functions for the *Journal of Speech and Hearing Disorders, Journal of Applied Behavior Analysis,* and *Analysis and Intervention in Developmental Disabilities.* McReynolds's interest in the application of behavior modification techniques to language impairments, especially articulation disorders, has been demonstrated in numerous articles, chapters in books, journal reviews, and workshops presented from coast to coast. Her current interests focus on articulation disorders and normal phonological development from the point of view of linguistics.

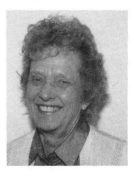

**G. Paul Moore** has been a recognized leader in the study of the voice and laryngeal function for more than 30 years. He was chairman of the Department of Speech at the University of Florida, where his career was capped by his appointment as Distinguished Service Professor in 1977. The Florida Chapter of the National Student Speech-Language and Hearing Association named their annual lecture series the G. Paul Moore Communication Symposium. The Voice Foundation in New York City established a G. Paul Moore lecture at its annual Symposium on the Care of the Professional Voice. A former president of the American Speech-Language-Hearing Association, American Speech-Language-Hearing Foundation, and Central States Speech Association, he has also been a member of several professional organizations, editorial boards, and government advisory committees. His many writings on voice and the larynx have appeared in professional journals in the United States, Europe, and Australia. He has also authored or coauthored nine films on laryngeal function and voice.

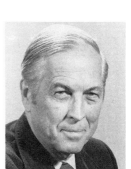

**Laurence B. Leonard** is a Professor in the Department of Audiology and Speech Sciences at Purdue University. Leonard's primary interests center on language development and language disorders in children. His work on these subjects has appeared in many professional journals and textbooks. Leonard is a member of several professional organizations and is a Fellow of the American Speech-Language-Hearing Association. He has served as editorial consultant for a number of scholarly journals, and as editor of the *Journal of Speech and Hearing Disorders.*

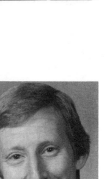

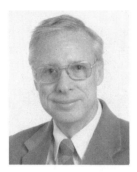

**Frederick N. Martin** is the Lillie Hage Jamail Centennial Professor in Speech Communication at the University of Texas—Austin. He is a Fellow of the American Speech-Language-Hearing Association, and is author or editor of over 200 books, book chapters, monographs, journal articles, and convention papers, including the popular text, *Introduction to Audiology*, published by Prentice-Hall. He has received the Award for Teaching Excellence from the College of Communication, and the Graduate Teaching Award from the Graduate School of the University of Texas.

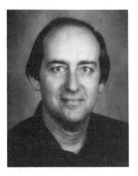

The distinguished career of **Betty Jane McWilliams** has been committed to individuals with cleft palate and related disorders. A past president of the American Cleft Palate Association and current Editor of the *Cleft Palate Journal,* she is Director of the Cleft Palate Center and Professor of Audiology and Speech Pathology at the University of Pittsburgh. She continues to be active in her community and at the university, along with writing numerous books, chapters, and articles focusing on both the technical and the interpersonal management of cleft palate. McWilliams has been honored as a Fellow of both the American Speech and Hearing Association and the American College of Dentists, and with the Service Award of the American Cleft Palate Association (1975) and the Herbert Cooper Memorial Award (1979).

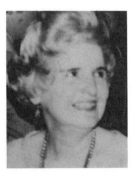

**Leonard L. (Chick) LaPointe** began his professional career as an itinerant speech-language clinician in 10 schools in Menasha, Wisconsin. During his graduate study at the University of Colorado, Boulder, he acquired his ongoing interest in brain function and communication by serving traineeships and internships at Rose Memorial Hospital, Denver Veterans Administration Medical Center, University of Colorado Medical School, and Fitzsimons Army Hospital. For 14 years, he worked at the Gainesville, Florida, Veterans Administration Medical Center and the University of Florida. He is presently Chair of the Department of Speech and Hearing Science at Arizona State University, in Tempe. LaPointe has authored, co-authored, or edited three books, fourteen book chapters, two films, a reading test for aphasia, and over 40 scientific articles. He has presented over 200 invited papers or workshops throughout the United States, Europe, and South America. His other interests include the crafts and culture of American Indians, humor and nonsense, and the cultivation of optimism.

A Professor of Speech Pathology and Chairman of the Department of Speech and Language Pathology and Audiology at Teachers College, Columbia University, **Edward D. Mysak** teaches and does research on stuttering, neurogenic speech problems, and cerebral palsy. He has been a leader in ASHA for many years, and holds both the CCC in Speech Pathology and the CCC in Audiology. Mysak has written five textbooks dealing with speech or cerebral palsy, along with numerous articles, chapters, and films. Since 1960, he has presented over 100 talks and short courses at conventions, colleges and universities, hospitals, and special schools on a wide range of topics, including language development and disorders, vocal aging, stuttering, cerebral palsy, feedback theory, cleft palate, articulation, dysarthria, and speech system theory.

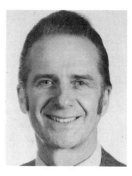

**Robert E. Owens, Jr.** is an Associate Professor and the Graduate Program Director in the Department of Speech Pathology and Audiology at the State University of New York at Geneseo. He has published several articles, made many presentations at professional conferences and workshops, and is the author of *Language Development: An Introduction,* published by Merrill Publishing Company. He received his doctorate from Ohio State University.

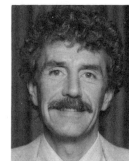

**Audrey L. Holland** is Professor of Speech and Research Assistant Professor of Psychiatry at the University of Pittsburgh, where she received her undergraduate and graduate training. An active member of her university community, she is also a leader in both the American Speech-Language-Hearing Association and the Academy of Aphasia. She has served in editorial roles for the *Journal of Speech and Hearing Disorders, Behavioral Sciences and Allied Health,* and *Journal of Speech and Hearing Research*. Holland has written many articles, reviews, and textbook chapters, as well as *Communicative Abilities in Daily Living: An Assessment Procedure for Aphasic Adults.* Her career is marked by a twofold interest in applied research and in clinical management, most particularly dealing with aphasia, neurogenic speech-language disorders, and neurolinguistics.

**O. M. Reinmuth, M.D.,** completed his undergraduate education at the University of Texas. He obtained his M.D. degree from Duke University, where he also completed his internship. This was followed by residencies in internal medicine at Yale University and in neurology at Harvard University (Boston City Hospital) and at Queen's Square Hospital, London, England. He served as Professor of Neurology at the University of Miami Medical School before becoming Professor and Chairman of the Department of Neurology at the University of Pittsburgh, a position he has held for the past 4 years. He is a Fellow of the American Academy of Neurology and the American College of Physicians, a member and past officer of the American Neurological Association, and is currently serving as Chairman of the Stroke Council of the American Heart Association.

**Carol S. Swindell** became interested in adult neurogenic communication disorders while completing her Ph.D. at the University of Pittsburgh. She is currently an Assistant Professor in the Department of Audiology and Speech Pathology at Memphis State University, and Adjunct Professor of Research at the University of Tennessee Center for Health Sciences. She has presented and published numerous articles on stroke recovery, and was recently awarded the Senior Research Investigator Award by the American Speech-Language-Hearing Foundation to study the usefulness of augmentative communication systems in the treatment of severe aphasia. Her other research interests include the cognitive, communicative, and emotional characteristics of normal and abnormal aging.

# SUBJECT INDEX